Pharmacology *for* Health Professionals

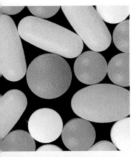
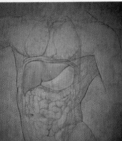

Pharmacology *for* Health Professionals

Sally Roach, MSN, RN

Associate Professor
University of Texas at Brownsville and Texas Southmost College
Brownsville, Texas

Tom Lochhaas

Contributing Writer

LIPPINCOTT WILLIAMS & WILKINS
A **Wolters Kluwer** Company

Philadelphia • Baltimore • New York • London
Buenos Aires • Hong Kong • Sydney • Tokyo

Acquisitions Editor: John Goucher
Managing Editor: Kevin C. Dietz
Marketing Manager: Hilary Henderson
Production Editor: Christina Remsberg
Compositor: Maryland Composition
Printer: RR Donnelley-Willard

Library of Congress Cataloging-in-Publication Data

Roach, Sally S.
    Pharmacology for health professionals/Sally Roach; Tom Lochhaas, Contributing
writer.—1st ed.
        p. ; cm.
    Includes bibliographical references and index.
    ISBN 13: 978-0-7817-5284-8
    ISBN 10: 0-7817-5284-1
1. Pharmacology.   I. Lochhaas, Thomas A.   II. Title.
[DNLM: 1. Pharmaceutical Preparations.   2. Pharmacology.   QV   55   R628p   2005]
RM300.R63 2005
615'.1—dc22   2004025212

*The publishers have made every effort to trace the copyright holders for borrowed material. If they
have inadvertently overlooked any, they will be pleased to make the necessary arrangements at the first
opportunity.*

To purchase additional copies of this book, call our customer service department at
(800) 638-3030 or fax orders to **(301) 824-7390.** International customers should call
(301) 714-2324.

Visit Lippincott Williams & Wilkins on the Internet: http://www.LWW.com. Lippincott Williams
& Wilkins customer service representatives are available from 8:30 am to 6:00 pm, EST.

06 07 08 09
2 3 4 5 6 7 8 9 10

List of Reviewers

Yvonne Beth Alles, MBA
Medical Language Specialist
Davenport University
Eastern Avenue Career Center
Grand Rapids, Michigan
Holland Campus
Holland, Michigan

Kathleen Bode, RN, BS, MS
Chair, Division of Health
Flint Hills Technical College
Emporia, Kansas

Jeff Kushner, Ph.D.
James Madison University
Harrisonburg, Virginia

Shirley Williams
Associate Dean
Allied Health Sciences
Trident Technical College
North Charleston, South Carolina

Jean Zorko, MT (ASCP)
Assistant Professor
Science Department
Stark State College of Technology
Canton, Ohio

Preface

Pharmacology for Health Professionals reflects the ever-changing science of pharmacology and the roles of health professionals related to pharmacologic agents. All information is based on the latest available information. The text prepares health care workers directly or indirectly involved in patient care to understand the uses of and issues related to most medications.

Purpose

This text is designed to provide students with a clear, concise introduction to pharmacology. The basic explanations presented in this text are not intended to suggest that pharmacology is an easy subject. Drug therapy is one of the most important and complicated treatment modalities in modern health care. Because of its importance and complexity, and the frequent additions and changes in the field of pharmacology, it is imperative that health care professionals constantly review and update their knowledge.

Current Drug Information

Students and practitioners should remember that information about drugs, such as dosages and new forms, is constantly changing. Likewise, there may be new drugs on the market that were not approved by the Federal Drug Administration (PDA) at the time of publication of this text. The reader may find that certain drugs or drug dosages available when this textbook was published may no longer be available. For the most current drug information and dosages, references should be consulted, such as the most current *Physician's Desk Reference* or *Facts and Comparison* and the package inserts that accompany most drugs. Pharmacists or physicians can also be contacted for information concerning a specific drug, including dosage, adverse reactions, contraindications, precautions, interactions, or administration.

Special Features

A number of features have proven useful for students in their study of basic pharmacology. The following features appear in this text:

- **Key Terms**—definitions are provided up front for important new words used in the chapter. These terms are boldfaced at their first use in the chapter to remind students of the earlier definitions.
- **Chapter Objectives**—clarify for students what information they are expected to learn while reading and studying each chapter.
- **Organizing Framework**—each chapter presents information in a similar order and format to facilitate learning. First, the class of drugs is introduced. Then, sections explain the drug class's actions and uses. Next, common adverse reactions are described, followed by a section on how these are typically managed. The next section briefly describes contraindications, precautions, and interactions of these drugs. Although space prevents every contraindication, precaution, and interaction to be listed, the more common ones are included in the text. Pregnancy categories are identified for many drugs discussed within the chapter. For health professionals involved in direct patient care activities, the next section discusses common patient management issues, followed by a section on educating the patient and family members as appropriate.
- **Alerts**—short segments that identify urgent considerations in the management of patients receiving a specific drug or drug category.
- **Gerontologic Alerts**—short segments about specific problems for which older adults are at increased risk. As the number of the older adults in our society increases, it becomes imperative to recognize the necessity of specialized care.
- **Home Health Care Checklists**—in appropriate chapters, these checklists highlight specific issues that the patient or family may encounter while undergoing drug therapy in the home setting. As more and more patients are cared for outside the hospital, it becomes increasingly important to know what information the patient or family needs to obtain an optimal response to the drug regimen.
- **Patient Education Boxes**—highlight teaching points relating to specific pharmacologic techniques and must-know information for the patient undergoing drug therapy. This empowers the family to participate knowledgeably and accurately in the patient's drug regimen.
- **Summary Drug Tables**—contain commonly used drugs representative of the class of drugs discussed in the chapter. Important drug information is provided, including the generic name, pronunciation

guide for generic names, trade names, adverse reactions, and dosage ranges. In these tables, generic names are followed by trade names; when a drug is available under several trade names, several of the available trade names are given. The more common or serious adverse reactions associated with the drug are listed in the table's adverse reaction section. It should be noted that any patient might exhibit adverse reactions not listed in this text. Because of this possibility, any sign or symptom should be considered a possible adverse reaction until the primary health care provider determines the cause of the problem. The dose ranges for the drug follow the adverse reactions. In most cases, the adult dose ranges are given in these tables because space does not permit the inclusion of all possible dosages for various types of disorders. Likewise, space limitation does not permit an inclusion of pediatric dose ranges because of the complexity of determining the pediatric dose of many drugs. Many drugs given to children are determined on the basis of body weight or body surface area and have a variety of dosage schedules.

- **Key Points**—are a quick summary at the conclusion of the chapter to provide an overview of critical information.
- **Natural Remedies**—are brief sections that describe common uses of herbals and other natural substances. As the general public increasingly uses such substances, health care professionals need to be aware of their effects and possible problems resulting from self-administration.
- **Case Study Exercise**—presents a patient situation followed by multiple-choice questions to help students recall and apply information learned in the chapter.
- **Website Activities**—encourage students to learn to use the Internet as a resource to obtain additional information about drugs and patient care related to pharmacology therapy.
- **Review Questions**—help students review key chapter content and assess their learning.
- **Answers to Case Study Questions and Review Questions**—appear in Appendix A to help students assess their responses to these exercises.
- **Abbreviations**—important pharmacological and general medical abbreviations that health care professionals need to know, related to drug therapy, are spelled out in Appendix B.
- **Glossary**—key terms and other drug-related terms are listed and defined in Appendix C.
- **Drugs and Health Care Information Sources on the World Wide Web**—are provided in Appendix E as a resource listing for more information about pharmacological issues.

- **Select Herbs and Natural Products Used for Medicinal Purposes**—are provided in a brief, tabular format for quick reference. Important common natural remedies are described in more detail within the appropriate chapters.
- **Four-Color Illustrations**—the text is beautifully illustrated throughout with four-color illustrations that highlight and explain important pharmacologic concepts, techniques, or ideas.

Organization

The text contains 32 chapters organized in eight units. The organization is based on the teaching method most commonly used for pharmacology: drugs affecting the different body systems. Although pharmacological agents are presented in specific units, a disease may be treated with more than one type of drug, which may require consulting one or more units.

Unit I presents a foundation for the study of pharmacology. These chapters cover the general principles of pharmacology, drug forms and methods of administration, and a review of the teaching learning process and general areas of consideration when educating the patient and family.

Unit II contains seven chapters that present drugs that affect the neurological system, grouped according to common classifications. Included are the various types of drugs used to manage pain.

Unit III contains three chapters on drugs that affect the respiratory system.

Unit IV contains five chapters on drugs that affect the cardiovascular system, including drugs for heart conditions and those related to the blood.

Unit V has three chapters concerning drugs that affect the gastrointestinal and urinary systems. Diuretic drugs are included here because of their primary effects on the urinary system.

Unit VI covers drugs that affect the endocrine and reproductive systems.

Unit VII consists of four chapters dealing with drugs that affect the immune system, including antibacterial and other anti-infective drugs, as well as antineoplastic agents.

Unit VIII has four chapters addressing drugs that affect other body systems, including the musculoskeletal system, skin, ears, and eyes, as well as fluids and electrolytes.

Chapter Content

As described, the body of each chapter focuses on the actions, uses, adverse reactions, contraindications, precautions, and interactions of drug classes or types along with patient management issues and patient and family education. The information is intended to be introductory and at a level appropriate for students in health professions who may not administer drugs directly to patients but who may be directly or indirectly involved in patient care or otherwise need to understand basic pharmacological principles and information about drug classes.

- Actions—a basic explanation of how the drug accomplishes its intended activity.
- Uses—the more common uses of the drug class or type are provided. No unlabeled or experimental uses of drugs are given in the text (unless specifically identified as an unlabeled use) because the FDA does not approve these uses. Students should be reminded that under certain circumstances, some physicians may prescribe drugs for a condition not approved by the FDA or may prescribe an experimental drug.

Note that when discussing the use of antibiotics, this text does not list specific microorganisms. Microorganisms can become resistant to antibiotic drugs very rapidly. Because of this, listing specific microorganisms or types of infections for an antibiotic may be misleading.

- Adverse Reactions—the most common adverse drug reactions are listed under this heading.
- Contraindications—contraindications for administration of the drug or drugs discussed in the chapter.
- Precautions—precautions that should be taken before, during, or after drug administration.
- Interactions—more common interactions between the drug(s) discussed in the chapter and other drugs or substances.
- Patient Management—includes assessments that need to be made of the patient related to the administration of the drugs discussed in the chapter. In addition, information is provided related to promoting an optimal response to therapy, monitoring and managing adverse reactions, and educating the patient and family.

Teaching/Learning Package

Study Guide for Pharmacology for Health Professionals

The study guide that accompanies the text is designed to reinforce the key words, drug classifications, generic and trade drug names, important pharmacologic facts, concepts, and clinical applications presented in the content of the text. It guides the student through progressively more difficult material by using the following types of questions:

- matching
- true and false
- multiple choice
- recall
- concept application

The goal of the study guide is to help the student and the instructor pinpoint areas of content that need additional study before the exam.

Instructor's Resource Material

This text includes the following instructor's resource material on a CD-ROM:

- PowerPoint Slideshows
- Answers to Study Guide Questions
- Test Generator
- Instructor Notes on Web Site Activities
- Teaching Strategies

There are other things that can make this course more engaging and entertaining. For example, many invite a guest speaker to enhance the learning experience. At times, the student will know of a person to invite or you may wish to check with pharmaceutical representatives, pharmacists, nurse practitioners, physician assistants, or even a physician and have them present a specific topic of interest. Be sure to inform the speaker of any time limitations, student's understanding level, and the scope of the topic for the presentation.

The use of visual aids for a pharmacology class is limitless. Drug literature is plentiful and medical journals are an excellent source of advertisements to scrutinize. It is also helpful to seek out empty vials, ampules, syringe cartridges, and other demonstration aids. Often a pharmaceutical representative can be very helpful in this area, using plastic replicas of many of their products for demonstration purposes. Outdated drug handbooks or periodicals are often available when a local hospital updates these on a yearly basis for their transcriptionists or other allied health staff.

Contents

Appendices

1 General Principles of Pharmacology

KEY TERMS

additive drug reaction—a reaction that occurs when the combined effect of two drugs is equal to the sum of each drug given alone

adverse reaction—undesirable drug effects

agonist—a drug that binds with a receptor to produce a therapeutic response

allergic reaction—a drug reaction that occurs because the individual's immune system views the drug as a foreign substance

anaphylactic shock—an extremely serious allergic drug reaction

antagonist—a drug that joins with a receptor to prevent the action of an agonist at that receptor

antibodies—immune system molecules produced in reaction with an antigen

antigen—a substance that the immune system perceives as foreign and that causes production of antibodies

controlled substances—drugs with a high potential for abuse that are controlled by special regulations

cumulative drug effect—a drug effect that occurs when the body has not fully metabolized a dose of a drug before the next dose is given

drug idiosyncrasy—any unusual or abnormal reaction to a drug

drug tolerance—a decreased response to a drug, requiring an increase in dosage to achieve the desired effect

hypersensitivity—being allergic to a drug

nonprescription drugs—drugs designated by the FDA to be obtained without a prescription

pharmaceutic phase—the dissolution of the drug

pharmacodynamics—a drug's actions and effects within the body

pharmacogenetic disorder—a genetically determined abnormal response to normal doses of a drug

pharmacokinetics— activities occurring within the body after a drug is administered, including absorption, distribution, metabolism, and excretion

pharmacology—the study of drugs and their action on living organisms

physical dependence—a compulsive need to use a substance repeatedly to avoid mild to severe withdrawal symptoms

polypharmacy—the taking of numerous drugs that can potentially react with one another

prescription drugs—drugs the federal government has designated as potentially harmful unless supervised by a licensed health care provider

psychological dependence—a compulsion to use a substance to obtain a pleasurable experience

receptor—a specialized macromolecule that binds to the drug molecule, altering the function of the cell and producing the therapeutic response

synergism—a drug interaction that occurs when drugs produce an effect that is greater than the sum of their separate actions

teratogen—any substance that causes abnormal development of the fetus

therapeutic response—the intended (beneficial) effect of a drug

toxic—harmful drug effect

CHAPTER OBJECTIVES

On completion of this chapter, students will be able to:

1 Define the chapter's key terms.

2 Identify the different names assigned to drugs.

3 Distinguish between prescription drugs, nonprescription drugs, and controlled substances.

4 Discuss the various types of drug reactions produced in the body.

5 Identify factors that influence drug action.

6 Discuss the types of drug interactions that may occur.

7 Discuss the use of herbal medicines.

Pharmacology is the study of drugs and their actions on living organisms. A sound knowledge of basic pharmacologic principles is essential for most health care professionals, especially those who interact with patients who receive medications. This chapter gives a basic overview of pharmacologic principles, drug development, federal legislation affecting the dispensing and use of drugs, and the use of herbal medicines.

Drug Development

Drug development is a long and arduous process, which takes anywhere from 7 to 12 years, and sometimes even longer. The United States Food and Drug Administration (FDA) has the responsibility of approving new drugs and monitoring drugs for adverse or toxic reactions. The development of a new drug is divided into the pre-FDA phase and the FDA phase (Fig. 1-1). During the pre-FDA phase, a manufacturer develops a drug that looks promising. In vitro testing (testing in an artificial environment, such as in a test tube) is performed using animal and human cells. This testing is followed by studies in live animals. The manufacturer then applies to the FDA for investigational new drug (IND) status.

With IND status, clinical testing of the new drug begins. Clinical testing involves three phases, each involving a larger number of people. All pharmacologic and biologic effects are noted. Phase I lasts 4 to 6 weeks and involves 20 to 100 individuals who are either "normal" volunteers or individuals in the intended treatment population. If phase I studies are successful, the testing moves to phase II, and if those results are positive, to phase III. Each successive phase has a larger subject population. Phase III studies generate more information on dosing and safety. The three phases last anywhere from 2 to 10 years, with an average of 5 years.

A new drug application (NDA) is submitted after the investigation of the drug in phases I, II, and III is complete and the drug is found to be safe and effective. With the NDA, the manufacturer submits all data collected during the clinical trials. A panel of experts, including pharmacologists, chemists, physicians, and other professionals, reviews the application and makes a

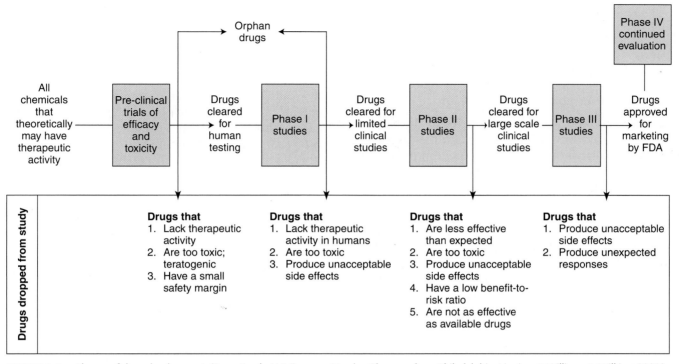

FIGURE 1-1. Phases of drug development. (From Karch AM. *Focus on Nursing Pharmacology*. Philadelphia: Lippincott Williams & Wilkins; 2000.)

recommendation to the FDA. The FDA then either approves or disapproves the drug for use. This process of review takes approximately 2 years.

After FDA approval, continued surveillance is performed to ensure safety after the manufacturer places the drug on the market. During this surveillance, an ongoing review of the drug occurs with particular attention given to adverse reactions. Health care professionals are encouraged to help with this surveillance by reporting adverse effects of drugs to the FDA by using the MedWatch system (Box 1-1).

Special FDA Programs

Although it takes considerable time for most drugs to get FDA approval, the FDA has special programs to meet certain needs, such as the orphan drug program, accelerated programs for urgent needs, and compassionate use programs.

Orphan Drug Program

The Orphan Drug Act of 1983 was passed to encourage the development and marketing of products used to treat rare diseases. The act defines a "rare disease" as a condition affecting fewer than 200,000 individuals in the United States. The National Organization of Rare Disorders reports that there are more than 6000 rare disorders that affect a total of approximately 25 million individuals. Examples of rare disorders include Tourette syndrome, ovarian cancer, acquired immunodeficiency syndrome (AIDS), Huntington disease, and certain forms of leukemia.

The act provides for incentives, such as research grants, protocol assistance by the FDA, and special tax credits, to encourage manufacturers to develop orphan drugs. If the drug is approved, then the manufacturer has 7 years of exclusive marketing rights. More than 100 new drugs have received FDA approval since the law was

---

Box 1-1 How Adverse Reactions Are Reported

A drug must be used and studied for many years before all of its adverse reactions are identified. The FDA established a reporting program called MedWatch, by which health care professionals can report observations of serious adverse drug effects by using a standard form (see Appendix D). The FDA protects the identity of those who voluntarily report adverse reactions. This form also is used to report an undesirable experience associated with the use of medical products (e.g., latex gloves, pacemakers, infusion pumps, anaphylaxis, blood, blood components, etc).

The FDA considers serious adverse reactions as those that may result in death, life-threatening illness, hospitalization, disability, or those that may require medical or surgical intervention.

Adverse drug reactions may be reported to the FDA by mail, fax, or e-mail. For more information, go to this website:

www.fda.gov/medwatch/index.html

passed. Examples of orphan drugs include thalidomide for leprosy, triptorelin pamoate for ovarian cancer, tetrabenazine for Huntington disease, and zidovudine for AIDS.

Accelerated Programs

Accelerated approval of drugs is offered by the FDA as a means to make promising products for life-threatening diseases available on the market, based on preliminary evidence, before complete testing has demonstrated benefits for patients. A "provisional approval" may be granted, with a written commitment from the pharmaceutical company to complete clinical studies that formally demonstrate patient benefit. This program seeks to make life-saving investigational drugs available to treat diseases that pose a significant health threat to the public. One example of a disease that qualifies as posing a significant health threat is AIDS. Because AIDS is so devastating to the individuals affected, and because of the danger the disease poses to public health, the FDA and pharmaceutical companies are working together to shorten the IND approval process for some drugs that show promise in treating AIDS. This accelerated process allows health care providers to administer a drug with positive results in early phase I and II clinical trials, rather than wait until final approval is granted. If the drug continues to prove beneficial, then the process of approval is accelerated.

Compassionate Access to Unapproved Drugs

The compassionate access program allows patients to receive drugs that have not yet been approved by the FDA. This program provides experimental drugs for patients who could benefit from new treatments but who probably would die before the drug is approved for use. These patients are often too sick to participate in controlled studies. Drug manufacturers make a proposal to the FDA to target patients with the disease. The company then provides the drug free to these patients. The pharmaceutical company analyzes and presents to the FDA data about this treatment. This program can be beneficial but is not without problems. Because the drug is not in full production, quantities may be limited; the number of patients may be limited, and patients may be selected at random. Because patients receiving compassionate access often are sicker, they have an increased risk for toxic reactions. Thus, a newly developed drug may gain a bad reputation even before marketing begins.

Drug Names

Throughout the process of development, drugs may have several names: a chemical name, a generic (nonproprietary) name, an official name, and a trade or brand name. These names can be confusing without a clear understanding of the different names used. Table 1-1 identifies the different names and explains each.

TABLE 1-1   Drug Names

Drug Name and Example	Explanation
Chemical Name Example: ethyl 4-(8-chloro-5,6-dihydro- 11H-benzo[5,6] cycloheptal[1,2-b]- pyridin-11-ylidene)-1- piperidinecardisplayylate	Gives the exact chemical makeup of the drug and placing of the atoms or molecular structure; it is not capitalized
Generic Name (nonproprietary) Example: loratadine	Name given to a drug before it becomes official; may be used in all countries, by all manufacturers; it is not capitalized
Official Name Example: loratadine	Name listed in *The United States Pharmacopeia-National Formulary*; may be the same as the generic name
Trade Name (brand name) Example: Claritin™	Name that is registered by the manufacturer and is followed by the trademark symbol; the name can be used only by the manufacturer; a drug may have several trade names, depending on the number of manufacturers; the first letter of the name is capitalized

Drug Categories

After approving a drug, the FDA assigns it to one of the following categories: prescription, nonprescription, or controlled substance.

Prescription Drugs

Prescription drugs are drugs that the federal government has designated to be potentially harmful unless their use is supervised by a licensed health care provider, such as a nurse practitioner, physician, or dentist. Although these drugs have been tested for safety and therapeutic effect, prescription drugs may cause different reactions in some individuals.

In hospitals and other institutional settings, patients are monitored for the therapeutic effect and adverse reactions of the drugs they are given. Some drugs have the potential to be **toxic** (harmful). When these drugs are prescribed to be taken at home, the patient and/or family members are educated about the drug.

Prescription drugs, also called legend drugs, are the largest category of drugs. Prescription drugs must be prescribed by a licensed health care provider. The prescription (Fig. 1-2) contains the name of the drug, the dosage, the method and times of administration, and the signature of the licensed health care provider prescribing the drug, along with other information.

Nonprescription Drugs

Nonprescription drugs are drugs that are designated by the FDA to be safe if taken as directed. They can be obtained without a prescription. These drugs are also referred to as over-the-counter (OTC) drugs and are available in many different settings, such as a pharmacy, drugstore, or supermarket. OTC drugs include those taken for symptoms of the common cold, headaches, constipation, diarrhea, and upset stomach.

Even nonprescription drugs, however, carry some risk and may produce adverse reactions. For example, acetylsalicylic acid, commonly known as aspirin, is potentially harmful and can cause gastrointestinal bleeding and salicylism (see Chapter 10). Product labels must give consumers important information regarding the drug, dosage, contraindications, precautions, and adverse reactions. Consumers are urged to read the directions carefully before taking OTC drugs.

Controlled Substances

Controlled substances are the most carefully monitored of all drugs. These drugs have a high potential for abuse and may cause physical or psychological dependence. **Physical dependence** is a compulsive need to use a substance repeatedly to avoid mild to severe with-

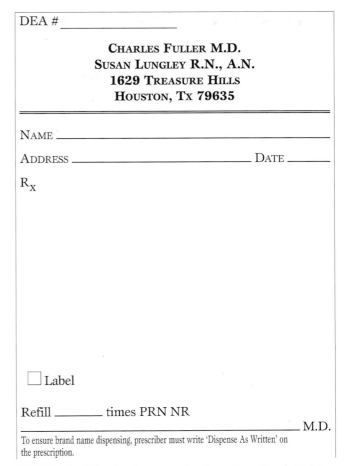

DEA # _____

CHARLES FULLER M.D.
SUSAN LUNGLEY R.N., A.N.
1629 TREASURE HILLS
HOUSTON, TX 79635

NAME _____

ADDRESS _____ DATE _____

Rx

☐ Label

Refill _____ times PRN NR

_____ M.D.

To ensure brand name dispensing, prescriber must write 'Dispense As Written' on the prescription.

FIGURE 1-2. Example of a prescription form. (From Roach SS. *Introductory Clinical Pharmacology*, 7th ed. Baltimore: Lippincott Williams & Wilkins; 2004.)

drawal symptoms; it is the body's dependence on repeated administration of a drug. **Psychological dependence** is a compulsion to use a substance to obtain a pleasurable experience; it is the mind's dependence on the repeated administration of a drug. One type of dependence may lead to the other.

The Controlled Substances Act of 1970 regulates the manufacture, distribution, and dispensing of drugs that have abuse potential. Drugs under the Controlled Substances Act are categorized in five schedules, based on their potential for abuse and physical and psychological dependence. Box 1-2 describes the five schedules.

Prescriptions for controlled substances must be written in ink and include the name and address of the patient and the Drug Enforcement Agency number of the health care provider. Prescriptions for these drugs cannot be filled more than 6 months after the prescription was written and cannot be refilled more than five times. Under federal law, limited quantities of certain schedule C-V drugs may be purchased without a prescription, with the purchase recorded by the dispensing pharmacist. In some cases, state laws are more restrictive than federal laws and impose additional

Box 1-2 Schedules of Controlled Substances

Schedule I (C-I)
- High abuse potential
- No accepted medical use in the United States
- Examples: heroin, marijuana, LSD (lysergic acid diethylamide), peyote

Schedule II (C-II)
- Potential for high abuse with severe physical or psychological dependence
- Examples: narcotics such as meperidine, methadone, morphine, oxycodone; amphetamines; and barbiturates

Schedule III (C-III)
- Less abuse potential than schedule II drugs
- Potential for moderate physical or psychological dependence
- Examples: nonbarbiturate sedatives, nonamphetamine stimulants, limited amounts of certain narcotics

Schedule IV (C-IV)
- Less abuse potential than schedule III drugs
- Limited dependence potential
- Examples: some sedatives and anxiety agents, nonnarcotic analgesics

Schedule V (C-V)*
- Limited abuse potential
- Examples: small amounts of narcotics (codeine) used as antitussives or antidiarrheals

---

* Under federal law, limited quantities of certain schedule V drugs may be purchased without a prescription directly from a pharmacist if allowed under state law. The purchaser must be at least 18 years of age and must furnish identification. All such transactions must be recorded by the dispensing pharmacist.

requirements for the sale and distribution of controlled substances. In hospitals or other agencies that dispense controlled substances, scheduled drugs are counted every 8 to 12 hours to account for each ampule, tablet, or other form of the drug. Any discrepancy in the number of drugs must be investigated and explained immediately.

Federal Drug Legislation And Enforcement

Many laws regarding drug distribution and administration have been enacted during the past century, including the Pure Food and Drug Act; Harrison Narcotic Act; Pure Food, Drug, and Cosmetic Act; and the Comprehensive Drug Abuse Prevention and Control Act. These laws control the use of prescription and nonprescription drugs and controlled substances.

Pure Food and Drug Act

The Pure Food and Drug Act, passed in 1906, was the first attempt by the government to regulate and control the manufacture, distribution, and sale of drugs. Before 1906, any substance could be called a drug, and no testing or research was required before placing a drug on the market. Before this time, the potency and purity of many drugs were questionable, and some were even dangerous for human use.

Harrison Narcotic Act

The Harrison Narcotic Act, passed in 1914, regulated the sale of narcotic drugs. Before the passage of this act, any narcotic could be purchased without a prescription. This law was amended many times. In 1970, the Harrison Narcotic Act was replaced by the Comprehensive Drug Abuse Prevention and Control Act.

Pure Food, Drug, and Cosmetic Act

In 1938, Congress passed the Pure Food, Drug, and Cosmetic Act, which gave the FDA control over the manufacture and sale of drugs, food, and cosmetics. Previously, some drugs, as well as foods and cosmetics, contained chemicals that were often harmful to humans. This law requires that these substances are safe for human use. It also requires pharmaceutical companies to perform toxicology tests before submitting a new drug to the FDA for approval. After FDA review of the tests performed on animals and other research data, approval may be given to market the drug, as described earlier.

Comprehensive Drug Abuse Prevention and Control Act

Congress passed the Comprehensive Drug Abuse Prevention and Control Act in 1970 because of the growing problem of drug abuse. It regulates the manufacture, distribution, and dispensation of drugs with a potential for abuse. Title II of this law, the Controlled Substances Act, deals with control and enforcement. The Drug Enforcement Agency within the US Department of Justice is the leading federal agency responsible for the enforcement of this act.

Drug Enforcement Administration

The Drug Enforcement Administration (DEA) within the US Department of Justice is the chief federal agency responsible for enforcing the Controlled Substances Act. Failure to comply with the Controlled Substances Act is punishable by fine and/or imprisonment. With drug abuse so prevalent, all health care workers must diligently adhere to FDA and state regulations.

Drug Use and Pregnancy

The use of any prescription or nonprescription medication carries a risk of causing birth defects in a developing fetus. Drugs administered to pregnant women, particularly during the first trimester (3 months), may cause teratogenic effects. A **teratogen** is any substance that causes abnormal development of the fetus, which may lead to a severely deformed fetus.

In an effort to prevent teratogenic effects, the FDA has established five drug categories based on the potential of a drug for causing birth defects (Box 1-3). Information regarding the pregnancy category of a specific drug is found in reliable drug literature, such as the inserts accompanying drugs and drug reference books. In general, most drugs are contraindicated during pregnancy or lactation unless the potential benefits of taking the drug outweigh the risks to the fetus or infant.

During pregnancy, no woman should consider taking any drug, legal or illegal, prescription or nonprescription, unless the drug is prescribed or recommended by her health care provider. Smoking and drinking alcoholic beverages also carry risks, such as low birth weight, premature birth, and fetal alcohol syndrome. Children born to mothers using addictive drugs, such as cocaine or heroin, often are born with an addiction to the drug, along with other health problems.

Drug Actions Within the Body

Drugs act in various ways in the body. Drugs taken by mouth (except liquids) go through three phases: the pharmaceutic phase, pharmacokinetic phase, and pharmacodynamic phase. Liquid and parenteral drugs (drugs given by injection) go through the latter two phases only.

Pharmaceutic Phase

The **pharmaceutic phase** of drug action is the dissolution of the drug. Drugs must be in solution to be absorbed. Drugs that are liquid or drugs given by injection (parenteral drugs) do not go through the pharmaceutic phase because they are already in solution. A tablet or capsule (solid forms of a drug) goes through this phase as it disintegrates into small particles and dissolves into body fluids within the gastrointestinal tract. Enteric-coated tablets do not disintegrate until reaching the alkaline environment of the small intestine.

Pharmacokinetic Phase

Pharmacokinetics refers to activities involving the drug within the body after it is administered. These activities include absorption, distribution, metabolism, and excretion. Another pharmacokinetic component, the drug's half-life, is a measure of the rate at which it is removed from the body.

Absorption

Absorption follows administration and is the process by which a drug becomes available for use in the body. It occurs after dissolution of a solid form of the drug or after the administration of a liquid or parenteral drug. In this process, the drug particles within the gastrointestinal tract are moved into body fluids. This movement can be accomplished in several ways: active absorption, passive absorption, and pinocytosis. In active absorption, a carrier molecule such as a protein or enzyme actively moves the drug across a membrane. Passive absorption occurs by diffusion (movement from a higher concentration to a lower concentration). In pinocytosis, cells engulf the drug particle causing movement across the cell.

As the body transfers the drug from body fluids to tissue sites, absorption into body tissues occurs. Several

---

Box 1-3 Pregnancy Categories

Pregnancy Category A
- Controlled studies show no risk to the fetus.
- Adequate well-controlled studies in pregnant women have not demonstrated risk to the fetus.

Pregnancy Category B
- There is no evidence of risk in humans.
- Animal studies show risk, but human findings do not.
- If no adequate human studies have been performed, then animal studies are negative.

Pregnancy Category C
- Risk cannot be ruled out.
- Human studies are lacking, and animal studies are either positive for fetal risk or lacking.
- The drug may be used during pregnancy if the potential benefits of the drug outweigh its possible risks.

Pregnancy Category D
- There is positive evidence of risk to the human fetus.
- Investigational or postmarketing data show risk to the fetus.
- However, potential benefits may outweigh the risk to the fetus. If needed in a life-threatening situation or a serious disease, then the drug may be acceptable if safer drugs cannot be used or are ineffective.

Pregnancy Category X
- Use of the drug is contraindicated in pregnancy.
- Studies in animals or humans or investigational or postmarketing reports have shown fetal risk that clearly outweighs any possible benefit to the patient.

Regardless of the pregnancy category or the presumed safety of the drug, no drug should be administered during pregnancy unless it is clearly needed and the potential benefits outweigh potential harm to the fetus.

factors influence the rate of absorption, including the route of administration, the solubility of the drug, and certain body conditions. Drugs are most rapidly absorbed when given by the intravenous route directly into the bloodstream, followed by the intramuscular route (injection into muscle tissue), the subcutaneous (injection under the skin), and, lastly, the oral route (Fig. 1-3). Some drugs are more soluble and thus are absorbed more rapidly than others. For example, water-soluble drugs are readily absorbed into the systemic circulation. Some body conditions, such as developing lipodystrophy (atrophy of the subcutaneous tissue) caused by repeated subcutaneous injections, inhibit absorption of a drug given in the site of lipodystrophy.

Distribution

The systemic circulation (blood flow throughout the body) distributes drugs to various body tissues or target sites. There, drugs interact with specific receptors. Some drugs travel by binding to protein (albumin) in the blood. Drugs bound to protein are pharmacologically

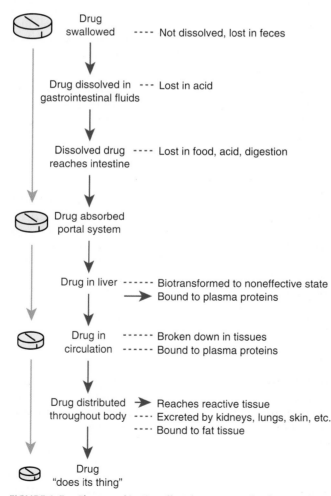

FIGURE 1-3. Pharmacokinetics affect the amount of a drug reaching reactive tissues. Very little of an oral dose of a drug actually reaches reactive sites. (From Karch AM. *Focus on Nursing Pharmacology.* Philadelphia: Lippincott Williams & Wilkins; 2000.)

inactive. Only when the protein molecules release the drug can it diffuse into the tissues, interact with receptors, and produce a therapeutic effect.

As the drug circulates in the blood, a certain blood level must be maintained for it to be effective. When the blood level decreases to below the therapeutic level, the drug will not produce the desired effect. Should the blood level increase significantly above the therapeutic level, toxic symptoms may develop.

Metabolism

Metabolism, sometimes called biotransformation, is the process of chemical reactions by which the liver converts a drug to inactive compounds. Patients with liver disease may require lower dosages of a drug, or the health care provider may select a drug that does not undergo biotransformation in the liver. Frequent liver function tests are necessary when a patient has liver disease. The kidneys, lungs, plasma, and intestinal mucosa also aid in the metabolism of drugs.

Excretion

The elimination of drugs from the body is called excretion. After the liver renders a drug inactive, the kidney excretes the inactive compounds from the body in the urine. Some drugs are excreted unchanged by the kidney without liver involvement. Patients with kidney disease may require a lower dosage and careful monitoring of their kidney function. Because children have immature kidney function, they too may require dosage reduction and kidney function tests. Similarly, older adults have diminished kidney function and require careful monitoring and lower dosages. Other drugs are eliminated from the body through sweat, breast milk, breathing, or feces.

Half-Life

Half-life is the time required for the body to eliminate 50% of the drug. Drugs with a short half-life (2–4 hours) need to be administered frequently, whereas a drug with a long half-life (21–24 hours) requires less frequent dosing. For example, digoxin (Lanoxin) has a long half-life (36 hours) and requires once-daily dosing. However, aspirin has a short half-life and requires frequent dosing. It takes five to six half-lives to eliminate approximately 98% of a drug from the body. Although a drug's half-life is the same in most people, patients with liver or kidney disease may have problems excreting a drug; this increases its half-life and increases the risk of toxicity. Older patients or patients with impaired kidney or liver function require frequent diagnostic tests of their renal or hepatic function.

Pharmacodynamic Phase

Pharmacodynamics are the drug's actions and effects within the body. After administration, most drugs enter the systemic circulation and expose almost all body tissues to their possible effects. All drugs produce more than one effect in the body. The primary effect of a drug is the desired or therapeutic effect. Secondary effects are all other effects, whether desirable or undesirable, produced by the drug.

Most drugs have an affinity for certain organs or tissues and exert their greatest action at the cellular level in those specific areas, which are called target sites. The two main mechanisms of action are an alteration in cellular environment or cellular function.

Alteration in Cellular Environment

Some drugs act on the body by changing the cellular environment physically or chemically. Physical changes in the cellular environment include changes in osmotic pressures, lubrication, absorption, or conditions on the surface of the cell membrane. An example of a drug that changes osmotic pressure is mannitol, which produces a change in the osmotic pressure in brain cells, reducing cerebral edema. A drug that acts by altering the cellular environment by lubrication is sunscreen. An example of a drug that acts by altering absorption is activated charcoal, which is administered orally to absorb a toxic chemical ingested into the gastrointestinal tract. The stool softener docusate is an example of a drug that acts by altering the surface of the cellular membrane. Docusate has emulsifying and lubricating activity that causes a lowering of the surface tension in the cells of the bowel, permitting water and fats to enter the stool. This softens the fecal mass, allowing easier passage of the stool.

Chemical changes in the cellular environment include inactivation of cellular functions or an alteration of the chemical components of body fluid, such as a change in the pH. For example, antacids neutralize gastric acidity in patients with peptic ulcers.

Alteration in Cellular Function

Most drugs act on the body by altering cellular function. A drug cannot completely change the function of a cell, but it can alter its function. A drug that alters cellular function can increase or decrease certain physiologic functions, such as increase heart rate, decrease blood pressure, or increase urine output.

Receptor-Mediated Drug Action. The function of a cell alters when a drug interacts with a receptor. A **receptor** is a specialized macromolecule (a large group of molecules linked together) that attaches or binds to the drug molecule. This alters the function of the cell and produces the drug's **therapeutic response.** For a drug–receptor reaction to occur, a drug must be attracted to a particular receptor. Drugs bind to a receptor much like a piece of a puzzle. The closer the shape, the better the fit, and the better the therapeutic response. The intensity of a drug response is related to how good the "fit"

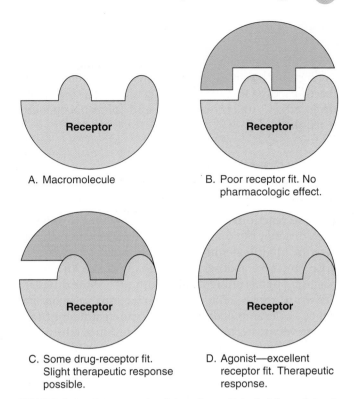

FIGURE 1-4. Drug–receptor interactions. (Adapted from Reiss & Evans. *Pharmacological Aspects of Nursing Care,* 3rd ed.)

of the drug molecule is and the number of receptor sites occupied.

Agonists are drugs that bind with a receptor to produce a therapeutic response. Drugs that bind only partially to the receptor generally have only a slight therapeutic response. Figure 1-4 identifies the different drug–receptor interactions. Partial agonists are drugs that have some drug receptor fit and produce a response but inhibit other responses.

Antagonists join with a receptor and thereby prevent the action of an agonist. When the antagonist binds more tightly than the agonist to the receptor, the action of the antagonist is strong. Drugs that act as antagonists produce no pharmacologic effect. An example of an antagonist is Narcan, a narcotic antagonist that completely blocks the effects of morphine. This drug is useful in reversing the effects of an overdose of narcotics (see Chapter 10).

Receptor-Mediated Drug Effects. The number of available receptor sites influences the effects of a drug. If a drug occupies only a few receptor sites when many sites are available, then the response will be small. If the drug dose is increased, then more receptor sites are involved and the response increases. If only a few receptor sites are available, then the response does not increase if more of the drug is administered. However, not all receptors on a cell need to be occupied for a drug to be effective. Some extremely potent drugs are effective even when the drug occupies few receptor sites.

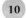

Drug Reactions

Drugs produce many reactions in the body. The following sections discuss adverse drug reactions, allergic drug reactions, drug idiosyncrasy, drug tolerance, cumulative drug effect, toxic reactions, and pharmacogenetic reactions.

Adverse Drug Reactions

Patients may experience one or more adverse reactions (side effects) when they are given a drug (Fig. 1-5). **Adverse reactions** are undesirable drug effects. Adverse reactions may be common or rare. They may be mild, severe, or life-threatening. They may occur after the first dose, after several doses, or after many doses. An adverse reaction often is unpredictable, although some drugs are known to cause certain adverse reactions in many patients. For example, drugs used in the treatment of cancer are very toxic and are known to produce adverse reactions in many patients receiving them. Other drugs produce adverse reactions in fewer patients. Some adverse reactions are predictable, but many adverse drug reactions occur without warning.

Some texts use both the terms "side effect" and "adverse reaction." Often "side effects" refer to mild, common, and nontoxic reactions; "adverse reactions" refer to more severe or life-threatening reactions. In this text, only the term "adverse reaction" is used, referring to reactions that may be mild, severe, or life-threatening.

Allergic Drug Reactions

An **allergic reaction** also is called a **hypersensitivity** reaction. Allergy to a drug usually begins to occur after more than one dose of the drug has been given. Sometimes an allergic reaction may occur the first time a drug is given if the patient had received or taken the drug in the past.

A drug allergy occurs because the individual's immune system views the drug as a foreign substance, or **antigen**. The recognition of an antigen stimulates the antigen–antibody response that prompts the body to produce **antibodies,** which are immune system molecules that react with the antigen. If the patient takes the drug after the antigen–antibody response has occurred, then an allergic reaction results.

Even a mild allergic reaction can produce serious effects if it goes unnoticed and the drug is given again. Any

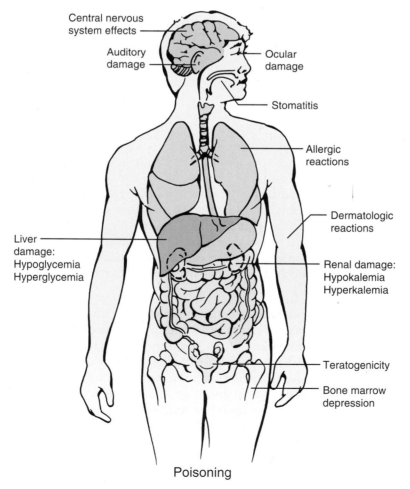

Poisoning

FIGURE 1-5. Various adverse effects may occur with drug use. (From Karch AM. *Focus on Nursing Pharmacology*. Philadelphia: Lippincott Williams & Wilkins, 2000.)

indication of an allergic reaction must be reported to the health care provider before the next dose of the drug is given. Serious allergic reactions must be reported immediately because emergency treatment may be necessary.

Some allergic reactions occur within minutes (even seconds) after the drug is given; others may be delayed for hours or days. Allergic reactions that occur immediately are often the most serious.

Allergic reactions cause a variety of signs and symptoms that may be observed by health care workers or reported by the patient. Examples of some allergic signs and symptoms include itching, skin rashes, and hives (urticaria). Other signs and symptoms include difficulty breathing, wheezing, cyanosis, a sudden loss of consciousness, and swelling of the eyes, lips, or tongue.

Anaphylactic shock is an extremely serious allergic drug reaction that usually occurs soon after the administration of a drug to which the individual is sensitive. This type of allergic reaction requires immediate medical attention. The signs and symptoms of anaphylactic shock are listed in Table 1-2.

All or only some of these signs and symptoms may be present. Anaphylactic shock can be fatal if it not recognized and treated immediately. The treatment is to raise the patient's blood pressure, improve breathing, restore cardiac function, and treat other problems as they occur. Epinephrine (adrenalin) may be given by subcutaneous or intramuscular injection. Hypotension and shock may be treated with fluids and vasopressors. Bronchodilators are given to relax the smooth muscles of the bronchial tubes to improve breathing. Antihistamines may be given to block the effects of histamine.

Angioedema (angioneurotic edema) is another type of allergic drug reaction. It is manifested by the collection of fluid in subcutaneous tissues. The most commonly affected areas are the eyelids, lips, mouth, and throat, although other areas also may be affected. Angioedema can be dangerous when the mouth is affected because the swelling may block the airway causing asphyxia. Difficulty breathing or swelling in any area of the body should be reported immediately to the health care provider.

Drug Idiosyncrasy

Drug idiosyncrasy refers to any unusual or abnormal reaction to a drug. It is any reaction that is different from the one normally expected from a specific drug and dose. For example, a patient may be given a drug to promote sleep (e.g., a hypnotic), but instead of falling asleep the patient remains wide awake and shows signs of nervousness or excitement. This response is an idiosyncratic response because it is different from what normally occurs with this type of drug. Another patient may receive the same drug and dose, fall asleep, and after 10 hours be difficult to awaken. This, too, is an abnormal over-response to the drug.

The cause of drug idiosyncrasies is not clear. They are believed to occur because of a genetic deficiency that makes a patient unable to tolerate certain chemicals, including drugs.

Drug Tolerance

Drug tolerance is a decreased response to a drug, requiring an increase in dosage to achieve the desired effect. Drug tolerance may develop when a patient takes a certain drug, such as a narcotic or tranquilizer, for a long time. Someone who takes the drug at home may increase the dose when the expected effect does not occur. Drug tolerance is a sign of drug dependence. Drug tolerance may also occur in hospitalized patients. When a patient receives a narcotic for more than 10 to 14 days, drug tolerance (and possibly drug dependence) may be occurring. The patient may also begin to ask for the drug more frequently.

Cumulative Drug Effect

A **cumulative drug effect** may occur in patients with liver or kidney disease because these organs are the major sites for the breakdown and excretion of most drugs. This drug effect occurs when the body does not metabolize and excrete one (normal) dose of a drug before the next dose is given. Thus, if a second dose of this drug is given, some drug from the first dose remains active in the body. A cumulative drug effect can be serious because too much of the drug can accumulate in the body and lead to toxicity.

Patients with liver or kidney disease are usually given drugs with caution because a cumulative effect may oc-

TABLE 1-2   Signs and Symptoms of Anaphylactic Shock

Respiratory	Bronchospasm Dyspnea (difficult breathing) Feeling of fullness in the throat Cough Wheezing
Cardiovascular	Extremely low blood pressure Tachycardia (heart rate >100 bpm) Palpations Syncope (fainting) Cardiac arrest
Integumentary	Urticaria (rash) Angioedema Pruritus (itching) Sweating
Gastrointestinal	Nausea Vomiting Abdominal pain

cur. When the patient is unable to excrete the drug at a normal rate, the drug accumulates in the body, causing a toxic reaction. Sometimes the health care provider lowers the dose of the drug to prevent a toxic drug reaction.

Toxic Reactions

Most drugs can produce **toxic** or harmful reactions if administered in large dosages or when blood concentration levels exceed the therapeutic level. Toxic levels may also build if the patient's kidneys are not functioning properly and cannot excrete the drug. Some toxic effects are immediately visible; others may not be seen for weeks or months. Some drugs, such as lithium or digoxin, have a narrow margin of safety, even when given in recommended dosages. It is important to monitor these drugs closely to avoid toxicity.

Drug toxicity can be reversible or irreversible, depending on the organs involved. Damage to the liver may be reversible because liver cells can regenerate. An example of irreversible damage is hearing loss caused by damage to the eighth cranial nerve caused by toxic reaction to the anti-infective drug streptomycin. Sometimes drug toxicity can be reversed by the administration of another drug that acts as an antidote. For example, in serious instances of digitalis toxicity, the drug Digibind may be given to counteract the effect of digoxin toxicity.

Because some drugs can cause toxic reactions even in recommended doses, health care workers involved in direct patient care should be aware of the signs and symptoms of toxicity of commonly prescribed drugs.

Pharmacogenetic Reactions

A **pharmacogenetic disorder** is a genetically caused abnormal response to normal doses of a drug. This abnormal response occurs because of inherited traits that cause abnormal metabolism of a drug. For example, individuals with glucose-6-phosphate dehydrogenase (G6PD) deficiency have abnormal reactions to a number of drugs. These patients experience varying degrees of hemolysis (destruction of red blood cells) if they take these drugs. More than 100 million people are affected by this disorder. Examples of drugs that cause hemolysis in patients with a G6PD deficiency include aspirin, chloramphenicol, and the sulfonamides.

Drug Interactions

Health care workers involved in patient care should be aware of the various drug interactions that can occur, most importantly drug–drug interactions and drug–food interactions. The following sections give a brief overview of drug interactions. Specific drug–drug and drug–food interactions are discussed in later chapters.

Drug–Drug Interactions

A drug–drug interaction occurs when one drug interacts with or interferes with the action of another drug. For example, taking an antacid with oral tetracycline causes a decrease in the effectiveness of the tetracycline. The antacid chemically interacts with the tetracycline and impairs its absorption into the bloodstream, thus reducing the effectiveness of the tetracycline. Drugs known to cause interactions include oral anticoagulants, oral hypoglycemics, anti-infectives, antiarrhythmics, cardiac glycosides, and alcohol. Drug–drug interactions can produce effects that are additive, synergistic, or antagonistic.

Additive Drug Reaction

An **additive drug reaction** occurs when the combined effect of two drugs is equal to the sum of each drug given alone. For example, taking the drug heparin with alcohol will increase bleeding. The equation "one + one = two" is sometimes used to illustrate the additive effect of drugs.

Synergistic Drug Reaction

Drug **synergism** occurs when drugs interact with each other and produce an effect that is greater than the sum of their separate actions. The equation "one + one = four" illustrates synergism. An example of drug synergism occurs when a person takes both a hypnotic and alcohol. When alcohol is taken simultaneously or soon before or after the hypnotic is taken, the action of the hypnotic increases. The individual experiences a drug effect that is much greater than that of either drug taken alone. A synergistic drug effect can be serious or even fatal.

Antagonistic Drug Reaction

An antagonistic drug reaction occurs when one drug interferes with the action of another, causing neutralization or a decrease in the effect of one drug. For example, protamine sulfate is a heparin antagonist. This means that the administration of protamine sulfate completely neutralizes the effects of heparin in the body.

Drug–Food Interactions

When a drug is given orally, food may impair or enhance its absorption. A drug taken on an empty stomach is absorbed into the bloodstream at a faster rate than when taken with food in the stomach. Some drugs must be taken on an empty stomach to achieve an optimal effect. Drugs that should be taken on an empty stomach are taken 1 hour before or 2 hours after meals. Other drugs, especially drugs that irritate the stomach, result in nausea or vomiting, or cause epigastric distress, are best given with food or meals to minimize gastric irritation. The nonsteroidal anti-inflammatory drugs and salicylates are examples of drugs given with food to decrease epigastric distress. Still other drugs combine with a food, forming an insoluble food–drug mixture. For example, when tetracycline is administered with dairy products, a drug–food mixture is formed that is unabsorbable by the body. When a drug cannot be absorbed by the body, no pharmacologic effect occurs.

Factors Influencing Drug Response

Various factors may influence a patient's drug response, including age, weight, gender, disease, and the route of administration.

Age

The age of the patient may influence the effects of a drug. Infants and children usually require smaller doses of a drug than adults do. Immature organ function, particularly the liver and kidneys, can affect the ability of infants and young children to metabolize drugs. An infant's immature kidneys are less able to eliminate drugs in the urine. Liver function is poorly developed in infants and young children. Drugs metabolized by the liver may produce more intense effects for longer periods. Parents must be taught the potential problems associated with administering drugs to their children. For example, a safe dose of a nonprescription drug for a 4-year-old child may be dangerous for a 6-month-old infant.

Elderly patients may also require smaller doses, although this depends also on the type of drug administered. For example, an elderly patient may take the same dose of an antibiotic as a younger adult. However, the same older adult may require a smaller dose of a drug that depresses the central nervous system, such as a narcotic. Changes that occur with aging affect the pharmacokinetics (absorption, distribution, metabolism, and excretion) of a drug. Any of these processes may be altered because of the physiologic changes of aging. Table 1-3 summarizes changes that occur with aging and possible pharmacokinetic effects.

Polypharmacy is the taking of multiple drugs, which can potentially react with one another. When practiced by the elderly, polypharmacy leads to an increased potential for adverse reactions. Although multiple drug therapy is necessary to treat certain disease states, it always increases the possibility of adverse reactions.

Weight

In general, dosages are based on an average weight of approximately 150 lb for both men and women. A drug dose may sometimes be increased or decreased because the patient's weight is significantly higher or lower than

TABLE 1-3   Factors Altering Drug Response in the Elderly

Age-Related Changes	Effect on Drug Therapy
Decreased gastric acidity; decreased gastric motility	Possible decreased or delayed absorption
Dry mouth and decreased saliva	Difficulty swallowing oral drugs
Decreased liver blood flow; decreased liver mass	Delayed and decreased metabolism of certain drugs; possible increased effect, leading to toxicity
Decreased lipid content of the skin	Possible decrease in absorption of transdermal drugs
Increased body fat; decreased body water	Possible increase in toxicity of water-soluble drugs; more prolonged effects of fat-soluble drugs
Decreased serum proteins	Possible increased effect and toxicity of highly protein-bound drugs
Decreased renal mass, blood flow, and glomerular filtration rate	Possible increased serum levels, leading to toxicity of drugs excreted by the kidney
Changes in sensitivity of certain drug receptors	Increase or decrease in drug effect

Adapted from Eisenhauer L, Nichols L, Spencer R, Bergan F. *Clinical pharmacology and nursing management*, 5th ed. Philadelphia: Lippincott-Raven; 1998:189. Used with permission.

this average. With narcotics, for example, higher or lower dosages may be necessary to produce relief of pain, depending on the patient's weight.

Gender

The person's gender may influence the action of some drugs. Women may require a smaller dose of some drugs than men because women have a body fat and water ratio different from that of men.

Disease

The presence of disease may influence the action of some drugs. Sometimes disease is a reason for not prescribing a drug or for reducing the dose of a certain drug. Both hepatic (liver) and renal (kidney) disease can greatly affect drug response.

In liver disease, for example, the ability to metabolize or detoxify a drug may be impaired. If the normal dose of the drug is given, then the liver may be unable to metabolize it at a normal rate. Consequently, the drug may be excreted from the body at a much slower rate than normal. The health care provider may then prescribe a lower dose and lengthen the time between doses.

Patients with kidney disease may experience drug toxicity and a longer duration of drug action. The dosage of drugs may be reduced to prevent the accumulation of toxic levels in the blood or further injury to the kidney.

Route of Administration

Intravenous administration of a drug produces the most rapid drug action. Next in order of time of action is the intramuscular route, followed by the subcutaneous route. Giving a drug orally usually produces the slowest drug action.

Some drugs can be given only by one route; for example, antacids are given only orally. Other drugs are available in oral and parenteral forms. The health care provider selects the route of administration based on many factors, including the desired rate of action. For example, a patient with a severe cardiac problem may require intravenous administration of a drug that affects the heart. Another patient with a mild cardiac problem may have a good response to oral administration of the same drug.

Herbal Therapy and Nutritional Supplements

Herbal therapy, also called botanical medicine, is a type of complementary or alternative therapy that uses plants or herbs to treat various disorders. People around the world use herbal therapy and nutritional supplements extensively. According to the World Health Organization (WHO), 80% of the world's population relies on herbs for a substantial part of their health care. Herbs have been used by virtually every culture in the world throughout known history. For example, Hippocrates prescribed St. Johns wort, an herbal remedy for depression that is still popular. Native Americans used plants such as coneflower, ginseng, and ginger for therapeutic purposes.

Herbal therapy is part of a group of nontraditional therapies commonly known as complementary/alternative medicine (CAM). Although CAM therapies have not been widely taught in medical schools, this is slowly changing. A 1998 survey revealed that 75 of 117 US medical schools offered elective courses in CAM or included CAM topics in required courses. Complementary therapies are therapies such as relaxation techniques, massage, dietary supplements, healing touch, and herbal therapy that can be used to "complement" traditional health care. Alternative therapies, however, are therapies used instead of conventional or Western medical therapies. The term "complementary/alternative therapy" often is used as an umbrella term for many therapies from all over the world.

Although herbs have been used for thousands of years, most of what we know has come from observation rather than clinical study. Most herbs have not been scientifically studied for safety and efficacy (effectiveness). Much of what we know about herbal therapy has come from Europe, particularly Germany. During the past several decades, European scientists have studied botanical plants in ways that seek to identify how they work at the cellular level, what chemicals are most effective, and what adverse effects are related to their use. Germany has compiled information on 300 herbs and has made recommendations for their use.

Dietary Supplement Health and Education Act

Because herbs cannot be sold and promoted in the United States as drugs, they are regulated as nutritional or dietary substances. Nutritional or dietary substances are terms used by the federal government to identify substances not regulated as drugs by the FDA but that are purported to promote health. Herbs, like vitamins and minerals, are classified as dietary or nutritional supplements. Because natural products cannot be patented in the United States, it is not profitable for drug manufacturers to spend millions of dollars and 8 to 12 years to study and develop these products as drugs.

In 1994, the US government passed the Dietary Supplement Health and Education Act (DSHEA). This act defines substances such as herbs, vitamins, minerals, amino acids, and other natural substances as "dietary supplements." The act permits general health claims such as "improves memory" or "promotes regularity" as long as the label also has a disclaimer stating that the supplements are not approved by the FDA and are not intended to diagnose, treat, cure, or prevent any disease.

The claims must be truthful and not misleading and must be supported by scientific evidence. Some have abused the law by making exaggerated claims, but the FDA has the power to enforce the law, which it has done, and such claims have decreased.

Center for Complementary and Alternative Health

In 1992, the National Institutes of Health established an Office of Alternative Medicine to facilitate the study of alternative medical treatments and to disseminate information to the public. In 1998, the name was changed to National Center for Complementary and Alternative Medicine (NCCAM). This office was established partly because of the increased interest and use of these therapies in the United States. An estimated 40% of all individuals in the United States use some form of CAM therapy. In 1997, Americans spent more that $27 billion on these therapies. Among the various purposes of NC-CAM, one is to evaluate the safety and efficacy of widely used natural products, such as herbal remedies and nutritional and food supplements. Although the scientific study of CAM is relatively new, the Center is dedicated to developing programs and encouraging scientists to investigate CAM treatments that show promise. NC-CAM's budget has steadily grown from $2 million in 1993 to more than $68.7 million in 2000. This funding increase reflects the public's interest and need for CAM information based on rigorous scientific research.

Educating Patients on the Use of Herbs and Nutritional Supplements

The use of herbs and nutritional supplements to treat various disorders is common. Herbs are used for various effects, such as to boost the immune system, treat depression, or promote relaxation. People are becoming more aware of the benefits of herbal therapies and nutritional supplements. Advertisements, books, magazines, and Internet sites abound concerning these topics. Eager to cure or control various disorders, people take herbs, teas, megadoses of vitamins, and various other natural products. Although much information is available on nutritional supplements and herbal therapy, obtaining the correct information sometimes is difficult. Medicinal herbs and nutritional substances are available at supermarkets, pharmacies, health food stores, and specialty herb stores, and through the Internet. Much misinformation has been made public. Because these substances are "natural products," many individuals may incorrectly assume that they are without adverse effects. When a patient uses any herbal remedy or dietary supplement, it should be reported to the health care provider. Many of these botanicals have strong pharmacological activity, and some may interact with prescription drugs or be toxic in the body. For example, comfrey, an herb that was once widely used to promote digestion, can cause liver damage. Although it may still be available in some areas, it is a dangerous herb and is not recommended for use as a supplement.

When a patient's drug history is obtained, the patient should always be questioned about the use of any herbs, teas, vitamins, or other nutritional or dietary supplements. Many patients consider herbs as natural and therefore safe. It is also difficult for some to think of their use of an herbal tea as a part of their health care regimen. Box 1-4 identifies teaching points to consider when discussing the use of herbs and nutritional supplements with patients. Although a complete discussion about the use of herbs is beyond the scope of this book, sections on herbal remedies, including alerts, are included in all drug chapters in this text as relevant. Ap-

---

Box 1-4 Teaching Points when Discussing the Use of Herbal Therapy

- If you regularly use herbal therapies, then get a good herbal reference book such as *Guide to Popular Natural Products*, edited by Ara DerMarderosian (Facts and Comparisons Publishing Group, 2001).
- Store clerks are not experts in herbal therapy. Your best choice is to select an herbal product manufactured by a reputable company.
- Check the label for the word "standardized." This means that the product has a specific percentage of a specific chemical.
- Some herbal tinctures are 50% alcohol, which could pose a problem to individuals with a history of alcohol abuse.
- Use products with more than six herbs cautiously. It is generally better to use the single herb than to use a diluted product with several herbs.

- Do not overmedicate with herbs. The adage "if one is good, two must be better" is definitely not true. Take only the recommended dosage.
- Herbs are generally safe when taken in recommended dosages. However, if you experience any different or unusual symptoms, such as heart palpitations, headaches, rashes, or difficulty breathing, stop taking the herb and contact your health care provider.
- Inform your health care provider of any natural products that you take (e.g., herbs, vitamins, minerals, teas, etc). Certain herbs can interact with the medications that you take, causing serious adverse reactions or toxic effects.
- Allow time for the herb to work. Generally, 30 days is sufficient. If your symptoms have not improved within 30 to 60 days, then discontinue use of the herb.

Adapted from Fontaine KL. *Healing practices: Alternative therapies for nursing.* Upper Saddle River, NJ: Prentice Hall; 2000:126–127. Used with permission.

pendix F also gives an overview of selected common herbs and nutritional supplements.

KEY POINTS

◉ Federal and sometimes state laws govern the development and sale of drugs to ensure public safety and to control prescription drugs and controlled substances whose effects could be harmful. Health care professionals are an important part of this process by monitoring patients' responses to drugs and reporting adverse reactions.

◉ Drugs may have several names: a chemical name, a generic (nonproprietary) name, an official name, and a trade or brand name.

◉ Drugs are categorized in a number of ways: (1) as prescription or nonprescription drugs; (2) in different classes of controlled substances; and (3) by pregnancy categories.

◉ After absorption and distribution in the body, drugs have therapeutic effects by binding to specific receptors on cells and altering cellular environment or function. Then the drug is metabolized and excreted.

◉ Possible drug reactions include adverse reactions, allergic reactions, idiosyncratic reactions, tolerance, cumulative drug effect, and toxic reactions. All such observed patient responses should be reported to the health care provider.

◉ Drug interactions include additive reactions, synergistic reactions, antagonist reactions, and interactions with food.

◉ How an individual patient responds to a drug depends on factors such as age, weight, gender, disease conditions present, and the route of administration. Dose size and frequency may have to be adjusted for the individual.

◉ Herbal therapy may be an important complementary or alternative to drug therapy, but herbs can have many effects and interactions and should be used as carefully as drugs, based on available information and safety warnings. Patients frequently view herbs as harmless and may need to be taught cautions to take with any herbal product.

WEBSITE ACTIVITIES

1. Go to the MedWatch website (www.fda.gov/medwatch/index.html). Navigate to the section on "Safety Information" and look for "Safety Alerts" for drugs. This information is organized by year; find the list of drugs for which safety alerts have been issued in the current year. Read the alerts for several different drugs and consider the following questions:
   a. Find a drug safety alert for which new adverse reactions are being reported. Look up that drug in this text or a drug reference such as the PDR. Does the alert add significant new information to what you would have known about the drug from only looking at this text or the reference?
   b. Explain the value of the alert for a health care provider who is prescribing this drug for a new patient.

2. Go the website of the National Center for Complementary and Alternative Medicine (http://nccam.nih.gov). Go to the "Health Information" section and then to Treatment Information "By Disease or Condition." Choose any medical condition (or a herb) and look for information on an herb used in treatment. Briefly answer these questions based on what you learn from this site:
   a. Name the herb and a medical condition for which it is used.
   b. How effective is this herb thought to be in the treatment of this condition?
   c. Are there any adverse effects of this herbal therapy?
   d. Does this herb interact with any drug or food to produce a negative effect?
   e. Are there any known problems with high doses of this herb?
   f. If this herb is recommended for treatment of this condition, are there certain patient types or other conditions that affect who should or should not use this herb?

CASE STUDY

Jenny Davis, age 25, is pregnant. Jenny's health care provider tells her that she may not take any medication without first checking with her health care provider during the pregnancy. Jenny is puzzled and questions you about this. Discuss how you would address Jenny's concerns.

REVIEW QUESTIONS

1. Mr. Carter has a rash and pruritus. You suspect an allergic reaction. What question would be most important to ask Mr. Carter?
   a. Are you having any difficulty breathing?
   b. Have you noticed any blood in your stool?
   c. Do you have a headache?
   d. Are you having difficulty with your vision?

2. Mr. Jones, a newly admitted patient, has a history of liver disease. Drug dosages must be based on the consideration that liver disease may result in a/an:
   a. increase in the excretion rate of a drug
   b. impaired ability to metabolize or detoxify a drug
   c. necessity to increase the dosage of a drug
   d. decrease in the rate of drug absorption

3. A patient asks you what a hypersensitivity reaction is. You might begin by telling the patient that a hypersensitivity reaction is also called a:
   a. synergistic reaction
   b. antagonistic reaction
   c. drug idiosyncrasy
   d. drug allergy

4. If a patient takes a drug on an empty stomach, the drug will be:
   a. absorbed more slowly
   b. neutralized by pancreatic enzymes
   c. affected by enzymes in the colon
   d. absorbed more rapidly

5. A synergistic drug effect may be defined as:
   a. an effect greater than the sum of the separate actions of two or more drugs
   b. a decrease in the action of one of the two drugs being given
   c. a neutralizing drug effect
   d. a comprehensive drug effect

6. An example of a schedule II controlled substance is:
   a. codeine cough medicine
   b. nonnarcotic analgesics
   c. morphine
   d. LSD

7. A drug's effect will occur most quickly if it is administered:
   a. subcutaneously
   b. intravenously
   c. orally
   d. intramuscularly

8. A drug that blocks the effect of another drug by binding to its receptors is called a/an:
   a. mediator
   b. receiver
   c. antagonist
   d. agonist

9. If you think a patient is experiencing anaphylactic shock, you should:
   a. write this in the patient's chart at the end of your shift
   b. ask the patient to call you in an hour if he/she feels the same
   c. report this to the health care provider as soon as you have a free moment
   d. call for help immediately

10. Health care providers care about patients' use of herbal remedies because:
    a. some herbs may interact with prescription drugs
    b. some patients may take herbs in too large a dose
    c. some herbs may be dangerous
    d. all of the above

2 The Administration of Drugs

KEY TERMS

buccal—within the cheek

drug error—any incident in which a patient receives the wrong dose, the wrong drug, a drug by the wrong route, or a drug given at the incorrect time

extravasation—the escape of fluid from a blood vessel into surrounding tissues

infiltration—the collection of fluid in a tissue

inhalation—route of administration in which drug droplets, vapor, or gas is inhaled and absorbed through the mucous membranes of the respiratory tract

intradermal—route of administration in which the drug is injected into skin tissue

intramuscular—route of administration in which the drug is injected into muscle tissue

intravenous—route of administration in which the drug is injected into a vein

parenteral—a general term for drug administration in which the drug is injected inside the body

standard precautions—a set of actions recommended by CDC for preventing contact with potentially infectious body fluids, such as wearing gloves

subcutaneous—route of administration in which the drug is injected just below the layer of skin

sublingual—route of administration in which the drug is placed under the tongue for absorption

transdermal—route of administration in which the drug is absorbed through the skin from a patch

unit dose—a single dose of a drug packaged ready for patient use

Z-track—a technique of intramuscular injection used with drugs that are irritating to subcutaneous tissues

CHAPTER OBJECTIVES

On completion of this chapter, students will be able to:

1 Define the chapter's key terms.

2 Name the six rights of drug administration.

3 Identify the different types of medication orders.

4 Describe the various types of medication dispensing systems.

5 List the various routes by which a drug may be given.

6 Describe the administration of oral and parenteral drugs.

7 Describe the administration of drugs through the skin and mucous membranes.

Although drugs are administered only by physicians, nurses, and, in some states, medical assistants or others, all health professionals who work with patients should understand the basics of drug administration to help ensure patient safety. The patient and often family members as well also need to understand how drugs are administered safely.

The Six Rights of Drug Administration

Six "rights" in the administration of drugs ensure that patients receive medications correctly and safely:

- Right patient
- Right drug
- Right dose
- Right route
- Right time
- Right documentation

Right Patient

The health care professional administering a drug must be certain that the patient receiving the drug is the patient for whom the drug has been ordered. With a hospitalized patient, this is accomplished by checking the patient's wristband containing the patient's name.

Right Drug

Drug names can be confused, especially when the names sound similar or the spellings are similar. Someone who hurriedly prepares a drug for administration or who fails to look up a questionable drug is more likely to administer the wrong drug. Table 2-1 gives examples of drugs that can easily be confused. The person administering the drug should compare the medication, container label, and medication record.

TABLE 2-1   Examples of Easily Confused Drugs

Accupril	Accutane
albuterol	atenolol
Alupent	Atrovent
Amikin	Amicar
Bentyl	Aventyl
Capitrol	captopril
Cefzil	Ceftin
Celebrex	Celexa
DiaBeta	Zebeta
dobutamine	dopamine
Elavil	Mellaril
Eurax	Serax
Flomax	Fosamax
Inderal	Isordil
K-Dur	Imdur
Klonopin	clonidine
Lodine	codeine
Nicobid	Nitro-Bid
nifedipine	nicardipine
prednisolone	prednisone
Prilosec	Prozac
Retrovir	ritonavir
Taxol	Paxil
TobraDex	Tobrex
Versed	VePesid
Zocor	Zoloft
Zyvox	Vioxx

Right Dose, Route, and Time

The health care professional prescribing drugs for patients should write an order for the administration of all drugs. This written order must include the patient's name, the drug name, the dosage form and route, the dosage to be administered, and the frequency of administration. The health care provider must sign the drug order. In an emergency, a nurse or other qualified health care professional may administer a drug with a verbal order from the health care provider, who must then write and sign the order as soon as the emergency is over.

Right Documentation

After any drug is administered, the health care professional who administered it must record the process immediately. Immediate documentation is particularly important when drugs are given on an as-needed basis (PRN drugs). For example, most analgesics require 20 to 30 minutes before the drug begins to relieve pain. Patients may forget that they received a drug for pain, may not have been told that the administered drug was for pain, or may not know that pain relief is not immediate—and may then ask another health care worker for the drug. If the first administration of the analgesic had not been recorded, then the patient might receive a second dose soon after the first dose. This kind of situation can be extremely serious, especially with narcotics or other central nervous system depressants. Immediate documentation prevents accidental administration of a drug by another individual. Proper documentation is essential to the process of administering drugs correctly.

Considerations in Drug Administration

Drug Errors

Drug errors are any occurrence that can cause a patient to receive the wrong dose, the wrong drug, a drug by the wrong route, or a drug given at the incorrect time. Errors may occur in transcribing drug orders, dispensing the drug, or administering the drug. When a drug error occurs, it must be reported immediately so that any necessary steps can be taken to counteract the action of the drug or observe the patient for adverse effects. It is important that errors are reported even if the patient suffers no harm.

Drug errors occur when one or more of the six "rights" has not been followed. Each time a drug is prepared and administered, the six rights must be a part of the procedure. In addition to consistently practicing the six rights, the person administering the drug should follow these precautions to help prevent drug errors:

- Confirm any questionable orders.
- When a dosage calculation is necessary, verify it with another person.
- Listen to the patient when he or she questions a drug, the dosage, or the drug regimen. Never administer the drug until the patient's questions have been adequately researched.
- Concentrate on only one task at a time.

Most drug errors are made during administration. The most common errors are a failure to administer a drug that has been ordered, administration of the wrong dose or strength of the drug, or administration of the wrong drug. Errors commonly occur, for example, with insulin and heparin.

The Medication Order

Before a medication can be administered to a patient, it must be ordered by a health care provider such as a physician, dentist, or, in some cases, a nurse practitioner. Common orders include the standing order, the single order, the PRN order, and the STAT order. Box 2-1 explains these types of orders.

Box 2-1 Types of Medication Orders

Standing order: This type of order is written when the patient is to receive the prescribed drug on a regular basis. The drug is administered until the physician discontinues it. Occasionally a drug may be ordered for a specified number of days, or in some cases a drug can only be given for a specified number of days before the order needs to be renewed.
Example: Lanoxin 0.25 mg PO QD.
Single order: An order to administer the drug one time only.
Example: Valium 10 mg IVP at 10:00 AM.
PRN order: An order to administer the drug as needed.
Example: Demerol 100 mg IM q4h PRN for pain.
STAT order: A one-time order given as soon as possible.
Example: Morphine 10 mg IV STAT.

Once-per-Week Drugs

Increasingly available are drugs in once-per-week, or even twice-per-month, forms. These are designed to replace daily doses of drugs. For example, in 2001 the FDA approved two new strengths for alendronate (Fosamax), a drug used to treat osteoporosis (see Chapter 29), to be given once per week. The 70-mg tablet is used to treat postmenopausal osteoporosis, and the 35-mg tablet is used for prevention of postmenopausal osteoporosis. Clinical trials showed that the once-per-week dosing caused no greater adverse reactions than the once-daily regimen. Once-per-week dosing may prove beneficial for those experiencing mild adverse reactions because they would experience the reactions only once per week rather than every day.

Drug Dispensing Systems

A number of drug dispensing systems are used to dispense medications after they have been ordered for patients. A brief description of three methods follows.

Computerized Dispensing System

Automated or computerized dispensing systems are used in many hospitals and other agencies dispensing drugs. Drugs are dispensed in the pharmacy for drug orders sent from the individual floors or units. Each floor or unit has a medication cart in which medications are placed for individual patients. Medication orders are filled in the hospital pharmacy and are placed in the drug dispensing cart. When orders are filled, the cart is delivered to the unit. The dispensing of the drugs is automatically recorded in the computerized system. After drugs are dispensed, the cart goes back to the pharmacy to be refilled and for new drug orders to be placed.

Unit Dose System

In the **unit dose** system, drug orders are filled and medications dispensed to fill each patient's medication order(s) for a 24-hour period. The pharmacist dispenses each dose (unit) in a package that is labeled with the drug name and dosage. The drug(s) are placed in drawers in a portable medication cart with a drawer for each patient. Many drugs are packaged by their manufacturers in unit doses; each package is labeled by the manufacturer and contains one tablet or capsule, a premeasured amount of a liquid drug, a prefilled syringe, or one suppository. Hospital pharmacists also may prepare unit doses. The pharmacist restocks the cart each day with the drugs patients need for the next 24-hour period (Fig. 2-1).

Some hospitals use a bar code scanner in the administration of unit dose drugs. A bar code is placed on the patient's hospital identification band when the patient is admitted to the hospital. This bar code, along with bar codes on the drug unit dose packages, is used to identify the patient and to record and charge routine and PRN drugs. The scanner also keeps an ongoing inventory of controlled substances, which eliminates the need for narcotic counts at the end of each shift.

Floor Stock

Some agencies, such as nursing homes or small hospitals, use a floor stock method to dispense drugs. Some special units in hospitals, such as the emergency department, may use this method. In this system, the drugs most frequently prescribed are kept on the unit in containers in a designated medication room or at the nurses' station. Medication are taken from the appropriate container and administered to patients and recorded in the patient's administration record.

General Principles of Drug Administration

Health care professionals involved in drug administration and patient care should know about each drug given, the reasons the drug is used, the drug's general action, its more common adverse reactions, special precautions in administration (if any), and the normal dose ranges.

With commonly used drugs, health care workers often become familiar with their pharmacologic properties. With less commonly used or new drugs, information can be obtained from reliable sources, such as the drug package insert or the hospital department of pharmacy.

Patient considerations are also important, such as allergy history, previous adverse reactions, the patient's comments, and any change in the patient's condition. Before a patient is given any drug for the first time, he or she should be asked about any known allergies and any family history of allergies. This includes allergies not only to drugs but also to food, pollen, animals, and so on. Patients with a personal or family history of allergies are more likely to experience additional allergies and must be monitored closely.

If the patient makes any statement about the drug or if the patient's condition changes, then the situation is carefully considered before the drug is given. Examples of such situations include:

- Problems that may be associated with the drug, such as nausea, dizziness, ringing in the ears, and difficulty walking. Any comments made by the patient may indicate the occurrence of an adverse reaction. The drug should be withheld until the health care provider is contacted.
- A patient's comment that the drug looks different from the one previously received, that the drug was just given by someone else, or that the health care provider had discontinued the drug therapy.
- A change in the patient's condition, a change in one or more vital signs (pulse, respiration, blood pressure, or temperature), or the appearance of new symptoms. Depending on the drug being given and the patient's diagnosis, such a change may indicate that the drug should be withheld and the health care provider contacted.

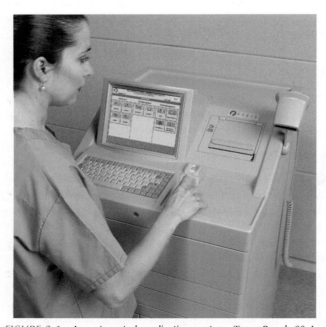

FIGURE 2-1   An automated medication system. (From Roach SS. *Introductory Clinical Pharmacology*, ed. 7. Baltimore: Lippincott Williams & Wilkins; 2004.)

Preparing a Drug for Administration

Preparing a drug for administration should follow these guidelines:

- The health care provider's written orders should be checked and any questions answered.
- Drugs should be prepared in a quiet, well-lit area.
- The label of the drug should be checked three times: (1) when the drug is taken from its storage area; (2) immediately before removing the drug from the container; and (3) before returning the drug to its storage area.
- A drug should never be removed from an unlabeled container or from a container whose label is illegible.
- The person preparing a drug for administration should wash hands immediately before the procedure.
- Capsules and tablets should not be touched with one's hands. The correct number of tablets or capsules is shaken into the cap of the container and from there into the medicine cup.
- Aseptic technique must be followed when handling syringes and needles.
- Some drugs have names that sound alike but are very different. Giving one drug when another is ordered could cause serious consequences. For example, digoxin and digitoxin sound alike but are different drugs.
- The caps of drug containers should be replaced immediately after the drug is removed.
- Drugs requiring special storage must be returned to the storage area immediately after being prepared for administration. This rule applies mainly to the refrigeration of drugs but may also apply to drugs that must be protected from exposure to light or heat.
- Tablets must never be crushed or capsules opened without first checking with the pharmacist. Some tablets can be crushed or capsules opened and the contents added to water or a tube feeding when the patient cannot swallow a whole tablet or capsule. Some tablets have a special coating that delays the absorption of the drug. Crushing the tablet may destroy this drug property and result in problems such as improper absorption of the drug or gastric irritation. Capsules are made of gelatin and dissolve on contact with a liquid. The contents of some capsules do not mix well with water and therefore are best left in the capsule. If the patient cannot take an oral tablet or capsule, then the health care provider should be consulted because the drug may be available in liquid form.
- No one should ever give a drug that someone else prepared. The individual preparing the drug must administer the drug.

- With a unit dose system, the wrappings of the unit dose should not be removed until the drug reaches the bedside of the patient who is to receive it. After the drug is administered, it is charted immediately on the unit dose drug form.

Administration of Drugs by the Oral Route

The oral route is the most frequent route of drug administration and rarely causes physical discomfort in patients. Oral drug forms include tablets, capsules, and liquids. Some capsules and tablets contain sustained-release drugs, which dissolve over an extended period of time. Administration of oral drugs is relatively easy for patients who are alert and can swallow.

Patient Care Considerations for Oral Drug Administration

- The patient should be in an upright position. It is difficult, as well as dangerous, to swallow a solid or liquid when lying down.
- A full glass of water should be available to the patient.
- The patient may need help removing the tablet or capsule from the container, holding the container, holding a medicine cup, or holding a glass of water. Some patients with physical disabilities cannot handle or hold these objects and may require assistance.
- The patient should be advised to take a few sips of water before placing a tablet or capsule in the mouth.
- The patient is instructed to place the pill or capsule on the back of the tongue and tilt the head back to swallow a tablet or slightly forward to swallow a capsule. The patient is encouraged to take a few sips of water to move the drug down the esophagus and into the stomach, and then to finish the whole glass.
- The patient is given any special instructions, such as drinking extra fluids or remaining in bed, that are pertinent to the drug being administered.
- A drug is never left at the patient's bedside to be taken later unless the health care provider has ordered this. A few drugs (e.g., antacids and nitroglycerin tablets) may be ordered to be left at the bedside.
- Patients with a nasogastric feeding tube may be given their oral drugs through the tube. Liquid drugs are diluted and then flushed through the tube. Tablets are crushed and dissolved in water before administering them through the tube. The tube should be checked first for correct placement.

Afterwards, the tube is flushed with water to completely clear the tubing.

- The patient is instructed to place a **buccal** drug against the mucous membranes of the cheek in either the upper or lower jaw. These drugs are given for a local, rather than systemic, effect. They are absorbed slowly from the mucous membranes of the mouth. Examples of drugs given buccally are lozenges.
- Certain drugs are given by the **sublingual** route (placed under the tongue). These drugs must not be swallowed or chewed and must be dissolved completely before the patient eats or drinks. Nitroglycerin is commonly given sublingually.

Administration of Drugs by the Parenteral Route

Parenteral drug administration means the giving of a drug by the **subcutaneous** (SC), **intramuscular** (IM), **intravenous** (IV), or **intradermal** route. Other routes of parenteral administration include intralesional (into a lesion), intra-arterial (into an artery), intracardiac (into the heart), and intra-articular (into a joint).

Patient Care Considerations for Parenteral Drug Administration

- Gloves must be worn for protection from a potential blood spill when giving parenteral drugs. The risk of exposure to infected blood is increasing for all health care workers. The Centers for Disease Control and Prevention (CDC) recommends that gloves be worn when touching blood or body fluids, mucous membranes, or any broken skin area. This recommendation is one of the **Standard Precautions**, which combine the Universal Precautions for Blood and Body Fluids with Body Substance Isolation guidelines.
- At the site for injection, the skin is cleansed. Most hospitals and medical offices have a policy regarding the type of skin antiseptic used for cleansing the skin before parenteral drug administration. The skin is cleansed with a circular motion, starting at an inner point and moving outward.
- After the needle is inserted for IM administration, the syringe barrel is pulled back to aspirate the drug. If blood appears in the syringe, the needle is removed so that the drug is not injected. The drug, needle, and syringe are discarded, and another injection prepared. If no blood appears in the syringe, the drug is injected. Aspiration is not necessary when giving an intradermal or SC injection.

- After the needle is inserted into a vein for IV drug administration, the syringe barrel is pulled back. Blood should flow back into the syringe. After a backflow of blood is obtained, it is safe to inject the drug.
- After the needle is removed from an IM, SC, or IV injection site, pressure is placed on the area. Patients with bleeding tendencies often require prolonged pressure on the area.
- Syringes are not recapped but are disposed of according to agency policy. Needles and syringes are discarded into clearly marked, appropriate containers. Most agencies have a "sharps" container located in each room for immediate disposal of needles and syringes after use (Fig. 2-2).
- Most hospitals and medical offices use needles designed to prevent accidental needle sticks. This needle has a plastic guard that slips over the needle as it is withdrawn from the injection site. The guard locks in place and eliminates the need to recap the syringe. Other models are available as well. These newer types of methods for administering parenteral fluids provide a greater margin of safety (see OSHA Guidelines).

Occupational Safety and Health Administration Guidelines

Each year between 600,000 and 1 million health care workers experience accidental needle sticks from conventional needles and sharps. Needle exposures can

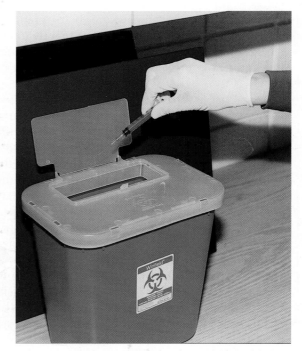

FIGURE 2-2　A sharps container for disposal of used hypodermic needles.

transmit hepatitis B, hepatitis C, and human immuno-deficiency virus. Other infections, such as tuberculosis, syphilis, and malaria, also can be transmitted through needle sticks. More than 80% of needle stick injuries can be prevented with the use of safe needle devices.

In 2001 the Occupational Safety and Health Administration (OSHA) announced new guidelines for needle stick prevention. The revisions clarify the need for employers to select safer needle devices as they become available and to involve employees in identifying and choosing the devices. Employers with 11 or more employees must also maintain a Sharps Injury Log to help employees and employers track all needle stick incidents to help identify problem areas. In addition, employers must have a written Exposure Control Plan that is updated annually. As new safer devices become available, they should be adopted for use in the agency. The new OSHA guidelines help reduce needle stick injuries among health care workers and others who handle medical sharps. Safety-engineered devices such as self-sheathing needles and needleless systems are now commonly used.

Administration of Drugs by the Subcutaneous Route

A subcutaneous (SC) injection places the drug into the tissues between the skin and the muscle. Drugs administered in this manner are absorbed more slowly than are intramuscular injections. Heparin and insulin are two drugs most commonly given by the SC route.

Patient Care Considerations for Subcutaneous Drug Administration

- A small volume of 0.5 to 1 mL is used for SC injection. Larger volumes are best given as IM injections.
- The sites for SC injection are the upper arms, the upper abdomen, and the upper back. Injection sites are rotated to ensure proper absorption and to minimize tissue damage.
- When a drug is given by the SC route, the needle is generally inserted at a 45-degree angle. The needle length and angle of insertion depend on the patient's body weight.

Administration of Drugs by the Intramuscular Route

An intramuscular (IM) injection is the administration of a drug into a muscle. Drugs that are irritating to SC tissue can be given via IM injection. Drugs given by this route are absorbed more rapidly than drugs given by the SC route because of the rich blood supply in the muscle. In addition, a larger volume (1–3 mL) of drug can be given at one site.

Patient Care Considerations for Intramuscular Drug Administration

- With a large drug volume, the drug is divided and given as two separate injections. Volumes larger than 3 mL will not be absorbed properly at one site.
- The sites for IM administration are the deltoid muscle (upper arm), the ventrogluteal or dorsogluteal sites (hip), and the vastus lateralis (thigh). The vastus lateralis site is frequently used for infants and small children because it is more developed than the gluteal or deltoid sites. In children who have been walking for more than 2 years, the ventrogluteal site may be used.
- When a drug is given by the IM route, the needle is inserted at a 90-degree angle. When a drug is injected into the ventrogluteal or dorsogluteal muscles, the patient should be in a comfortable position, preferably in a prone position with the toes pointing inward. When the deltoid site is used, a sitting or lying down position may be used. The patient is placed in a recumbent position for injection of a drug into the vastus lateralis.
- The **Z-track** method of IM injection is used when a drug is highly irritating to SC tissues or may permanently stain the skin. In this technique, the skin and subcutaneous tissues are pulled to one side before the injection and an air bubble is injected from the syringe after the drug. This technique prevents the drug from oozing up through the small pathway created by the needle into the SC tissue.

Administration of Drugs by the Intravenous Route

A drug administered by the intravenous (IV) route is given directly into the blood by a needle inserted into a vein. Drug action occurs almost immediately. Drugs administered via the IV route may be given in a number of ways:

- Slowly, over 1 or more minutes
- Rapidly (IV push)
- By piggyback infusions (drugs are mixed with a compatible IV fluid and administered over 30–60 minutes piggybacked onto the primary IV line)
- Into an existing IV line (the IV port)
- Into an intermittent venous access device called a heparin lock (a small IV catheter in the patient's vein connected to a small fluid reservoir with a rubber cap through which the needle is inserted to administer the drug)
- By being added to an IV solution and allowed to infuse into the vein over a longer period

When a drug is administered into a vein by a venipuncture, a tourniquet is placed above the vein and tightened so that venous blood flow is blocked but arterial blood flow is not. The vein is allowed to fill (distend) and the needle is inserted into the vein at a short angle to the skin. Blood should immediately flow into the syringe if the needle is properly inserted into the vein.

Some drugs are added to an IV solution, such as 1000 mL of dextrose 5% and water. The drug is usually added to the IV fluid container immediately before the fluid is added to the IV line. Whenever a drug is added to an IV fluid, the bottle must have an attached label indicating the drug and drug dose added to the IV fluid.

Intravenous Infusion Controllers and Pumps

Electronic infusion devices include infusion controllers and infusion pumps. The primary difference between the two is that an infusion pump administers the infused drug under pressure, whereas an infusion controller does not add pressure. An infusion pump can be set to deliver the desired number of drops of medication per minute. An alarm sounds if the IV rate is more than or less than the preset rate. Controllers and pumps have detectors and alarms that alert health care workers to problems such as air in the line, an occlusion, a low battery, the completion of an infusion, or an inability to deliver the drug at the preset rate. Whenever an alarm is activated, the device must be checked.

Patient Care Considerations for Intravenous Drug Administration

After an IV infusion is started, the type of IV fluid and the drug added to the IV solution are documented in the patient's chart. The infusion rate must be checked every 15 to 30 minutes. The needle site is inspected for signs of redness, swelling, or other problems. Swelling around the needle may indicate extravasation or infiltration. **Extravasation** is the escape of fluid from a blood vessel into surrounding tissues while the needle or catheter is in the vein. **Infiltration** is the collection of fluid in tissues (usually SC tissue) when the needle or catheter is out of the vein. Either problem necessitates stopping the infusion and inserting an IV line in another vein. Some drugs can cause severe tissue damage if extravasation or infiltration occurs. The health care provider should be contacted if such a drug escapes into the tissues surrounding the needle insertion site.

Administration of Drugs by the Intradermal Route

The intradermal route is usually used for sensitivity tests (e.g., the tuberculin test or allergy skin testing). Absorption is slow from this route, providing good results when testing for allergies or administering local anesthetics. The needle is inserted at a 15-degree angle between the upper layers of the skin. Injection produces a small wheal (raised area) on the outer surface of the skin. If a wheal does not appear, then the drug may have entered the SC tissue, making test results inaccurate.

Patient Care Considerations for Intradermal Drug Administration

- The inner part of the forearm and the upper back are used for intradermal injections. A hairless area should be chosen; areas near moles, scars, or pigmented skin areas should be avoided. The area is cleansed in the same manner as for SC and IM injections.
- Small volumes (usually <0.1 mL) are used for intradermal injections.

Other Parenteral Routes of Drug Administration

The health care provider may administer a drug by the intracardiac, intralesional, intra-arterial, or intra-articular routes. Special devices and materials are required for these routes of administration.

Venous access ports are implanted self-sealing ports attached to a catheter leading to a large vessel, usually the vena cava. These devices are most commonly used for chemotherapy or other long-term therapy. They require surgical insertion and removal. Drugs are administered through injections made into the portal through the skin.

Administration of Drugs Through the Skin and Mucous Membranes

Drugs may be applied to the skin and mucous membranes using several routes: topically (on the outer layers of skin), **transdermally** through a patch in which the drug has been implanted, or inhaled through the membranes of the upper respiratory tract.

Administration of Drugs by the Topical Route

Most topical drugs act on the skin but are not absorbed through the skin. These drugs are used to soften, disinfect, or lubricate the skin. A few topical drugs are enzymes that remove superficial debris, such as the dead skin and purulent matter present in skin ulcerations. Other topical drugs are used to treat minor superficial skin infections. The various forms of topical applications are described in Box 2-2.

Patient Care Considerations for Topical Drug Administration

- The health care provider may write special instructions for the application of a topical drug, such as

Box 2-2 Topical Applications and Locations of Use

- Creams, lotions, or ointments applied to the skin with a tongue blade, gloved fingers, or gauze
- Sprays applied to the skin or into the nose or oral cavity
- Liquids inserted into body cavities, such as fistulas
- Liquids inserted into the bladder or urethra
- Solids (e.g., suppositories) or jellies inserted into the urethra
- Liquids dropped into the eyes, ears, or nose
- Ophthalmic ointments applied to the eyelids or dropped into the lower conjunctival sac
- Solids (e.g., suppositories, tablets), foams, liquids, and creams inserted into the vagina
- Continuous or intermittent wet dressings applied to skin surfaces
- Solids (e.g., tablets, lozenges) dissolved in the mouth
- Sprays or mists inhaled into the lungs
- Liquids, creams, or ointments applied to the scalp
- Solids (e.g., suppositories), liquids, or foams inserted into the rectum

to apply the drug in a thin even layer or to cover the area after the drug is applied to the skin.

- The manufacturer sometimes provides special instructions for drug administration, such as to apply the drug to a clean hairless area or to let the drug dissolve slowly in the mouth. All such instructions are important because drug action may depend on correct administration of the drug.

Administration of Drugs by the Transdermal Route

Drugs administered by the transdermal route are readily absorbed from the skin and have systemic effects. The drug dose is implanted in a small patch-type bandage. The backing is removed, and the patch is applied to the skin, where the drug is gradually absorbed into the systemic circulation. This drug administration system maintains a relatively constant blood concentration and reduces the possibility of toxicity. In addition, drugs administered transdermally cause fewer adverse reactions. Nitroglycerin (used to treat cardiac problems) and scopolamine (used to treat dizziness and nausea) are two drugs commonly given by the transdermal route.

Patient Care Considerations for Transdermal Drug Administration

- Transdermal patches are applied to clean, dry, non-hairy areas of intact skin.
- The old patch is removed when the next dose is applied in a new site.

- Sites for transdermal patches are rotated to prevent skin irritation. The chest, flank, and upper arm are the most commonly used sites. The area of application should not be shaved because this may cause skin irritation.
- Ointments are sometimes used. They come with a special paper marked in inches. The correct length of ointment is measured onto the paper, and the paper is placed with the drug ointment side down on the skin and secured with tape. Before the next dose, the paper and tape are removed and the skin cleansed.

Administration of Drugs Through Inhalation

Drug droplets, vapor, and gas are administered through the mucous membranes of the respiratory tract. The patient breathes the drug in through a face mask, a nebulizer, or a positive-pressure breathing machine. Examples of drugs administered through **inhalation** include bronchodilators, mucolytics, and some anti-inflammatory drugs. These drugs primarily have a local effect in the lungs.

Patient Care Considerations for Drug Administration by Inhalation

The patient must be provided with proper instructions for taking the drug. For example, many patients with asthma use a metered-dose inhaler to dilate the bronchi and make breathing easier. Without proper instruction on how to use the inhaler, much of the drug may be deposited on the tongue rather than in the respiratory tract; this would decrease the therapeutic effect of the drug. The specific instructions are provided with the inhaler. Figure 2-3 illustrates the proper use of one type of inhaler.

Patient Care Considerations After Drug Administration

- The administration of a drug to a patient is always documented. This should be performed as soon as possible.
- Other information concerning the administration of the drug is also often recorded, including information such as the IV flow rate, the site used for parenteral administration, any problems with administration, and the patient's vital signs taken immediately before administration.
- The patient's response to the drug is monitored and, when applicable, recorded. This evaluation may include such facts as relief of pain, decrease in body temperature, relief of itching, and decrease in the number of stools passed.

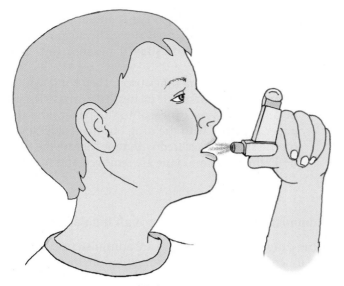

FIGURE 2-3   A respiratory inhalant is used to deliver a drug directly into the lungs. To deliver a dose of the drug, the patient takes a slow, deep breath while depressing the top of the canister. (See Chapter 12 for more information on drugs given by inhalation.) (From Roach SS. *Introductory Clinical Pharmacology*, ed. 7, Lippincott Williams & Wilkins; 2004.)

Box 2-3 Administering Drugs Safely in the Home

Patients are often prescribed drugs to be taken at home. Because the home is not as controlled an environment as a health care facility, the patient's home environment should be considered:

- Does the home have a space that is relatively free of clutter and easily accessible to the patient or a caregiver?
- Do any small children live in or visit the home? If so, is there a place where drugs can be stored safely out of their reach?
- Does the drug require refrigeration? If so, does the refrigerator work?
- Does the patient need special equipment, such as needles and syringes? If so, where and how can the equipment be stored for safety and convenience? Does the patient have an appropriate disposal container? Will disposed items be safe from children and pets? Plastic storage containers with snap-on lids or clean, dry glass jars with screw tops can be used for needle disposal. A plastic milk jug with a lid or a heavy-duty, clean, cardboard milk or juice carton may be used if necessary. Patients should understand the importance of precautions to make sure discarded needles do not puncture the container.
- If the patient needs several drugs, can the patient or caregiver identify which drugs are used and when? Do they know how to use them and why?

- The patient is observed for adverse reactions. The frequency of observation depends on the drug administered. All suspected adverse reactions are documented and reported to the health care provider. Serious adverse reactions must be reported immediately.

Administration of Drugs in the Home

Often drugs are taken by patients in their homes or are administered by family members acting as caregivers. The patient or caregivers need to understand the treatment regimen and to be able to ask questions about their drug therapy, such as why the drug was prescribed, how to give or take it, and possible adverse reactions that may occur (see Chapter 3 on patient and family education). Box 2-3 gives guidelines for drug use in the home by the patient or caregiver rather than by health care providers.

KEY POINTS

◎ Six "rights" in the administration of drugs ensure that patients receive medications correctly and safely: right patient, right drug, right dose, right route, right time, and right documentation.

◎ Drug errors are any occurrence that can cause a patient to receive the wrong dose, the wrong drug, a drug by the wrong route, or a drug given at the incorrect time. Errors may occur in transcribing drug orders, dispensing the drug, or administering the drug. When a drug error occurs, it must be reported immediately.

◎ Common medication orders include the standing order, the single order, the PRN order, and the STAT order.

◎ Drug dispensing systems include computerized dispensing systems, unit dose systems, and floor stock systems.

◎ Health care professionals involved in drug administration and patient care should know about each drug given, the reasons the drug is used, the drug's general action, its more common adverse reactions, special precautions in administration, and the normal dose ranges.

◎ In drug administration, patient considerations are important, such as allergy history, previous adverse reactions, the patient's comments, and any change in the patient's condition.

◎ Drugs may be administered by any of the following routes, each with its own patient care considerations: the oral, parenteral (subcutaneous, intramuscular, intravenous, or intradermal), topical, transdermal, and inhalation routes.

◎ When drugs are taken by patients in their homes, the patients or caregivers need to understand the treatment regimen, such as why the drug was prescribed, how to give or take it, and possible adverse reactions that may occur.

WEBSITE ACTIVITIES

1. Go to the website of the U.S. Department of Labor Occupational Safety & Health Administration (OSHA) (http://www.osha.gov). Under "Safety/Health Topics" navigate to the section on Bloodborne Pathogens. Explore this page and find the OSHA material addressing the question, "What are some examples of possible solutions for workplace hazards?" In each of the following categories of how to prevent problems with infectious materials in the workplace, write in one example of a solution for control programs, safer needle devices, and decontamination.

REVIEW QUESTIONS

1. To ensure a drug is given correctly, it should be administered:
   a. to the right patient
   b. at the right time
   c. by the right route
   d. all of the above

2. If a patient reports that the pill just given to him/her is a different color from the last one he/she received, you should:
   a. explain they should not worry because many pills come in different colors
   b. pretend you will check on it so he/she stop worrying
   c. report this to the health care provider
   d. try to get the patient to vomit up the pill as quickly as possible

3. A STAT medication order means the drug should be given:
   a. as soon as possible
   b. whenever the patient is having symptoms and requests it
   c. first thing in the morning
   d. following the daily staff meeting

4. Drugs can be administered to patients from the drug cart on the floor by:
   a. only the pharmacist
   b. only those allowed by law, such as physicians, nurses, some medical assistants, etc.
   c. any health care worker authorized by a nurse
   d. any staff person on duty at the time

5. True or false: the administration of topical medications need not follow the "6 rights" of medication administration because the medication can be wiped off the skin if given incorrectly.
   a. true
   b. false

6. Why do health care workers watch patients for potential allergic reactions?
   a. allergic reactions can be uncomfortable for patients
   b. a different drug may need to be prescribed
   c. allergic reactions can be life-threatening
   d. all of the above

7. Which statement is true about the administration of oral medications?
   a. The patient should be in an upright position.
   b. The patient should not be allowed to drink water before a tablet or capsule is placed in the mouth.
   c. The pill or capsule to be swallowed should be placed under the tongue and the patient's head tilted forward.
   d. The patient should drink at least 3 glasses of water after taking the medication.

3 Patient and Family Teaching

The Teaching/Learning Process

The Three Domains of Learning
Cognitive Domain
Affective Domain
Psychomotor Domain

Adult Learning

Developing a Teaching Plan
Assessing the Patient's Learning Needs
Developing an Individualized Teaching Plan
Information to Consider for the Teaching Plan

Teaching the Patient

Evaluating Patient Learning

Key Points

Case Study

Review Questions

KEY TERMS 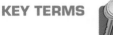 **affective domain**—refers to one's attitudes, feelings, beliefs, and opinions
cognitive domain—refers to intellectual activities such as thought, recall, decision making, and drawing conclusions
learning—acquiring new knowledge or skills
motivation—the desire for, or seeing the need for, something
psychomotor domain—refers to physical skills or tasks
teaching—an interactive process that promotes learning

CHAPTER OBJECTIVES

On completion of this chapter, students will be able to:

1 Define the chapter's key terms.

2 Identify important aspects of the teaching/learning process.

3 Describe the three domains of learning.

4 List important aspects of adult learning.

5 Explain how a teaching plan can be developed.

6 Identify basic information that may be included in a teaching plan.

7 Discuss suggestions that may be made to patients for drug administration in the home.

Patient teaching is an integral part of patient care involving many health care professionals. When a drug is prescribed, the patient and the family need information about the drug. The teaching/learning process is the means through which the patient is made aware of the drug regimen.

The Teaching/Learning Process

Teaching is an interactive process that promotes learning. Both the patient and the health care professional doing the teaching must be actively involved for the teaching to be effective. **Learning** is acquiring new knowledge or skills. When learning occurs, the patient's behavior and/or thinking changes.

A patient must have **motivation** (the desire or seeing the need) to learn. Motivation depends on the patient's perception of a need to learn. The patient may need to understand the disease process to become motivated to learn about drug treatment for the disease. Encouraging patients' participation in the teaching/learning process helps them be more motivated. Patients who have no motivation are likely not to comply well with their drug treatment.

An accepting and positive atmosphere also enhances learning (Fig. 3-1). Physical discomfort negatively affects patients' concentration and their ability to learn. Making sure the patient is not in pain is vital to the teaching/learning process.

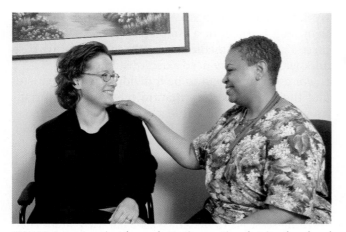

FIGURE 3-1   A patient learns better in a setting that is relaxed and positive.

The Three Domains of Learning

Learning occurs in three domains: cognitive, affective, and psychomotor. A domain is a set of related human characteristics and skills. When developing a teaching plan for the patient, each domain should be considered.

Cognitive Domain

The **cognitive domain** refers to intellectual activities such as thought, recall, decision-making, and drawing conclusions. Based on their previous experiences, knowledge, and perceptions, people give meaning to new information or modify their previous thinking. Health care professionals consider patients' cognitive abilities when giving them information about their disease process, their medication regimen, and adverse reactions that may occur. The patient processes this information, asks questions, and makes decisions.

Affective Domain

The **affective domain** includes attitudes, feelings, beliefs, and opinions. Health care providers too often ignore these aspects of patient teaching. It is easy to hand a patient printed material about a drug or therapeutic regimen and forget that the patient's feelings and attitudes are also important—not just their knowledge.

The best way to learn about a patient's affective behavior is to develop a therapeutic relationship with the patient based on trust and caring. When health care workers take the time to develop a therapeutic relationship, the patient and family members have confidence in them and therefore more confidence in the information they are provided. All health care workers should respect patients and encourage the expression of their thoughts and feelings.

Psychomotor Domain

The **psychomotor domain** involves learning physical skills (such as injection of insulin) or tasks (such as taking an oral medication). Such tasks or skills are taught using a step-by-step method. Patients first take the medication under supervision, and their abilities to do so correctly by themselves are assessed.

Adult Learning

Generally, adults learn only what they feel they need to learn. Adults learn best when they have a strong inner motivation to learn a new skill or acquire new knowledge. They learn less if they are passive recipients of "canned" information. Adults have a vast array of experiences and knowledge to bring to a new learning experience. Teachers who consider this experience bring about the greatest behavior change. Although 83% of adults are visual learners, only 11% learn by listening. Most adults remember information they are taught if they are able to "do" something with that new knowledge immediately. For example, when patients are taught how to administer their own insulin, the technique is first demonstrated, patients are given time for supervised practice, and, when they are ready, patients then prepare and inject the insulin. Most adults prefer an informal learning environment where there is mutual exchange and freedom of expression.

Developing a Teaching Plan

Teaching patients about medication involves a process of identifying the patient's knowledge and skill needs, devising a plan of care to meet the identified needs, performing the teaching, and evaluating its effectiveness. Generally, patients need to know the proper way to take their drugs, the possibility of adverse reactions, and the signs and symptoms of toxicity (when applicable).

Assessing the Patient's Learning Needs

Assessing the patient's learning needs is important for choosing the best teaching methods and individualizing the teaching plan for the individual patient. Patients' learning needs may involve three areas: (1) information the patient or family needs to know about a particular drug; (2) the patient's or family member's ability to learn, accept, and use this information; and (3) any barriers or obstacles to learning.

Some drugs have simple uses and therefore require relatively little patient teaching. For example, applying a nonprescription ointment to the skin requires only minimal teaching. Other drugs, such as insulin, require detailed information that may need to be given over several days.

Assessing an individual patient's ability to learn may be difficult. Not all adults have the same literacy level. The presentation of information must be geared to the patient's educational and reading level. Some patients cannot read well. The patient's ability to communicate is also important because without accurate communication, learning will not occur. If the patient has a learning impairment, then a family member or friend should be included in the teaching process. Most people readily understand what is being taught them, but some cannot. For example, a visually impaired patient may be unable to read a label or printed directions, and another means of teaching will have to be used.

It is also important to determine what barriers or obstacles (if any) may prevent a patient or family member from fully understanding the drug information presented. The patient's cultural background should be taken into account when planning a teaching session. For example, for some patients an interpreter is needed. In some cultures a certain individual (for example, the mother or the grandmother) is the decision-maker in the family. The decision-maker should be included with the patient in the teaching session.

Developing an Individualized Teaching Plan

After assessment, one plans the specific strategies to be used in the teaching and what information is to be taught. Box 3-1 identifies important information that may need to be included in the teaching plan.

Teaching plans are individualized because all patients' needs are not identical. Subjects covered in the individualized teaching plan may depend on the drug prescribed, the health care provider's preference for including or excluding specific facts about the drug, and what the patient needs to know to take the drug correctly. Teaching strategies to be used depend on the individual's learning needs and abilities. For example, a patient who speaks and reads only Spanish will not benefit from instructions given or written in English. Different strategies must be implemented, such as providing instructions written in Spanish or communicating through another health care worker fluent in Spanish. As another example, one patient may learn from a simple explanation of how to place a sublingual medication under the tongue, whereas another patient may need a demonstration.

For a teaching plan to be individualized for patients and their families, information relevant to a specific drug must be selected, the teaching strategies adapted to the individual's level of understanding, and medical terminology avoided unless terms are explained or defined. Standardized forms are often used by those developing a teaching plan. As a general principle, repetition enhances learning. With more complicated aspects of drug administration, it may be helpful to use several teaching sessions to better-assess what the patient is actually learning and to allow time for clarification. Patients should be encouraged to ask questions and express their feelings.

Information to Consider for the Teaching Plan

The teaching plan typically includes information on the dosage regimen, possible adverse reactions, the role of family members, and basic information about drugs, drug containers, and drug storage. These topics are described in the next sections.

Dosage Regimen

The dosage regimen is an important aspect of the teaching plan, including the following general points:

- Capsules or tablets should be taken with water unless the health care provider or pharmacist directs otherwise (e.g., take with food, milk, or an antacid). Some liquids, such as coffee, tea, fruit juice, and carbonated beverages, may interfere with the action of certain drugs.
- The patient usually drinks a full glass of water when taking an oral drug. It may be necessary to drink extra fluids during the day while taking certain drugs.
- It is important not to chew capsules before swallowing; they must be swallowed whole. The patient also should not chew tablets unless they are labeled as "chewable." Some tablets have special coatings that are required for specific purposes, such as proper absorption of the drug or prevention of irritation of the lining of the stomach.
- The patient should never increase or decrease the dose of a drug or the time interval between doses unless directed by the health care provider.
- A prescribed drug or nonprescription drug should not be stopped or omitted except on the advice of the health care provider.
- If the patient's symptoms for which a drug was prescribed do not improve, or if the symptoms become worse, then the health care provider must be contacted as soon as possible because a change in dosage or a different drug may be necessary.

Box 3-1 Important Information to Include in the Teaching Plan

1. Therapeutic response expected from the drug
2. Adverse reactions to expect when taking the drug
3. Adverse reactions to report to the health care provider
4. Dosage and route
5. Any special considerations or precautions associated with the particular drug
6. Additional education regarding special considerations of certain drugs, such as techniques for giving injections, applying topical patches, or instilling eye drops

- If a dose of a drug is omitted or forgotten, then the patient should not double the next dose or take the drug at more frequent intervals unless advised to do so by the health care provider.
- All health care workers should always be informed of all drugs (prescription and nonprescription) the patient is currently taking on a regular or occasional basis.
- The patient should keep the exact names of all prescription and nonprescription drugs currently being taken in a wallet or purse for reference when seeing a physician, dentist, or other health care provider.
- Refilled prescriptions from the pharmacy should be carefully checked and any changes in the prescription (e.g., changes in color, size, shape) should be reported to the pharmacist or health care provider before taking the drug, because an error may have occurred.
- The patient should wear a Medic-Alert bracelet or other type of identification when taking a drug for a long time. This is especially important for drugs such as anticoagulants, steroids, oral hypoglycemic agents, insulin, or digitalis. In case of an emergency, the bracelet ensures that medical personnel are aware of the patient's health problems and current drug therapy.

Adverse Drug Effects

Information about potential adverse drug effects of prescribed drugs must be included in the teaching plan for a patient, including the following general points:

- All drugs potentially cause adverse reactions (side effects). Examples of some of the more common adverse reactions are nausea, vomiting, diarrhea, constipation, skin rash, dizziness, drowsiness, and dry mouth. Some may be mild and disappear with time or with a dosage adjustment by the health care provider. In some instances, mild reactions, such as dry mouth, may have to be tolerated. Some adverse reactions are potentially serious and even life-threatening.
- Adverse effects should always be reported to the health care provider as soon as possible.
- Medical personnel must be informed of all drug allergies before any treatment or drug is given.

Family Members

The following points concerning family members should be considered for the teaching plan:

- A drug prescribed for one family member is never given to another family member, relative, or friend unless directed by the health care provider.
- All family members or relatives should be aware of all prescription and nonprescription drugs that the patient is currently taking.

Drugs, Drug Containers, and Drug Storage

The following important facts about drugs, drug containers, and the storage of drugs should be considered:

- The term "drug" applies to nonprescription and prescription drugs.
- A drug should be kept in the container in which it was dispensed or purchased. Some drugs require special containers, such as light-resistant (brown) bottles to prevent deterioration that may occur with exposure to light.
- If a drug changes color or develops a new odor, then the pharmacist should be consulted immediately.
- The original label on the drug container must not be removed.
- Two or more different drugs must never be mixed in one container, even for a brief time, because one drug may chemically affect another. Mixing drugs can also lead to mistaking one drug for another, especially when their size and color are similar.
- The lid or cap of the container must be replaced immediately after the drug is removed from the container. The lid or cap must be firmly snapped or screwed in place because exposure to air or moisture shortens the life of most drugs.
- Drugs requiring refrigeration are labeled with that information. The container must be returned to the refrigerator immediately after the drug is removed.
- All drugs must be kept out of the reach of children.
- Unless otherwise directed, drugs must be stored in a cool, dry place.
- A drug should not be exposed to excessive sunlight, heat, cold, or moisture because it may deteriorate.
- The patient or family member should read the entire label on the prescription or nonprescription drug container, including the recommended dosage and warnings.
- All directions printed on the label (e.g., "shake well before using," "keep refrigerated," "take before meals") must be followed to ensure the drug's effectiveness.
- In some instances, especially with an ointment or liquid drug, some of the drug may remain in the container after it has been used or taken for the prescribed time. Some drugs have a short life (a few weeks to a few months) and may deteriorate or change chemically after a time. A prescription drug must never be saved for later use unless the health care provider so advises.

Teaching the Patient

Teaching proceeds after the teaching plan has been developed. Teaching at an appropriate time for each patient fosters learning. For example, hospitalized patients should not be taught when they have visitors present (unless they are to be involved in the administration of the patient's drugs), immediately before they are discharged from the hospital, or if they have been sedated or are in pain.

Teaching of hospitalized patients is begun a day or more before discharge, at a time when the patient is alone and alert, and continued as needed each day until discharge. The teaching is adapted to the patient's level of understanding and, when necessary, includes both written and oral instructions. If there is much information to be given, then it is often best to present the material in two or more sessions. Modifications in the plan for drug administration may be necessary for patients at home (Box 3-2).

Evaluating Patient Learning

To determine that the teaching has been effective, the patient's knowledge of the material is evaluated. Evaluation can be performed in several ways, depending on the nature of the information.

For example, if the patient is being taught a skill such as administering insulin, demonstrations can be scheduled, followed by a return demonstration by the patient with the health care provider observing to evaluate the patient's technique.

Questions such as "Do you understand?" or "Is there anything you do not understand?" should be avoided, because patients may feel uncomfortable admitting their lack of understanding. When factual material is being evaluated, the patient should periodically be asked to list or repeat some of the information presented.

KEY POINTS

◉ When a drug is prescribed, the patient and the family need information about the drug. The teaching/learning process is the means through which the patient is made aware of the drug regimen.

◉ A patient must have **motivation** (the desire or seeing the need) to learn. Motivation depends on the patient's perception of a need to learn. The patient may need to understand the disease process to become motivated to learn about drug treatment for the disease.

◉ An accepting and positive atmosphere also enhances learning. Physical discomfort negatively affects patients' concentration and their ability to learn.

◉ Learning occurs in three domains: cognitive, affective, and psychomotor. A domain is a set of related

---

Box 3-2 Modifying Drug Administration in the Home

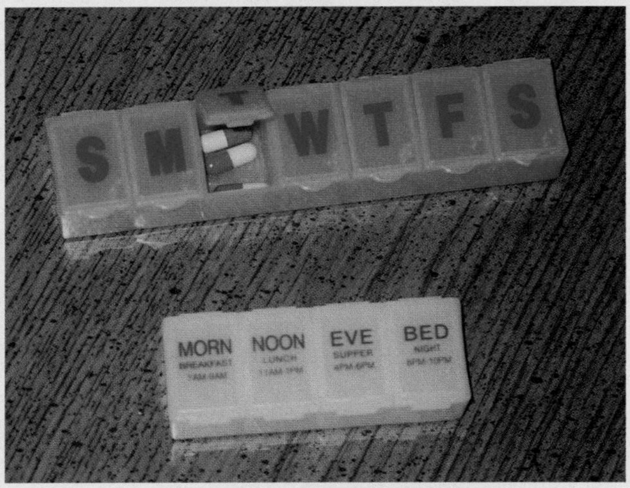

Once the patient is at home, some modifications may be necessary to ensure safe drug administration. Written instructions should be provided, using large print (if necessary), nonglare paper, and words that the patient and caregiver can understand. Following are additional teaching suggestions:

· For patients taking more than one drug, develop a clear, easy-to-read drug schedule or a chart resembling a clock for the patient or caregiver to consult.
· Try using a daily calendar as an inexpensive, yet effective, means for scheduling.
· If the patient or caregiver has a problem with drug names, then refer to the drug by shape or color. Another idea is to number bottles and use this number on the drug chart.
· If financially feasible, then suggest the use of commercially available drug organizers (Fig. 3-2). If the patient cannot afford a drug organizer, then an egg carton or a muffin tin can be labeled and used as a drug organizer.
· If the patient finds it helpful to keep all drugs together, then suggest using a bowl, tray, or small box to hold all the containers.
· If temporary refrigeration is necessary, then suggest the use of a small cooler or insulated bag.
· If equipment items such as needles and syringes are used, then suggest keeping all the supplies in one area.
· If the supplies came in a delivery box, then suggest that the patient use it for storage. Other suggestions include using plastic storage containers with snap-on lids or clean, dry glass jars with screw tops.

FIGURE 3-2   Commercially available drug organizers.

· Advise the patient to use an impervious container with a properly fitting lid, such as a coffee can, for safe disposal. A plastic milk jug with a lid or a heavy-duty, clean, cardboard milk or juice carton may be used if necessary.
· Explain the importance of taking precautions to make sure discarded needles do not puncture the container.

uman characteristics and skills. When developing a teaching plan for the patient, each domain should be considered.

○ Teaching patients about medication involves a process of identifying the patient's knowledge and skill needs, devising a plan of care to meet the identified needs, performing the teaching, and evaluating its effectiveness.

○ Subjects covered in the individualized teaching plan may depend on the drug prescribed, the health care provider's preference for including or excluding specific facts about the drug, and what the patient needs to know to take the drug correctly.

○ Teaching strategies to be used depend on the individual's learning needs and abilities.

○ The teaching plan typically includes information on the dosage regimen, possible adverse reactions, the role of family members, and basic information about drugs, drug containers, and drug storage.

CASE STUDY

Mrs. Miller, age 85, is being discharged from the hospital after being treated for a broken hip. Her physician has prescribed several drugs for her to take at home, including pain medication and a stool softener, for the time she will be bedridden.

1. To manage her multiple medications, Mrs. Miller should be taught to:
   a. empty all the medications together into a jar for ease of administration
   b. keep each of the medications in its original container
   c. take all the drugs at the same time, regardless of what the labels say, so that she does not forget any of them
   d. keep the drug containers open on her bedroom window sill where she can see them at all times

2. On her second day at home Mrs. Miller notices a skin rash that is very itchy has developed. She should:
   a. accept it as inevitable and try to ignore it
   b. buy some ointment to put on the rash
   c. report it to her health care provider
   d. all of the above

3. To help Mrs. Miller remember to take all her drugs, she might use:
   a. a daily calendar with the schedule written on it
   b. a commercially available drug organizer
   c. a homemade labeled organizer such as an egg carton
   d. any of the above

REVIEW QUESTIONS

1. An interactive process that promotes learning is defined as:
   a. motivation
   b. cognitive ability
   c. the psychomotor domain
   d. teaching

2. When developing a teaching plan, the patient's affective learning domain should be assessed, which means consideration of the patient's:
   a. attitudes, feelings, beliefs, and opinions
   b. ability to perform a return demonstration
   c. intellectual ability
   d. home environment

3. Unless the health care provider or pharmacist directs otherwise, the patient should take oral medications with:
   a. fruit juice
   b. milk
   c. water
   d. food

4. True or false: the patient or helping family member should read the entire label of a pre-scription drug, including the dosage and warnings.
   a. true
   b. false

5. True or false: only drugs with life-threatening potential adverse reactions need to be kept out of children's reach.
   a. true
   b. false

4 Adrenergic and Cholinergic Drugs

KEY TERMS

acetylcholine—a neurotransmitter in the parasympathetic nervous system
acetylcholinesterase—a neurotransmitter that inactivates acetylcholine
adrenergic blocking drugs—drugs that impede certain sympathetic nervous system functions
adrenergic drugs—drugs with effects similar to those that occur in the body when the adrenergic nerves are stimulated
autonomic nervous system—the branch of the peripheral nervous system that controls functions essential for survival

cardiac arrhythmia—irregular heartbeat

central nervous system—consists of the brain and the spinal cord

cholinergic blocking drugs—drugs that impede certain parasympathetic nervous system functions

cholinergic drugs—drugs that mimic the activity of the parasympathetic nervous system

cholinergic crisis—cholinergic drug toxicity

first dose effect—an unusually strong therapeutic effect experienced by some patients with the first doses of a medication

glaucoma—an eye condition in which a blockage of drainage channels within the eye results in increased intraocular pressure that may lead to blindness

myasthenia gravis—a disease that causes fatigue of skeletal muscles because of the lack of acetylcholine released at the nerve endings of parasympathetic nerve fibers

neurotransmitter—a chemical substance, also called a neurohormone, released at nerve endings to help transmit nerve impulses

orthostatic hypotension—a feeling of light-headedness and dizziness after suddenly changing position, caused by a decrease in blood pressure when a person sits or stands up

parasympathetic nervous system—a branch of the autonomic nervous system partly responsible for activities such as slowing the heart rate, digesting food, and eliminating body wastes

peripheral nervous system—all nerves outside of the brain and spinal cord, connecting all parts of the body with the central nervous system

postural hypotension—a feeling of light-headedness and dizziness after suddenly changing from a lying to a sitting or standing position, or from a sitting to a standing position

shock—a life-threatening condition occurring when the supply of arterial blood flow and oxygen to the cells and tissues is inadequate

somatic nervous system—branch of the peripheral nervous system that controls sensation and voluntary movement

sympathetic nervous system—branch of the autonomic nervous system that regulates the expenditure of energy and has key effects in stressful situations

vasopressor—a drug that raises the blood pressure because it constricts blood vessels

CHAPTER OBJECTIVES

On completion of this chapter, students will be able to:

1 Define the chapter's key terms.

2 Discuss the activity of the central nervous system, the peripheral nervous system, and the sympathetic and parasympathetic nervous systems.

3 Discuss the uses, general drug actions, contraindications, precautions, interactions, and adverse reactions associated with the administration of adrenergic drugs, adrenergic blocking drugs, cholinergic drugs, and cholinergic blocking drugs.

4 Discuss important points to keep in mind when educating patients about the use of adrenergic drugs, adrenergic blocking drugs, cholinergic drugs, and cholinergic blocking drugs.

This chapter describes four groups of drugs: adrenergic drugs, adrenergic blocking drugs, cholinergic drugs, and cholinergic blocking drugs. As described herein, these drug groups are named in relation to their different effects within the neurological systems of the body.

Adrenergic drugs have effects similar to those that occur in the body when the adrenergic nerves are stimulated. Adrenergic nerves are nerves in the autonomic nervous system that use norepinephrine as a neurotransmitter. The primary effects of these drugs occur in the heart, the blood vessels, and the smooth muscles, such as the bronchi. Adrenergic drugs mimic the activity of the sympathetic nervous system and therefore are also called sympathomimetic drugs. Epinephrine and norepinephrine are neurohormones produced naturally by the body. Synthetic preparations of these two neurohormones, which are identical to those naturally produced by the body, are used in medicine. Adrenergic drugs such as metaraminol (Aramine), isoproterenol (Isuprel), and ephedrine are synthetic adrenergic drugs.

Adrenergic blocking drugs, also called sympathomimetic blocking drugs, have generally the opposite effects of adrenergic drugs. They impede sympathetic nervous system functions. The four classes of adrenergic blocking drugs block four different sets of nervous system receptors and therefore have four related but different actions in the body.

Cholinergic drugs, however, mimic the activity of the parasympathetic nervous system. They also are called parasympathomimetic drugs. Cholinergic drugs have limited usefulness in medicine, partly because of their adverse reactions, but are used for certain diseases or conditions.

Like adrenergic blocking drugs, **cholinergic blocking drugs** also have effects on the autonomic nervous system. These drugs block the action of the neurotransmitter acetylcholine in the parasympathetic nervous system. Because parasympathetic nerves control many areas of the body, cholinergic blocking drugs have numerous effects. Cholinergic blocking drugs also are called anticholinergics or parasympathomimetic blocking drugs.

A basic knowledge of the nervous system is necessary to understand these four classes of drugs and how they work in the body.

The Nervous System

The nervous system is a complex part of the human body that regulates and coordinates body activities such as movement, digestion of food, sleep, and elimination of waste products. The nervous system has two main divisions: the central nervous system and the peripheral nervous system. Figure 4-1 illustrates the divisions of the nervous system.

The **central nervous system** consists of the brain and the spinal cord, which receive, integrate, and interpret nerve impulses from the body. The **peripheral nervous system** encompasses all nerves outside of the brain and

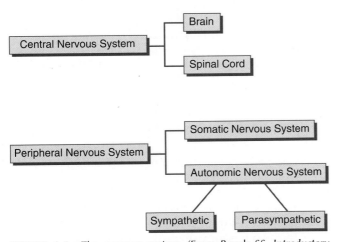

FIGURE 4-1   The nervous system. (From Roach SS. *Introductory Clinical Pharmacology*, 7th ed. Baltimore: Lippincott Williams & Wilkins; 2004.)

spinal cord. The peripheral nervous system connects all parts of the body with the central nervous system.

Peripheral Nervous System

The peripheral nervous system is further divided into the **somatic nervous system** and the autonomic nervous system. The somatic branch of the peripheral nervous system controls sensation and voluntary movement. The sensory part of the somatic nervous system sends messages to the brain about the internal and external environment, such as sensations of heat, pain, cold, and pressure. The voluntary part of the somatic nervous system controls the voluntary movement of skeletal muscles, such as walking, chewing food, or writing a letter.

Autonomic Branch of the Peripheral Nervous System

The autonomic branch of the peripheral nervous system controls functions essential for survival. Functional activity of the **autonomic nervous system** is not consciously controlled (i.e., the activity is automatic). This system controls blood pressure, heart rate, gastrointestinal activity, and glandular secretions. Table 4-1 describes the main actions of the autonomic nervous system in the body.

The autonomic nervous system is divided into the sympathetic and parasympathetic nervous systems. The sympathetic nervous system generally regulates the expenditure of energy and has key effects when one is confronted with stressful situations, such as danger, intense emotion, or severe illness.

The **parasympathetic nervous system** helps conserve body energy and is partly responsible for activities such as slowing the heart rate, digesting food, and eliminating body wastes.

Neurotransmitters

Neurotransmitters are chemical substances called neurohormones. They are released at the nerve endings to help transmit nerve impulses. Electron microscopes show a minuscule space between nerve endings and the effector organ (e.g., the muscle, cell, or gland) that the nerve innervates (controls). For a nerve impulse to be transmitted from the nerve ending across the space to the effector organ, a neurohormone is needed.

The two neurohormones (neurotransmitters) of the sympathetic nervous system are epinephrine and norepinephrine. Epinephrine is secreted by the adrenal medulla. Norepinephrine is secreted mainly at nerve endings of sympathetic (also called adrenergic) nerve fibers (Fig. 4-2).

The parasympathetic nervous system has two different neurotransmitters: **acetylcholine** (ACh) and **acetylcholinesterase** (AChE). These two neurohormones are released at nerve endings of parasympathetic nerve

TABLE 4-1   Action of the Autonomic Nervous System on Body Organs and Structures

Organs or Structures	Sympathetic (Adrenergic) Effects	Types of Sympathetic (Adrenergic) Receptor	Parasympathetic (Cholinergic) Effects
Heart	Increase in heart rate, heart muscle contractility, increase in speed of atrioventricular conduction	β	Decrease in heart rate, decrease in heart muscle contractility
Blood Vessels Skin, mucous membranes Skeletal muscle	Constriction Usually dilatation	α Cholinergic, *β	
Bronchial Muscles	Relaxation	β	Contraction
Gastrointestinal Muscle motility, tone decrease Sphincters Gallbladder	Usually contraction Relaxation	β α	Increase Usually relaxation Contraction
Urinary Bladder Detrusor muscle Trigone, sphincter muscles	Relaxation Contraction	β α	Contraction Relaxation
Eye Radial muscle of iris Sphincter muscle of iris Ciliary muscle	Contraction (pupil dilates)	α	Contraction (pupil constricts) Contraction
Skin Sweat glands Pilomotor muscles	Increased activity in localized areas Contraction (gooseflesh)	Cholinergic* α	
Uterus	Relaxation	β	
Salivary Glands	Thickened secretions	α	Copious, watery secretions
Liver	Glycogenolysis	β	
Lacrimal and Nasopharyngeal Glands		α	Increased secretion
Male Sex Organs	Emission	α	Erection

*Cholinergic transmission, but nerve cell chain originates in the thoracolumbar part of the spinal cord and is therefore sympathetic. alpha, α; beta, β.

fibers, at some nerve endings in the sympathetic nervous system, and at nerve endings of skeletal muscles. When a parasympathetic nerve fiber is stimulated, the nerve fiber releases ACh, and the nerve impulse travels from the nerve fiber to the effector organ or structure. After the impulse has crossed over to the effector organ or structure, ACh is inactivated (destroyed) by AChE. When the next nerve impulse is ready to travel along the nerve fiber, ACh is again released and then inactivated by AChE.

Actions of Adrenergic Drugs

Generally, adrenergic drugs produce one or more of the following responses:

- In the central nervous system: wakefulness, quickened reaction to stimuli, and quickened reflexes
- In the parasympathetic nervous system: relaxation of the smooth muscles of the bronchi, constriction of blood vessels and the sphincters of the stomach,

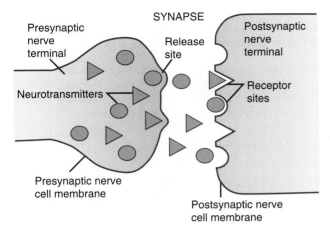

SYNAPSE

Presynaptic nerve terminal

Neurotransmitters

Presynaptic nerve cell membrane

Release site

Postsynaptic nerve terminal

Receptor sites

Postsynaptic nerve cell membrane

FIGURE 4-2   Neurotransmission in the central nervous system. Neurotransmitter molecules (e.g., norepinephrine), released by the presynaptic nerve, cross the synapse and bind with receptors in the cell membrane of the postsynaptic nerve, resulting in the transmission of the nerve impulse. (From Roach SS. *Introductory Clinical Pharmacology*, 7the ed. Baltimore: Lippincott Williams & Wilkins; 2004.)

dilation of coronary blood vessels, and decrease in gastric motility
- Heart: increase in the heart rate
- Metabolism: increased use of glucose (sugar) and liberation of fatty acids from adipose tissue

Figure 4-3 shows additional sites of action.

Adrenergic Nerve Receptors

Adrenergic nerve fibers have either alpha (α) or beta (β) receptors. Adrenergic drugs may act on α receptors only, on β receptors only, or on both α and β receptors. For example, phenylephrine (Neo-Synephrine) acts chiefly on α receptors, isoproterenol acts chiefly on β receptors, and epinephrine acts on both α and β receptors. Whether an adrenergic drug acts on α, β, or α and β receptors accounts for variations in the effects of adrenergic drugs. Table 4-1 lists the type of adrenergic nerve fiber receptors that corresponds with each action of the autonomic nervous system on the body.

Uses of Adrenergic Drugs

Adrenergic drugs have a wide variety of uses. They may be used to treat:

- Hypovolemic and septic shock
- Moderately severe to severe episodes of hypotension
- Control of superficial bleeding during surgical and dental procedures of the mouth, nose, throat, and skin
- Bronchial asthma
- Cardiac decompensation and arrest
- Allergic reactions (anaphylactic shock, angioneurotic edema)

- Temporary treatment of heart block
- Ventricular arrhythmias (under certain conditions)
- Nasal congestion (applied topically)
- Along with local anesthetics to prolong anesthetic action

Other adrenergic drugs have specific uses. Isoproterenol may be used in the treatment of some **cardiac arrhythmias** (irregular heartbeat), cardiac arrest, Adams–Stokes syndrome, or as a systemic bronchodilator (see Chapter 12). Midodrine is used to treat **orthostatic hypotension** (a feeling of light-headedness and dizziness after suddenly changing position after standing in one place for a long period). The uses of various adrenergic drugs are given in the Summary Drug Table: Adrenergic Drugs.

Treatment of Shock

The adrenergic drugs are an important treatment for patients in shock. **Shock** is a life-threatening condition of inadequate perfusion. In shock, the supply of arterial blood flow and oxygen to the cells and tissues is inadequate. The body uses compensatory mechanisms to counteract the symptoms of shock, including the release of epinephrine and norepinephrine. In some situations, the body can compensate and maintain blood pressure. However, if shock is untreated and the body's compensatory mechanisms fail, then death will occur.

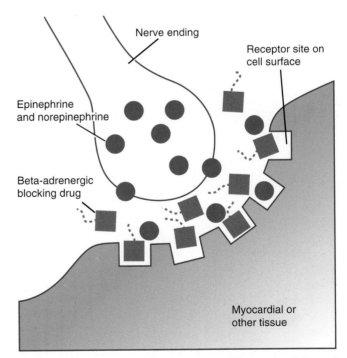

Nerve ending

Receptor site on cell surface

Epinephrine and norepinephrine

Beta-adrenergic blocking drug

Myocardial or other tissue

FIGURE 4-3   Beta–adrenergic blocking drugs prevent epinephrine and norepinephrine from occupying receptor sites on cell membranes. This action alters cell functions normally stimulated by epinephrine and norepinephrine, according to the number of receptor sites occupied by the beta-blocking drugs. (Adapted by Harley J. Encyclopedia Britannica Medical and Health Annual. Chicago: Encyclopedia Britannica; 1983.)

SUMMARY DRUG TABLE   Adrenergic Drugs

Generic Name	Trade Name*	Uses	Adverse Reactions	Dosage Ranges
dobutamine HCL *doe'-byoo-ta-meen*	Dobutrex, *generic*	Cardiac decompensation caused by decreased contractility caused by organic heart disease or cardiac surgical procedures	Headache, nausea, increased heart rate, increase in systolic blood pressure, palpitations, anginal and nonspecific chest pain	2.5–15 mcg/kg/min IV (up to 40 mcg/kg/min); titrate to patient's hemodynamic and renal status
dopamine *doe'-pa-meen*	Intropin, *generic*	Shock caused by MI, trauma, open-heart surgery, renal failure, and chronic cardiac decompensation in CHF	Nausea, vomiting, ectopic beats, tachycardia, anginal pain, palpitations, hypotension, dyspnea	2–50 mcg/kg/min IV (infusion rate determined by patient's response)
ephedrine sulfate *e-fed'-rin*	*Generic*	Hypotension, relief of acute bronchospasm, allergic disorders, nasal and nasopharyngeal mucosal congestion, adjunctive treatment of middle ear infection	Anxiety, insomnia, tenseness, restlessness, headache, light-headedness, dizziness, nausea, dysuria, pallor	Hypotension and allergic disorders, asthma: 25 –50 mg IM, SC, or IV; topical nasal decongestant: instill in each nostril q4h
epinephrine *ep-i-nef'-rin*	Adrenalin chloride, AsthmaHaler, Bronkaid, *generic*	Ventricular standstill; treatment and prophylaxis of cardiac arrest, heart block; muscosal congestion of hay fever, rhinitis, and acute sinusitis; relief of bronchial asthmatic paroxysms; simple open-angle glaucoma	Anxiety, insomnia, tenseness, restlessness, headache, light-headedness, dizziness, nausea, dysuria, pallor	Cardiac arrest: 0.5–1.0 mg IV; respiratory distress (eg, asthma, anaphylaxis): 0.3–0.5 mL of 1:1000 solution, SC or IM q20 min for 4 h or 0.1–0.3mL/ SC of 1:200 suspension; 1 inhalation q3h; 1–3 deep inhalation by nebulizer 4–6 times/d; ophthalmic, 1–2 gtts times daily
isoproterenol *eye-sew-proe-tear'- e-nall*	Isuprel, Medihaler-Iso	Injection: shock, bronchospasm during anesthesia, cardiac standstill and arrhythmias Inhalation: acute bronchial asthma, emphysema, bronchitis, bronchiectasis	Anxiety, insomnia, tenseness, restlessness, headache, light-headedness, dizziness, nausea, dysuria, pallor, pulmonary edema	Injection shock: 2 mcg/mL diluted solution IV; bronchospasm during anesthesia: 0.01–0.02 mg of diluted solution IV; cardiac arrhythmias, cardiac standstill: 0.02–0.06 mg of diluted solution IV, 5 µg/ min IV infusion; 0.2 mg of undiluted 1:5000 solution IM, SC; inhalation bronchial spasm: hand bulb nebulizer 1:200 solution 5–15 deep inhalations or 1:100 solution in 3–7 inhalations; for metered-dose inhaler, 1–2 inhalations 4–6 times/d

Generic Name	Trade Name*	Uses	Adverse Reactions	Dosage Ranges
levalbuterol *lev-al-byoo'-ter-ole*	Xopenex	Treatment or prevention of bronchospasm in adults and adolescents 12 years and older with reversible obstructive airway disease	Restlessness, apprehension, anxiety, fear, CNS stimulation, cardiac arrhythmias, sweating, pallor, flushing, nausea	0.63–1.25 mg TID by nebulization
metaraminol *met-a-ram-i-nole*	Aramine	Hypotension with spinal anesthesia, hypotension caused by hemorrhage, drug reactions, surgical complication, shock associated with brain damage	Headache, flushing sinus or ventricular tachycardia, arrhythmias, nausea, apprehension, palpitation	2–10 mg IM, SC; 15–100 mg in 250-mL or 500-mL solution IV
midodrine *mid'-oh-dryn*	ProAmatine	Orthostatic hypotension	Paresthesias, headache, pain, dizziness, supine hypertension, bradycardia, piloerection, pruritus, dysuria, chills	10 mg PO TID during daylight hours when upright
norepinephrine *nor-ep-i-nef'-rin* (levarterenol)	Levophed	Shock, hypotension, cardiac arrest	Restlessness, headache, dizziness, bradycardia, hypertension	1 mg/mL in 1000 mL 5% dextrose solution, 2–3 mL/min IV, rate adjusted to maintain desired blood pressure; average dose, 2–4 g/min

*The term *generic* indicates the drug is available in generic form.

There are five types of shock: hypovolemic shock, cardiogenic shock, septic shock, obstructive shock, and neurogenic shock. Table 4-2 describes the various types of shock.

Shock causes a number of clinical manifestations:

- Pallor, cyanosis, cold and clammy skin, sweating
- Agitation, confusion, disorientation, coma
- Hypotension, tachycardia, arrhythmias, wide pulse pressure, gallop rhythm
- Tachypnea, pulmonary edema
- Urinary output less than 20 mL per hour
- Acidosis

Regardless of the type, shock results in decreased cardiac output, decreased arterial blood pressure (hypotension), hypoxia (decreased oxygen reaching the cells), and other problems. The functioning of vital organs, such as the heart, brain, and kidneys, is compromised. Adrenergic drugs improve the patient's hemodynamic status by improving myocardial contractility and increasing heart rate, which increase cardiac output. Peripheral resistance is increased by vasoconstriction, making more blood available for vital organs. In cardiogenic shock or advanced shock associated with low cardiac output, an adrenergic drug may be used with a va-sodilating drug. A vasodilator such as nitroprusside (Chapter 16) or nitroglycerin (Chapter 15) improves myocardial performance as the adrenergic drug maintains blood pressure.

Adverse Reactions of Adrenergic Drugs

The adverse reactions of adrenergic drugs depend on the specific drug, the dose used, and the individual patient's response. The more common adverse reactions include cardiac arrhythmias, such as bradycardia and tachycardia, headache, insomnia, nervousness, anorexia, and increased blood pressure (which may reach dangerously high levels). Additional adverse reactions for specific adrenergic drugs are listed in the Summary Drug Table: Adrenergic Drugs.

Managing Adverse Reactions of Adrenergic Drugs

Any symptom the patient has while taking an adrenergic drug should be reported. Particularly important are ensuring adequate tissue perfusion and cardiac output, managing anorexia, and managing sleep disorders.

TABLE 4-2 Types of Shock

Type*	Description
Hypovolemic	Occurs when extracellular fluid volume is significantly diminished, such as with hemorrhage, fluid loss caused by burns, diarrhea, vomiting, or excess diuresis
Cardiogenic	Occurs when cardiac output is inadequate to maintain perfusion to the vital organs, such as with an acute myocardial infarction, ventricular arrhythmias, congestive heart failure, or severe cardiomyopathy
Septic	Occurs as a result of circulatory insufficiency associated with overwhelming infection
Obstructive	Occurs when obstruction of blood flow results in inadequate tissue perfusion, such as with a massive pulmonary embolism, pericardial tamponade, restrictive pericarditis, or severe cardiac valve dysfunction
Neurogenic (rare)	Occurs as a result of blockade of neurohumoral outflow such as caused by spinal anesthesia or direct injury to the spinal cord.

*Other causes of shock include anaphylaxis, hypoglycemia, hypothyroidism, or Addison disease.

ALERT

Supine hypertension (high blood pressure when lying down) is a potentially dangerous adverse reaction of midodrine. This reaction can be minimized if the medication is given during the day while the patient is upright. Also, the patient may sleep with the head of the bed elevated.

Older adults are particularly vulnerable to adverse reactions of adrenergic drugs, particularly epinephrine. Older adults are also more likely to have cardiovascular problems that predispose them to potentially serious cardiac arrhythmias. All elderly patients taking an adrenergic drug should be monitored, and any changes in pulse rate or rhythm must be reported immediately.

Ensuring Adequate Tissue Perfusion and Cardiac Output

Adrenergic drugs may cause hypertension or tachycardia, which may cause decreased oxygenation at the cellular level. A patient who is given an adrenergic drug for hypotension already has a potential problem with tissue perfusion; the adrenergic drug may correct the problem or, if the blood pressure becomes too high, tissue perfusion may again be a problem. These patients' pulse and blood pressure must be monitored.

Managing Anorexia

Adrenergic drugs may cause anorexia (lack of appetite). The patient's food preferences should be considered and modifications made in the diet. An easily digested diet high in carbohydrates and protein and low in fat is usually well-tolerated. Several small meals may be better-tolerated than three large meals. The patient should be monitored for weight loss.

Managing Sleep Disturbances

Patients taking an adrenergic drug may experience insomnia and nervousness, which can cause considerable stress. The care of hospitalized patients may have to be modified to prevent disturbing their sleep. Caffeinated beverages should be avoided, especially after late afternoon. Other sleep aids may be used (e.g., warm milk, back rub, progressive relaxation, or a bedtime snack). The patient should be assured that the sleeplessness and nervousness will pass when the drug therapy is over.

Contraindications, Precautions, and Interactions of Adrenergic Drugs

Adrenergic drugs are contraindicated in patients with known hypersensitivity. Isoproterenol is contraindicated in patients with tachyarrhythmias, tachycardia, or heart block caused by digitalis toxicity, ventricular arrhythmias, and angina pectoris. Dopamine is contraindicated in patients with pheochromocytoma (tumor of adrenal gland), unmanaged arrhythmias, and ventricular fibrillation. Epinephrine is contraindicated in patients with narrow-angle glaucoma, cerebral arteriosclerosis, or cardiac insufficiency. Norepinephrine and ephedrine are contraindicated in patients with hypotension cause by a loss of blood volume. Midodrine is contraindicated in patients with severe organic heart disease, acute renal disease, pheochromocytoma, or supine hypertension.

Adrenergic drugs are used cautiously for patients with coronary insufficiency, cardiac arrhythmias, angina pectoris, diabetes, hyperthyroidism, occlusive vascular disease, or prostatic hypertrophy, and for those taking digoxin. Patients with diabetes may require a higher dosage of insulin. Epinephrine is used cautiously in patients with Parkinson disease or ventricular fibrillation, and in the elderly. Ephedrine is used cautiously in patients with acute-closure glaucoma. Midodrine is used cautiously in patients with urinary problems or hepatic disease, and during lactation. Adrenergic drugs are classified as pregnancy category C and are used with extreme caution during pregnancy.

Patients face an increased risk of hypertension when dobutamine is given along with a β-adrenergic blocking drug. When dopamine is given with a monoamine oxidase inhibitor (see Chapter 5) or tricyclic antidepressant (see Chapter 5), the effects of dopamine may be increased. There is an increased risk of seizures, hypotension, and bradycardia when dopamine is administered with phenytoin. When epinephrine is administered with a tricyclic antidepressant, the patient has an increased risk of sympathomimetic effects. Excessive hypertension can occur when epinephrine is administered with propranolol. A decreased bronchodilating effect occurs when epinephrine is administered with the β-adrenergic drugs. Metaraminol must be used cautiously in patients taking digoxin because of an increased risk for cardiac arrhythmias. When midodrine is administered with cardiac glycosides, psychotropic drugs, or β blockers, bradycardia, heart block, or arrhythmias can occur.

Adrenergic Blocking Drug Classifications

Adrenergic blocking drugs may be divided into four groups. Their actions, uses, adverse reactions, and contraindications and precautions vary according to the group:

- Alpha (α)-adrenergic blocking drugs—drugs that block α-adrenergic receptors. These drugs have their greatest effect in the vascular system.
- Beta (β)-adrenergic blocking drugs—drugs that block β-adrenergic receptors. These drugs produce their greatest effect on adrenergic nerves in the heart.
- Antiadrenergic drugs—drugs that block adrenergic nerve fibers. These drugs have effects within the central nervous system and the peripheral nervous system.
- α/β-Adrenergic blocking drugs—drugs that block both α- and β-adrenergic receptors. These drugs have a wider range of effects.

α-Adrenergic Blocking Drugs

Actions of α-Adrenergic Blocking Drugs

Stimulation of α-adrenergic fibers results in vasoconstriction (see Table 4-1). If stimulation of these α-adrenergic fibers is blocked, then the result instead is vasodilation—the directly opposite effect. Phentolamine (Regitine) is an example of an α-adrenergic blocking drug.

Uses of α-Adrenergic Blocking Drugs

Phentolamine (Regitine) is used for its vasodilating effect on peripheral blood vessels. It can be beneficial in the treatment of hypertension caused by pheochromocytoma, a tumor of the adrenal gland that produces excessive amounts of epinephrine and norepinephrine. This drug is used to control hypertension before surgical excision of pheochromocytoma.

Some drugs such as norepinephrine or dopamine are particularly damaging to surrounding tissues if extravasation (infiltration) occurs when they are given intravenously. Phentolamine is also used to prevent or treat tissue damage caused by extravasation of these drugs.

Adverse Reactions of α-Adrenergic Blocking Drugs

α-Adrenergic blocking drugs may result in weakness, orthostatic hypotension, cardiac arrhythmias, hypotension, and tachycardia.

Contraindications, Precautions, and Interactions of α-Adrenergic Blocking Drugs

α-Adrenergic blocking drugs are contraindicated in patients who are hypersensitive to them and in patients with coronary artery disease. These drugs are used cautiously during pregnancy (pregnancy category C) and lactation, after a recent myocardial infarction, and in patients with renal failure or Raynaud disease. When phentolamine is given with epinephrine or ephedrine, the vasoconstrictor and hypertensive effects are decreased.

β-Adrenergic Blocking Drugs

Actions of β-Adrenergic Blocking Drugs

β-Adrenergic blocking drugs, also called β blockers, decrease the activity of the sympathetic nervous system in certain tissues. β-Adrenergic receptors are found mainly in the heart. Stimulation of β receptors of the heart results in an increase in the heart rate. If stimulation of these β-adrenergic fibers is blocked, then the heart rate decreases and blood vessels dilate. Examples of β-adrenergic blocking drugs are esmolol (Brevibloc), metoprolol (Lopressor), nadolol (Corgard), and propranolol (Inderal).

β-Adrenergic blocking drugs, such as betaxolol (Betoptic) and timolol (Timoptic), when used topically as eye drops, appear to reduce the production of aqueous humor in the anterior chamber of the eye.

Uses of β-Adrenergic Blocking Drugs

These drugs are primarily used in the treatment of hypertension (see the Summary Drug Table: Adrenergic Blocking Drugs; also see Chapter 14) and certain cardiac

SUMMARY DRUG TABLE   Adrenergic Blocking Drugs

Generic Name	Trade Name*	Uses	Adverse Reactions	Dosage Ranges
α-Adrenergic Blocking Agents phentolamine *fen-tole-a-meen*	Regitine	Diagnosis of pheochromocytoma, hypertensive episodes before and during surgery, prevention/treatment of dermal necrosis after IV administration of norepinephrine or dopamine	Weakness, dizziness, flushing, nausea, vomiting, orthostatic hypotension	5 mg IV, IM for tissue necrosis: 5–10 mg in 10 mL saline infiltrated into affected area
β-Adrenergic Blocking Drugs acebutolol HCl *a-se-byoo'-toe-lol*	Sectral, *generic*	Hypertension, ventricular arrhythmias	Bradycardia, dizziness, weakness, hypotension, nausea, vomiting, diarrhea, nervousness	Hypertension: 400 mg PO in 1–2 doses; arrhythmias: 400–1200 mg/d PO in divided doses
atenolol *a-ten'-oh-lol*	Tenormin, *generic*	Hypertension, angina, acute MI	Bradycardia, dizziness, fatigue, weakness, hypotension, nausea, vomiting, diarrhea, nervousness	50–200 mg/d PO; 5 mg IV
betaxolol HCL *beh-tax'-oh-lol*	Kerlone	Hypertension	Bradycardia, dizziness, hypotension, bronchospasm, nausea, vomiting, diarrhea, nervousness	5–20 mg/d PO
betaxolol HCL *beh-tax'-oh-lol* (ophthalmic)	Betoptic	Glaucoma	Brief ocular discomfort, tearing	I gtt BID
bisoprolol *bye-sew'-proe-lol*	Zebeta	Hypertension	Bradycardia, dizziness, weakness, hypotension, nausea, vomiting, diarrhea, nervousness	5 mg PO QD; maximum dose, 20 mg PO QD
carteolol *kar'-tee-oh-lol*	Cartrol	Hypertension	Bradycardia, dizziness, weakness, hypotension, nausea, vomiting, diarrhea, nervousness	2.5 mg–10 mg/d PO
esmolol HCL *ess'-moe-lol*	Brevibloc	Supraventricular tachycardia, noncompensatory tachycardia	Hypotension, weakness, light-headedness, urinary retention	25–500 mcg/kg/min IV
metoprolol *me-toe'-proe-lol*	Lopressor, Toprol-XL, *generic*	Hypertension, angina, MI	Dizziness, hypotension, CHF, arrhythmia, nausea, vomiting, diarrhea	100–450 mg/d PO; 5 mg IV; extended release: 50–100 mg/d PO
nadolol *nay-doe'-lol*	Corgard, *generic*	Angina, hypertension	Dizziness, hypotension, nausea, vomiting, diarrhea, CHF, cardiac arrhythmias	40–320 mg/d PO

Generic Name	Trade Name*	Uses	Adverse Reactions	Dosage Ranges
penbutolol *pen-byoo'-toe-lol*	Levatol	Hypertension	Bradycardia, dizziness, hypotension, nausea, vomiting, diarrhea	20 mg PO QD
pindolol *pen'-doe-lol*	Visken, *generic*	Hypertension	Bradycardia, dizziness, hypotension, nausea, vomiting, diarrhea	5–60 mg/d PO in divided doses
propranolol *pro-pran'-oh-lol*	Inderal, *generic*	Cardiac arrhythmias, MI, angina, hypertension, migraine prophylaxis	Bradycardia, dizziness, hypotension, nausea, vomiting, diarrhea, bronchospasm, hyperglycemia, pulmonary edema	Arrhythmias: 10–30 mg PO TID, QID; hypertension: 40–640 mg/d PO in divided doses; angina: 10–320 mg/d PO in divided doses; life-threatening arrhythmias: up to 1–3 mg IV; migraine: 80–240 mg/d PO in divided doses
sotalol HCl *soh'-tal-lole*	Betapace, *generic*	Ventricular arrhythmias	Dizziness, hypotension, nausea, vomiting, diarrhea, respiratory distress	80–320 mg/d PO in divided doses
timolol maleate *tye-moe'-lole*	Blocadren, *generic*	Hypertension, MI, migraine prophylaxis	Dizziness, hypotension, nausea, vomiting, diarrhea, pulmonary edema	Hypertension: 10–60 mg/d PO in divided doses; MI: 10 mg PO BID; migraine: 10–30 mg/d PO
timolol maleate (ophthalmic) *tye-moe'-lole*	Timoptic	Glaucoma	Ocular irritation, tearing	1 gtt BID
α/β-Adrenergic Blocking Agents carvedilol *car-veh'-dih-lol*	Coreg	Hypertension, CHF	Bradycardia, hypotension, cardiac insufficiency, fatigue, dizziness, diarrhea	Hypertension: 6.25–50 mg PO BID; CHF: dose individualized based on patient response; initial dose 3.125 mg PO BID, increased gradually to a maximum dose of 50 mg PO BID
labetalol *lah-bet'-ah-lol*	Normodyne, Trandate, *generic*	Hypertension	Fatigue, drowsiness, insomnia, hypotension, impotence, diarrhea	100–400 mg/d PO in divided doses; 20–300 mg IV
Antiadrenergic Drugs: Centrally Acting clonidine HCl *kloe'-ni-deen*	Catapres, Catapres-TTS, *generic*	Severe pain in patients with cancer, hypertension	Drowsiness, dizziness, sedation, dry mouth, constipation, syncope, dreams, rash	100–2400 mg/d PO; transdermal: 0.1–0.3 mg/24 h

Generic Name	Trade Name*	Uses	Adverse Reactions	Dosage Ranges
guanabenz acetate *gwan'-ah-benz*	Wytensin, *generic*	Hypertension	Dry mouth, sedation, dizziness, headache, weakness, arrhythmias	4–32 mg BID
guanfacine HCL *gwan'-fa-sine*	Tenex	Hypertension	Dry mouth, somnolence, asthenia, dizziness, headache, constipation, fatigue	1–3 mg/d PO at hs
methyldopa OR methyldopate HCL *meth'-ill-doe-pa- meth'-ill-doe-pate*	Aldomet, *generic*	Hypertension, hypertensive crisis	Bradycardia, aggravation of angina pectoris, heart failure, sedation, headache, rash, nausea, vomiting nasal stuffiness	250 mg PO BID–TID; maintenance dose, 3 g/d; 250–500 mg q6h IV
guanadrel *gwan'-ah-drel*	Hylorel	Hypertension	Palpitation, chest pain, fatigue, gas, headache, faintness, drowsiness, nocturia, shortness of breath on exertion, weight gain or loss, aching limbs, urination urgency	5–75 mg PO BID
guanethidine monosulfate *gwahn-eth'i-deen*	Ismelin	Hypertension, renal hypertension	Bradycardia, fluid retention, dizziness, weakness, diarrhea, nausea, dry mouth	10–50 mg/d PO
prazosin *pray-zoe'-sin*	Minipress, *generic*	Hypertension	Dizziness, postural hypotension, drowsiness, headache, loss of strength, palpitation, nausea	1–20 mg/d PO in divided doses
terazosin *tear-aye'-zoe-sin*	Hytrin	Hypertension, benign prostatic hyperplasia (BPH)	Dizziness, postural hypotension, headache, dyspnea, nasal congestion	1–20 mg/d PO

*The term *generic* indicates the drug is available in generic form.

arrhythmias. They are used to prevent another heart attack in patients with a recent myocardial infarction (heart attack). Some of these drugs have additional uses, such as the use of propranolol for migraine headaches and nadolol for angina pectoris.

β-Adrenergic blocking drugs also can be used topically as eye drops. For example, betaxolol (Betoptic) and timolol (Timoptic) are used in the treatment of glaucoma. **Glaucoma** is a narrowing or blockage of the drainage channels (canals of Schlemm) between the anterior and posterior chambers of the eye. This results in increased intraocular pressure in the eye. Blindness may occur if glaucoma is left untreated.

Adverse Reactions of β-Adrenergic Blocking Drugs

The adverse reactions of β-adrenergic blocking drugs include orthostatic hypotension, bradycardia, dizziness, vertigo, bronchospasm (especially in those with a history of asthma), hyperglycemia, nausea, vomiting, and diarrhea. Many of these reactions are mild and may disappear as therapy continues. More serious adverse reactions include symptoms of congestive heart failure (dyspnea, weight gain, peripheral edema). Adverse reactions of β-adrenergic ophthalmic preparations include headache, depression, cardiac arrhythmias, and bronchospasm.

Contraindications, Precautions, and Interactions of β-Adrenergic Blocking Drugs

These drugs are contraindicated in patients with an allergy to them and patients with sinus bradycardia, second-degree or third-degree heart block, heart failure, asthma, emphysema, or hypotension. The drugs are used cautiously in patients with diabetes, thyrotoxicosis, and peptic ulcer.

When used with verapamil, the effects of the β blockers are increased. When the β blockers are used with indomethacin, ibuprofen, sulindac, or barbiturates, the effects of the β blockers may decrease. Diuretics may increase the hypotensive effects of the β-adrenergic blocking drugs. A paradoxical hypertensive effect may occur when clonidine is given with a β-adrenergic blocking drug. When given with lidocaine and cimetidine, β-adrenergic blocking drugs may have increased serum levels and cause toxic effects.

Antiadrenergic Blocking Drugs

Actions of Antiadrenergic Blocking Drugs

One group of antiadrenergic drugs inhibits the release of norepinephrine from certain adrenergic nerve endings in the peripheral nervous system. This group is composed of antiadrenergic drugs that act on peripheral structures. An example of a peripherally acting antiadrenergic drug is guanethidine (Ismelin). The other antiadrenergic drugs are called centrally acting antiadrenergic drugs because they act on the central nervous system, rather than on the peripheral nervous system. This group affects specific central nervous system centers and decreases some of the activity of the sympathetic nervous system. Although the actions of these types of antiadrenergic drugs are somewhat different, the results are basically the same. An example of a centrally acting antiadrenergic drug is clonidine (Catapres-TTS).

Uses of Antiadrenergic Blocking Drugs

Antiadrenergic drugs are used mainly for the treatment of certain cardiac arrhythmias and hypertension (see the Summary Drug Table: Adrenergic Blocking Drugs).

Adverse Reactions of Antiadrenergic Blocking Drugs

The adverse reactions of centrally acting antiadrenergic drugs include dry mouth, drowsiness, sedation, anorexia, rash, malaise, and weakness. Adverse reactions of peripherally acting antiadrenergic drugs include hypotension, weakness, light-headedness, and bradycardia.

Contraindications, Precautions, and Interactions of Antiadrenergic Blocking Drugs

The centrally acting antiadrenergic drugs are contraindicated in patients with active hepatic disease such as acute hepatitis or active cirrhosis and in patients with a history of hypersensitivity. They are used cautiously in patients with a history of liver disease or renal function impairment, and during pregnancy and lactation. If methyldopa is administered with anesthetics, then the effect of the anesthetic is increased. The centrally acting antiadrenergic drugs increase the activity of sympathomimetics, possibly causing hypertension. Clonidine decreases the effectiveness of levodopa. When clonidine is given along with a β-adrenergic blocking drug, a potentially life-threatening hypertensive episode may occur.

The peripherally acting antiadrenergic drugs are contraindicated in patients with a known hypersensitivity. Reserpine is contraindicated in patients with active peptic ulcer or ulcerative colitis or depression. Reserpine is used cautiously in patients with renal impairment or cardiovascular disease, and during pregnancy and lactation. Guanethidine, another peripherally acting antiadrenergic drug, is contraindicated in patients with pheochromocytoma or congestive heart failure. The drug is used cautiously in patients with bronchial asthma or renal impairment, and during pregnancy and lactation. Anorexiants, haloperidol, monoamine oxidase inhibitors, tricyclic antidepressants, and phenothiazines decrease the hypotensive effects of guanethidine.

α/β-Adrenergic Blocking Drugs

Actions of α/β-Adrenergic Blocking Drugs

α/β-Adrenergic blocking drugs block the stimulation of both α- and β-adrenergic receptors, resulting in peripheral vasodilation. The two drugs in this category are carvedilol (Coreg) and labetalol (Normodyne).

Uses of α/β-Adrenergic Blocking Drugs

Labetalol is used to treat hypertension, either alone or in combination with another drug such as a diuretic. Carvedilol is used to treat essential hypertension and to reduce progression of congestive heart failure.

Adverse Reactions of α/β-Adrenergic Blocking Drugs

The adverse reactions of labetalol include fatigue, drowsiness, insomnia, weakness, hypotension, diarrhea, dyspnea, and skin rash. Most adverse effects are mild and do not require discontinuation of therapy. Adverse reactions of carvedilol include fatigue, hypotension, cardiac insufficiency, chest pain, bradycardia, dizziness, diarrhea, hypotension, and fatigue.

Contraindications, Precautions, and Interactions of α/β-Adrenergic Blocking Drugs

Both carvedilol and labetalol are contraindicated in patients with hypersensitivity and in patients with bronchial asthma, decompensated heart failure, or severe bradycardia. The drugs are used cautiously in patients with drug-controlled congestive heart failure, chronic bronchitis, impaired hepatic or cardiac function, or diabetes, and during pregnancy (category C) and lactation.

When either drug is taken along with a diuretic or other hypotensive drug, an increased hypotensive effect may occur. When labetalol is given with cimetidine, the effects of labetalol are increased. Halothane increases the effects of labetalol. When carvedilol is given with an antidiabetic drug, the antidiabetic drug has increased effect. Clonidine taken with carvedilol has increased effectiveness. Digoxin has an increased serum level when taken with carvedilol.

Managing Adverse Reactions of Adrenergic Blocking Drugs

Some patients may experience one or more adverse drug reactions during treatment with adrenergic blocking drugs. As with any drug, adverse reactions must be reported to the health care provider. Some adverse reactions are serious, and the health care provider must be informed immediately. The patient may have to tolerate adverse reactions that pose no serious threat to the patient's well-being, such as dry mouth or mild constipation. The patient should be assured that these less serious reactions often disappear or lessen after a time.

Even minor adverse drug reactions can be distressing to the patient, especially when they persist. When possible, minor adverse reactions can be relieved with simple measures. For example, a patient with dry mouth can take frequent sips of water or suck on a piece of hard candy (assuming the patient does not have diabetes or is not on a special diet with limited sugar intake). Constipation can be relieved with increased fluid intake, unless extra fluids are contraindicated. The health care provider also may order a laxative or stool softener. The patient may experience minimal gastrointestinal side effects, such as anorexia, diarrhea, and constipation, if the drug

is given at a specific time in relation to meals, with food, or with an antacid.

Managing Hypotension

Adrenergic blocking drugs may cause hypotension. If the drug is administered for hypertension, then a blood pressure decrease is expected.

Some adrenergic blocking drugs (such as prazosin and tera-zosin) may cause a "first dose" effect. A **first dose effect** occurs when the patient experiences marked hypotension and syncope (fainting) with the first few doses of the drug. The first dose effect may be minimized if the initial dose is decreased and the drug given at bedtime. The dosage is then slowly increased until a full therapeutic effect is achieved. A patient who experiences syncope should lie down. This effect is self-limiting and in most cases does not recur after the initial period of therapy. Light-headedness and dizziness are more common, however, than fainting.

ALERT

Blood Pressure Drop

If a patient has significant decrease in blood pressure (a drop of 20 mm Hg systolic or a systolic pressure below 90 mm Hg) after a dose of an adrenergic blocking drug, then the health care provider should be notified immediately. A dosage reduction or discontinuation of the drug may be necessary.

Decreasing the Patient's Risk for Injury

Some patients receiving an adrenergic blocking drug may experience postural or orthostatic hypotension. **Postural hypotension** is a feeling of light-headedness and dizziness after suddenly changing from a lying to a sitting or standing position, or from a sitting to a standing position. Orthostatic hypotension is similar to postural hypotension but occurs when the patient changes or shifts position after standing in one place for a long period. The following measures help minimize these adverse reactions:

- Instruct patients to rise slowly from a sitting or lying position.
- Help the patients get out of a bed or a chair if symptoms of postural hypotension are severe. Place the call light nearby and instruct patients to ask for assistance each time they get in and out of a bed or a chair.
- Assist patients in bed to a sitting position, and have the patients sit on the edge of the bed for approximately 1 minute before standing.
- Help seated patients to a standing position and instruct them to stand in one place for approximately 1 minute before walking.

- Stay with the patients while they are standing in one place and when walking.
- Instruct the patients to avoid standing in one place for prolonged periods.
- Teach the patients to avoid taking hot showers or baths, which may increase these symptoms.

Symptoms of postural or orthostatic hypotension often lessen with time, but patients should be allowed to get out of bed or a chair without assistance only when it is clear they have no danger of falling.

Actions of Cholinergic Drugs

Cholinergic drugs may act like the neurohormone ACh or may inhibit the release of the neurohormone AChE. Cholinergic drugs that act like ACh are called direct-acting cholinergics. A cholinergic drug that inhibits the release of AChE prolongs the activity of the ACh produced naturally by the body. Cholinergic drugs that prolong the activity of ACh by inhibiting the release of AChE are called indirect-acting cholinergics. The results of these different drug actions, however, are basically the same.

Uses of Cholinergic Drugs

The major uses of cholinergic drugs are for treating glaucoma, myasthenia gravis, and urinary retention.

Glaucoma is a disorder of increased pressure within the eye caused by an obstruction of the outflow of aqueous humor through the canal of Schlemm. The normal flow of aqueous humor keeps the pressure within the eye within normal limits. Glaucoma may be treated by topical application (eye drops) of a cholinergic drug, such as carbachol or pilocarpine (Isopto Carpine). Treating glaucoma with a cholinergic drug produces miosis (constriction of the iris). This opens the blocked channels and allows the normal flow of aqueous humor, thus reducing intraocular pressure.

Myasthenia gravis is a disease that causes fatigue of skeletal muscles because of the lack of ACh released at the nerve endings of parasympathetic nerve fibers. Drugs used to treat this disorder include ambenonium (Mytelase) and pyridostigmine (Mestinon).

Urinary retention results when urination is impaired. Urination is a voluntary and an involuntary act. The parasympathetic nervous system partly controls the process of urination by constricting the detrusor muscle and relaxing the bladder sphincter (Table 4-1). Treatment of urinary retention with cholinergic drugs, such as ambenonium, bethanechol chloride (Urecholine), or pyridostigmine, results in the spontaneous passage of urine.

Adverse Reactions of Cholinergic Drugs

Unless applied topically, as in the treatment of glaucoma, cholinergic drugs are not selective in their action. This means they may affect many different organs and structures in the body and cause a variety of adverse effects. Oral or parenteral administration can result in nausea, diarrhea, abdominal cramping, salivation, flushing of the skin, cardiac arrhythmias, and muscle weakness. Topical administration usually produces few adverse effects, but a temporary reduction of visual acuity (sharpness of vision) and headache may occur. The Summary Drug Table: Cholinergic Drugs lists the adverse reactions that may occur with specific cholinergic drugs.

Managing Adverse Reactions of Cholinergic Drugs

Adverse drug reactions may affect the heart, respiratory and gastrointestinal tracts, and the central nervous system. The patient is monitored for adverse drug reactions such as a change in vital signs or an increase in other symptoms. The health care provider should be notified.

Managing Disturbed Visual Perception

Because drug-induced myopia (near-sightedness) may occur after cholinergic eyedrops are given to treat glaucoma, the patient may need help getting out of bed or walking. Obstacles that might not be seen and trip a patient, such as slippers, chairs, and tables, should be placed out of the way, especially at night.

Managing Diarrhea

Oral forms of these drugs sometimes cause excessive salivation, abdominal cramping, flatus (gas), and diarrhea. The patient is informed that these reactions will continue until tolerance develops, usually within a few weeks. Until then, hospitalized patients need proper facilities, such as a bedside commode, bedpan, or bathroom, readily available. Walking can help the patient pass flatus. The health care provider should be informed if the patient has excessive diarrhea because this may be an indication of the drug's toxicity.

Contraindications, Precautions, and Interactions of Cholinergic Drugs

These drugs are contraindicated in patients with a known hypersensitivity and in patients with asthma, peptic ulcer disease, coronary artery disease, or hyperthyroidism. Bethanecol is contraindicated in patients with mechanical obstruction of the gastrointestinal or

SUMMARY DRUG TABLE   Cholinergic Drugs

Generic Name	Trade Name*	Uses	Adverse Reactions	Dosage Ranges
ambenonium *am-be-noe'-nee-um*	Mytelase	Myasthenia gravis	Increased bronchial secretions, cardiac arrhythmias, muscle weakness, urinary frequency	5–75 mg PO TID, QID
bethanechol chloride *be-than'-e-kole*	Duvoid, Urecholine, *generic*	Acute nonobstructive urinary retention, neurogenic atony of urinary bladder with urinary retention	Abdominal discomfort, diarrhea, nausea, vomiting, salivation, urgency, flushing, sweating	10–50 mg PO BID to QID; 2.5–5 mg SC TID to QID
carbachol, topical *kar'-ba-kole*	Isopto Carbachol, Miostat	Glaucoma	Temporary reduction of visual acuity, headache	1–2 drops in eye up to 3 times/d
edrophonium *ed-roe-fone'-ee-yum*	Enlon, Tensilon	Diagnosis of myasthenia gravis	Increased bronchial secretions, cardiac arrhythmias, muscle weakness, urinary frequency	2–10 mg IV, look for cholinergic reaction
neostigmine *nee-oh-stig'-meen*	Prostigmin, *generic*	Myasthenia gravis, urinary retention	Cardiac arrhythmias, vomiting, bowel cramps, increased peristalsis, urinary frequency, flushing, weakness, diaphoresis, nausea, diarrhea, salivation	Myasthenia gravis: maintenance dose 15–375 mg/d PO; 0.5–1 mg IM, SC q4–6h PRN
pilocarpine hydrochloride *pye-loe-kar'-peen*	Isopto Carpine, Pilocar, generic	Glaucoma	Temporary reduction in visual acuity, headache	1–2 gtts TID in eye 1–6 times/d
pilocarpine ocular therapeutic system *pye-loe-kar'-peen*	Ocusert	Elevated intraocular pressure	Temporary reduction in visual acuity, headache, redness, burning, iris cysts	1 U placed in the conjunctival sac, replaced as directed by the physician (usually every 7 d)
pyridostigmine bromide *peer-id-oh-stig'-meen*	Mestinon, Regonol	Myasthenia gravis	Increased bronchial secretions, cardiac arrhythmias, muscle weakness	Average dose is 600 mg/d PO at spaced intervals, with doses as low as 60 mg/d and as high as 1500 mg/d

*The term *generic* indicates the drug is available in generic form.

genitourinary tract. Patients with secondary glaucoma, iritis, corneal abrasion, or any acute inflammatory disease of the eye should not use cholinergic eyedrops.

These drugs are used cautiously in patients with hypertension, epilepsy, cardiac arrhythmias, bradycardia, recent coronary occlusion, or megacolon. The safety of these drugs has not been established for use during pregnancy (pregnancy category C) or lactation, or in children.

When a cholinergic drug is given along with another cholinergic, the effects of the drugs are increased and the patient has a greater risk for toxicity. Concurrent use of an anticholinergic drug with a cholinergic drug minimizes the effects of cholinergic drug. Because of this, atropine is used as an antidote for an overdosage of cholinergic drugs. Carbachol and pilocarpine have an additive effect when used together. The effects of cholinergic drugs, particularly edrophonium, neostigmine, and pyridostigmine, are decreased, along with possible muscular depression, when given with a corticosteroid.

Actions of Cholinergic Blocking Drugs

Cholinergic blocking drugs inhibit the activity of acetylcholine in parasympathetic nerve fibers. When the activity of acetylcholine is inhibited, nerve impulses traveling along parasympathetic nerve fibers cannot pass to the effector organ or structure. Because of the wide distribution of parasympathetic nerves, these drugs affect many organs and structures in the body, including the eyes, the respiratory and gastrointestinal tracts, the heart, and the bladder (see Box 4-1).

Patients' responses to cholinergic blocking drugs vary, often depending on the drug and the dosage. For example, scopolamine may occasionally cause excitement, delirium, and restlessness. This reaction is considered a drug idiosyncrasy (an unexpected or unusual drug effect).

Uses of Cholinergic Blocking Drugs

Because of their widespread effects on many organs and structures, cholinergic blocking drugs have a variety of uses. The uses of atropine include treatment of pylorospasm, peptic ulcer, ureteral and biliary colic, vagal-induced bradycardia, and parkinsonism; preoperatively, it is given to reduce secretions of the upper respiratory tract before the administration of a general anesthetic. The action of some other cholinergic blocking drugs is more selective, affecting principally one structure of the body. An example of this type of drug is clidinium bromide (Quarzan), which is used only to treat peptic ulcer. The Summary Drug Table: Cholinergic Blocking Drugs lists the uses of specific cholinergic blocking drugs.

Adverse Reactions of Cholinergic Blocking Drugs

Dryness of the mouth with difficulty in swallowing, blurred vision, and photophobia (aversion to bright light) commonly occur with cholinergic blocking drugs. The severity of many adverse reactions often depends on the dose: the larger the dose, the more intense the reaction. Even in normal doses, some degree of dryness of the mouth almost always occurs.

Constipation may occur in patients taking one of these drugs regularly. Drowsiness may occur with these drugs, but sometimes this adverse reaction is desirable, such as when atropine is used preoperatively to reduce respiratory secretions.

Elderly patients may experience confusion or excitement, even at small doses.

Other adverse reactions that may occur with cholinergic blocking drugs include:

- Central nervous system—headache, flushing, nervousness, drowsiness, weakness, insomnia, nasal congestion, fever
- Eyes—blurred vision, mydriasis (dilated pupils), photophobia, increased ocular tension
- Gastrointestinal tract—nausea, vomiting, difficulty swallowing, heartburn
- Urinary tract—urinary hesitancy and retention, dysuria (difficult or painful urination)
- Cardiovascular system—palpitations, bradycardia (after low doses of atropine), tachycardia (after higher doses of atropine)
- Other—urticaria (skin rash) or other skin manifestations, anaphylactic shock

Managing Adverse Reactions of Cholinergic Blocking Drugs

Because these drugs may have widespread effects, patients should be observed closely for adverse drug reactions. In hot weather, sweating may be decreased, causing heat prostration. Patients should be observed for signs of heat prostration (fever, tachycardia, flushing, warm dry skin, mental confusion), especially if the patient is elderly or debilitated. The health care provider should be notified immediately if heat prostration is suspected. Elderly patients receiving a cholinergic blocking drug should be observed for agitation, mental con-

---

Box 4-1 **Effects of Cholinergic Blocking Drugs**

Cholinergic blocking drugs produce the following responses:
- *Central nervous system*—dreamless sleep, drowsiness; atropine may produce mild stimulation in some patients
- *Eye*—mydriasis (dilatation of the pupil), cycloplegia (paralysis of accommodation or inability to focus the eye)
- *Respiratory tract*—drying of the secretions of the mouth, nose, throat, bronchi, relaxation of smooth muscles of the bronchi resulting in slight bronchodilatation
- *Gastrointestinal tract*—decrease in secretions of the stomach, decrease in gastric and intestinal movement (motility)
- *Cardiovascular system*—increase in pulse rate (most pronounced with atropine)
- *Urinary tract*—dilatation of smooth muscles of the ureters and kidney pelvis, contraction of the detrusor muscle of the bladder

SUMMARY DRUG TABLE   Cholinergic Blocking Drugs

Generic Name	Trade Name*	Uses	Adverse Reactions	Dosage Ranges
atropine *a'-troe-peen*	*Generic*	Pylorospasm, reduction of bronchial and oral secretions, excessive vagal-induced bradycardia, ureteral and biliary colic	Drowsiness, blurred vision, tachycardia, dry mouth, urinary hesitancy	0.4–0.6 mg PO IM, SC, IV
belladonna alkaloids *bel'-ah-dohn-a*	*Generic*	Adjunctive therapy for peptic ulcer, digestive disorders, diverticulitis, pancreatitis, diarrhea	Drowsiness, blurred vision, tachycardia, dry mouth, urinary hesitancy	0.25–0.5 mg PO TID
clidinium bromide *klih'-dih-nee-uhm*	Quarzan	Adjunctive therapy for peptic ulcer	Drowsiness, blurred vision, tachycardia, dry mouth, urinary hesitancy	2.5–5 mg PO 3–4 times/d
dicyclomine HCl *dye-sye'-kloe-meen*	Bentyl, Di-Spasz, *generic*	Functional bowel/irritable bowel syndrome	Drowsiness, blurred vision, tachycardia, dry mouth, urinary hesitancy	80–160 mg PO QID
flavoxate *fla-vox'-ate*	Urispas	Relieves dysuria, urgency, frequency, and pain of cystitis and prostatitis	Nausea, vomiting, dry mouth, nervousness, vertigo, headache, drowsiness, blurred vision	100–200 mg PO 3–4 times/d
glycopyrrolate *glye-koe-pye'-roe-late*	Robinul	Oral: peptic ulcer Parenteral: in conjunction with anesthesia to reduce bronchial and oral secretions, to block cardiac vagal inhibitory reflexes during induction of anesthesia and intubation; protection against the peripheral muscarinic effects of cholinergic agents (eg, neostigmine)	Blurred vision, dry mouth, altered taste perception, nausea, vomiting, dysphagia, urinary hesitancy and retention	PO: 1–2 mg BID, TID Parenteral: peptic ulcer, 0.1–0.2 mg IM, IV TID, QID; preanesthesia, 0.002 mg/Ib IM Intraoperative: 0.1 mg IV
l-hyoscyamine sulfate *high-oh-sigh'-ah-meen*	Anaspaz, Donnamar, Levbid	Aids in control of gastric secretions, visceral spasm, hypermotility in spastic colitis, spastic bladder, pylorospasm, relief of symptoms in functional intestinal disorders, biliar and renal colic, peptic ulcer, irritable bowel syndrome, neurogenic colon, pancreatitis	Drowsiness, blurred vision, tachycardia, dry mouth, urinary hesitancy	0.125–0.25 mg PO or sublingually 3 or 4 times/d; 0.375–0.75 mg sustained-release form q12h; 0.25–0.5 mg SC, IM, or IV 2–4 times/d
mepenzolate bromide *meh-pen'-zoe-late*	Cantil	Adjunctive treatment of peptic ulcer	Drowsiness, blurred vision, tachycardia, dry mouth, urinary hesitancy	25–50 mg PO TID–QID with meals and at bedtime

Generic Name	Trade Name*	Uses	Adverse Reactions	Dosage Ranges
methantheline bromide *mehth-an'-the-leen*	Banthine	Adjunctive treatment for peptic ulcer, hypertonic neurogenic bladder	Drowsiness, blurred vision, tachycardia, dry mouth, urinary hesitancy	50–100 mg PO q6h
methscopolamine *mehth-scoe-pol'-a-meen*	Pamine	Adjunctive therapy for peptic ulcer	Drowsiness, blurred vision, tachycardia, dry mouth, urinary hesitancy	2.5 mg 30 minutes AC and 2.5–5 mg HS PO
propantheline bromide *proe-pan'-the-leen*	Pro-Banthine, *generic*	Adjunctive therapy for peptic ulcer	Dry mouth, constipation, hesitancy, urinary retention, blurred vision	15 mg PO 30 minutes AC and HS
scopolamine hydrobromide *scoe-pol'-a-meen*	*Generic*	Preanesthetic sedation, motion sickness	Confusion, dry mouth, constipation, hesitancy, urinary retention, blurred vision	0.32–0.65 mg IM, SQ, IV, and diluted with sterile water for injections; apply 1 patch 4h before travel every 3 d
tridihexethyl chloride *trye-hex-eth'-el*	Pathilon	Adjunctive therapy for peptic ulcers	Drowsiness, blurred vision, tachycardia, dry mouth, urinary hesitancy	25–50 mg PO 3 or 4 times/d AC and HS
trihexyphenidyl *trye-hex-ee-fen'-i-dill*	Artane	Parkinsonism, extrapyramidal effects caused by antipsychotic drugs	Disorientation, confusion, light-headedness, dizziness, blurred vision, mydriasis, dry mouth, urinary retention, flushing	1–2 mg/d; increase by 2 mg q3–5d, to a total of 6–10 mg/d; divide dose into 3–4 times/d

*The term *generic* indicates the drug is available in generic form.

fusion, drowsiness, urinary retention, or other adverse effects. If any of these occur, then the health care provider should be informed and the patient's safety ensured.

Managing Alterations in Visual Acuity

Blurred vision and photophobia commonly occur with cholinergic blocking drugs. The patient may need help walking. If photophobia is a problem, then the patient may need to wear sunglasses outside, even on cloudy days. The patient's room should be dimly lit and curtains or blinds closed to keep bright sunlight from the room.

Managing Dry Mouth

Patients who take these drugs daily may experience severe and very uncomfortable mouth dryness. Patients may have difficulty swallowing oral drugs and food. The patient should take a few sips of water before and with an oral drug, and sip water at intervals during meals. If allowed, hard candy slowly dissolved in the mouth and frequent sips of water during the day may help relieve a dry mouth.

Minimizing Risk for Injury

Cholinergic blocking drugs may cause drowsiness, dizziness, and blurred vision. Patients (especially the elderly) may need help walking.

GERONTOLOGIC ALERT
Visual Difficulties

For elderly patients, as well as all patients experiencing visual difficulties, any furniture (e.g., footstools, chairs, stands) that may obstruct walking should be moved out of the way. Throw rugs should be removed.

Managing Constipation

Constipation can be a problem with cholinergic blocking drugs. The patient may obtain relief by increasing fluid intake up to 2000 mL daily (if health conditions permit), eating a diet high in fiber, and getting adequate exercise. The health care provider may prescribe a stool softener, if necessary, to prevent constipation.

Contraindications, Precautions, and Interactions of Cholinergic Blocking Drugs

Cholinergic blocking drugs are contraindicated for patients with glaucoma because these drugs may cause an attack of acute glaucoma. Unfortunately, glaucoma in an early stage may have few or no symptoms, and patients may be unaware of this disorder until they have an eye examination. Other contraindications for the anticholinergics include tachyarrhythmias, myocardial infarction (heart attack), and congestive heart failure (unless bradycardia is present).

These drugs can cause urinary retention and are given with great caution to patients with an enlarged prostate. This caution applies also to some over-the-counter medications for allergy and cold symptoms and for aiding sleep. Some of these products contain atropine, scopolamine, or other cholinergic blocking drugs. Although this warning is printed on the drug's container or package, many users fail to carefully read drug labels.

These drugs are also used with caution in patients with gastrointestinal infections, benign prostatic hypertrophy, hyperthyroidism, hepatic or renal disease, or hypertension. Atropine must be used with caution in patients with asthma. The anticholinergic drugs are classified as pregnancy category C drugs and are used only when the benefit to the woman outweighs the risk to the fetus.

Giving atropine with meperidine (Demerol), flurazepam (Dalmane), diphenhydramine (Benadryl), phenothiazines, or tricyclic antidepressants may increase the effects of atropine. The effectiveness of haloperidol is decreased when it is administered with an anticholinergic drug.

Patient Management Issues with Adrenergic and Cholinergic Drugs

Adrenergic Drugs

Because adrenergic drugs are powerful and potentially dangerous, proper supervision and patient management before, during, and after administration of the drug is needed to minimize any serious problems.

Caring for a Patient in Shock

When an adrenergic drug is to be given for shock, the patient's blood pressure, pulse rate and quality, and respiratory rate and rhythm are first assessed. This information is important for treatment.

Management of shock is aimed at providing basic life support (airway, breathing, and circulation) while attempting to correct the underlying cause. The initial pharmacologic intervention is aimed at supporting the circulation with a **vasopressor** (a drug that raises the blood pressure because it constricts blood vessels).

Some hypotensive episodes require the use of a less potent vasopressor, such as metaraminol, whereas at other times a more potent vasopressor, such as dobutamine (Dobutrex), dopamine (Intropin), or norepinephrine (Levophed), is necessary. The patient's heart rate, blood pressure, and ECG are monitored continuously.

The less potent vasopressors, such as metaraminol, also require close patient supervision during use. Blood pressure and pulse assessments are also made.

Caring for Patients Taking Midodrine

When midodrine is prescribed for orthostatic hypotension, the patient's blood pressure should be checked before therapy with the patient both lying down and sitting. This is important because midodrine is contraindicated in patients with supine hypertension.

This drug is given only when the patient is out of bed. Bedridden patients should not receive the drug. Patients taking midodrine need frequent monitoring of blood pressure and heart rate. Bradycardia is common at the beginning of therapy. Persistent bradycardia should be reported to the health care provider. Because the drug can cause dysuria, the patient is asked to urinate before being given the drug.

ALERT

Blood Pressure Drops with Adrenergic Drugs

Regardless of the actual numerical reading, any continuing fall of blood pressure is serious. Any progressive fall of the blood pressure, or a fall in systolic blood pressure below 100 mm Hg, should be reported to the health care provider.

Adrenergic Blocking Drugs

An accurate patient database is needed before any adrenergic blocking drug is first given. For example, patients with hypertension have their blood pressure and pulse taken on both arms in sitting, standing, and supine positions. Patients with a cardiac arrhythmia have their pulse taken and their pulse rhythm determined. Once drug therapy is started, the effects of therapy can be evaluated by comparing the patient's current symptoms with the symptoms before therapy started.

Patients receiving adrenergic drug therapy are continually observed for adverse reactions. Some adverse reactions are mild, whereas others, such as diarrhea, may cause a problem, especially if the patient is elderly or debilitated.

During therapy for hypertension with an adrenergic blocking drug, the patient's blood pressure is measured before each dose is given. Some patients have an unusual response to the drugs. In addition, some drugs may decrease the blood pressure in some patients more rapidly than other drugs. The patient's blood pressure is measured in both arms and in sitting, standing, and lying positions for the first week or more of therapy.

Patients receiving adrenergic blocking drugs for cardiac arrhythmias also require monitoring. Some cardiac arrhythmias, such as ventricular fibrillation, are life-threatening and require immediate attention. A patient with a life-threatening arrhythmia may receive an adrenergic blocking drug, such as propranolol, by the intravenous route, in which case specialized cardiac monitoring is necessary.

When adrenergic blocking drugs are given to patients to control hypertension, angina, or cardiac arrhythmias, the health care provider must stay informed about the patient's response to therapy. When given for a cardiac arrhythmia, these drugs can provoke new or worsen existing ventricular arrhythmias. If angina worsens or does not appear to be controlled by the drug, then the health care provider must be notified immediately. When the drug is administered for hypertension, the patient's blood pressure is monitored.

Most adrenergic blocking drugs can be given without regard to food. Propranolol and metoprolol, however, should be given at the same time each day because food may affect their absorption. Sotalol is given on an empty stomach because food may reduce its absorption.

When β-adrenergic blocking eyedrops, such as timolol, are administered to patients with glaucoma, they need periodic follow-up examinations by an ophthalmologist. The intraocular pressure should be measured to determine the effectiveness of drug therapy.

Cholinergic Drugs

Patients receiving a cholinergic drug should be monitored for drug toxicity or **cholinergic crisis**. Specific patient management issues apply also to patients with glaucoma, myasthenia gravis, or urinary retention.

ALERT

Cholinergic Crisis

Symptoms of cholinergic crisis (cholinergic drug toxicity) include severe abdominal cramping, diarrhea, excessive salivation, muscle weakness, rigidity and spasm, and clenching of the jaw. Patients with these symptoms require immediate medical treatment, and their condition must be immediately reported to the health care provider. An antidote such as atropine may be given in case of an overdose.

Caring for Patients with Glaucoma

Before therapy for glaucoma is started, the patient needs an eye examination. The patient is also assessed for the ability to perform the activities of daily living, especially if the patient is elderly or has limited vision.

The health care provider's order and the drug label must be checked carefully before instilling eyedrops. The drug label must indicate that the preparation is for ophthalmic use. A patient or family member may be taught to instill the eyedrops correctly. The tip of the dropper must never touch the eye. Hospitalized patients who use the eyedrops themselves should be checked periodically to ensure the drug being used at the prescribed times using the correct technique.

Caring for Patients with Myasthenia Gravis

Once drug therapy is underway, the patient must be checked for any increase in the symptoms of the disease or adverse drug reactions before each dose is given. This patient assessment is important because the dosage often must be increased or decreased early in therapy, depending on the patient's response, to keep the symptoms of myasthenia gravis from incapacitating the patient. For many patients, the symptoms are fairly well-controlled with drug therapy once the optimal drug dose is determined.

Patients with severe symptoms of the disease require the drug every 2 to 4 hours, even during the night. Sustained-released tablets may be used that allow less frequent dosing and give the patient longer undisturbed periods at night.

ALERT

Cholinergic Drugs for Myasthenia Gravis

Because dosage adjustments may be frequent, the patient must be observed closely for symptoms of drug overdosage or underdosage. Signs of drug overdosage include muscle rigidity and spasm, salivation, and clenching of the jaw. Signs of drug underdosage are the signs of the disease itself: rapid fatigability of the muscles, drooping of the eyelids, and difficulty breathing. If symptoms of drug over–dosage or underdosage develop, the health care provider must be notified immediately.

Caring for Patients with Urinary Retention

Patients with urinary retention must be monitored for fluid intake and output. The health care provider should be notified if the patient fails to urinate after taking the drug.

Urination usually occurs 5 to 15 minutes after subcutaneous drug administration and 30 to 90 minutes after oral administration. With a hospitalized patient, the call light and any other items the patient might need, such as a urinal or the bedpan, should be within easy reach.

Cholinergic Blocking Drugs

Patients taking a cholinergic blocking drug should be closely observed. Vital signs are monitored and the patient observed for adverse reactions. Any increase in the severity of symptoms of the condition for which the patient is being treated must be reported to the health care provider immediately.

Caring for Patients with Heart Block

Patient receiving atropine for third-degree heart block are placed on a cardiac monitor during and after administration of the drug to monitor for changes in pulse rate or rhythm. Tachycardia or other arrhythmias must be immediately reported, as well as a failure of the drug to increase the patient's heart rate. Other drugs or medical management may be necessary.

Caring for Patients Receiving a Preoperative Drug

If a cholinergic blocking drug is to be given before surgery, the patient is asked to urinate before the drug is given. Patients are told that their mouth will become very dry but that they cannot drink any fluid before the surgery.

Educating the Patient and Family with Adrenergic and Cholinergic Drugs

Adrenergic Drugs

Some adrenergic drugs, such as the vasopressors, are given only by medical personnel. In this case the drug must be explained to the patient or family, along with what results are expected and what effects may occur.

Patient Education Box 4-1 includes key points about adrenergic drugs given for nasal congestion, bronchodilation, or orthostatic hypotension that the patient or family members should know.

Adrenergic Blocking Drugs

Patients need to know why they are taking these drugs and why therapy must be continuous to attain and maintain an optimal state of health and well-being. Patient Education Box 4-2 includes key points about adrenergic blocking drugs for specific conditions that the patient or family members should know.

Cholinergic Drugs

The purpose of the drug therapy should be explained to the patient and family members, along with the adverse reactions that may occur. Patient Education Box 4-3 includes key points about cholinergic drugs the patient or family members should know.

Cholinergic Blocking Drugs

A cholinergic blocking drug may be prescribed for a prolonged period. Some patients may discontinue drug use, especially if their original symptoms have been relieved.

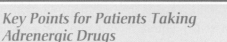

PATIENT EDUCATION BOX 4-1

Key Points for Patients Taking Adrenergic Drugs

NASAL DECONGESTANTS
- ❏ The patient or family member needs to be shown the correct method of using nasal decongestants.
- ❏ Over-the-counter nasal decongestants should not be used by patients with high blood pressure.
- ❏ Overuse of nasal decongestants can actually increase nasal congestion (rebound congestion).

BRONCHODILATORS
- ❏ Adverse reactions must be reported to the health care provider as soon as possible.
- ❏ For drugs prescribed in sublingual form, the technique of placing the drug under the tongue is demonstrated and explained.

MIDODRINE
- ❏ Patients with severe orthostatic hypotension need to take this drug during daytime hours when they are upright.
- ❏ Take doses in 3-hour intervals if needed to control symptoms.
- ❏ Do not take the drug within 4 hours of bedtime.
- ❏ Do not lie down soon after taking the drug.
- ❏ It may be necessary to sleep with the head of the bed elevated.
- ❏ If urinary retention is a problem, then urinate before taking the drug.
- ❏ See the health care provider regularly for medical evaluation.
- ❏ Report any changes in vision, pounding in the head when lying down, slow heart rate, or difficulty urinating.

The patient and family need to understand the prescribed drug must still be taken even though symptoms have been relieved. Patient Education Box 4-4 includes key points about cholinergic blocking drugs the patient or family members should know.

GERONTOLOGIC ALERT

Cholinergic Blocking Drugs

Family members of an elderly patient should be told about possible visual and mental impairments (blurred vision, confusion, agitation) that may occur during therapy with cholinergic blocking drugs. Objects or situations that may cause falls, such as throw rugs, footstools, and wet or newly waxed floors, should be removed or avoided whenever possible. The patient must be closely observed during the first few days of therapy and the health care provider notified if mental changes occur.

Key Points for Patients Taking Adrenergic Blocking Drugs

PATIENTS WITH HYPERTENSION, CARDIAC ARRHYTHMIA, OR ANGINA

Some hypertensive patients may be advised to lose weight or eat a special diet, such as a low-salt diet. Patients with angina or a cardiac arrhythmia may also need a special diet. Some patients with hypertension may be taught to monitor their own blood pressure between office visits. In addition:

❑ Do not stop taking the drug abruptly except as advised by your health care provider. Most of these drugs require gradually decreasing the dosage to prevent worsening the adverse effects.
❑ Notify your health care provider promptly if adverse drug reactions occur.
❑ Be cautious while driving or performing other hazardous tasks because these drugs (β-adrenergic blockers) may cause drowsiness, dizziness, or light-headedness.
❑ Immediately report any signs of congestive heart failure (weight gain, difficulty breathing, or edema of the extremities).
❑ Do not use any nonprescription drug (e.g., cold or flu preparations or nasal decongestants) unless it is approved by the health care provider.
❑ Inform dentists and other care providers you are taking this drug.
❑ Keep all health care appointments because close monitoring of therapy is essential with these drugs.

MONITORING BLOOD PRESSURE

The patient and family member are taught how to take an accurate blood pressure reading. This involves choosing the correct instrument and the steps to taking a blood pressure reading. The patient and family member are supervised during several trial blood pressure readings to ensure accuracy of the measurements.

❑ Use the same arm and body position each time to take the blood pressure.
❑ Blood pressure can vary slightly with emotion, the time of day, and the position of your body.
❑ Slight changes in readings are normal, but if a drastic change occurs in either or both the systolic or diastolic readings, then contact your health care provider as soon as possible.

PATIENTS WITH GLAUCOMA

When an adrenergic blocking drug is prescribed for glaucoma, the patient needs a demonstration of how to correctly use eye drops. In addition:

❑ Stay on the eye drop instillation schedule, because delaying or discontinuing the drug may result in a marked increase in intraocular pressure, which can lead to blindness.
❑ Contact your health care provider if you experience eye pain, excessive tearing, or any change in vision.

Key Points for Patients Taking Cholinergic Drugs

PATIENT'S WITH GLAUCOMA

When a cholinergic drug is prescribed for glaucoma, the patient and family member are shown how to correctly instill the eye drops.

❑ The eye drops may sting when put in the eye; this is normal but usually temporary.
❑ Be cautious while driving or performing any task that requires visual acuity.
❑ Local irritation and headache may occur at the beginning of therapy.
❑ Notify your health care provider if you experience abdominal cramping, diarrhea, or excessive salivation.

INSTILLING LIQUID EYE MEDICATION

❑ It is important to keep the bottle tightly closed.
❑ Do not wash the tip of the dropper.
❑ Do not put the dropper down on a table or other surface.
❑ Support your hand holding the dropper against your forehead.
❑ Do not let the tip of the dropper touch the eye.
❑ Put the dropper back in the bottle immediately after use.
❑ Tilt your head back to instill the prescribed number of drops in the inner lower eyelid.
❑ If you or a family member cannot instill the eye drops, then contact your health care provider immediately.

THE PILOCARPINE OCULAR SYSTEM

If the pilocarpine ocular system is prescribed, then the patient must be able to insert and remove the system. A package insert is provided with the system, which should be reviewed with the patient. In addition:

❑ Remove and replace the system every 7 days or as instructed by your health care provider.
❑ Do the replacement at bedtime (unless ordered otherwise) because there is some impairment of vision for a short time after insertion.
❑ Check for unit placement before going to bed and after getting up in the morning.
❑ Notify your health care provider if you have excessive eye secretions or irritation.

PATIENTS WITH MYASTHENIA GRAVIS

Many patients with myasthenia gravis learn to adjust their drug dosage according to their needs because dosages may vary slightly from day to day. The patient and family members are taught to recognize symptoms of overdosage and underdosage and what steps to take if either occurs. The patient should be given a written or printed description of the signs and symptoms of drug overdosage or underdosage. In addition:

❑ Keep a record of your response to drug therapy (e.g., time of day, increased or decreased muscle strength, fatigue), and bring this to each provider or clinic visit until your symptoms are well-controlled and the drug dosage is stabilized.
❑ Wear or carry identification (such as a Medic-Alert tag) indicating that you have myasthenia gravis.

PATIENT EDUCATION BOX 4-4

Key Points for Patients Taking Cholinergic Blocking Drugs

❑ If you experience drowsiness, dizziness, or blurred vision, then avoid driving or performing other tasks requiring alertness and good vision.

❑ If you experience photophobia, then wear sunglasses when outside, even on cloudy days, keep rooms dimly lit, and close curtains or blinds to eliminate bright sunlight in the room. Schedule outdoor activities (when necessary) before taking the first dose of the drug, such as early in the morning.

❑ For constipation, drink plenty of fluids during the day, exercise if approved by your health care provider, and eat foods high in fiber.

❑ To prevent heat prostration, avoid going outside on hot, sunny days; use fans to stay cool if the day is extremely warm; sponge your skin with cool water if other cooling measures are not available; and wear loose-fitting clothes in warm weather.

FOR DRY MOUTH

❑ Perform frequent mouth care, including brushing, rinsing, and flossing.

❑ Keep a glass or sports bottle filled with fluid on hand at all times.

❑ Sip small amounts of cool water or fluids throughout the day and with meals.

❑ Take a few sips of water before taking any oral drugs.

❑ Suck on ice chips or frozen ices, such as popsicles.

❑ Chew gum.

❑ Suck on sugar-free hard candies.

❑ Avoid alcohol-based mouthwashes.

PATIENTS RECEIVING A PREOPERATIVE DRUG

❑ Urinate before the preoperative drug is administered.

❑ Drowsiness and extreme dryness of the mouth and nose will occur approximately 20 to 30 minutes after the drug is given.

❑ Stay in bed with the side rails raised after the drug is administered.

PATIENTS WITH PEPTIC ULCER

❑ A special diet may be ordered by the health care provider; following this diet is important.

❑ Take the drug exactly as prescribed (e.g., 30 minutes before meals or between meals) to obtain the desired results.

KEY POINTS

⬤ Adrenergic drugs mimic the activity of the sympathetic nervous system and have many effects throughout the body and many uses, including the treatment of shock, asthma, and nasal congestion. Common adverse effects include anxiety or restlessness, dizziness, headache, and cardiac arrhythmias.

⬤ Adrenergic blocking drugs inhibit actions in the sympathetic nervous system. The four classes of these drugs have many uses, including the treatment of hypertension, glaucoma, and cardiac arrhythmias. Common adverse effects include bradycardia, dizziness, hypotension, and nausea and vomiting.

⬤ Cholinergic drugs mimic the activity of the parasympathetic nervous system. They are used primarily for treatment of glaucoma, myasthenia gravis, and urinary retention. Common adverse effects include cardiac arrhythmias, abdominal discomfort, temporary reduction in visual acuity, and headache.

⬤ Cholinergic blocking drugs inhibit actions in the parasympathetic nervous system and have widespread effects throughout the body. Common uses are the treatment of pylorospasm, peptic ulcer, and parkinsonism. Common adverse effects include drowsiness, blurred vision, dry mouth, and tachycardia.

⬤ Patient management and teaching for all these drugs focus on the need for strict dosage control and the management of common adverse reactions.

CASE STUDY

Ms. Martin has been prescribed propranolol (Inderal) for hypertension. A few days later she says that she is feeling dizzy and sometimes feels as if she is going to faint.

1. Ms. Martin needs to know:
   a. dizziness is a rare, life-threatening adverse reaction that must be reported immediately to her health care provider
   b. dizziness is a common adverse effect that may disappear with continued therapy
   c. she can stop taking the drug whenever the adverse reactions bother her
   d. taking the drug only with meals will make this adverse effect go away

2. Ms. Martin also has diabetes. This means:
   a. she should not be taking propranolol at all
   b. the propranolol will likely cure her diabetes
   c. the propranolol has been prescribed with caution
   d. she should take the propranolol only when her blood sugar is low

3. To lower the risk that Ms. Martin may be injured when she feels dizzy, her family members should:
   a. discourage her from taking hot showers
   b. ask her to get up slowly from a sitting or lying position
   c. help her walk when necessary
   d. all of the above

WEBSITE ACTIVITIES

1. Go to the website of the National High Blood Pressure Education Program (NHBPEP) (http://www.nhlbi.nih.gov/about/nhbpep/index.htm). Navigate to the document titled "Your Guide to Lowering High Blood Pressure." Go to the section on Treatment and find the discussion of lifestyle modifications that people can use to help lower their blood pressure. Write down five things that help lower blood pressure.

   1. _____
   2. _____
   3. _____
   4. _____
   5. _____

2. In the Treatment section of this website, look at the Medication section for the document "Tips to Help You Remember to Take Your Medicine." Write down five tips that can be shared with patients to help them remember to take any medication.

   1. _____
   2. _____
   3. _____
   4. _____
   5. _____

REVIEW QUESTIONS

1. Which of the following is a common adverse reaction of **adrenergic drugs**?
   a. bradycardia
   b. increase in appetite
   c. nausea
   d. skin rashes

2. A patient with glaucoma will likely receive a(n):
   a. adrenergic blocking drug
   b. adrenergic drug

   c. cholinergic blocking drug
   d. any of the above

3. Pilocarpine eye drops may be prescribed to treat:
   a. near-sightedness
   b. glaucoma
   c. eye infection
   d. mydriasis of the eyes

4. A patient taking clidinium for a peptic ulcer complains of dry mouth. This patient should be told:
   a. this effect is unusual and the health care provider should be notified
   b. to take frequent sips of water
   c. to rinse the mouth with salt water
   d. to ignore this reaction because it is only temporary

5. Because of the effect of cholinergic blocking drugs on intestinal motility, patients taking these drugs should be monitored for the development of:
   a. esophageal ulcers
   b. diarrhea
   c. heartburn
   d. constipation

5 Psychiatric Drugs

Review Questions
KEY TERMS

addiction—physical drug dependence
akathisia—extreme restlessness and increased motor activity
antianxiety drugs—drugs used to treat anxiety
antidepressants—drugs used to treat depression
antipsychotic drugs—drugs used to treat psychotic disorders
anxiety—a feeling of apprehension, worry, or uneasiness that may or may not be based
    on reality
anxiolytics—another term that refers to antianxiety drugs
ataxia—a loss of control of voluntary movements, especially producing an unsteady gait
bipolar disorder—a psychiatric disorder characterized by severe mood swings from ex-
    treme hyperactivity to depression (manic–depressive disease)
depression—a common psychiatric disorder characterized by feelings of intense sadness,
    helplessness, and worthlessness and by impaired functioning
dysphoric—extreme or exaggerated sadness, anxiety, or unhappiness
dystonia—facial grimacing and twisting of the neck into unnatural positions
endogenous—made within the body
extrapyramidal effects—a group of adverse reactions occurring in the extrapyramidal por-
    tion of the nervous system, causing abnormal muscle movements
hypnotic—a drug that induces sleep
neuroleptic drugs—another term for antipsychotic drugs
neuroleptic malignant syndrome—a rare reaction to antipsychotic drugs characterized
    by a combination of extrapyramidal effects, hyperthermia, and autonomic
    disturbance

orthostatic hypotension—a feeling of light-headedness and dizziness after suddenly changing position after standing in one place for a long period, caused by a drop in blood pressure when a person sits or stands up

photophobia—an intolerance to light

photosensitivity—abnormally heightened reactivity of the skin to sunlight

psychotherapeutic drug—used to treat disorders of the mind

psychotic disorder—a disorder, such as schizophrenia, characterized by extreme personality disorganization and a loss of contact with reality

psychotropic drug—another term for psychotherapeutic drugs

sedative—a drug that produces a relaxing, calming effect

soporific—another term for a hypnotic drug

tardive dyskinesia—a syndrome consisting of potentially irreversible, involuntary dyskinetic movements

tolerance—patient condition in which increasingly larger dosages are required to obtain the desired effect

withdrawal—a syndrome of physical and psychological symptoms caused by abruptly stopping use of a drug in a dependent patient

CHAPTER OBJECTIVES

On completion of this chapter, students will be able to:

1 Define the chapter's key terms.

2 Discuss the uses, general drug actions, contraindications, precautions, interactions, and adverse reactions associated with the administration of sedatives and hypnotics, antianxiety drugs, antidepressants, and antipsychotic drugs.

3 Discuss important points to keep in mind when educating patients and family members about the use of sedatives and hypnotics, antianxiety drugs, antidepressants, and antipsychotic drugs.

A wide range of drugs are used to treat patients with mental symptoms or disorders. These include psychotherapeutic drugs, also called **psychotropic** drugs, which are used to treat disorders of the mind. The types of psychotherapeutic drugs used to treat mental illness include:

- Antianxiety drugs (tranquilizers)
- Antidepressant drugs
- Antipsychotic drugs

Sedatives and hypnotics are also discussed in this chapter because they may also be used for patients experiencing anxiety, although they are used for other medical purposes, also, such as to induce sleep the night before surgery.

Sedatives and Hypnotics

A **sedative** is a drug that produces a relaxing, calming effect. Sedatives are usually given during daytime hours, and although they may make the patient drowsy, they usually do not produce sleep. A **hypnotic** is a drug that induces sleep, that is, it allows the patient to fall asleep and stay asleep. Hypnotics are also called **soporifics**. Hypnotics are given at night or when the patient needs to go to sleep.

Sedatives and hypnotics can be divided into two classes: barbiturates and miscellaneous sedatives and hypnotics. The barbiturates are divided into several groups, depending on their duration of action.

- Ultrashort-acting. The ultrashort-acting barbiturates are used as anesthetics (see Chapter 9). Single doses have a duration of 20 minutes or less.
- Short-acting. The average duration of action of short-acting barbiturates is 3 to 4 hours.
- Intermediate-acting. The average duration of action of intermediate-acting barbiturates is 6 to 8 hours.
- Long-acting. The average duration of action of the long-acting barbiturates is 10 to 16 hours.

The Summary Drug Table: Sedatives and Hypnotics gives examples of the short-, intermediate-, and long-acting barbiturate sedatives and hypnotics.

The miscellaneous sedatives and hypnotics are a group of unrelated drugs and a second group called the benzodiazepines. The benzodiazepines are also called antianxiety drugs (see later section). The miscellaneous

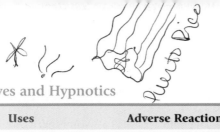

SUMMARY DRUG TABLE   Sedatives and Hypnotics

Generic Name	Trade Name*	Uses	Adverse Reactions	Dosage Ranges
Barbiturates amobarbital sodium *am-oh-bar'-bi-tal*	Amytal Sodium	Sedative, hypnotic, preoperative sedation	Respiratory and central nervous system depression, nausea, vomiting, constipation, diarrhea, bradycardia, hypotension, syncope, hypersensitivity reactions, headache	Sedative: 200 mg 1–2 h before surgery IM; IV: 65–500 mg
aprobarbital *a-pro-bar'-bi-tal*	Alurate	Sedative, hypnotic	Same as amobarbital sodium	Sedative: 40 mg PO TID
butabarbital *byoo-ta-bar'-bi-tal*	Butisol sodium, *generic*	Sedative, hypnotic, preoperative sedation	Same as amobarbital sodium	Sedative: 15–30 mg PO TID, QID; hypnotic: 50–100 mg PO; preoperative sedation: 50–100 mg PO 60–90 min before surgery
mephobarbital *me-foe-bar'-bi-tal*	Mebaral	Sedative, epilepsy	Same as amobarbital sodium	Sedative: 32–100 mg PO TID, QID; epilepsy: 400–600 mg/d
pentobarbital sodium *pen-toe-bar'-bi-tal*	Nembutal Sodium, *generic*	Sedative, hypnotic, preoperative sedation	Same as amobarbital sodium	Sedative: 200 mg TID–QID; hypnotic: 100 mg HS
phenobarbital *fee-noe-bar'-bi-tal*	Bellatal, Luminal, Solfoton, (parenteral)	Insomnia, seizures, convulsive episodes, preanesthetic	Somnolence, agitation, confusion, ataxia, vertigo, CNS depression, nightmares, nausea, constipation, bradycardia, hypotension, respiratory depression	30–200 mg/d PO; 30–320 mg/d IM or IV
secobarbital sodium *see-koe-bar'-bi-tal*	*Generic*	Hypnotic, preoperative sedation	Same as amobarbital sodium	Hypnotic: 100 mg HS; sedation: 200–300 mg
Miscellaneous Sedatives and Hypnotics chloral hydrate *klor-al hye'-drate*	Aquachloral, Noctec, *generic*	Hypnotic, sedative	Disorientation, gastric irritation, nausea, vomiting, delirium, light-headedness, vertigo, hypersensitivity reactions	Sedative: 250 mg PO TID; hypnotic: 500 mg–1 g PO
dexmedetomidine HCL *dex-meh-dih-toe'-mih-deen*	Precedex	Sedation of intubated and mechanically ventilated patients	Hypotension, nausea, bradycardia, hypoxia, dizziness, headache, apnea, blood pressure fluctuations	0.2–0.7 mcg/kg/h (rate adjusted to achieve the desired level of sedation)

Generic Name	Trade Name*	Uses	Adverse Reactions	Dosage Ranges
ethchlorvynol *eth-klor-vi'-nole*	Placidyl	Hypnotic	Vomiting, gastric upset, dizziness, blurred vision, hypotension	500–1000 mg PO
glutethimide *gloo-teth'-i-mide*	*Generic*	Hypnotic	Drowsiness, skin rash, vertigo, headache, depression	250–500 mg PO
paraldehyde *par-al'-de-hyde*	Paral, *generic*	Sedative, hypnotic, delirium tremens	Strong unpleasant breath, GI upset, rash	Sedative: 5–10 mL PO, rectal; hypnotic: 10–30 mL PO, 10–20 mL rectal; delirium tremens: 10–35 mL PO
zaleplon *zal'-ah-plahn*	Sonata	Insomnia	Dizziness, headache, drowsiness, anxiety, rebound insomnia, nausea, visual impairment, myalgia	10 mg PO HS
zolpidem tartrate *zol'-pih-dem*	Ambien	Hypnotic	Drowsiness, amnesia, dizziness, nausea, vomiting, diarrhea	10 mg PO
Benzodiazepines estazolam *es-taz'-e-lam*	ProSom	Hypnotic	Headache, heartburn, nausea, palpitations, rash, somnolence, vomiting, weakness, body and joint pain	1–2 mg PO
flurazepam *flur-az'-e-pam*	Dalmane, generic	Hypnotic	Same as estazolam	15–30 mg PO
quazepam *kwa'-ze-pam*	Doral	Hypnotic	Same as estazolam	7.5–15 mg PO
temazepam *te-maz'-e-pam*	Restoril, *generic*	Hypnotic	Same as estazolam	15–30 mg PO
triazolam *trye-ay'-zoe-lam*	Halcion, *generic*	Sedative, hypnotic	Same as estazolam	0.125–0.5 mg PO HS

*The term *generic* indicates the drug is available in generic form.

sedatives and hypnotics are listed in the Summary Drug Table: Sedatives and Hypnotics.

Actions of Sedatives and Hypnotics

All barbiturates have essentially the same mode of action. Depending on the dose given, these drugs produce central nervous system depression and mood alteration ranging from mild excitation to mild sedation, hypnosis (sleep), or deep coma. These drugs also are respiratory depressants, with the degree of depression usually depending on the dose given. When these drugs are used as hypnotics, their respiratory depressant effect is usually similar to that normally occurring during sleep. The sedative or hypnotic effects of the barbiturates diminish after

approximately 2 weeks. Outpatients taking these drugs for periods longer than 2 weeks may increase the dose to produce the desired effects (e.g., sleep, sedation). Physical and psychological dependence may occur, especially after prolonged use of high doses. Discontinuing use of a barbiturate after prolonged use may result in severe, and sometimes fatal, withdrawal symptoms. **Withdrawal** is a syndrome of physical and psychological symptoms caused by abruptly stopping use of a drug in a dependent patient, as discussed later in this chapter.

Miscellaneous or nonbarbiturate sedatives and hypnotics have essentially the same mode of action as the barbiturates, that is, they depress the central nervous system. However, the miscellaneous sedatives and hypnotics have a lesser effect on the respiratory rate.

Effect of Barbiturates on Sleep

Sleep occurs in four stages. People experience varying degrees of wakefulness followed by deeper sleep throughout the sleep cycle. These stages fall into two areas: rapid eye movement (REM) sleep and nonrapid eye movement (NREM) sleep. NREM sleep occurs mostly in the early hours of sleep; REM sleep tends to lengthen progressively during the later sleep period.

Dreaming occurs mostly during REM sleep. Dreams appear to be a necessary part of sleep, and when an individual is deprived of dreaming for a prolonged period, a psychosis can develop. Sleep induced by a barbiturate involves reduced time in the REM stage (the dreaming stage) of sleep. Abrupt discontinuation of a barbiturate can cause increased dreaming, nightmares, or insomnia.

Uses of Sedatives and Hypnotics

Sedatives and hypnotics are primarily used to treat insomnia.

FACTS ABOUT INSOMNIA

- Insomnia affects nearly 84 million people. Forty-eight percent of Americans report insomnia occasionally, whereas 22% experience insomnia every or almost every night.
- Insomnia may be caused by lifestyle changes, such as a new job or moving to a new town, or returning to school.
- Other common causes include jet lag, pain from arthritis or headaches, stress, or anxiety.
- Women are more likely to report insomnia than are men.
- People older than age 65 are more likely to report insomnia than are younger people.
- Divorced, widowed, and separated people report more insomnia.
- Lack of sleep because of insomnia may contribute to illness, including heart disease.

Source: The National Sleep Foundation.

Helping hospitalized patients sleep is an important part of the management of illness. Hospitalized patients are in unfamiliar surroundings unlike their home situation. Noises and lights at night often interfere with or interrupt their sleep. Because sleep deprivation can interfere with the healing process, a hypnotic may be given. These drugs also may be prescribed for short-term use after discharge from the hospital.

Zaleplon, a miscellaneous sedative, is a prescription sleep preparation a patient can take later in the night if at least 4 hours remain before the patient will become active again. With zaleplon, the patient will fall asleep quickly and wake up with little or no aftereffects of the drug.

A hypnotic may be given the night before an operation to prepare the patient for surgery. On the day of surgery, a barbiturate or miscellaneous sedative and hypnotic may be used either alone or with other drugs as part of the preoperative regimen. The anesthesiologist or surgeon selects a drug tailored to the patient's needs. When a barbiturate or miscellaneous sedative and hypnotic are used as a hypnotic, a dose larger than that required to produce sedation is given.

GERONTOLOGIC ALERT
Sedatives and Hypnotics
Elderly patients may require a smaller hypnotic dose. In some instances, a sedative dose produces sleep.

Although barbiturates and miscellaneous sedatives and hypnotics used for sedation have largely been replaced by the antianxiety drugs (see following section), they occasionally may be used to provide sedation before certain types of procedures, such as cardiac catheterization or the administration of a local or general anesthesia. Sedative doses, usually given during daytime hours, may be used to treat anxiety and apprehension. Patients with chronic disease may require sedation to reduce anxiety and as an adjunct in the treatment of their disease.

Paraldehyde, a miscellaneous sedative and hypnotic, may be used to treat delirium tremens and other psychiatric conditions. In addition, some barbiturates are used as anticonvulsants (see Chapter 6).

A hypnotic or sedative should never be left at the patient's bedside to be taken at a later hour, because these are controlled substances (see Chapter 1). In addition, these drugs should never be left unattended in a nurses' station, hallway, or other areas to which patients, visitors, or hospital personnel have direct access. If these drugs are prepared in advance, then they must be kept in a locked cupboard until the time of administration.

Adverse Reactions of Sedatives and Hypnotics

Adverse reactions associated with the use of barbiturates include:

- Central nervous system symptoms: somnolence, agitation, confusion, central nervous system depression, ataxia (unsteady gait), nightmares, lethargy, residual sedation (drug hangover), hallucinations, paradoxical excitement
- Respiratory symptoms: hypoventilation, apnea, respiratory depression, bronchospasm, laryngospasm
- Gastrointestinal symptoms: nausea, vomiting, constipation, diarrhea, epigastric pain

- Cardiovascular symptoms: bradycardia, hypotension, syncope
- Hypersensitivity symptoms: rash, angioneurotic edema, fever, urticaria (skin rash)
- Other: headache and liver damage.

Adverse reactions associated with the use of the miscellaneous sedatives and hypnotics vary depending on the drug used. Common adverse reactions include dizziness, drowsiness, headache, and nausea. Other adverse reactions of miscellaneous sedatives and hypnotics are listed in the Summary Drug Table: Sedatives and Hypnotics.

Managing Adverse Reactions of Sedatives and Hypnotics

During periods of excitement or confusion, the patient must be protected from harm and provided supportive care and a safe environment. The health care provider should be informed if the patient fails to sleep, awakens one or more times during the night, or develops an adverse drug reaction. In some instances, supplemental doses of a hypnotic may be ordered if the patient awakens during the night.

Excessive drowsiness and headache the morning after a hypnotic has been given (drug hangover) may occur in some patients. This problem should be reported to the health care provider because a smaller dose or a different drug may be necessary. The patient should be assisted when walking if necessary. When getting out of bed, the patient is encouraged to rise to a sitting position first, wait a few minutes, and then rise to a standing position.

GERONTOLOGIC ALERT

Adverse Effects of Sedatives and Hypnotics

Older adults are at greater risk for oversedation, dizziness, confusion, or ataxia (unsteady gait) when taking a sedative or hypnotic. Elderly and debilitated patients are observed for marked excitement, central nervous system depression, and confusion. If excitement or confusion occurs, then the patient is observed frequently (as often as every 5–10 minutes may be necessary) and safety measures are used to prevent injury. If oversedation, extreme dizziness, or ataxia occurs, then the health care provider is notified.

Monitoring and Managing Respiratory Depression. These drugs depress the central nervous system and can cause respiratory depression. The patient's respiratory function (rate, depth, and quality) is monitored before a sedative is given, 30 minutes to 1 hour after the drug is given, and frequently thereafter. A toxic reaction of a barbiturate can cause severe respiratory depression, hypoventilation, and circulatory collapse.

ALERT

Barbiturate Toxicity

The onset of symptoms of barbiturate toxicity may occur several hours after the drug is administered. Symptoms of acute toxicity include central nervous system and respiratory depression, constriction or paralytic dilation of the pupils, tachycardia, hypotension, lowered body temperature, oliguria (scanty urine production), circulatory collapse, and coma. Any symptoms of toxicity should be reported to the health care provider immediately.

The treatment of barbiturate toxicity is mainly supportive and involves maintaining a patent airway, giving oxygen if needed, and monitoring the patient's vital signs and fluid balance. The patient may require treatment for shock, respiratory assistance, administration of activated charcoal, and, in severe cases of toxicity, hemodialysis.

Managing Drug Dependency. Sedatives and hypnotics are not usually given longer than 2 weeks and preferably for a shorter time. Barbiturates and miscellaneous sedatives and hypnotics can cause drug dependency. The drug should not be suddenly discontinued when there is a question of possible dependency. Patients who have been taking a sedative or hypnotic for several weeks are gradually withdrawn from the drug to prevent withdrawal symptoms. Symptoms of withdrawal include restlessness, excitement, euphoria, and confusion. Withdrawal can have serious consequences, especially in those with existing diseases or disorders.

Contraindications, Precautions, and Interactions of Sedatives and Hypnotics

These drugs are contraindicated in patients with known hypersensitivity to sedatives or hypnotics. They are not administered to comatose patients, those with severe respiratory problems, those with a history of drug and alcohol abuse, or pregnant or lactating women. The barbiturates are classified as pregnancy category D drugs. Most miscellaneous sedatives and hypnotics are pregnancy category C drugs. Some benzodiazepines (e.g., estazolam, quazepam, temazepam, triazolam) are classified as pregnancy category X drugs and can cause damage to the developing fetus if given during pregnancy.

ALERT

Pregnancy and Sedatives and Hypnotics

Women taking a barbiturate or benzodiazepine should be warned of the potential risk to the fetus so that contraceptive methods may be used, if necessary. A child born to a mother taking benzodiazepines may develop withdrawal symptoms during the postnatal period.

All drugs entering the body ultimately leave the body. Some leave virtually unchanged, whereas others are transformed into other less potent chemicals or detoxified compounds before they are eliminated. Barbiturates and miscellaneous sedatives and hypnotics are detoxified by the liver and ultimately excreted by the kidney. These drugs are given with great caution to patients with liver or kidney disease because their diseased organs will not be able to detoxify or eliminate the drug, and a drug build-up will occur. Barbiturates should be administered only with extreme caution to patients with a history of drug abuse (e.g., alcoholics and opiate abusers) or mental illness. If the drugs are prescribed to an outpatient, then the amount dispensed is limited to the amount needed until the next appointment. These drugs should be used with great caution during lactation. Drowsiness in infants of breastfeeding mothers who have taken the barbiturates has been reported.

Sedatives and hypnotics have an additive effect when administered with alcohol, antidepressants, narcotic analgesics, antihistamines, or phenothiazines.

ALERT

Sedatives and Hypnotics with Narcotic Analgesics

Because narcotic analgesics depress the central nervous system, a barbiturate or miscellaneous sedatives and hypnotics should not be given approximately 2 hours before or after administration of a narcotic analgesic or other central nervous system depressant. If the time interval between administration of a narcotic analgesic and a sedative or hypnotic is less than 2 hours, then the patient may experience severe respiratory depression, bradycardia, and unresponsiveness.

Patient Management Issues with Sedatives and Hypnotics

Before a barbiturate or miscellaneous sedative and hypnotic are given, the patient's blood pressure, pulse, and respiratory rate are checked and recorded. In addition, the following patient needs are assessed:

- Is the patient uncomfortable? If the reason for discomfort is pain, then an analgesic, rather than a hypnotic, may be required.
- Is it too early for the patient to receive the drug? Is a later hour preferred?
- Does the patient receive a narcotic analgesic every 4 to 6 hours? A hypnotic may not be necessary because a narcotic analgesic can also cause drowsiness and sleep.
- Are there disturbances in the environment that may keep the patient awake and decrease the effectiveness of the drug?

Barbiturates have little or no analgesic action and are not used if the patient cannot sleep because of pain. Barbiturates given to a patient with pain may cause restlessness, excitement, and delirium.

If the patient is receiving one of these drugs for daytime sedation, the patient's general mental state and level of consciousness are monitored. If the patient appears sedated and is difficult to awaken, the drug may be withheld and the health care provider consulted as soon as possible.

After the drug is first used, the patient is checked for response. Did it help the patient sleep? If not, then a different drug or dose may be needed, and the health care provider should be informed about the drug's ineffectiveness. In addition, it is important to determine if any factors such as noise, lights, pain, or discomfort are interfering with the patient's sleep and whether these can be controlled or eliminated.

If the patient has an order for a PRN (as needed) narcotic analgesic or other central nervous system depressant and a hypnotic, then the health care provider must specify the time interval between administration of these drugs. Usually at least 2 hours should elapse between administration of a hypnotic and any other central nervous system, but this interval may vary, depending on factors such as the patient's age and diagnosis.

ALERT

Central Nervous System Depression with Sedatives and Hypnotics

The drug should be withheld and the health care provider consulted if any one of the patient's vital signs changes significantly, if the respiratory rate is 10/min or less, or if the patient appears lethargic.

Enhancing Sleep Patterns

To promote the effects of the sedative or hypnotic, the patient should be given supportive care, such as back rubs, night lights or a darkened room, and a quiet atmosphere. The patient is discouraged from drinking beverages containing caffeine, such as coffee, tea, or cola drinks, which can contribute to wakefulness.

When these drugs are given orally, the patient should be encouraged to drink a full glass of water with the drug. Oral paraldehyde can be mixed with cold orange or tomato juice to eliminate some of its pungent taste.

Preventing Injury

After a hypnotic is given to a hospitalized patient, the bed's side rails are raised and the patient asked to remain in bed and to call for assistance when getting out of bed. Patients receiving sedative doses may or may not require this safety measure, depending on their response to the drug.

Natural Remedies: Melatonin

Melatonin is a hormone produced by the pineal gland in the brain. Melatonin has been used in treating insomnia, overcoming jet lag, improving the effectiveness of the immune system, and as an antioxidant. The most significant use is for the short-term treatment of insomnia at low doses.

Melatonin has been available in a form obtained from animal pineal tissue and a synthetic form. The animal derivative is not recommended because of the risk of contamination. The synthetic form of melatonin does not carry this risk. However, melatonin is an over-the-counter dietary supplement and has not been evaluated for safety, effectiveness, and purity by the Food and Drug Administration (FDA). Like all supplements, melatonin should be purchased from a reliable source to minimize the risk of contamination.

Few scientific studies have been conducted about melatonin's long-term effects, safety, adverse effects, or interactions with other drugs. The potential risks and benefits are not fully known. Possible adverse reactions include headache and depression. According to the National Sleep Foundation, fatigue and depression, constriction of cardiac arteries (which could increase the risk of heart attack), and possible effects on fertility have been reported.

Individuals wishing to use melatonin should consult with their primary health care provider or a pharmacist before using the supplement. The most effective dosage level is not known, however. Drowsiness may occur within 30 minutes after taking melatonin. The drowsiness may persist for an hour or more, affecting any activity that requires mental alertness, such as driving.

Although uncommon, allergic reactions to melatonin have been reported. The supplement should be stopped and emergency care sought if symptoms of an allergic reaction (e.g., difficulty breathing, hives, or swelling of lips, tongue, or face) occur.

Natural Remedies: Valerian

Valerian, an herb, first arrived in America with the landing of the Mayflower. In Europe, it is widely used for its sedative effects, including the treatment of insomnia, nervousness, and anxiety, and is growing in popularity in the United States as a sleep aid. Valerian works by relaxing muscles and improves the quality of sleep by shortening the length of time it takes to fall asleep and reducing the number of awakenings through the night. Unlike sedative drugs, valerian does not cause sluggishness on awakening and does not lead to dependence. In the United States it is classified by the FDA as a dietary supplement rather than a drug. It is commercially available over the counter in tea, tablet, capsule, or tincture form.

When treating anxiety, it is safe and potentially more effective to combine valerian with other calming herbs such as chamomile or lemon balm. It may take 2 to 4 weeks before an improvement in symptoms is noticeable.

Although potential serious side effects are rare, valerian can cause digestive problems, and with long-term use, headache, sleeplessness, restlessness, and pupil dilation may occur. Some people may find the smell of valerian overpowering and unpleasant. The odor has been compared to that of dirty socks, and cats and rats are especially drawn to its scent. It has been said that the Pied Piper of Hamelin was able to charm the rats because of the scent of valerian emanating from his body.

Educating the Patient and Family About Sedatives and Hypnotics

Sedatives and hypnotics are subject to abuse by outpatients. The most common abuses are increasing the dose of the drug and drinking an alcohol beverage soon before, with, or soon after taking the sedative or hypnotic.

Because sedatives and hypnotics can become less effective after they are taken for a period of time, patients may be tempted to increase the dose without consulting their health care provider. The importance of not increasing or decreasing the dose unless a change in dosage is recommended by the health care provider should be emphasized. In addition, the dose should not be repeated during the night if sleep is interrupted or sleep only lasts a few hours, unless the health care provider has approved taking the drug more than once per night.

Alcohol is a central nervous system depressant, as are sedatives and hypnotics. When alcohol and a sedative or hypnotic are taken together, because of the additive effect there is an increase in central nervous system depression, which has sometimes resulted in death. Patients must understand the importance of not drinking alcohol while taking this drug because of the serious effects.

Patient Education Box 5-1 includes additional key points that the patient or family members should know about sedatives and hypnotics.

Antianxiety Drugs

Anxiety is a feeling of apprehension, worry, or uneasiness that may or may not be based on reality. Anxiety may occur in many types of situations, ranging from chronic anxiety related to one's job to acute anxiety that may occur during withdrawal from alcohol. Although it is normal for most people to feel some anxiety, excess anxiety interferes with day-to-day functioning and can cause undue stress. Drugs used to treat anxiety are called **antianxiety drugs**, or **anxiolytics**.

Antianxiety drugs include the benzodiazepines and the nonbenzodiazepines. Examples of the benzodiazepines are alprazolam (Xanax), chlordiazepoxide

(Librium), diazepam (Valium), and lorazepam (Ativan). All benzodiazepines are classified as schedule IV controlled substances (see Chapter 1). Nonbenzodiazepines that are useful as antianxiety drugs are buspirone (BuSpar), hydroxyzine (Atarax), and zolpidem (Ambien).

Actions of Antianxiety Drugs

The exact mechanism of action of antianxiety drugs is not fully understood. The benzodiazepines are thought to exert their tranquilizing effect by potentiating the effects of gamma-aminobutyric acid (GABA), an inhibitory transmitter, by binding to the specific benzodiazepine receptor sites. Nonbenzodiazepines exert their action in various other ways. For example, buspirone is thought to act on the brain's dopamine and serotonin receptors. Hydroxyzine (Atarax) produces its antianxiety effect by acting on the hypothalamus and brain stem reticular formation.

Uses of Antianxiety Drugs

Antianxiety drugs are used in the management of anxiety disorders and for short-term treatment of the symptoms of anxiety. Long-term use of these drugs is usually not recommended because prolonged therapy can result in drug dependence and serious withdrawal symptoms.

Some of these drugs have additional uses as sedatives, muscle relaxants, or anticonvulsants and in the treatment of alcohol withdrawal. For example, clorazepate (Tranxene) and diazepam (Valium) are used as anticonvulsants (see Chapter 6). Additional uses of individual antianxiety drugs are included in the Summary Drug Table: Antianxiety Drugs.

Lorazepam and oxazepam are relatively safe for older adults when given in normal dosages. Buspirone (BuSpar) also is a safe choice for older adults with anxiety because it does not cause excessive sedation, and there is less risk of falling. Buspirone, unlike most of the benzodiazepines, must be taken regularly and is not effective on an as-needed basis.

Adverse Reactions of Antianxiety Drugs

Transient, mild drowsiness commonly occurs during the first few days of treatment with antianxiety drugs. It is rare to have to discontinue therapy, however, because of the undesirable effects of the antianxiety agent. Depending on the severity of the patient's anxiety or other circumstances, it may be desirable to allow some degree of sedation to occur during early therapy. Other adverse reactions include lethargy, apathy, fatigue, disorientation, anger, restlessness, constipation, diarrhea, dry mouth, nausea, visual disturbances, and incontinence. Some adverse reactions occur only when higher dosages are used.

The long-term use of antianxiety drugs may result in **addiction** (physical drug dependence) and **tolerance** (increasingly larger dosages required to obtain the desired effect). The withdrawal syndrome may occur after as little as 4 to 6 weeks of therapy with a benzodiazepine. The withdrawal syndrome is more likely to occur when the benzodiazepine is taken for 3 months or more and is abruptly discontinued. Antianxiety drugs must never be discontinued abruptly because withdrawal symptoms, which can be extremely severe, may occur. Withdrawal symptoms usually begin within 1 to 10 days after discontinuing the drug, and last from 5 days to 1 month. Symptoms of withdrawal are listed in Box 5-1.

When discontinuing the use of an antianxiety drug in patients who have used the drug for a prolonged period, the health care provider prescribes a decreasing dosage gradually for a period of 4 to 8 weeks to prevent withdrawal symptoms.

SUMMARY DRUG TABLE   Antianxiety Drugs

Generic Name	Trade Name*	Uses	Adverse Reactions	Dosage Ranges
Benzodiazepines alprazolam *al-prah-zoe-lam*	Xanax, *generic*	Anxiety disorders, short-term relief of anxiety	Transient mild drowsiness, sedation, nausea, depression, lethargy, apathy, confusion, constipation, diarrhea, dry mouth, incontinence, visual disturbances	0.25–0.5 mg PO TID, may be increased to 4 mg/d in divided doses
chlordiazepoxide *klor-dye-az-e-pox'-ide*	Librium, Libritabs, *generic*	Anxiety disorders, short-term relief of anxiety, acute alcohol withdrawal	Transient mild drowsiness, sedation, nausea, depression, lethargy, apathy, confusion, constipation, diarrhea, dry mouth, incontinence, visual disturbances	Anxiety: 5–25 mg PO 3 or 4 times/d, 50–100 mg IM, IV, then 25–50 mg IM, IV 3 or 4 times/d; acute alcohol withdrawal: up to 300 mg/d PO in divided doses, 50–100 mg IM, IV may repeat in 2–4 h
clorazepate *klor-az'-eh-pate*	Tranxene SD, Tranxene T, *generic*	Anxiety disorders, short-term relief of anxiety, acute alcohol withdrawal	Transient mild drowsiness, sedation, nausea, depression, lethargy, apathy, confusion, constipation, diarrhea, dry mouth, incontinence, visual disturbances	7.5–60 mg PO in divided doses (average dose, 7.5 mg PO TID)
diazepam *dye-az'-e-pam*	Valium, *generic*	Anxiety disorders, short-term relief of anxiety, acute alcohol withdrawal, anticonvulsant, preoperative muscle relaxant	Transient mild drowsiness, sedation, nausea, depression, lethargy, apathy, confusion, constipation, diarrhea, dry mouth, incontinence, visual disturbances	Individualize dosage: 2–10 mg PO 2–4 times/d (15–30 mg/d), 2–10 mg IM or IV; may repeat in 3–4 h if needed
halazepam *hal-az'-e-pam*	Paxipam	Anxiety disorders, short-term relief of anxiety	Transient mild drowsiness, sedation, nausea, depression, lethargy, apathy, confusion, constipation, diarrhea, dry mouth, incontinence, visual disturbances	20–40 mg PO 3–4 times/d; increase dosage according to need and tolerance
lorazepam *lor-a'-ze-pam*	Ativan, *generic*	Anxiety disorders, short-term relief of anxiety	Transient mild drowsiness, sedation, nausea, depression, lethargy, apathy, confusion, constipation, diarrhea, dry mouth, incontinence, visual disturbances	1–10 mg/d PO in divided doses; up to 4 mg IM, IV
oxazepam *ox-a'-ze-pam*	Serax, *generic*	Anxiety disorders, short-term relief of anxiety	Transient mild drowsiness, sedation, nausea, depression, lethargy, apathy, confusion, constipation, diarrhea, dry mouth, incontinence, visual disturbances	10–30 mg PO 3–4 times/d

Generic Name	Trade Name*	Uses	Adverse Reactions	Dosage Ranges
NonBenzodiazepine				
buspirone hydrochloride *byoo-spye-rone*	BuSpar	Anxiety disorders, short-term relief of anxiety	Dizziness, nausea, headache, nervousness, light-headedness, excitement	15–60 mg/d PO in divided doses
hydroxyzine *high-drox'-ih-zeen*	Atarax, Vistaril, *generic*	Symptomatic relief of anxiety and tension associated with psychoneurosis, pruritus, premedication sedative	Dry mouth, transitory drowsiness, involuntary motor activity	25–100 mg PO QID, 50–100 mg IM q4–6h PRN; premedication: 50–100 mg PO, 25–100 mg IM
meprobamate *me-pro-ba'-mate*	Equanil, Miltown, *generic*	Anxiety disorders, short-term relief of anxiety	Drowsiness, ataxia, nausea, dizziness, slurred speech, headache, weakness, vomiting, diarrhea	1.2–1.6 g/d PO in 3–4 doses

*The term *generic* indicates the drug is available in generic form.

Some antianxiety drugs, such as buspirone (BuSpar), seem to have less abuse potential and less effect on motor ability and cognition than other antianxiety drugs.

Managing Adverse Reactions of Antianxiety Drugs

At the start of drug therapy the patient is watched closely for adverse drug reactions. Some adverse reactions, such as dry mouth, episodes of postural hypotension, and drowsiness, may need to be tolerated because the drug therapy must continue. Some of these reactions may be relieved by offering frequent sips of water, helping the patient out of the bed or chair, and supervising the patient's activities when standing or walking (Fig. 5-1). Patients experiencing extreme sedation need help eating, dressing, and walking.

Although rare, benzodiazepine toxicity may occur with an overdose of the drug. Benzodiazepine toxicity causes sedation, respiratory depression, and coma. Flumazenil (Romazicon) is an antidote (antagonist) for benzodiazepine toxicity and acts to reverse the sedation, respiratory depression, and coma within 6 to 10 minutes after intravenous administration. The adverse reactions of flumazenil include agitation, confusion, seizures, and, in some cases, symptoms of benzodiazepine withdrawal. The adverse reactions of flumazenil related to the symptoms of benzodiazepine withdrawal are relieved by the administration of the benzodiazepine.

Contraindications, Precautions, and Interactions of Antianxiety Drugs

Antianxiety drugs are contraindicated in patients with a known hypersensitivity, psychoses, acute narrow-angle glaucoma, or shock. These drugs are also contraindicated in patients in a coma or with acute alcoholic intoxication and depressed vital signs.

The benzodiazepines are pregnancy category D drugs, and the drug metabolite freely crosses the placenta. Use of these drugs during pregnancy is contraindicated because of the risk of birth defects or neonatal withdrawal syndrome manifested by irritability tremors and respiratory problems. The benzodiazepines are contraindicated during labor because of reports of floppy infant syndrome manifested by sucking difficulties, lethargy, and hypotonia. Lactating women should also avoid the benzodiazepines because of the effect on the infant, who becomes lethargic and loses weight.

Antianxiety drugs are used cautiously in patients with impaired liver or kidney function and in elderly and debilitated patients. The metabolism of the benzodiazepines is slowed in the liver, increasing the risk of benzodiazepine toxicity. Lorazepam and oxazepam are the only benzodiazepines whose elimination is not significantly affected by liver metabolism. Two nonbenzodiazepines (buspirone and zolpidem) are pregnancy

Box 5-1 **Symptoms of Withdrawal**	
Increased anxiety	Numbness in the extremities
Fatigue	Nausea
Hypersomnia	Sweating
Metallic taste	Muscle tension and cramps
Concentration difficulties	Psychoses
Fatigue	Hallucinations
Headache	Memory impairment
Tremors	Convulsions (possible)

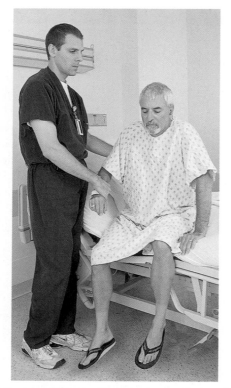

FIGURE 5-1   A hospitalized patient experiencing dizziness because of an antianxiety drug needs assistance getting up and walking.

category B drugs; hydroxyzine is a pregnancy category C drug. No adequate studies have been performed in pregnant women. These drugs should be used during pregnancy only when clearly needed and when the potential good would outweigh any harm to the fetus.

Central nervous system depressants, such as alcohol, narcotic analgesics, tricyclic antidepressants (see next section), and antipsychotic drugs (see later section), increase the sedative effects of antianxiety drugs. Combining any of these drugs with an antianxiety drug is dangerous and can cause serious respiratory depression and profound sedation. Drinking alcohol with an antianxiety drug can cause convulsions and coma.

Buspirone causes less additive central nervous system depression than other antianxiety drugs but should still be avoided with concurrent of a central nervous system depressant. Buspirone may increase serum digoxin levels, increasing the risk of digitalis toxicity.

Patient Management Issues with Antianxiety Drugs

Both outpatients and hospitalized patients may receive antianxiety drugs. Before starting therapy, a complete medical history is obtained, including the patient's mental status and anxiety level. When severe anxiety is present, the history should be obtained from a family member or friend. The patient is observed for behavioral symptoms indicating anxiety, such as extreme restlessness, facial grimaces, and a tense posture. The physio-

logic manifestations of anxiety include increased blood pressure and pulse rate, increased rate and depth of respiration, and increased muscle tension. An anxious patient generally has cool, pale skin.

In addition, if possible, a history of any past drug or alcohol abuse should be obtained. Individuals with a history of previous abuse are more likely to abuse other drugs such as an antianxiety drug.

The patient's mental status and anxiety level should be periodically monitored during therapy to check for improvement or worsening of the behavioral and physical symptoms identified before the drug therapy was begun.

The patient is also monitored for adverse reactions. The sedation and drowsiness that sometimes occur with an antianxiety drug may decrease as therapy continues. Prolonged therapy (more than 3–4 months) may lead to dependence.

Antianxiety drugs are not recommended for longterm use. When the antianxiety drugs are used for short periods (1–2 weeks), tolerance, dependence, or withdrawal symptoms usually do not develop. Any signs of tolerance or dependence must be reported, such as the patient requesting larger doses of drug or increased anxiety and agitation (see Box 5-1).

With hospitalized patients, the vital signs are monitored frequently, usually 3 or 4 times daily. In some instances, such as when hypotensive episodes occur, the patient's vital signs are taken still more often. Any significant change in the patient's vital signs should be reported to the health care provider.

Antianxiety drugs are given parenterally primarily in acute situations. The patient is observed closely for at least 3 hours after parenteral administration. The patient should lie down for 30 minutes to 3 hours after the drug is given.

GERONTOLOGIC ALERT
Antianxiety Drugs

Parenteral administration of antianxiety drugs to older adults, debilitated patients, or those with limited pulmonary reserve requires extreme care because the patient may experience apnea (stopped breathing) and cardiac arrest. Resuscitative equipment should be readily available during parenteral (particularly intravenous) administration.

Oral antianxiety drugs may be taken with food or meals to decrease the possibility of gastrointestinal upset. Some patients have difficulty swallowing the drug (because of a dry mouth, a common adverse effect, or other causes). The patient may chew sugarless gum, suck on hard candy, or take frequent sips of water to reduce the discomfort of dry mouth.

Benzodiazepines

Benzodiazepines are excreted more slowly in older adults and therefore may have a prolonged effect. The drug may accumulate in the blood, resulting in increased adverse reactions or toxicity. For this reason, the initial dose is usually small, and the dosage is increased gradually until a therapeutic response is obtained.

Natural Remedies: Kava

Kava, an herb, has been used by many Pacific Island cultures for thousands of years as a psychoactive beverage. It is currently available over the counter in pill, tincture, tea, and topical forms. Kava is a popular treatment for reducing stress, anxiety, and depression, for promoting sleep, and for relieving menstrual symptoms. In the United States, it is classified by the FDA as a dietary supplement rather than a drug. Kava is promoted as a natural alternative to anxiety drugs, including Xanax and Valium, and also has a reputation as an aid to feeling "high" and for being an aphrodisiac.

The FDA has issued an alert that the use of kava may cause liver damage. Because kava-containing products have been associated with liver-related injuries such as hepatitis, cirrhosis, and liver failure, the safest use of kava seems to be using the herb occasionally for episodes of anxiety rather than on a regular basis. Individuals using a kava-containing dietary supplement who experience symptoms of liver disease should immediately consult their health care provider. Symptoms of liver disease include jaundice, urine with a brown discoloration, nausea, vomiting, light-colored stools, weakness, and loss of appetite.

Kava may increase one's drowsiness when taken with other substances that cause drowsiness, such as antidepressants, sedatives, pain relievers, antianxiety drugs, seizure medications, muscle relaxants, and others.

Identifying kava-containing products can be difficult (see Fig. 5-2). Careful reading of the "Supplement Facts" information on the label may identify kava by any of the following names: ava, ava pepper, awa, kava root, kava-kava, kew, piper methysticum, sakau, tonga, or yanggona. Using multiple forms of kava simultaneously increases the risk of adverse effects and overdose.

Kava should not be used for longer than 3 months without supervision by a health care provider. Long-term use of kava has reportedly led to "kawaism." The symptoms of "kawaism" include dry, flaking, discolored skin, a scaly skin rash, red eyes, puffy face, muscle weakness, blood abnormalities, and general feelings of poor health.

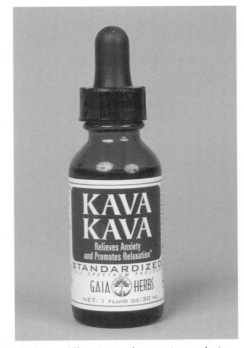

FIGURE 5-2 Many different over-the-counter products contain kava. (D. Weinstein/Custom Medical Stock Photo.)

Educating the Patient and Family About Antianxiety Drugs

Adverse reactions that may occur with a specific antianxiety drug should be explained to the patient, who should be encouraged to contact the health care provider immediately if a serious drug reaction occurs. Patient Education Box 5-2 includes key points the patient or family members should know about antianxiety drugs.

Antidepressants

FACTS ABOUT DEPRESSION

- An estimated 20 million Americans have depression.
- Twice as many women experience depression as men.
- Although depression can occur at any age, it is more common in older people.
- Most people with depression do not seek treatment, but the majority could be helped by treatment.

Source: The National Institutes of Health

Depression is one of the most common psychiatric disorders. It is characterized by feelings of intense sadness, helplessness, worthlessness, and impaired functioning. Those experiencing a major depressive episode exhibit physical and psychological symptoms, such as appetite

PATIENT EDUCATION BOX 5-2

Key Points for Patients Taking Antianxiety Drugs

❑ Take the drug exactly as directed. Do not increase, decrease, or omit a dose or stop taking this drug unless directed to do so by your health care provider.

❑ Do not stop using the drug abruptly because withdrawal symptoms may occur.

❑ Do not drive or perform other hazardous tasks if you feel drowsy.

❑ Do not take any nonprescription drug unless it has been approved by your health care provider.

❑ Inform physicians, dentists, and other health care providers of your therapy with this drug.

❑ Do not drink alcoholic beverages unless your health care provider approves.

❑ If you feel dizzy when changing position, rise slowly when getting out of bed or a chair. For severe dizziness, always ask for help when changing positions.

❑ If you experience dry mouth, take frequent sips of water, suck on hard candy, or chew gum (preferably sugarless).

❑ If you experience constipation, eat foods high in fiber, increase your fluid intake, and exercise if your condition permits.

❑ Keep all appointments with your health care provider because close monitoring of therapy is essential.

❑ Report any unusual changes or physical effects to your health care provider.

disturbances, sleep disturbances, and diminished interest in their job, family, and other activities they usually enjoy. A major depressive episode is a depressed or **dysphoric** (extreme or exaggerated sadness, anxiety, or unhappiness) mood that interferes with daily functioning and includes five or more of the following symptoms:

- Depressed mood
- Diminished interest in life activities
- Significant weight loss or gain (without dieting)
- Insomnia (inability to sleep) or hypersomnia (excessive sleeping)
- Fatigue or loss of energy
- Feelings of worthlessness
- Excessive or inappropriate guilt feelings
- Diminished ability to think or concentrate or indecisiveness
- Recurrent thoughts or death or suicide (or suicide attempt)

A patient is said to have major depression if their symptoms occur daily or nearly every day for a period of 2 weeks or more. A normal bereavement over the loss of a loved one or the effects of a disease such as hypothyroidism are not classified as major depression.

Depression is treated with the use of **antidepressant drugs**. Psychotherapy is often also used with antidepressant drugs to treat major depressive episodes. The four types of antidepressants are:

- Tricyclic antidepressants (TCAs)
- Monoamine oxidase inhibitors (MAOIs)
- Selective serotonin reuptake inhibitors (SSRIs)
- Miscellaneous, unrelated drugs

Actions of Antidepressants

It was previously thought that antidepressants blocked the reuptake of the neurohormones, norepinephrine and serotonin, thereby stimulating the central nervous system. Although their exact action is unknown, this theory is now being questioned. New research indicates that the antidepressants cause changes in the brain's receptors for norepinephrine and serotonin and normalize neurotransmission activity.

The tricyclic antidepressants (TCAs), for example, amitriptyline (Elavil) and doxepin (Sinequan), inhibit reuptake of norepinephrine or serotonin at the presynaptic neuron. Drugs classified as MAOIs inhibit the activity of monoamine oxidase, resulting in an increase in the **endogenous** (made within the body) neurohormones epinephrine, norepinephrine, and serotonin in the nervous system. This increase stimulates the central nervous system. The action of the SSRIs is linked to their inhibition of neuronal uptake of the central nervous system neurotransmitter serotonin. The increase in serotonin levels is thought to act as a stimulant to reverse depression.

The mechanism of action of most of the miscellaneous antidepressants is not clearly understood.

Uses of Antidepressants

Antidepressants are used to manage major depression or depression accompanied by anxiety. The SSRIs also are used to treat obsessive–compulsive disorders. The uses of individual antidepressants are given in Summary Drug Table: Antidepressant Drugs. Treatment is usually continued for 9 months after recovery from the first major depressive episode. If the patient later has another major depressive episode, then treatment is continued up to 5 years. If a third episode occurs, then treatment is continued indefinitely.

Tricyclic Antidepressants (TCAs)

ALERT

Cardiac Reactions with Tricylics

The tricyclics can cause cardiac-related adverse reactions, such as tachycardia and heart block. For this reason, these drugs are given with caution to patients with preexisting cardiac disease and to the elderly.

SUMMARY DRUG TABLE   Antidepressants

Generic Name	Trade Name*	Uses	Adverse Reactions	Dosage Ranges
Tricyclics amitriptyline *am-ee-trip'-ti-leen*	Elavil, *generic*	Depression	Sedation, anticholinergic effects (dry mouth, dry eyes, urinary retention), nausea, nasal congestion, blurred vision, orthostatic hypotension, lethargy, confusion, constipation, diarrhea	Up to 300 mg/d PO in divided doses; 20–30 mg IM QID
amoxapine *a-mox'-a-peen*	Asendin, *generic*	Depression accompanied by anxiety	Sedation, anticholinergic effects (dry mouth, dry eyes, urinary retention), nausea, nasal congestion, blurred vision, orthostatic hypotension, lethargy, confusion, constipation, diarrhea	Up to 600 mg/d PO in divided doses
clomipramine *kloe-mi'-pra-meen*	Anafranil	Obsessive compulsive disorder (OCD)	Sedation, anticholinergic effects (dry mouth, dry eyes, urinary retention), nausea, nasal congestion, blurred vision, orthostatic hypotension, lethargy, confusion, constipation, diarrhea	25–250 mg/d PO in divided doses
desipramine *dess-ip'-ra-meen*	Norpramin, *generic*	Depression	Sedation, anticholinergic effects (dry mouth, dry eyes, urinary retention), nausea, nasal congestion, blurred vision, orthostatic hypotension, lethargy, confusion, constipation, diarrhea	100–300 mg/d PO
doxepin *dox'-e-pin*	Sinequan, *generic*	Anxiety or depression, emotional symptoms accompanying organic disease	Sedation, anticholinergic effects (dry mouth, dry eyes, urinary retention), nausea, nasal congestion, blurred vision, orthostatic hypotension, lethargy, confusion, constipation, diarrhea	25–300 mg/d PO in divided doses
imipramine *im-ip'-ra-meen*	Tofranil, *generic*	Depression	Sedation, anticholinergic effects (dry mouth, dry eyes, urinary retention), nausea, nasal congestion, blurred vision, orthostatic hypotension, lethargy, confusion, constipation, diarrhea	75–300 mg/d PO in divided doses
nortriptyline *nor-trip'-ti-leen*	Aventyl, Pamelor, *generic*	Depression	Sedation, anticholinergic effects (dry mouth, dry eyes, urinary retention), nausea, nasal congestion,	25 mg PO TID, QID; do not exceed 150 mg/d

Generic Name	Trade Name*	Uses	Adverse Reactions	Dosage Ranges
			blurred vision, orthostatic hypotension, lethargy, confusion, constipation, diarrhea	
protriptyline *proe-trip'-ti-leen*	Vivactil *generic*	Depression	Sedation, anticholinergic effects (dry mouth, dry eyes, urinary retention), nausea, nasal congestion, blurred vision, orthostatic hypotension, lethargy, confusion, constipation, diarrhea	15–60 mg/d PO in 3–4 doses
trimipramine *trye-mi'-pra-meen*	Surmontil	Depression	Sedation, anticholinergic effects (dry mouth, dry eyes, urinary retention), nausea, nasal congestion, blurred vision, orthostatic hypotension, lethargy, confusion, constipation, diarrhea	100–300 mg/d PO in divided doses
Monoamine Oxidase Inhibitors phenelzine *fen'-el-zeen*	Nardil	Neurotic or atypical depression	Orthostatic hypotension, vertigo, dizziness, nausea, constipation, dry mouth, diarrhea, headache, restlessness, blurred vision, hypertensive crisis	Up to 90 mg/d PO in divided doses
tranylcypromine *tran-ill-sip'-roe meen*	Parnate	Neurotic or atypical depression	Orthostatic hypotension, vertigo, dizziness, nausea, constipation, dry mouth, diarrhea, headache, restlessness, blurred vision, hypertensive crisis	Up to 60 mg/d PO in divided doses
Selective Serotonin Reuptake Inhibitors citalopram *si-tal'-oh-pram*	Celexa	Depression	Nausea, dry mouth, postural hypotension, sweating, somnolence, dizziness, insomnia, tremor, ejaculatory disorders	20–40 mg/d PO
fluoxetine *floo-ox'-e-teen*	Prozac, Prozac Weekly, Sarafem, generic	Depression, bulimia, OCD, premenstrual dysphoric disorder (Sarafem only)	Anxiety, nervousness, insomnia, drowsiness, fatigue, asthenia, tremor, sweating, dizziness, headache, sexual dysfunction, nausea, diarrhea, constipation, lightheadedness, anorexia	20 mg/d PO in the morning or 40–80 mg/d PO in divided doses; weekly dose: 1 capsule weekly; premenstrual dysphoric disorder: 20–60 mg/d PO

Generic Name	Trade Name*	Uses	Adverse Reactions	Dosage Ranges
fluvoxamine *floo-voks'-a-meen*	Luvox, *generic*	OCD, depression	Headache, nervousness, insomnia, drowsiness, anxiety, tremor, dizziness, light-headedness, nausea, vomiting, diarrhea, dry mouth, anorexia, constipation, dyspepsia, sweating, rash, pharyngitis, sexual dysfunction, urinary frequency	50–300 mg/d PO in divided doses
paroxetine *par-ox'-e-teen*	Paxil	Depression, OCD, panic disorder, general anxiety disorder, social anxiety disorder, post-traumatic stress syndrome	Headache, tremors, nervousness, dizziness, insomnia, nausea, diarrhea, visual disturbances, sweating	20–50 mg/d PO
sertraline *sir'-trah-leen*	Zoloft	Depression, OCD, panic disorders, post-traumatic stress disorder	Headache, nervousness, drowsiness, anxiety, tremor, dizziness, insomnia, vision changes, fatigue, nausea, diarrhea, dry mouth, rhinitis, painful menstruation, sweating	50–200 mg/d PO
Miscellaneous Drugs bupropion HCL *byoo-proe'-pee-on*	Wellbutrin, Wellbutrin SR, *generic* Zyban (smoking cessation)	Depression, smoking cessation (Zyban)	Agitation, dry mouth, insomnia, headache, nausea, vomiting, tremor, constipation, weight loss, anorexia, seizures	100–450 mg/d PO in divided doses; sustained release, 1 tablet twice daily PO
maprotiline *map-roe'-ti-leen*	Ludiomil, *generic*	Depression	Sedation, anticholinergic effects, confusion, disturbed concentration, dry mouth, constipation, orthostatic hypotension	75–225 mg/d PO
mirtazapine *mer-tah'-zah-peen*	Remeron	Depression	Sedation, anticholinergic effects, confusion, disturbed concentration, dry mouth, constipation, orthostatic hypotension	15–45 mg/d PO
nefazodone *ne-faz'-oh-done*	Serzone	Depression	Somnolence, insomnia, dizziness, nausea, dry mouth, constipation, blurred vision	200–600 mg/d PO in divided doses
trazodone *traz'-oh-done*	Desyrel *generic*	Depression	Drowsiness, skin disorders, tinnitus, anger, hostility, anemia, priapism, hypertension, blurred vision, hypotension, dry mouth, nausea, vomiting, diarrhea	150–600 mg/d PO in divided doses

Generic Name	Trade Name*	Uses	Adverse Reactions	Dosage Ranges
venlafaxine *ven-la-fax'-een*	Effexor, Effexor XR	Depression, anxiety disorders	Headache, abnormal dreams, dizziness, anxiety, nervousness, weakness, visual disturbances, rhinitis, anorexia, nausea, constipation hypertension, diarrhea, abnormal taste, weight loss, paresthesia, chills	75–225 mg/d PO in divided doses

*The term *generic* indicates the drug is available in generic form.

Adverse Reactions of Tricyclics

The tricyclics cause anticholinergic effects (see Chapter 4) such as dry mouth, blurred vision, postural hypotension, urinary retention, and constipation. Sedation and dry mouth are the most common adverse reactions. With continued use the patient develops tolerance to these effects. Orthostatic hypotension can result from the TCAs. **Orthostatic hypotension** is a decrease in blood pressure of 20 to 30 points when a person changes position, such as going from a lying position to a standing position, and may cause sudden dizziness. Mental confusion, lethargy, disorientation, rash, nausea, vomiting, constipation, urinary retention, visual disturbances, **photosensitivity** (abnormally heightened reactivity of the skin to sunlight), and nasal congestion also may occur. Sexual dysfunction may result from clomipramine.

GERONTOLOGIC ALERT

Tricylics
Older men with prostatic enlargement are at increased risk for urinary retention when taking a tricyclic antidepressant.

Contraindications, Precautions, and Interactions of Tricyclics

The TCAs are contraindicated in patients with known hypersensitivity to the drugs. Doxepin is contraindicated in patients with glaucoma or a tendency for urinary retention. The TCAs are not given within 14 days of using MAOI, in patients with a recent myocardial infarction, or during pregnancy or lactation. TCAs are contraindicated in patients scheduled to have a myelogram (x-ray of the spinal cord and associated nerves) in the next 48 hours or within 24 hours of having a myelogram.

Like all antidepressants, the TCAs are used cautiously in patients with hepatic or renal impairment. They are also used cautiously in patients with heart disease, angina, paroxysmal tachycardia, increased intraocular pressure, prostatic hypertrophy, or a history of seizures.

Adverse drug interactions may occur with TCAs if the patient is also taking an MAOI, many antihypertensive drugs, dicumarol, the adrenergic drugs, or clonidine.

Specific Patient Management Issues with Tricyclics

TCAs may be administered in a single daily dose at night because sedative effects promote sleep and adverse reactions are less troublesome. Because protriptyline may produce a mild stimulation, it is usually not taken at bedtime.

Monoamine Oxidase Inhibitors (MAOIs)

Adverse Reactions of MAOIs

Orthostatic hypotension is a common adverse reaction of MAOIs. Other common adverse reactions include dizziness, vertigo, nausea, constipation, dry mouth, diarrhea, headache, and over-activity.

Contraindications, Precautions, and Interactions of MAOIs

MAOI drugs are contraindicated in patients with known hypersensitivity to the drugs; in patients with liver and kidney disease, cerebrovascular disease, hypertension, and congestive heart failure; and in the elderly. These drugs are given cautiously to patients with impaired liver function, history of seizures, Parkinsonian symptoms, diabetes, or hyperthyroidism.

A serious hypertensive crisis (extremely high blood pressure) can occur if a patient taking MAOI eats a food containing tyramine (an amino acid present in some foods). A hypertensive crisis typically begins with a headache (usually occipital), followed by a stiff or sore neck, nausea, vomiting, sweating, fever, chest pain, dilated pupils, and bradycardia or tachycardia. Immediate medical intervention is necessary to reduce the blood pressure. Stroke (cerebrovascular accident) or death may occur. (See Patient Education Box 5-3).

Adverse drug interactions may occur with MAOIs if the patient is also taking an opiate drug, a thiazide diuretic, or adrenergic drug. MAOIs should be discontinued several weeks before surgery because they can cause unpredictable reactions.

Specific Patient Management Issues with MAOIs

The MAOIs are not widely used because of their potential for serious adverse reactions. Patients receiving MAOIs require strict dietary control.

ALERT

Headache in MAOI Patients

A headache in a patient taking a MAOI may indicate a hypertensive crisis. The patient's blood pressure should be checked and, if it is elevated, the health care provider must be notified immediately.

Serotonin Reuptake Inhibitors (SSRIs)

Adverse Reactions of SSRIs

Common adverse reactions associated with SSRIs include headache, nervousness, dizziness, insomnia, nausea, vomiting, weight loss, sweating, rash, pharyngitis, and painful menstruation. Fluoxetine may cause headache, activation of mania or hypomania, insomnia, anxiety, nervousness, nausea, vomiting, and sexual dysfunction.

Contraindications, Precautions, and Interactions of SSRIs

SSRIs are contraindicated in patients with hypersensitivity to the drugs and during pregnancy. SSRIs are used cautiously in patients with diabetes mellitus, impaired liver or kidney function, and during lactation.

Adverse drug interactions may occur with SSRIs if the patient is also taking MAOI, TCA, or St. John's wort. If sertraline is taken with MAOI, then a potentially fatal reaction can occur. Sertraline blood levels are increased when administered with cimetidine. Fluoxetine is less effective in patients who smoke cigarettes. Fluoxetine is not given with lithium.

Specific Patient Management Issues with SSRIs

SSRIs can cause weight loss. The patient's dietary intake may need to be monitored.

Miscellaneous Antidepressants

Adverse Reactions of Miscellaneous Antidepressants

Adverse reactions of bupropion include agitation, dry mouth, insomnia, headache, nausea, constipation, anorexia, weight loss, and seizures. Trazodone may cause drowsiness, skin disorders, anger, hostility, anemia, priapism, nausea, and vomiting. The adverse reactions of the other miscellaneous antidepressant drugs are listed in Summary Drug Table: Antidepressant Drugs.

Contraindications, Precautions, and Interactions of Miscellaneous Antidepressants

The miscellaneous antidepressant drugs are contraindicated in patients with known hypersensitivity to the drugs. Safe use of the antidepressants during pregnancy has not been established. These drugs are used cautiously in patients with liver or kidney impairment, taking alcohol or other central nervous system depressants, and during lactation.

Adverse drug interactions may occur with buspirone if the patient is also taking fluoxetine, erythromycin, or itraconazole. Venlafaxine adversely reacts with MAOIs or cimetidine. Trazadone adversely reacts with the phenothiazines, carbamazepine, digoxin, or phenytoin.

Specific Patient Management Issues with Miscellaneous Antidepressants

High doses of bupropion may cause seizure. Because trazodone may cause drowsiness or sedation, most of the dose is usually taken at bedtime. An uncommon but potentially serious adverse reaction of trazodone is priapism (a persistent erection of the penis); if not treated immediately, then priapism can result in impotence.

General Patient Management Issues with Antidepressants

Health care workers should be alert for any signs of suicidal thoughts in depressed patients. Any expressions of guilt, hopelessness, helplessness, insomnia, weight loss, and direct or indirect threats of suicide should be reported to the primary health care provider. It is also important for the patient's vital signs to be monitored and any changes reported. Some antidepressants cause excessive drowsiness initially, and patients may need help walking or caring for themselves.

The patient or a family member may mention an adverse drug reaction or other problem occurring during antidepressant therapy. These reactions or problems should be reported to the primary health care provider.

Natural Remedies: St. John's Wort

St. John's wort, an herb, has been used for centuries for medicinal purposes, including the treatment of depression, as a sedative, and as a balm for burns, wounds, and insect bites. In Europe it is prescribed widely as a treatment for depression. In the US it is classified by the FDA as a dietary supplement rather than a drug and is one of the top-selling herbal products. People also use St. John's wort for anxiety and sleep disorders. It is commercially available over the counter in capsules, a dried form used to make teas, and in concentrated extracts.

Scientific studies have shown that St. John's wort is useful for treating mild to moderate depression but is ineffective for more severe depression. Its mechanism of action is not precisely known, but it is thought that the compounds in this plant may prevent nerve cells in the brain from reabsorbing serotonin.

This herb has become popular for a number of reasons. Some people do not experience relief from prescribed antidepressants and turn to St. John's wort instead. Others who experience adverse effects from prescribed antidepressants prefer to use St. John's wort because of its fewer or lesser side effects. It is also less expensive than prescribed drugs. Some people believe that natural products like St. John's wort are automatically better or safer than prescribed drugs; this belief is more of a myth than reality. Many natural substances can have harmful effects, particularly if they are taken in large quantities or if they interact with other medications. The side effects of St. John's wort can include dry mouth, dizziness, fatigue, increased sensitivity to sunlight, and gastrointestinal symptoms. Because the FDA does not regulate herbal supplements as strenuously as drugs, the strength and quality of a particular product is also unpredictable.

In 2001 the National Institute of Mental Health issued a public alert that warned about serious adverse interactions that have been reported between St. John's wort and a number of drugs. Potentially dangerous effects can occur in patients taking indinavir (a protease inhibitor used to treat HIV), cyclosporine (used to reduce the risk of organ transplant rejection), digoxin, and warfarin.

A L E R T

Interactions with St. John's Wort

None of the antidepressants should be administered with herbal preparations containing St. John's Wort because of the potential for adverse reactions.

Educating the Patient and Family about Antidepressants

Some outpatients may not take their antidepressant drug as prescribed. Family members may need to assist. Family members also need to know to report any adverse reaction that occurs. Patient Education Box 5-4 includes key points about antidepressants the patient or family members should know.

PATIENT EDUCATION BOX 5-4

Key Points for Patients Taking Antidepressants

❑ Take the drug exactly as directed. Do *not* increase, decrease, or omit a dose or discontinue this drug unless your health care provider directs.
❑ Do not drive or perform other hazardous tasks if you feel drowsy.
❑ Do not take any nonprescription drug unless your health care provider approves it.
❑ Inform other health care providers, your dentist, and other medical personnel that you are taking this drug.
❑ Do not drink alcoholic beverages without approval from your health care provider.
❑ If you feel dizzy when changing position, rise slowly when getting out of bed or a chair. If you feel very dizzy, get help when changing positions.
❑ Relieve dry mouth by taking frequent sips of water, sucking on hard candy, or chewing gum (preferably sugarless).
❑ Do not take the antidepressants during pregnancy. Notify your health care provider if you are pregnant or you wish to become pregnant.
❑ Report any unusual changes or physical effects to your health care provider.

Antipsychotic Drugs

Antipsychotic drugs, also called **neuroleptic drugs**, are given to patients with a psychotic disorder, such as schizophrenia. A **psychotic disorder** is characterized by extreme personality disorganization and the loss of contact with reality. The patient usually has hallucinations (a false perception having no basis in reality) or delusions (false beliefs that cannot be changed with reason). Other symptoms include disorganized speech, behavior disturbances, social withdrawal, flattened affect (reduced or absent emotional response to any situation or condition), and anhedonia (finding no pleasure in activities that are normally pleasurable).

Although lithium is not a true antipsychotic drug, it is considered here with the antipsychotics because of its use in regulating the severe fluctuations of the manic phase of **bipolar disorder** (a psychiatric disorder characterized by severe mood swings of extreme hyperactivity to depression). During the manic phase, the person experiences altered thought processes, which can lead to bizarre delusions. The drug diminishes the frequency and intensity of hyperactive (manic) episodes.

Actions of Antipsychotic Drugs

The exact mechanism of action of antipsychotic drugs is not well-understood. These drugs are thought to act by inhibiting or blocking the release of the neurohormone dopamine in the brain and possibly increasing the firing of nerve cells in certain areas of the brain. These effects may suppress the symptoms of certain psychotic disorders. Examples of antipsychotic drugs include chlorpromazine (Thorazine), haloperidol (Haldol), and lithium. Lithium is an antimanic drug. Although its exact mechanism is unknown, it appears to alter sodium transport in nerve and muscle cells and inhibit the release of norepinephrine and dopamine. The Summary Drug Table: Antipsychotic Drugs gives a more complete listing of the antipsychotic drugs.

Uses of Antipsychotic Drugs

Antipsychotic drugs are used to manage acute and chronic psychoses. In addition to its antipsychotic properties, chlorpromazine (Thorazine) is used to treat uncontrollable hiccoughs. Clozapine (Clozaril) is used only in patients with schizophrenia that is unresponsive to other antipsychotic drugs. Lithium is effective in the management of bipolar (manic–depressive) illness. Some of these drugs, such as chlorpromazine (Thorazine) and prochlorperazine (Compazine), are also used as antiemetics (see Chapter 8). When given in small doses, neuroleptics effectively control acute agitation in the elderly. Additional specific uses of these drugs are given in the Summary Drug Table: Antipsychotic Drugs.

Adverse Reactions of Antipsychotic Drugs

These drugs may result in a wide variety of adverse reactions, including sedation, hypotension, postural hypotension, dry mouth, nasal congestion, **photophobia** (an intolerance to light), urticaria, **photosensitivity** (abnormal skin response or sensitivity when exposed to light), behavioral changes, and headache. Photosensitivity can result in severe sunburn when patients taking antipsychotic drugs are exposed to the sun or ultraviolet light.

Behavioral changes may also occur with the use of antipsychotic drugs. These changes include an increase in the intensity of the psychotic symptoms, lethargy, hyperactivity, paranoid reactions, agitation, and confusion. A decreased dosage may eliminate some of these symptoms, but it also may be necessary to try another drug.

Three important adverse reactions, extrapyramidal effects, tardive dyskinesia, and neuroleptic malignant syndrome, are described in the following sections.

Extrapyramidal Effects

Among the most significant adverse reactions of antipsychotic drugs are extrapyramidal effects. The term **extrapyramidal effects** refers to a group of adverse reactions occurring in the extrapyramidal portion of the nervous system. This part of the nervous system affects body posture and coordinates smooth and uninterrupted movement of various muscle groups. Antipsychotics disturb the function of the extrapyramidal portion of the nervous system, causing abnormal muscle movements. Extrapyramidal effects include three main sets of effects:

- Parkinson-like symptoms: fine tremors, muscle rigidity, a mask-like appearance of the face, slowness of movement, slurred speech, and unsteady gait
- **Akathisia**: extreme restlessness and increased motor activity
- Dystonia: facial grimacing and twisting of the neck into unnatural positions

Extrapyramidal effects usually diminish with a reduced dosage of the antipsychotic drug. The health care provider may also prescribe an antiparkinsonism drug, such as benztropine (see Chapter 6) to reduce the Parkinson-like symptoms.

Tardive Dyskinesia

Tardive dyskinesia is a syndrome consisting of potentially irreversible, involuntary dyskinetic movements. Tardive dyskinesia is characterized by rhythmic, involuntary movements of the tongue, face, mouth, or jaw, and sometimes the extremities. The patient's tongue may protrude, and the patient may make chewing movements, pucker the mouth, and grimace (Fig. 5-3).

SUMMARY DRUG TABLE   Antipsychotic Drugs

Generic Name	Trade Name*	Uses	Adverse Reactions	Dosage Ranges
chlorpromazine HCL *klor-proe'-ma-zeen*	Thorazine, *generic*	Psychotic disorders, nausea, vomiting, intractable hiccups	Hypotension, postural hypotension, tardive dyskinesia, photophobia, urticaria, nasal congestion, dry mouth, akathisia, dystonia, pseudoparkinsonism, behavioral changes, headache, photosensitivity	Psychiatric disorders: up to 2000 mg/d PO in divided doses, 25 IM; nausea and vomiting: 10–25 mg PO, 25–50 mg IM, 50–100 rectal; hiccups: 25–50 mg PO, IM, IV TID–QID
clozapine *kloe'-za-peen*	Clozaril, *generic*	Severely ill schizophrenic patients with no response to other therapies	Drowsiness, sedation, akathisia, seizures, dizziness, syncope, tachycardia, hypotension, nausea, vomiting	Up to 900 mg/d PO in divided doses
fluphenazine HCL *floo-fen'-a-zeen*	Permitil, Prolixin, *generic*	Psychotic disorders	Drowsiness, extrapyramidal effects, dystonia, akathisia, hypotension	0.5–10 mg/PO in divided doses up to 20 mg/d; 2.5–10 mg/d IM in divided doses
haloperidol *ha-loe-per'-i-dole*	Haldol	Psychotic disorders; Tourette syndrome, behavior problems in children	Extrapyramidal symptoms, akathisia, dystonia, tardive dyskinesia, drowsiness, headache, dry mouth, orthostatic hypotension	0.5–5 mg PO BID, TID with dosages up to 100 mg/d in divided doses; 2–5 mg IM; children 0.05–0.075 mg/kg/d PO
lithium *lith'-ee-um*	Eskalith, Lithobid, Lithonate, *generic*	Manic episodes of bipolar disorder	Headache, drowsiness, tremors, nausea, polyuria (see Table 32-1)	Based on lithium serum levels; average dose range is 900–1800 mg/d PO in divided doses
loxapine *lox'-a-peen*	Loxitane	Psychotic disorders	Extrapyramidal symptoms, akathisia, dystonia, tardive dyskinesia, drowsiness, headache, dry mouth, orthostatic hypotension	60–250 mg/d PO in divided doses; 12.5–50 mg IM
olanzapine *oh-lan'-za-peen*	Zyprexa	Schizophrenia, short-term treatment of manic episodes of bipolar disorder	Agitation, dizziness, nervousness, akathisia, constipation, fever, weight gain	5–20 mg/d PO
perphenazine *per-fen'-a-zeen*	Trilafon, *generic*	Psychotic disorders	Hypotension, postural hypotension, tardive dyskinesia, photophobia, urticaria, nasal congestion, dry mouth, akathisia,	Psychotic disorders: 4–16 mg PO BID to QID, 5–10 mg IM

Generic Name	Trade Name*	Uses	Adverse Reactions	Dosage Ranges
			dystonia, pseudoparkinsonism, behavioral changes, headache, photosensitivity	
pimozide *pi'-moe-zide*	Orap	Tourette syndrome	Parkinson-like symptoms, motor restlessness, dystonia, oculogyric crisis, tardive dyskinesia, dry mouth, diarrhea, headache, rash, drowsiness	Initial dose: 1–2 mg/d PO; maintenance dose: up to 10 mg/d PO
prochlorperazine *proe-klor-per'-a-zeen*	Compazine, *generic*	Psychotic disorders, nausea, vomiting, anxiety	Extrapyramidal effects, sedation, tardive dyskinesia, dry eyes, blurred vision, constipation, dry mouth, photosensitivity	Psychotic disorders: up to 150 mg PO, 10–20 mg IM; nausea, vomiting: 15–40 mg/d PO in divided doses; anxiety: 5 mg TID, PO
promazine HCL *proe'-ma-zeen*	Sparine, *generic*	Psychotic disorders	Drowsiness, extrapyramidal effects, dystonia, akathisia, hypotension	10–200 mg PO, IM q4–6h QID
quetiapine fumarate *kwe-tie'-ah-pine*	Seroquel	Psychotic disorders	Orthostatic hypotension, dizziness, vertigo, nausea, constipation, dry mouth, diarrhea, headache, restlessness, blurred vision	Up to 800 mg/d PO in divided doses
risperidone *ris-per'-i-done*	Risperdal	Psychotic disorders	Agitation, dizziness, nervousness, akathisia, constipation, fever, weight gain	1–3 mg BID PO
trifluoperazine HCL *try-floo-oh-per'-a-zeen*	Stelazine, *generic*	Psychotic disorders, anxiety	Drowsiness, pseudoparkinsonism, dystonia, akathisia, tardive dyskinesia, photophobia, blurred vision, dry mouth, salivation, nasal congestion, nausea, urine discolored pink to red-brown	Psychosis: 4–20 mg/d PO in divided doses; anxiety: 1–2 mg BID PO
ziprasidone HCL *zih-pray'-sih-dohn*	Geodon	Schizophrenia	Somnolence, drowsiness, sedation, headache, arrhythmias, dyspepsia, fever, constipation, extrapyramidal effects	80 mg BID PO

*The term *generic* indicates that the drug is available in generic form.

Tardive dyskinesia may occur in patients receiving an antipsychotic drug or after discontinuation of antipsychotic drug therapy. When symptoms of tardive dyskinesia occur during the course of therapy, the drug must be discontinued. Depending on the severity of the condition being treated, the health care provider may slowly taper the drug dose because abrupt discontinuation may result in a return of the psychotic symptoms. There is no known treatment for tardive dyskinesia, although partial or complete remission may occur if the antipsy-

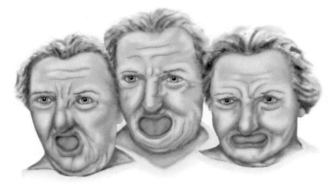

FIGURE 5-3   The characteristic signs of tardive dyskinesia include a protruding tongue, puckered mouth, and facial grimace.

chotic drug is withdrawn. The risk of tardive dyskinesia and the likelihood that it will become irreversible increase as the duration of treatment and total cumulative dosage administered increase. The highest incidence of tardive dyskinesia occurs in patients receiving an antiparkinson drug for extrapyramidal effects along with an antipsychotic drug. Although any patient taking an antipsychotic can experience tardive dyskinesia, elderly women are at highest risk.

Neuroleptic Malignant Syndrome

Neuroleptic malignant syndrome is a rare reaction characterized by a combination of extrapyramidal effects, hyperthermia, and autonomic disturbance. It may occur hours to months after the antipsychotic drug regimen is begun. Once neuroleptic malignant syndrome begins, it progresses rapidly during the next 24 to 72 hours. The syndrome most often occurs in patients taking haloperidol but has occurred also with thiothixene, thioridazine, and clozapine. Neuroleptic malignant syndrome is potentially fatal and requires intensive symptomatic treatment and immediate discontinuation of the causative drug.

Adverse Reactions of Lithium

Lithium carbonate is rapidly absorbed after oral administration. The most common adverse reactions include tremors, nausea, vomiting, thirst, and polyuria (frequent urination). Because some toxic reactions are potentially serious, the patient's lithium blood levels are usually measured during therapy, and the dosage adjusted accordingly.

Managing Adverse Reactions of Antipsychotic Drugs

During initial therapy or whenever the dosage is increased or decreased, the patient should be closely observed for adverse drug reactions, including tardive dyskinesia and any behavioral changes. Any change in behavior or adverse reactions must be reported to the

health care provider. A dosage change may be necessary, or the drug may need to be discontinued.

ALERT

‼ Extrapyramidal Effects

The patient is observed for extrapyramidal effects, which include muscular spasms of the face and neck, an inability to sleep or sit still, tremors, rigidity, or involuntary rhythmic movements. The health care provider is notified of any of these symptoms because they may indicate a need for dosage adjustment.

Patients may need to tolerate some adverse reactions, such as dry mouth, episodes of orthostatic hypotension (feeling dizzy when standing), and drowsiness, because their drug therapy must continue. Some of these reactions may be relieved by offering frequent sips of water, helping the patient out of bed or a chair, and supervising walking. A patient experiencing extreme sedation may need help with eating, dressing, and walking. Extremely hyperactive patients may need protection from injury to themselves or others.

ALERT

‼ Extreme Drowsiness

Antipsychotic drugs may cause extreme drowsiness and sedation, especially during the first or second weeks of therapy. This reaction may impair the patient's mental or physical abilities. Drowsiness usually diminishes after 2 to 3 weeks of therapy. However, if the patient continues to be troubled by drowsiness and sedation, a lower dosage may be used.

ALERT

‼ Tardive Dyskinesia

Because there is no known treatment for tardive dyskinesia and because it is irreversible in some patients, its symptoms occurring in a patient must be immediately reported. These include rhythmic, involuntary movements of the tongue, face, mouth, jaw, or the extremities.

Adverse Effects of Clozapine. This drug is available only through the Clozaril Patient Management System, a program involving white blood cell (WBC) testing, patient monitoring, and other services. Only 1 week of this drug is dispensed at a time. Patients taking clozapine have a higher risk of bone marrow suppression. A weekly WBC count is made throughout the period of therapy and for 4 weeks after its end. In addition, the patient is monitored for the symptoms of bone marrow suppression: lethargy, weakness, fever, sore throat, malaise, mucous membrane ulceration, or flu-like symptoms.

Adverse Effects of Lithium. Lithium toxicity can occur even when the drug is administered at therapeutic doses. Patients taking lithium are observed for signs of toxicity, such as diarrhea, vomiting, nausea, drowsiness, muscular weakness, and lack of coordination. For early symptoms, the health care provider may reduce the patient's dosage or discontinue the drug for 24 to 48 hours and then gradually restart the drug therapy at a lower dosage.

Patients receiving lithium often need more fluids. Fluids should be readily available to the patient, and extra fluids should be offered throughout waking hours.

GERONTOLOGIC ALERT

Lithium Toxicity
Older adults have an increased risk for toxicity because of a decreased rate of excretion. Lower dosages may be necessary to decrease the risk of toxicity.

Contraindications, Precautions, and Interactions of Antipsychotic Drugs

Antipsychotics are contraindicated in patients with a known hypersensitivity, in comatose patients, and in those who are severely depressed or have bone marrow depression, blood dyscrasias, Parkinson disease (haloperidol), liver impairment, coronary artery disease, or severe hypotension or hypertension.

Antipsychotic drugs are classified as pregnancy category C drugs (except for clozapine, which is pregnancy category B). Safe use of these drugs during pregnancy and lactation has not been established. They should be used only when clearly needed and when the potential good outweighs any potential harm to the fetus.

Lithium is contraindicated in patients who have hypersensitivity to tartrazine, renal or cardiovascular disease, sodium depletion, or dehydration, and in patients receiving diuretics. Lithium is a pregnancy category D drug and is contraindicated during pregnancy and lactation. Women of childbearing age may choose to use contraceptives while taking lithium.

Antipsychotic drugs are used cautiously in patients exposed to extreme heat or phosphorous insecticides and in those with respiratory disorders, glaucoma, prostatic hypertrophy, epilepsy, decreased renal function, lactation, or peptic ulcer. Antipsychotic drugs are used cautiously in elderly and debilitated patients because these patients are more sensitive to their effects. Lithium is used cautiously in patients in situations in which they may sweat profusely and in those who are suicidal, have diarrhea, or who have an infection or fever.

Taking an antipsychotic drug with alcohol may result in additive central nervous system depression. Anticholinergics (see Chapter 4) may reduce the therapeutic effects of the antipsychotic, causing worsening of the psychotic symptoms and an increased risk of tardive dyskinesia. Clozapine acts synergistically with other drugs that suppress bone marrow, resulting in increased severity of bone marrow suppression. When lithium is administered with another antipsychotic drug, lithium renal clearance may be reduced, making a decreased dosage necessary to prevent lithium toxicity. Lithium may have decreased effectiveness when taken with antacids. When thiazide or loop diuretics are administered with lithium, serum lithium levels increase, resulting in a greater risk for lithium toxicity.

Patient Management Issues with Antipsychotic Drugs

A patient receiving an antipsychotic drug may be treated in the hospital or as an outpatient. The patient's mental status is assessed before and periodically throughout therapy. Any hallucinations or delusions are documented in the patient's record. Patients with psychosis often are unable to give a reliable history of their illness, and the psychiatric history is obtained from a family member or friend. The patient is observed for any behavior patterns that appear to be deviations from normal, such as poor eye contact, a failure to answer questions completely, inappropriate answers to questions, a monotone speech pattern, and inappropriate laughter, sadness, or crying. The patient's vital signs are also taken.

Because antipsychotic drugs are often given for a long time, ongoing assessment is an important part of determining therapeutic drug effects and monitoring for adverse reactions, particularly extrapyramidal effects and tardive dyskinesia. Frequent assessments are necessary because dosage adjustments may be necessary during therapy. It is important to watch for the appearance of adverse drug effects because the patient may not be able to communicate physical changes to the health care provider.

With hospitalized patients, vital signs are taken at least daily. In some instances, such as when hypotensive episodes occur, vital signs are taken more frequently. Any significant changes are reported to health care provider.

Antipsychotic drugs may be given orally as a single daily dose or in divided doses several times per day. Divided daily doses are recommended when beginning drug therapy, but once-daily doses may be used with continued therapy. Taking the drug at bedtime helps to minimize the effects of postural hypotension and sedation.

Oral administration requires great care because some patients have difficulty swallowing (because of a dry mouth or other causes). Other patients may refuse to take the drug. The patient should never be forced to take an oral drug. If the patient refuses the drug, then the health care provider is notified because parenteral administration of the drug may be necessary.

After giving an oral drug, the patient's mouth is checked to be sure the drug was swallowed.

Oral liquid concentrates are available for patients who can more easily swallow a liquid. These concentrates are light-sensitive and dispensed in amber or opaque bottles to help protect the concentrate. They are administered mixed in liquids such as fruit juices, tomato juice, milk, or carbonated beverages. Semisolid foods, such as soups or puddings, may also be used. Perphenazine (Trilafon) concentrate should not be mixed with beverages containing caffeine (coffee, cola), tea, or apple juice because of the risk of incompatibility.

When these drugs are given parenterally, the patient should remain lying down for approximately 30 minutes after the drug is given.

With outpatients, at each visit to the health care provider, the patient is observed for a response to therapy. Questions asked depend on the patient and the diagnosis and may include questions such as:

- How are you feeling?
- Do you seem to be less nervous?
- Would you like to tell me how everything is going?

The patient or a family member is asked about adverse drug reactions or any other problems occurring during therapy, which are reported to the health care provider.

Educating the Patient and Family About Antipsychotics

Noncompliance with the drug therapy is a problem with some patients after discharge. The administration of antipsychotic drugs becomes a family responsibility if the outpatient appears to be unable to manage his or her own drug therapy.

Any adverse reactions that may occur with a specific antipsychotic drug are explained to the patient and family, who are encouraged to contact the health care provider immediately if a serious drug reaction occurs. Patient Education Box 5-5 includes key points the patient or family members should know about antipsychotic drugs.

KEY POINTS

● Sedatives and hypnotics act on the central nervous system and are used primarily to treat insomnia. Common adverse reactions include drowsiness, dizziness, lethargy, headache, and nausea.

PATIENT EDUCATION BOX 5-5

Key Points for Patients Taking Antipsychotic Drugs

- ❑ Keep all appointments with your health care provider because close monitoring of therapy is essential.
- ❑ Report any unusual changes or physical effects to your health care provider.
- ❑ Take the drug exactly as directed. Do not increase, decrease, or omit a dose or stop using this drug unless directed to do so by your health care provider.
- ❑ Do not drive or perform other hazardous tasks if you feel drowsy.
- ❑ Do not take any nonprescription drug unless the health care provider approves it.
- ❑ Inform physicians, dentists, and other medical personnel about your therapy with this drug.
- ❑ Do not drink alcoholic beverages without approval from your health care provider.
- ❑ If you become dizzy when changing position, rise slowly when getting out of bed or a chair. If the dizziness is severe, get help when changing positions.
- ❑ If you are bothered by dry mouth, relieve it by taking frequent sips of water, sucking on hard candy, or chewing gum (preferably sugarless).
- ❑ Notify your health care provider if you become pregnant or intend to become pregnant during therapy.
- ❑ Immediately report any of the following adverse reactions: restlessness, inability to sit still, muscle spasms,

mask-like expression, rigidity, tremors, drooling, or involuntary rhythmic movements of the mouth, face, or extremities. Avoid exposure to the sun. If exposure is unavoidable, wear sunblock, keep your arms and legs covered, and wear a sun hat.

- ❑ Note that only a 1-week supply of clozapine is dispensed at a time. The drug is obtained through a special program designed to ensure the required blood monitoring. Weekly blood tests are required. Immediately report any signs of weakness, fever, sore throat, malaise, or flu-like symptoms to your health care provider.
- ❑ Note that olanzapine is available either as a tablet to swallow or in a form to be dissolved in the mouth. When using the dissolving tablet, peel back the foil on the blister. With dry hands, remove the tablet and place the entire tablet in your mouth. The tablet will disintegrate with or without liquid.
- ❑ Remember to take lithium with food or immediately after meals to avoid stomach upset. Drink at least 10 large glasses of fluid each day and add extra salt to food. Prolonged exposure to the sun may lead to dehydration. If any of the following symptoms occur, do not take the next dose but immediately notify your health care provider: diarrhea, vomiting, fever, tremors, drowsiness, lack of muscle coordination, or muscle weakness.

◉ Antianxiety drugs exert tranquilizing effects through various actions in the brain. They are used primarily to treat anxiety disorders and secondarily for specific purposes such as treatment of acute alcohol withdrawal. Common adverse reactions include drowsiness, sedation, confusion, dry mouth, depression, and nausea.

◉ Antidepressants act on the central nervous system and are used to treat depression. Common adverse reactions include sedation, dry mouth, nausea, orthostatic hypotension, and constipation.

◉ Antipsychotics have actions that are not perfectly known. Different antipsychotics are used to treat various psychotic disorders ranging from schizophrenia to manic–depressive disorder and other specific disorders, as well as some medical conditions. Common adverse effects include extrapyramidal symptoms, tardive dyskinesia, headache, and photosensitivity.

◉ Patient management and teaching for all these drugs focus on the need for strict dosage control and the management of common adverse reactions.

CASE STUDY

Mr. Hopkins has been severely depressed for several months. Two weeks ago his physician prescribed amitriptyline 30 mg orally four times per day. His family is concerned because he is still depressed and wants to use some other medication. The physician decides to prescribe a higher dose of amitriptyline.

1. Mr. Hopkins will be more likely to experience which side effect?
   a. tinnitus
   b. dry mouth
   c. insomnia
   d. diarrhea

2. The family needs to be aware that Mr. Hopkins may experience sudden dizziness:
   a. after eating
   b. if he misses a dose
   c. when getting out of bed
   d. from drinking too much water

3. Mr. Hopkins is later discovered to have liver impairment. Which of these statements is true of his situation?
   a. amitriptyline should be used only with caution
   b. all antidepressants are safe in patients with liver impairment
   c. he should be given both amitriptyline and a MAOI
   d. his dose of amitriptyline should be doubled

WEBSITE ACTIVITIES

1. Go to the website of The National Sleep Foundation (http://www.sleepfoundation.org) and navigate to the section on tips for getting to sleep without using medication. List five of their tips.

   1. _____

   2. _____

   3. _____

   4. _____

   5. _____

2. Go to the website for the Merck Manual, a leading commercial reference book for medical practitioners (http://www.merck.com/pubs/mmanual/), and navigate to the section on Depression in the chapter on Mood Disorders (in the section on Psychiatric Disorders). Read the paragraph about the drug bupropion. Answer these questions:
   a. Bupropion may be used for patients with depression and what other concurrent conditions?
   b. What dangerous adverse reaction may occur at very high doses?

REVIEW QUESTIONS

1. Ms. Brown has arthritis in her lower back, and the pain keeps her awake at night. She asks if she can have a "sleeping pill." In considering her request, what must be taken into account?
   a. barbiturates, if given in the presence of pain, may cause excitement or delirium
   b. a hypnotic may be given instead of an analgesic to relieve her pain
   c. hypnotics often increase the pain threshold
   d. a hypnotic plus an analgesic is best given in this situation

2. When a hypnotic is given to Ms. Green, age 82 years, it is important to know that:
   a. elderly patients usually require larger doses of a hypnotic
   b. smaller doses of the drug are usually given to older patients
   c. older adults excrete the drug faster than younger adults
   d. dosages of the hypnotic may be increased each night until the desired effect is achieved

3. Which adverse effects are common with antianxiety drugs?
   a. skin rash, blurry vision
   b. tinnitus, hypertension
   c. anger, combativeness
   d. transient mild drowsiness, nausea, depression

4. Which statement is true about long-term use of antianxiety drugs?
   a. long-term use may result in dependence but not tolerance
   b. long-term use may result in tolerance but not dependence
   c. long-term use may result in both dependence and tolerance
   d. long-term use may result in neither dependence nor tolerance

5. Antidepressant drugs are thought to work by changing the brain's receptor sites for:
   a. histamine
   b. glucose
   c. leukocytes
   d. serotonin

6. A patient taking a monoamine oxidase inhibitor should not eat foods containing:
   a. glutamine
   b. sugar
   c. tyramine
   d. large amounts of iron

7. Patient education related to taking antidepressant medications includes which of the following?
   a. slowly increase your dose until all symptoms of depression are relieved
   b. avoid drinking too much water
   c. do not drink alcoholic beverages without approval from the health care provider
   d. avoid exercise during the first hour after taking any medication

8. Which of the following reactions would be expected in a patient experiencing tardive dyskinesia?
   a. muscle rigidity, dry mouth, insomnia
   b. arrhythmic, involuntary movements of the tongue, face, mouth, or jaw
   c. muscle weakness, paralysis of the eyelids, diarrhea
   d. dyspnea, somnolence, muscle spasms

9. Which of the following symptoms would indicate that a patient taking lithium is experiencing toxicity?
   a. constipation, abdominal cramps, rash
   b. stupor, oliguria, hypertension
   c. nausea, vomiting, diarrhea
   d. dry mouth, blurred vision, difficulty swallowing

10. Antipsychotic drugs are likely to cause drug interactions with:
    a. alcohol
    b. caffeine
    c. sugar
    d. tyramine

Central Nervous System Stimulants, Anticonvulsants, and Antiparkinsonism Drugs

Central Nervous System Stimulants
  Actions of Central Nervous System Stimulants
  Uses of Central Nervous System Stimulants
  Adverse Reactions of Central Nervous System Stimulants
  Contraindications, Precautions, and Interactions of Central Nervous System Stimulants
  Patient Management Issues with Central Nervous System Stimulants
  Educating the Patient and Family about Central Nervous System Stimulants

Anticonvulsants
  Actions of Anticonvulsants
  Uses of Anticonvulsants
  Adverse Reactions of Anticonvulsants
  Contraindications, Precautions, and Interactions of Anticonvulsants

Patient Management Issues with Anticonvulsants
Educating the Patient and Family about Anticonvulsants

Antiparkinsonism Drugs
  Dopaminergic Drugs
  Anticholinergic Drugs
  COMT Inhibitors
  Dopamine Receptor Agonists
  Patient Management Issues with Antiparkinsonism Drugs
  Educating the Patient and Family about Antiparkinsonism Drugs

Key Points

Case Study

Website Activities

Review Questions

KEY TERMS

absence seizures—previously referred to as petit mal seizures; are characterized by a brief loss of consciousness, during which physical activity ceases, and may last a few seconds and happen multiple times a day

analeptics—drugs that stimulate the respiratory center

anorexiants—drugs used to suppress the appetite

anticonvulsants—drugs used for the management of convulsive disorders

ataxia—a loss of control of voluntary movements, especially producing an unsteady gait

attention deficit hyperactivity disorder—a disorder manifested by a short attention span, hyperactivity, impulsiveness, and emotional lability

blood–brain barrier—a meshwork of tightly packed cells in the walls of the brain's capillaries that screen out certain substances

choreiform movements—the involuntary twitching of the limbs or facial muscles

convulsion—another term for seizure

dyscrasia—a morbid general state resulting from the presence of abnormal material in the blood

dystonic movements—muscular spasms most often affecting the tongue, jaw, eyes, and neck

epilepsy—a permanent, recurrent seizure disorder

epilepticus—an emergency situation characterized by continual seizure activity with no interruptions

gingival hyperplasia—overgrowth of gum tissue

jacksonian seizure—a focal seizure that begins with an uncontrolled stiffening or jerking of the body such as the finger, mouth, hand, or foot that may progress to a generalized seizure

myoclonic seizures—sudden, forceful contractions involving the musculature of the trunk, neck, and extremities

narcolepsy—disorder causing an uncontrollable desire to sleep during normal waking hours

nystagmus—constant, involuntary movement of the eyeball

on–off phenomenon—associated with long-term levodopa treatment, a patient may alternate suddenly between improved clinical status and loss of therapeutic effect

pancytopenia—a decrease in all of the cellular components of the blood

Parkinsonism— refers to the symptoms of Parkinson disease, as well as Parkinson-like symptoms that may be seen with the use of certain drugs, head injuries, and encephalitis

Parkinson disease—a degenerative disorder of the central nervous system; also known as paralysis agitans

psychomotor seizures—most often occur in children younger than 3 years of age through adolescence; may involve an aura with perceptual alterations, such as hallucinations or a strong sense of fear

seizure—a periodic attack of disturbed cerebral function

status epilepticus—an emergency situation characterized by continual seizure activity with no interruptions

tonic–clonic seizure—an alternate contraction (tonic phase) and relaxation (clonic phase) of muscles, a loss of consciousness, and abnormal behavior

---

CHAPTER OBJECTIVES

On completion of this chapter, students will be able to:

1 Define the chapter's key terms.

2 Describe the uses, general drug actions, adverse reactions, contraindications, precautions, and interactions of central nervous system stimulants, anticonvulsants, and antiparkinsonism drugs.

3 Discuss important points to keep in mind when educating the patient and family members about the use of a central nervous system stimulant, anticonvulsant, or antiparkinsonism drug.

This chapter describes three different groupings of drugs that act on the central nervous system:

- central nervous system stimulants
- anticonvulsants
- antiparkinsonism drugs

Central Nervous System Stimulants

The central nervous system is composed of the brain and the spinal cord. The central nervous system processes information to and from the peripheral nervous system and is the center of coordination and control for the entire body. Many drugs stimulate the central nervous system, but only a few are used therapeutically. This chapter discusses drugs that stimulate the central nervous system.

Central nervous system stimulants include **analeptics**, drugs that stimulate the respiratory center; amphetamines, drugs with a high abuse potential because of their ability to produce euphoria and wakefulness; and **anorexiants**, drugs used to suppress the appetite.

Actions of Central Nervous System Stimulants

Actions of Analeptics

Doxapram (Dopram) and caffeine (a combination of caffeine and sodium benzoate) are two analeptics used in medicine. Doxapram increases the depth of respirations by stimulating receptors located in the carotid arteries and upper aorta. These special receptors, called chemoreceptors, are sensitive to the amount of oxygen in arterial blood. Stimulation of these receptors results in an increase in the depth of the respirations. In larger doses, doxapram increases the respiratory rate by stimulating the medulla.

Caffeine is a mild to potent central nervous system stimulant. The extent of its stimulating effect depends on the dose. Caffeine stimulates the central nervous system at all levels, including the cerebral cortex, the medulla, and the spinal cord. Caffeine also has mild analeptic (respiratory stimulating) activity. Other actions include cardiac stimulation (which may lead to tachycardia), dilation of coronary and peripheral blood vessels, constriction of cerebral blood vessels, and skeletal muscle stimulation. Caffeine also has mild diuretic (promoting urination) activity.

Modafinil is an analeptic used to treat **narcolepsy**, a disorder causing an uncontrollable desire to sleep during normal waking hours even though the individual has a normal nighttime sleeping pattern. Its exact mechanism of action is not known, but the drug is thought to bind to dopamine reuptake carrier sites, increasing alpha activity in the brain and decreasing delta, theta, and beta activity, thereby reducing the number of sleepiness episodes. Modafinil does not cause the same cardiac and other systemic stimulatory effects as other central nervous system stimulants.

Actions of Amphetamines

Amphetamine, dextroamphetamine (Dexedrine), and methamphetamine (Desoxyn) are sympathomimetic (adrenergic) drugs that stimulate the central nervous system (see Chapter 4). Their action raises blood pressure, causes wakefulness, and may increase or decrease the pulse rate. Their anorexiant effect of suppressing the appetite is thought to be caused by their action on the appetite center in the hypothalamus.

Actions of Anorexiants

Anorexiants, such as phentermine and phendimetrazine, are nonamphetamine drugs that are pharmacologically similar to the amphetamines. Like the amphetamines, they are thought to suppress the appetite because of their action on the appetite center in the hypothalamus.

Uses of Central Nervous System Stimulants

Central nervous system stimulants have limited medical use. Primary uses are described in the following sections. Other uses of these drugs are given in the Summary Drug Table: Central Nervous System Stimulants.

Uses of Analeptics

Doxapram is used to treat drug-induced respiratory depression and to temporarily treat respiratory depression in patients with chronic pulmonary disease. This drug also may be used during the postanesthesia period when respiratory depression results from the anesthesia. It also is used to stimulate deep breathing in patients after anesthesia.

Caffeine and sodium benzoate are administered intramuscularly or intravenously as part of the treatment of respiratory depression caused by central nervous system depressants, such as narcotic analgesics and alcohol. Because caffeine also has other effects, such as constriction of cerebral arteries and stimulation of skeletal muscles, it is seldom used now for this purpose. Instead, narcotic antagonists are used for respiratory depression caused by narcotic overdose, and other drugs with greater analeptic activity (e.g., doxapram) are used more commonly. Orally, caffeine ingested as a beverage (coffee, tea) or taken in nonprescription tablet form is used by some individuals to relieve fatigue. Caffeine is also an ingredient in some nonprescription analgesics. Modafinil is used to treat narcolepsy and decreases the number of sleepiness episodes during the day.

Uses of Amphetamines

Amphetamines may be used in the short-term treatment of exogenous obesity (obesity caused by eating more than needed by the body). This use of amphetamines has declined, however, because long-term use carries the potential for addiction and abuse.

These drugs are also sometimes used for narcolepsy. An individual with narcolepsy may fall asleep for a few minutes to a few hours many times in one day. This disorder begins in adolescence or young adulthood and persists throughout life.

Amphetamines are also sometimes used to manage **attention deficit hyperactivity disorder** (ADHD) in children. Children with this disorder have a short attention span, hyperactivity, impulsiveness, and emotional lability. The condition is more common in boys than in girls and causes problems with school and learning, although these children usually have normal or above average intelligence. How amphetamines, which are central nervous system stimulants, calm a hyperactive child is unknown. These drugs reduce motor restlessness, increase mental alertness, elevate mood and produce mild euphoria, and reduce feelings of fatigue. In addition, children with ADHD also commonly receive psychotherapeutic counseling.

FACTS ABOUT ATTENTION DEFICIT HYPERACTIVITY DISORDER (ADHD)

- 3% to 5% of all children are afflicted.
- As many as 2 million American children have ADHD.
- Two to three times as many boys are affected as girls.
- The cause of ADHD is unknown.
- ADHD often continues into adolescence and adulthood.

Source: The National Institute of Mental Health

Uses of Anorexiants

Phendimetrazine and phentermine are chemically related to amphetamines and are also used for short-term treatment of exogenous obesity. These prescription drugs have addiction and abuse potential. Some nonprescription diet aids contain phenylpropanolamine, an adrenergic drug with actions similar to those of the adrenergic drug ephedrine. These diet aids are not true anorexiants, and those containing phenylpropanolamine have limited appetite-suppressing ability compared to the anorexiants. Phenylpropanolamine has little abuse potential and no addiction potential.

Adverse Reactions of Central Nervous System Stimulants

The adverse reactions of doxapram include excessive central nervous system stimulation, causing headache, dizziness, apprehension, disorientation, and hyperactivity. Other adverse reactions include nausea, vomiting, cough, dyspnea, urinary retention, and variations in heart rate. Caffeine and sodium benzoate may result in tachycardia, palpitations, nausea, and vomiting.

One of the chief adverse reactions of amphetamines and anorexiants is overstimulation of the central

SUMMARY DRUG TABLE   Central Nervous System Stimulants

Generic Name	Trade Name*	Uses	Adverse Reactions	Dosage Ranges
Analeptics caffeine *kaf-een'*	Caffedrine, Stay Awake, *generic*	Fatigue, drowsiness, as adjunct in analgesic formulation, respiratory depression	Palpitations, nausea, vomiting, insomnia, tachycardia, restlessness	100–200 mg PO q3–4h; caffeine and sodium benzoate: 500 mg–1g IM, IV
doxapram HCL *docks'-a-pram*	Dopram	Drug-induced postanesthesia, drug-induced respiratory depression, acute respiratory insufficiency superimposed on COPD	Dizziness, headache, apprehension, disorientation, nausea, cough, dyspnea, urinary retention	0.5–1 mg/kg IV
modafinil *moe-daf'-in-ill*	Provigil	Narcolepsy	Insomnia, nervousness, headache, tachycardia, anorexia, dizziness, excitement	200–400 mg/d PO
Amphetamines amphetamine sulfate *am-fet'-a-meen*	*Generic*	Narcolepsy, attention deficit hyperactivity disorder (ADHD), exogenous obesity	Insomnia, nervousness, headache, tachycardia, anorexia, dizziness, excitement	Narcolepsy: 5–60 mg/d PO in divided doses; ADD: 5 mg BID, increase by 10 mg/wk until desired effect; Obesity: 5–30 mg/d PO in divided doses
dexmethylphenidate *dex-meth-thyl-fen-i-date*	Focalin	ADHD	Nervousness, insomnia, loss of appetite, abdominal pain, weight loss, tachycardia, skin rash	2.5 mg PO BID; maximum dosage, 20 mg/d
dextroamphetamine sulfate *dex-troe-am-fet'-a-meen*	Dexedrine, *generic*	Narcolepsy, ADHD, exogenous obesity	Insomnia, nervousness, headache, tachycardia, anorexia, dizziness, excitement	Narcolepsy: 5–60 mg/d PO in divided doses; ADD: up to 40 mg/d PO; obesity: 5–30 mg/d PO in divided doses
methamphetamine *meth-am-fet'-a-meen*	Desoxyn	ADHD	Insomnia, nervousness, headache, tachycardia, anorexia, dizziness, excitement	Up to 25 mg/d PO
methylphenidate HCL *meh-thyl-fen'-ih-date*	Concerta, Metadate ER, Ritalin, *generic*	ADHD, narcolepsy	Nervousness, insomnia, anorexia, dizziness, drowsiness, headache	5–60 mg/day PO
pemoline *pem'-oh-leen*	Cylert	ADHD	Insomnia, nervousness, headache, tachycardia, anorexia, dizziness, excitement	37.5–112.5 mg/d PO

Generic Name	Trade Name*	Uses	Adverse Reactions	Dosage Ranges
Anorexiants benzphetamine HCL *benz-fe-ta-meen*	Didrex	Obesity	Insomnia, nervousness, headache, dry mouth, palpitations, tachycardia, anorexia, dizziness, excitement	25–50 mg PO 1–3 times/d
diethylpropion HCl *die-eth'-uhl-pro'-pee-ahn*	Tenuate, *generic*	Obesity	Insomnia, nervousness, headache, palpitations, tachycardia, anorexia, dizziness, excitement	Immediate release: 25 mg PO 3 times/d; Sustained release: 75 mg once daily
phentermine HCl *fen-ter'-meen*	Ionamin, Pro-Fast, *generic*	Obesity	Insomnia, nervousness, headache, tachycardia, anorexia, dizziness, excitement	8 mg PO TID or 15–37.5 mg PO as a single daily dose
sibutramine HCl *si-byoo-tra-meen*	Meridia	Obesity	Insomnia, palpitations, headache, dry mouth, nervousness, tachycardia, anorexia, dizziness, excitement	5–15 mg PO once daily

*The term *generic* indicates the drug is available in generic form.

nervous system, which may cause insomnia, tachycardia, nervousness, headache, anorexia, dizziness, and excitement. In some instances, the intensity of these reactions depends on the dose, but some patients may experience these symptoms intensely even at low doses. Other individuals experience few symptoms of central nervous system stimulation.

ALERT

Addiction with Central Nervous System Stimulants

Amphetamines and anorexiants may be abused and can result in addiction. Long-term use of amphetamines for obesity may result in tolerance to the drug and a tendency to increase the dose. Extreme psychological dependence may also occur.

Amphetamines and anorexiants are recommended only for short-term use in selected patients for the treatment of exogenous obesity. When used in children to treat ADHD, long-term use must be followed by gradual withdrawal of the drug.

Managing Adverse Reactions of Central Nervous System Stimulants

The adverse drug reactions of amphetamines, such as insomnia and a significant increase in blood pressure and pulse rate, may be serious enough to require discontin-

uing the drug. In other instances, the adverse drug effects are mild and may disappear during therapy.

When a central nervous system stimulant causes insomnia, the drug should be taken early in the day (when possible) to diminish sleep disturbances. The patient is encouraged not to nap during the day. The patient should avoid other stimulants, such as coffee, tea, or cola drinks. Some patients may experience nervousness, restlessness, and palpitations. In hospitalized patients, the vital signs are checked every 6 to 8 hours or more often if tachycardia, hypertension, or palpitations occurs. Often these adverse reactions diminish with continued use as tolerance develops. If tolerance develops, then the dosage is not increased.

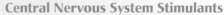

GERONTOLOGIC ALERT

Central Nervous System Stimulants

Older adults are especially sensitive to the effects of central nervous system stimulants and may experience excessive anxiety, nervousness, insomnia, and mental confusion. Cardiovascular disorders, which are more common in older adults, may be worsened by these drugs. Careful monitoring is important because such reactions may require discontinuing the drug.

Because nausea and vomiting may occur with use of an analeptic, health care workers should make appropriate preparations. If a hospitalized patient is at risk for urinary retention with the use of doxapram, then the patient's fluid intake and output are measured and the health care provider is notified if the patient does not urinate regularly.

Long-term treatment with central nervous system stimulants can retard growth in children. Children using these drugs long-term require frequent height and weight measurements to monitor their growth. Intermittent therapy is usually advised to prevent drug tolerance and to minimize the drug's effect on growth.

Contraindications, Precautions, and Interactions of Central Nervous System Stimulants

Central nervous system stimulants are contraindicated in patients with a known hypersensitivity or severe hypertension, in newborns, and in patients with epilepsy or convulsive states, pneumothorax, acute bronchial asthma, head injury, or stroke. In addition, amphetamines are contraindicated in patients with hyperthyroidism or glaucoma. Anorexiants are classified as pregnancy category X and should not be used during pregnancy.

These drugs are given with caution in all patients because of the risk of physical dependence. Some individuals are especially sensitive to the effects of central nervous system stimulants. Analeptics and amphetamines are pregnancy category B drugs and are not recommended during pregnancy, except when clearly needed. These drugs are used only with extreme caution in patients with cardiovascular disease and in women during the early stages of pregnancy.

Amphetamines and the anorexiants should not be given during or within 14 days after giving a monoamine oxidase inhibitor (see Chapter 5) because the patient may experience a hypertensive crisis and intracranial hemorrhage. When guanethidine is administered with an amphetamine or anorexiant, the antihypertensive effect of guanethidine may be diminished. Administration of an amphetamine or anorexiant with a tricyclic antidepressant may decrease the effects of the amphetamine or anorexiant.

Patient Management Issues with Central Nervous System Stimulants

Analeptics

When a central nervous system stimulant is prescribed for respiratory depression, the patient's blood pressure, pulse, and respiratory rate are first measured. The patient's airway must be patent. Oxygen is usually given before, during, and after the drug administration.

The patient's respiratory rate and pattern are then carefully monitored until they return to normal. The patient's level of consciousness, blood pressure, and pulse rate are checked at 5- to 15-minute intervals or as ordered by the health care provider. The patient is observed for any adverse drug reactions, which are reported immediately to the health care provider.

Amphetamines

When an amphetamine is prescribed for any reason, the patient is weighed and the blood pressure, pulse, and respiratory rate measured before starting drug therapy. A child with ADHD is observed for abnormal behavior, which is recorded in the patient's chart for comparison with changes that later occur during therapy. The drug regimen is periodically interrupted to determine if the child still has the symptoms of ADHD.

A hospitalized patient with narcolepsy is observed through the daytime hours. Any periods of sleep are recorded along with the time of day and the length of sleep.

Anorexiants

When an anorexiant or amphetamine is used to treat obesity, the drug is usually prescribed for outpatient use. Before therapy is started, the patient's blood pressure, pulse, respiratory rate, and weight are measured and recorded, Thereafter, the patient's weight and vital signs are measured at each outpatient visit.

Educating the Patient and Family About Central Nervous System Stimulants

The information given to the patient and family depend on the specific drug and the reason for its use. It is important to emphasize the importance of following the recommended dosage schedule. Patient Education Box 6-1 includes key points about central nervous system stimulants the patient or family members should know.

Anticonvulsants

The terms **convulsion** and seizure are often used interchangeably and basically have the same meaning. A **seizure** is a periodic attack of disturbed cerebral function. A seizure may also be described as an abnormal disturbance in the electrical activity in one or more areas of the brain. Seizures may be classified as partial (focal) or generalized. Each different type of seizure disorder is characterized by a specific pattern of events, as well as a different pattern of motor or sensory manifestation.

Partial or focal seizures arise from a localized area in the brain and cause specific symptoms. A partial seizure can spread to the entire brain and cause a generalized seizure. Partial seizures include simple seizures in which consciousness is not impaired, **jacksonian seizures** (a focal seizure that begins with an uncontrolled stiffening or jerking in one part of the body such as finger, mouth, hand, or foot that may progress to a generalized seizure), and psychomotor seizures.

PATIENT EDUCATION BOX 6-1.

Key Points for Patients Taking Central Nervous System Stimulants

ATTENTION DEFICIT HYPERACTIVITY DISORDER

❑ Take the drug in the morning 30 to 45 minutes before breakfast and before lunch. Do not take the drug in the afternoon.

❑ The therapeutic response of pemoline may take 3 to 4 weeks.

❑ Insomnia and anorexia usually disappear during continued therapy.

❑ Write a daily summary of the child's behavior, including periods of hyperactivity, general pattern of behavior, socialization with others, and attention span. Bring this record to each health care provider visit because the drug dosage may need to be adjusted or additional treatments given.

❑ The health care provider may prescribe the drug to be given only on school days when high levels of attention and performance are necessary.

NARCOLEPSY

❑ Keep a record of the number of times per day that periods of sleepiness occur, and bring this record to each visit to the health care provider.

AMPHETAMINES AND ANOREXIANTS

❑ Take the drug early in the day to avoid insomnia.

❑ Do not increase the dose or take the drug more frequently, except on the advice of your health care provider.

❑ These drugs may impair your ability to drive or perform hazardous tasks and may mask extreme fatigue.

❑ If you experience dizziness, light-headedness, anxiety, nervousness, or tremors, contact your health care provider.

❑ Avoid or decrease your use of coffee, tea, and carbonated beverages containing caffeine (see Patient Education Box 6-2).

CAFFEINE (ORAL, NONPRESCRIPTION)

❑ Do not use products with caffeine to stay awake if you have a history of heart disease, high blood pressure, or stomach ulcers.

❑ These products are intended for occasional use and should not be used if you experience heart palpitations, dizziness, or light-headedness.

Psychomotor seizures occur most often in children 3 years of age through adolescence. The individual may experience an aura with perceptual alterations, such as hallucinations or a strong sense of fear. Repeated coordinated but inappropriate movements, such as clutching, kicking, picking at clothes, walking in circles, and licking are characteristic. The most common motor symptom is drawing or jerking of the mouth and face.

Generalized seizures include absence, myoclonic, and tonic–clonic. Manifestations of a generalized **tonic–clonic** seizure include alternate contraction (tonic phase) and relaxation (clonic phase) of muscles, a loss of consciousness, and abnormal behavior. **Myoclonic seizures** involve sudden, forceful contractions involving the musculature of the trunk, neck, and extremities. **Absence seizures**, previously referred to as petit mal seizures, are seizures characterized by a brief loss of consciousness during which physical activity ceases. The seizures typically last a few seconds, occur many times per day, and may go unnoticed by others.

Seizure disorders are generally categorized as idiopathic or acquired. Idiopathic seizures have no known cause; acquired seizure disorders have a known cause, including high fever, electrolyte imbalances, uremia, hypoglycemia, hypoxia, brain tumors, and some drug withdrawal reactions. Once the cause is removed (if it can be removed), the seizures theoretically cease.

Epilepsy is a permanent, recurrent seizure disorder. Examples of the known causes of epilepsy include brain injury at birth, head injuries, and inborn errors of metabolism. In some patients, the cause of epilepsy is never determined.

Drugs used for the management of convulsive disorders are called **anticonvulsants**. Most anticonvulsants have specific uses, that is, they are of value only in the treatment of certain types of seizure disorders. There are five types of drugs used as anticonvulsants: barbiturates, benzodiazepines, hydantoins, oxazolidinediones, and the succinimides. In addition, several miscellaneous drugs are used as anticonvulsants. All can depress abnormal neural discharges in the central nervous system (CNS), resulting in an inhibition of seizure activity. Drugs that control generalized tonic–clonic seizures are not effective for absence (petit mal) seizures. If both conditions are present, then combined drug therapy is required.

Actions of Anticonvulsants

Generally, anticonvulsants reduce the excitability of the neurons (nerve cells) of the brain. When neuron excitability is decreased, seizures are theoretically reduced in intensity and frequency of occurrence or, in some instances, are virtually eliminated. For some patients, only partial control of the seizure disorder may be obtained with anticonvulsant drug therapy.

Uses of Anticonvulsants

Drugs for the more common types of seizures, which respond to a specific anticonvulsant, are listed in the Summary Drug Table: Anticonvulsants. In some cases, the

PATIENT EDUCATION BOX 6-2.

Using Anorexiants for Weight Loss

❑ It is important to take the drug exactly as prescribed. Do not increase the dose or take it more frequently unless your health care provider so instructs.
❑ This drug is for short-term therapy only. It can lead to possible addiction, drug tolerance, or psychological dependency.
❑ Notify your health care provider immediately should any adverse reaction occur.
❑ Take the drug early in the day to prevent insomnia.
❑ Do not drive or perform hazardous tasks if you feel dizzy or disoriented.
❑ Avoid other stimulants, including those containing caffeine such as coffee, tea, and cola drinks.
❑ Read the labels of foods and nonprescription drugs you are taking to avoid other possible stimulants.
❑ Follow your prescribed dietary and exercise program for weight reduction.

patient does not respond well to one drug, and another drug or a combination of anticonvulsants must be tried. Dosage increases and decreases are often necessary during the initial period of treatment. Dosage adjustment also may be necessary during times of stress, severe illness, or when other drugs are being taken for treatment of conditions other than a seizure disorder. The miscellaneous anticonvulsants are adjuncts to the more widely used anticonvulsants. They are used in patients who have an inadequate response to other anticonvulsants.

Occasionally, status **epilepticus** (an emergency situation characterized by continual seizure activity with no interruptions) can occur. Diazepam (Valium) is most often the initial drug prescribed for this condition. However, because the effects of diazepam last less than 1 hour, a longer-lasting anticonvulsant, such as phenytoin or phenobarbital, also must be given to control the seizure activity.

Adverse Reactions of Anticonvulsants

Adverse Reactions of Barbiturates

The most common adverse reaction associated with phenobarbital is sedation, which can range from mild sleepiness or drowsiness to somnolence. These drugs may also cause nausea, vomiting, constipation, bradycardia, hypoventilation, skin rash, headache, fever, and diarrhea. Agitation, rather than sedation, may occur in some patients. Some of these adverse effects may be reduced or eliminated as therapy continues. Occasionally, a slight dosage reduction, without reducing the ability of the drug to control the seizures, will reduce or eliminate some of these adverse reactions.

The barbiturates can produce a hypersensitivity rash. Should a skin rash occur, the health care provider must be notified immediately because he or she may choose to discontinue the drug.

Adverse Reactions of Benzodiazepines

As with the barbiturates, the most common adverse reaction seen with the use of clonazepam (Klonopin), clorazepate (Tranxene), and diazepam (Valium) is sedation in varying degrees. Additional adverse effects may include anorexia, constipation, or diarrhea. Some adverse reactions are dose-dependent, whereas others may diminish in intensity or cause few problems after several weeks of therapy.

Unusual bruising or unusual bleeding, fever, sore throat, rash, or mouth ulcers sometimes occur with the use of benzodiazepines and should be reported to the health care provider.

Adverse Reactions of Hydantoins

Phenytoin is the most commonly prescribed anticonvulsant. Many adverse reactions are associated with the use of phenytoin (Dilantin). The most common adverse reactions associated with the hydantoins are related to the central nervous system and include **nystagmus** (constant, involuntary movement of the eyeball), **ataxia** (loss of control of voluntary movements, especially gait), slurred speech, and mental changes. Other adverse reactions include various types of skin rashes, nausea, vomiting, **gingival hyperplasia** (overgrowth of gum tissue), hematologic changes (changes relating to the blood or blood-forming tissue), and hepatotoxicity. Some of these adverse reactions diminish with continuous use of the hydantoins.

Signs of blood **dyscrasias**, such as sore throat, fever, general malaise, bleeding of the mucous membranes, epistaxis (bleeding from the nose), and easy bruising are serious reactions that must be reported to the health care provider immediately. When a blood dyscrasia is present, the skin and mucous membranes are protected from bleeding and easy bruising by using a soft-bristled toothbrush, and the extremities are protected from trauma or injury.

ALERT

Anticonvulsants in Pregnancy

Research suggests an association between the use of anticonvulsants by pregnant women with epilepsy and an increased incidence of birth defects in children born to these women. The use of anticonvulsants generally is not discontinued in pregnant women with a history of major seizures because of the danger of precipitating status epilepticus. However, when seizure activity poses no serious threat to the pregnant woman, the health care provider will consider discontinuing use of the drug during pregnancy.

SUMMARY DRUG TABLE Anticonvulsants

Generic Name	Trade Name*	Uses	Adverse Reactions	Dosage Ranges
Barbiturates phenobarbital *fee-noe-bar'-bi-tal*	*Generic*	Status epilepticus, cortical focal seizures, tonic-clonic seizures	Somnolence, agitation, confusion, ataxia, CNS depression, nervousness, nausea, vomiting, constipation, diarrhea, rash	30–200 mg/d PO BID, TID
phenobarbital sodium *fee-noe-bar'-bi-tal*	Luminal Sodium, *generic*	Status epilepticus, cortical focal seizures, tonic-clonic seizures	Somnolence, agitation, confusion, ataxia, CNS depression, nervousness, nausea, vomiting, constipation, diarrhea, rash	30–320 mg IM, IV; may repeat in 6 h
Hydantoins ethotoin *eth'-i-toe-in*	Peganone	Tonic-clonic seizures, psychomotor seizures	Ataxia, CNS depression, hypotension, nystagmus, mental confusion, slurred speech, dizziness, drowsiness, gingival hyperplasia, rash, hematopoietic complications	1–3 g/d PO in 4–6 divided doses
mephenytoin *me-fen'-i-toyn*	Mesantoin	Tonic-clonic seizures, psychomotor seizures, focal seizures, jacksonian seizures	Ataxia, CNS depression, hypotension, nystagmus, mental confusion, slurred speech, dizziness, drowsiness, gingival hyperplasia, rash, hematopoietic complications	50–800 mg/d PO in divided doses
phenytoin sodium, parenteral *fen'-i-toe-in*	Dilantin, *generic*	Tonic-clonic seizures, psychomotor seizures, status epilepticus	Ataxia, CNS depression, hypotension, nystagmus, mental confusion, slurred speech, dizziness, drowsiness, gingival hyperplasia, rash, hematopoietic complications	10–15 mg/kg IV
phenytoin sodium, oral *fen'-i-toe-in*	Dilantin, *generic*	Tonic-clonic seizures, psychomotor seizures, status epilepticus	Ataxia, CNS depression, hypotension, nystagmus, mental confusion, slurred speech, dizziness, drowsiness, gingival hyperplasia, rash, hematopoietic complications	Loading dose: 1 g divided into three doses (400 mg, 300 mg, 300 mg) PO q2h; maintenance dose: started 24 h after loading dose, 300–400 mg/d PO
Succinimides ethosuximide *eth-oh-sux'-i-mide*	Zarontin, *generic*	Absence seizures	Drowsiness, ataxia, dizziness, irritability, hematologic changes, mental confusion, nervousness, blurred vision, nausea, vomiting, gastric cramps, urinary frequency, anorexia, pruritus, urticaria	Up to 1.5 g/d PO in divided doses; children, 250/mg/d PO

Generic Name	Trade Name*	Uses	Adverse Reactions	Dosage Ranges
methsuximide *meth-sux'-i-mide*	Celontin Kapseals	Absence seizures	Drowsiness, ataxia, mental confusion, dizziness, irritability, nervousness, blurred vision, nausea, vomiting, gastric cramps, anorexia, pruritus, urticaria	300 mg/d–1.2 g/d PO
phensuximide *fen-sux'-i-mide*	Milontin Kapseals	Absence seizures	Drowsiness, ataxia, mental confusion, dizziness, irritability, nervousness, blurred vision, nausea, vomiting, gastric cramps, anorexia, pruritus, urticaria	1–3 g/d PO in divided doses
Oxazolidinedione trimethadione *trye-meth-a-dye'-on*	Tridione	Absence seizures	Precipitation of clonic–tonic seizure, diplopia, drowsiness, vomiting, photosensitivity, blurred vision, personality changes, increased irritability, headache, fatigue, exfoliate dermatitis, skin rash, nephrosis, hematologic effects	900 mg–2.4 g/d PO in equally divided doses
Benzodiazepines clonazepam *clo-nay'-zeh-pam*	Klonopin, *generic*	Absence seizures, myoclonic and akinetic seizures	Drowsiness, depression, lethargy, apathy, diarrhea, constipation, dry mouth, bradycardia, tachycardia, fatigue, visual disturbances, urticaria, anorexia, rash, pruritus	Initial dose up to 1.5 mg/d PO in 3 divided doses; increase in increments of 0.5–1mg q3d; maximum dose, 20 mg/d
clorazepate *klor-az'-e-pate*	Tranxene SD, *generic*	Partial seizures, anxiety disorders	Drowsiness, depression, lethargy, apathy, diarrhea, constipation, dry mouth, bradycardia, tachycardia, fatigue, visual disturbances, urticaria, anorexia, rash, pruritus	7.5 mg PO TID; increase by increments of 7.5 mg or less weekly; maximum dose, 90 mg/d
diazepam *dye-az'-e-pam*	Valium, *generic*	Status epilepticus, convulsive disorders (all forms), anxiety disorders	Drowsiness, depression, lethargy, apathy, diarrhea, constipation, dry mouth, bradycardia, tachycardia, fatigue, visual disturbances, urticaria, anorexia, rash, pruritus	2–10 mg/d PO 2–4 times/d status epilepticus/severe recurrent convulsive seizures: 5–10 mg initially; may repeat at 5–10 min intervals to a maximum dose of 30 mg IV
Miscellaneous Preparations carbamazepine *kar-ba-maz'-e-peen*	Tegretol, Tegretol-XR, *generic*	Tonic-clonic, mixed seizures, psychomotor seizures	Dizziness, nausea, drowsiness, vomiting, aplastic anemia and other blood cell abnormalities	Maintenance: 800–1200 mg/d PO in divided doses

Generic Name	Trade Name*	Uses	Adverse Reactions	Dosage Ranges
felbamate *fell'-ba-mate*	Felbatol	Partial seizures (adults)	Insomnia, headache, anxiety, acne, rash, dyspepsia, vomiting, constipation, diarrhea, upper respiratory tract infection, fatigue, rhinitis	1200–3600 mg/d PO in divided doses
gabapentin *gab-ah-pen'-tin*	Neurontin	Partial seizures (adults)	Somnolence, dizziness, ataxia, Stevens-Johnson syndrome, nystagmus, tremor, rhinitis, diplopia	900–3600 mg/d PO TID
lamotrigine *la mo' tri geen*	Lamictal, Lamictal Chewable Dispersible Tablets	Partial seizures (adults)	Dizziness, insomnia, rash, somnolence, ataxia, nausea, vomiting, diplopia, headache	50–500 mg/d PO in 2 divided doses
magnesium sulfate *mag-nee'-zhum*	Epsom Salt, *generic*	Hypomagnesemia toxemia, evacuation of colon for rectal and bowel examinations	High magnesium levels, flushing, sweating, depressed reflexes, hypotension, cardiac and CNS depression	IM: 4–5 g of a 50% solution q4h IV: 4 g of a 10%–20% solution, not exceeding 1.5 mL/min of a 10% solution; IV infusion: 4–5 g in 250 mL of 5% dextrose, not exceeding 3 mL/min
oxcarbazepine *ox-car-baz'-e-peen*	Trileptal	Epilepsy	Headache, dizziness, somnolence, ataxia, nystagmus, abnormal gait, insomnia, abdominal pain, diarrhea, dyspepsia, nausea, vomiting	600–1200 mg PO BID
primidone *pri'-mi-done*	Mysoline	Grand mal, psychomotor or focal epileptic seizures	Somnolence, agitation, confusion, ataxia, CNS depression, nervousness, nausea, vomiting, constipation, diarrhea, rash	Up to 500 mg PO QID
valproic acid *val-proe'-ik*	Depakene, Depakote, *generic*	Absence seizures	Nausea, vomiting, rash, sedative effects, indigestion, nystagmus, diplopia	10–60 mg/kg/d PO; if dosage is >250 mg/d, give in divided doses
zonisamide *zoh-niss'-ah-mide*	Zonegran	Epilepsy	Agitation, somnolence, anorexia, nausea, dizziness, headache, diplopia, tiredness, abdominal pain	>16 years 100–600 mg/d PO

*The term *generic* indicates the drug is available in generic form.

Hypersensitivity reactions and Stevens-Johnson syndrome (a serious, sometimes fatal inflammatory disease) have been reported with the use of phenytoin.

The health care provider should be notified immediately if a skin rash occurs. The use of phenytoin is usually discontinued if a skin rash occurs. If the rash is ex-foliative (red rash with scaling of the skin), purpuric (small hemorrhages or bruising on the skin), or bullous (skin vesicle filled with fluid, i.e., a blister) then use of the drug is not resumed. If the rash is milder (e.g., measles-like), then therapy may be resumed after the rash has completely disappeared.

Signs of phenytoin drug toxicity include slurred speech, ataxia, lethargy, dizziness, nausea, and vomiting, and at concentrations greater than 30 mcg/mL, ataxia and mental changes are usually seen. These symptoms must be reported to the health care provider as well.

The hydantoins may affect the blood glucose levels. In some patients these drugs have an inhibitory effect on the release of insulin in the body, causing hyperglycemia. Blood glucose levels must be closely monitored, particularly in patients with diabetes. Any abnormalities are reported to the health care provider.

Long-term administration of the hydantoins can cause gingivitis and gingival hyperplasia (overgrowth of gum tissue). It is important that the teeth and gums of patients in a hospital or long-term clinical setting who are receiving one of these drugs have an oral examination periodically. Any changes in the gums or teeth are reported to the health care provider. In outpatient settings, it is important that oral care be given after each meal and that the mouth and gums be inspected routinely.

ALERT

Phenytoin

Phenytoin can cause hematologic changes (e.g., aplastic anemia, leukopenia, and thrombocytopenia). The following should be immediately reported to a health care provider: signs of thrombocytopenia (e.g., bleeding gums, easy bruising, increased menstrual bleeding, tarry stools) or leukopenia (e.g., sore throat, chills, swollen glands, excessive fatigue, or shortness of breath).

Adverse Reactions of Oxazolidinediones

Administration of trimethadione (Tridione) may result in hematologic changes, such as pancytopenia (decrease in all the cellular components of the blood), leukopenia, aplastic anemia, and thrombocytopenia. Also reported are various types of skin rashes, diplopia (double vision), vomiting, changes in blood pressure, central nervous system depression, photosensitivity, and fatal nephrosis. Because these drugs have been associated with serious adverse reactions and fetal malformations, they should be used only when other less toxic drugs are not effective in controlling seizures. The oxazolidinediones may precipitate a tonic–clonic seizure.

Drowsiness is the most common adverse reaction and, as with the other anticonvulsants, tends to subside with continued use. Visual disturbances may also occur. A patient with a visual disturbance is helped to walk and oriented carefully to the environment. A patient may be especially sensitive to bright lights and may want the room light to be kept dim. Because photosensitivity can occur, a patient must stay out of the sun. A patient

should be instructed to use sunscreens and protective clothing until the individual effects of the drug are known.

Adverse Reactions of Succinimides

Gastrointestinal symptoms occur frequently with the administration of ethosuximide (Zarontin), methsuximide (Celontin Kapseals), and phensuximide (Milontin Kapseals). Mental confusion and other personality changes, pruritus, urticaria, urinary frequency, weight loss, and hematologic changes may also be seen.

The succinimides are particularly toxic. Signs of blood dyscrasias, such as the presence of fever, sore throat, and general malaise should be reported immediately because fatal blood dyscrasias have occurred. Routine blood tests may be performed, such as complete blood counts and differential counts.

ALERT

Succinimide Overdosage

Symptoms of succinimide overdosage must be reported immediately. Symptoms of overdosage include confusion, sleepiness, unsteadiness, flaccid muscles, slow shallow respirations, nausea, vomiting, hypotension, absent reflexes, and central nervous system depression leading to coma. It is important to report symptoms to the health care provider immediately.

Adverse Reactions of Miscellaneous Anticonvulsants

The adverse reactions seen with the various miscellaneous anticonvulsants are listed in the Summary Drug Table: Anticonvulsants.

A severe and potentially fatal rash can occur in patients taking lamotrigine. Before the next dose is due, any rash must be reported to the health care provider. Discontinuation of the drug may be required.

Managing Adverse Reactions of Anticonvulsants

To prevent gastric upset, oral anticonvulsants are taken with food or soon after eating. Oral suspensions are shaken well before measuring. If a patient appears drowsy, then caution must be used when giving an oral preparation because aspiration of the tablet, capsule, or liquid may occur. The patient's swallowing ability should be checked by taking small sips of water before taking the drug. If a patient has difficulty swallowing, then the drug should not be taken, and the health care provider should be notified as soon as possible. A different route of administration may be necessary. Injury may occur when the patient has a seizure. Precautions to prevent falls and other injuries until seizures are controlled by the drug are essential.

Drowsiness is a common adverse reaction of the anticonvulsant drugs, especially early in therapy. Therefore, a patient needs help with all walking activities. A patient should rise from bed slowly and sit for a few minutes before standing. Drowsiness decreases with continued use.

GERONTOLOGIC ALERT

Barbiturates

The barbiturates may produce marked excitement, depression, and confusion in the elderly. In some individuals the barbiturates produce excitement rather than depression. Older adults should be carefully monitored during therapy with the barbiturates and any unusual effects reported to the health care provider.

GERONTOLOGIC ALERT

Diazepam

Older or debilitated adults may require a reduced dosage of diazepam to reduce ataxia and oversedation. These patients must be observed carefully. Apnea and cardiac arrest have occurred when diazepam is administered to older adults, very ill patients, and individuals with limited pulmonary reserve.

Contraindications, Precautions, and Interactions of Anticonvulsants

Contraindications, Precautions, and Interactions of Barbiturates

Barbiturates are contraindicated in patients with known hypersensitivity to the drugs. Barbiturates are used cautiously in patients with liver or kidney disease and those with neurological disorders. Barbiturates (e.g., phenobarbital) are used with caution in patients with pulmonary disease and in hyperactive children. When barbiturates are used with other central nervous system depressants (e.g., alcohol, narcotic analgesics, and antidepressants), an additive central nervous system depressant effect may occur. See Chapter 5 for additional information on the barbiturates.

Contraindications, Precautions, and Interactions of Benzodiazepines

Benzodiazepines are contraindicated in patients with known hypersensitivity to the drugs. Benzodiazepines are used cautiously during pregnancy (category D) and in patients with psychoses, acute narrow-angle glaucoma, liver or kidney disease, and neurologic disorders. Benzodiazepines are used cautiously in elderly or debilitated patients. When benzodiazepines are used with other central nervous system depressants (e.g., alcohol, narcotic analgesics, and antidepressants), an additive central nervous system depressant effect may occur. Increased effects of benzodiazepines are seen when the drugs are administered with cimetidine, disulfiram, and oral contraceptives. When a benzodiazepine is given with theophylline, there is a decreased effect of the benzodiazepine. See Chapter 5 for additional information on the benzodiazepines.

Contraindications, Precautions, and Interactions of Hydantoins

The hydantoins are contraindicated in patients with known hypersensitivity to the drugs. Phenytoin is contraindicated in patients with sinus bradycardia, sinoatrial block, second- and third-degree atrioventricular (AV) block, and Adams-Stokes syndrome; it also is contraindicated during pregnancy (ethotoin and phenytoin are pregnancy category D) and lactation. Ethotoin is contraindicated in patients with hepatic abnormalities.

When the hydantoins are used with other central nervous system depressants (e.g., alcohol, narcotic analgesics, and antidepressants), an additive central nervous system depressant effect may occur. The hydantoins are used cautiously in patients with liver or kidney disease and neurologic disorders. Phenytoin is used cautiously in patients with hypotension, severe myocardial insufficiency, and hepatic impairment.

Phenytoin interacts with many different drugs. For example, isoniazid, chloramphenicol, sulfonamides, benzodiazepines, succinimides, and cimetidine all increase phenytoin blood levels. The barbiturates, rifampin, theophylline, and warfarin decrease phenytoin blood levels. When a hydantoin is given with meperidine, the analgesic effect of meperidine is decreased.

Contraindications, Precautions, and Interactions of Oxazolidinediones.

The oxazolidinediones are contraindicated in patients with known hypersensitivity to the drugs. Trimethadione is classified as a pregnancy category D drug and is contraindicated during pregnancy and lactation. Trimethadione is used with caution in patients with eye disorders (e.g., retinal or optic nerve disease), liver or kidney disease, and neurologic disorders. When trimethadione is used with other nervous system depressants (e.g., alcohol, narcotic analgesics, and antidepressants), an additive central nervous system depressant effect may occur.

Contraindications, Precautions, and Interactions of Succinimides

The succinimides are contraindicated in patients with known hypersensitivity to the drugs. The succinimides are contraindicated in patients with bone marrow depression or hepatic or renal impairment and during lactation. Ethosuximide is classified as a pregnancy category C drug and is used with caution during pregnancy.

As with all anticonvulsants, when the succinimides are used with other central nervous system depressants (e.g., alcohol, narcotic analgesics, and antidepressants), an additive central nervous system depressant effect may occur.

When the hydantoins are administered with the succinimides, there may be an increase in the hydantoin blood levels. Concurrent administration of valproic acid and the succinimides may result in either a decrease or an increase in succinimide blood levels. When primidone is administered with the succinimides, lower primidone levels may occur.

Contraindications, Precautions, and Interactions of Miscellaneous Anticonvulsants

The miscellaneous anticonvulsants are contraindicated in patients with known hypersensitivity to any of the drugs. Carbamazepine is contraindicated in patients with bone marrow depression or hepatic or renal impairment and during pregnancy (category D). Valproic acid is not administered to patients with renal impairment or during pregnancy (category D). Oxcarbazepine (Trileptal), a miscellaneous anticonvulsant, may exacerbate dementia.

The miscellaneous anticonvulsants are used cautiously in patients with glaucoma or increased intraocular pressure; a history of cardiac, renal or liver dysfunction; or psychiatric disorders. When the miscellaneous anticonvulsants are used with other central nervous system depressants (e.g., alcohol, narcotic analgesics, and antidepressants), an additive central nervous system depressant effect may occur.

When carbamazepine is administered with primidone, decreased primidone levels and higher carbamazepine serum levels may result. Cimetidine administered with carbamazepine may result in an increase in plasma levels of carbamazepine that can lead to toxicity. Blood levels of lamotrigine increase when the agent is administered with valproic acid, requiring a lower dosage of lamotrigine.

Patient Management Issues with Anticonvulsants

Seizures that occur in the outpatient setting are almost always seen first by family members or friends, rather than by a member of the medical profession. The occurrence of abnormal behavior patterns or convulsive movements usually prompts the patient to visit a health care provider's office or a neurologic clinic. A family history of seizures (if any) and recent drug therapy (all drugs currently being used) are also important considerations, because either or both could contribute to seizure activity. Depending on the type of seizure disorder, other information may be needed, such as a history of a head injury or a thorough medical history.

A health care provider may order many laboratory and diagnostic tests, such as an electroencephalogram, computed tomographic scan, complete blood count, and hepatic and renal function tests to confirm the diagnosis and identify a possible cause of the seizure disorder, as well as to provide a baseline during therapy with anticonvulsants.

Anticonvulsants control, but do not cure, epilepsy. An accurate ongoing assessment is important to obtain the desired effect of the anticonvulsant. The dosage of the anticonvulsant may require frequent adjustments during the initial treatment period. Dosage adjustments are based on the patient's response to therapy (e.g., the control of the seizures), as well as the occurrence of adverse reactions. Depending on the patient's response to therapy, a second anticonvulsant may be added to the therapeutic regimen, or one anticonvulsant may be changed to another. Regular serum plasma levels of the anticonvulsant are taken to monitor for toxicity.

A patient's seizures, as well as response to drug therapy, must be observed when a hospitalized patient is receiving an anticonvulsant. Most seizures occur without warning, and a health care provider may not see a patient until after the seizure begins or after the seizure is over. However, any observations made during and after the seizure are important and may aid in the diagnosis of the type of seizure, as well as assist the health care provider in evaluating the effectiveness of drug therapy.

> **ALERT**
>
> **Discontinuing an Anticonvulsant**
> Status epilepticus may result from abrupt discontinuation of the drug, even when the anticonvulsant is being administered in small daily doses.

A patient must not omit or miss a dose (except by order of the health care provider). An abrupt interruption in therapy by omitting a dose may result in a recurrence of the seizures. In some instances, abrupt withdrawal of an anticonvulsant can result in status epilepticus. If the health care provider discontinues the anticonvulsant therapy, then the dosage is gradually withdrawn or another drug is gradually substituted.

Educating the Patient and Family About Anticonvulsants

When the patient receives a diagnosis of epilepsy, the health care provider must assist the patient and the family to adjust to the diagnosis. The health care provider should instruct family members in the care of a patient before, during, and after a seizure. The health care provider explains the importance of restricting some activities until the seizures are controlled by drugs. Restriction of activities often depend on the age, sex, and occupation of the patient. For example, the health care provider should advise a mother with a seizure disorder who has a newborn infant to have help when caring for her child. The health care provider would also warn a carpenter about climbing ladders or using power tools. For some patients, the restriction of activities may create problems with employment, management of the home environment, or child care. If a problem is recognized, then a referral may be needed to a social worker, discharge planning coordinator, or public health nurse.

The health care provider reviews adverse drug reactions associated with the prescribed anticonvulsant with a patient and family members. The patient and family members are instructed to contact the health care provider if any adverse reactions occur before the next dose of the drug is due. A patient must not stop taking the drug until the problem is discussed with the health care provider.

Some patients, once their seizures are under control (e.g., stop occurring or occur less frequently), may have a tendency to stop the drug abruptly or begin to omit a dose occasionally. The drug must never be abruptly discontinued or doses omitted. If a patient experiences drowsiness during initial therapy, then a family member should be responsible for administration of the drug.

Patient Education Box 6-3 includes key points about anticonvulsants a patient or family should know.

Antiparkinsonism Drugs

Parkinson disease, also called paralysis agitans, is a degenerative disorder of the central nervous system. The disease is thought to be caused by a deficiency of dopamine and an excess of acetylcholine within the cen-

---

tral nervous system. Parkinson disease affects the part of the brain that controls muscle movement, causing such symptoms as trembling, rigidity, difficulty walking, and problems in balance. It is characterized by fine tremors and rigidity of some muscle groups and weakness of others. Parkinson disease is progressive, with the symptoms becoming worse over time. As the disease progresses, speech becomes slurred, the face has a mask-like and emotionless expression, and the patient may have difficulty chewing and swallowing. The patient may have a shuffling and unsteady gait, and the upper part of the body bends forward. Fine tremors begin in the fingers with a pill-rolling movement, increase with stress, and decrease with purposeful movement. Depression or dementia may occur, causing memory impairment and alterations in thinking.

Parkinson disease has no cure, but the antiparkinsonism drugs are used to relieve the symptoms and assist in maintaining the patient's mobility and functioning capability as long as possible. For years, levodopa was the drug that provided the mainstay of treatment. Now, there are new drugs that are used either alone or in combination with levodopa. Entacapone (Comtan), pramipexole (Mirapex), and ropinirole (Requip) are newer drugs used in the treatment of Parkinson disease. Drug-induced parkinsonism is treated with the anticholinergics benztropine (Cogentin) and trihexyphenidyl (Artane).

Parkinsonism is a term that refers to the symptoms of Parkinson disease, as well as the Parkinson-like symptoms that may be seen with the use of certain drugs, head injuries, and encephalitis. Drugs used to treat the symptoms associated with parkinsonism are called antiparkinsonism drugs. As with some other types of drugs, it may be necessary to change from one antiparkinsonism drug to another or to increase or decrease the dosage until maximum response is obtained. The Summary Drug Table: Antiparkinsonism Drugs lists the drugs used to treat Parkinson disease. Antiparkinsonism drugs discussed in the chapter are classified as dopaminergic agents, anticholinergic drugs, COMT inhibitors, and dopamine receptor agonists (non-ergot).

Dopaminergic Drugs

Actions of Dopaminergic Drugs

Dopaminergic drugs are drugs that affect the dopamine content of the brain. These drugs include levodopa (Larodopa), carbidopa (Ladosyn), amantadine (Symmetrel), and pergolide mesylate (Permax). (See Summary Drug Table: Antiparkinsonism Drugs.)

SUMMARY DRUG TABLE   Antiparkinsonism Drugs

Generic Name	Trade Name*	Uses	Adverse Reactions	Dosage Ranges
Dopaminergic Agents amantadine *a-man'-ta-deen*	Symmetrel, *generic*	Parkinson disease/ drug-induced extrapyramidal reactions, prevention and treatment of influenza A virus	Light-headedness, dizziness, insomnia, confusion, nausea, constipation, dry mouth, orthostatic hypotension, depression	100–400 mg/d PO in divided doses
bromocriptine *broe-moe-krip'-tine*	Parlodel, Parlodel Snap Tabs	Parkinson disease	Drowsiness, sedation, dizziness, faintness, epigastric distress, anorexia	1.25–100 mg/d PO
carbidopa *kar'-bi-doe-pa*	Lodosyn	Used with levodopa in the treatment of Parkinson disease	None when given alone; when administered with levodopa, adverse reactions of levodopa	Up to 200 mg/d PO
carbidopa/ levodopa *kar'-bi-doe-pa/ lee'-voe-doe-pa*	Sinemet CR, Sinemet 10/100, Sinemet 25/100, Sinemet 25/250, *generic*	Parkinson disease	Same as levodopa	Dosages individualized to obtain therapeutic effect; average dose is 1 tablet PO TID

Generic Name	Trade Name*	Uses	Adverse Reactions	Dosage Ranges
levodopa *lee'-voe-doe-pa*	Dopar, Larodopa, *generic*	Parkinson disease	Choreiform or dystonic movements, anorexia, nausea, vomiting, abdominal pain, dysphagia, dry mouth, mental changes, headache, dizziness, increased hand tremor	0.5–8 g/d
pergolide *per'-goe-lide*	Permax	As adjunct to levodopa/carbidopa in Parkinson disease	Nausea, dyskinesia, dizziness, hallucinations, somnolence, insomnia, peripheral edema, constipation	0.05–3 mg/d PO TID
selegiline *sell-eh'-geh-leen*	Carbex, Eldepryl, *generic*	As adjunct to levodopa/carbidopa in Parkinson disease	Nausea, hallucinations, confusion, depression, loss of balance, dizziness, nausea	10 mg/d PO in divided doses
Anticholinergic Agents benztropine mesylate *benz'-tro-peen*	Cogentin, *generic*	Adjunct therapy in Parkinson disease	Dry mouth, blurred vision, dizziness, nausea, nervousness, skin rash, urinary retention, dysuria, tachycardia, muscle weakness, disorientation, confusion	0.5–6 mg/d PO, IM, IV
biperiden *by-per'-i-den*	Akineton	Adjunct therapy in Parkinson disease	Same as benztropine mesylate	2 mg PO 3–4 times/d; maximum dose, 16 mg/24 h; 2 mg IM or IV
diphenhydramine *dye-fen-hye'-dra-meen*	Benadryl, *generic*	Drug-induced extrapyramidal reactions in Parkinson disease, allergies	Same as benztropine mesylate	25–50 mg PO q4–6h; 10–400 mg IM, IV
procyclidine *pro-sye'-kli-deen*	Kemadrin	Parkinson disease	Same as benztropine mesylate	2.5–5 mg PO TID
trihexyphenidyl *trye-hex-ee-fen'-i-dill*	Artane, Trihexy-2, *generic*	Adjunct in the treatment of Parkinson disease	Same as benztropine mesylate	1–15 mg/d PO in divided doses
COMT Inhibitors entacapone *en-tah-kap'-own*	Comtan	As adjunct to levodopa/carbidopa in Parkinson disease	Orthostatic hypotension, dyskinesia, sleep disorders, dystonia, excessive dreaming, somnolence, confusion, dizziness, nausea, anorexia, diarrhea, muscle cramps	200–1600 mg/d PO

Generic Name	Trade Name*	Uses	Adverse Reactions	Dosage Ranges
tolcapone *toll-kap'-own*	Tasmar	As adjunct to levodopa/carbidopa in Parkinson disease	Orthostatic hypotension, dyskinesia, sleep disorders, dystonia, excessive dreaming, somnolence, confusion, dizziness, nausea, anorexia, diarrhea, muscle cramps	100–200 mg PO TID
Dopamine Receptor Agonists, Non-Ergot pramipexole *pram-ah-pex'-ole*	Mirapex	Parkinson disease	Dizziness, somnolence, insomnia, hallucinations, confusion, nausea, dyspepsia, syncope	0.125–1.5 mg PO TID
ropinirole HCL *roe-pin'-o-role*	Requip	Parkinson disease	Dizziness, somnolence, insomnia, hallucinations, confusion, nausea, dyspepsia, syncope	0.25–1 mg PO TID; maximum dose, 24 mg/d

*The term *generic* indicates the drug is available in generic form.

The symptoms of parkinsonism are caused by a depletion of dopamine in the central nervous system. Dopamine, when given orally, does not cross the blood–brain barrier and therefore is ineffective. The body's **blood–brain barrier** is a meshwork of tightly packed cells in the walls of the brain's capillaries that screen out certain substances. This unique meshwork of cells in the central nervous system prohibits large and potentially harmful molecules from crossing into the brain. This ability to screen out certain substances has important implications for drug therapy because some drugs are able to pass through the blood–brain barrier more easily than others.

Levodopa is a chemical formulation found in plants and animals that is converted into dopamine by nerve cells in the brain. Levodopa does cross the blood–brain barrier, and a small amount is then converted to dopamine. This allows the drug to have a pharmacologic effect in patients with Parkinson disease (Fig. 6-1). Combining levodopa with another drug (carbidopa) causes more levodopa to reach the brain. When more levodopa is available, the dosage of levodopa may be reduced. Carbidopa has no effect when given alone. Sinemet is a combination of carbidopa and levodopa and is available in several combinations (e.g., Sinemet 10/100 has 10 mg of carbidopa and 100 mg of levodopa; Sinemet CR is a time-released version of the combined drugs).

The mechanism of action of amantadine (Symmetrel) and selegiline (Eldepryl) in the treatment of parkinsonism is not fully understood.

Uses of Dopaminergic Drugs

The dopaminergic drugs are used to treat the signs and symptoms of parkinsonism. As with some other types of

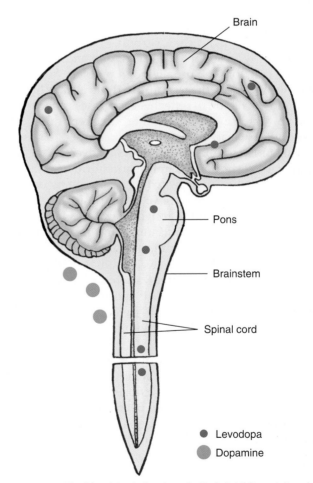

FIGURE 6-1   The blood–brain barrier selectively inhibits certain substances from entering the interstitial spaces of the brain and spinal fluid. It is thought that certain cells within the brain form tight junctions that prevent or slow the passage of certain substances. Levodopa passes the blood–brain barrier, whereas dopamine is unable to pass. (From Roach SS. *Introductory Clinical Pharmacology,* 7th ed. Baltimore: Lippincott Williams & Wilkins; 2004.)

drugs, it may be necessary to change from one antiparkinsonism drug to another or to increase or decrease the dosage until maximum response is obtained.

Levodopa has been considered the gold standard drug therapy for Parkinson disease since it was first used in the 1960s. Carbidopa is always given with levodopa, combined either as one drug or as two separate drugs. When it is necessary to titrate the dose of carbidopa, both carbidopa and levodopa may be given at the same time, but as separate drugs. Sometimes the response with these two drugs can be enhanced by the addition of another drug. For example, selegiline or pergolide may be added to the drug regimen of those being treated with carbidopa and levodopa but who have had a decreased response to therapy with these two drugs.

Amantadine is less effective than levodopa in the treatment of Parkinson disease but more effective than the anticholinergics. Amantadine may be given alone or in combination with an antiparkinsonism drug with anticholinergic activity. Amantadine is also used as an antiviral drug (see Chapter 26).

Adverse Reactions of Dopaminergic Drugs

During early treatment with levodopa and carbidopa, adverse reactions are usually not a problem. But as the disease progresses, the response to the drug may become less, and the period of time that each dose is effective begins to decrease, leading to more frequent doses, and more adverse reactions.

The most serious and frequent adverse reactions seen with levodopa include choreiform movements (involuntary muscular twitching of the limbs or facial muscles) and dystonic movements (muscular spasms most often affecting the tongue, jaw, eyes, and neck). Less common but serious reactions include mental changes, such as depression, psychotic episodes, paranoia, and suicidal tendencies. Common and less serious adverse reactions include anorexia, nausea, vomiting, abdominal pain, dry mouth, difficulty in swallowing, increased hand tremor, headache, and dizziness. Carbidopa is used with levodopa and has no effect when given alone.

The most common serious adverse reactions to amantadine are orthostatic hypotension, depression, congestive heart failure, psychosis, urinary retention, convulsions, leukopenia, and neutropenia. Less serious reactions include hallucinations, confusion, anxiety, anorexia, nausea, and constipation. Adverse reactions with selegiline include nausea, hallucinations, confusion, depression, loss of balance, and dizziness.

Contraindications, Precautions, and Interactions of Dopaminergic Drugs

The dopaminergic drugs are contraindicated in patients with known hypersensitivity to the drugs. Levodopa is contraindicated in patients with narrow-angle glaucoma, those receiving a monoamine oxidase inhibitor (see Chapter 5), and during lactation. Levodopa is used cautiously in patients with cardiovascular disease, bronchial asthma, emphysema, peptic ulcer disease, renal or hepatic disease, and psychosis. Levodopa and combination antiparkinsonism drugs (e.g., carbidopa/levodopa) are classified as pregnancy category C and are used with caution during pregnancy and lactation.

Levodopa interacts with many different drugs. When levodopa is used with phenytoin, reserpine, and papaverine, there is a decrease in response to levodopa. The risk of a hypertensive crisis increases when levodopa is used with the monoamine oxidase inhibitors (see Chapter 5). Foods high in pyridoxine (vitamin B_6) or vitamin B_6 preparations reverse the effect of levodopa. However, when carbidopa is used with levodopa, pyridoxine has no effect on the action of levodopa. In fact, when levodopa and carbidopa are given together, pyridoxine may be prescribed to decrease the adverse effects associated with levodopa.

Selegiline is used cautiously in patients with psychosis, dementia, or excessive tremor. When selegiline is administered with levodopa, the effectiveness of levodopa increases. This effect allows for a decrease in the dosage of levodopa. If selegiline is given in higher doses, then there is an increased risk of hypertension, particularly if tyramine-containing foods (e.g., beer, wine, aged cheese, yeast products, chicken livers, and pickled herring) are ingested. A potentially serious reaction (confusion, agitation, hypertension, and seizures) can occur when fluoxetine is administered with selegiline. Fluoxetine therapy is discontinued for a least 1 week before treatment with selegiline is initiated.

Amantadine is used cautiously in patients with seizure disorders, hepatic disease, psychosis, cardiac disease, and renal disease. The antihistamines, phenothiazines, disopyramide, and alcohol, increase the risk of adverse reactions when administered with amantadine.

Anticholinergic Drugs

Actions of Anticholinergic Drugs

Drugs with anticholinergic activity inhibit acetylcholine (a neurohormone produced in excess in Parkinson disease) in the central nervous system. Drugs with anticholinergic activity are generally less effective than levodopa.

Uses of Anticholinergic Drugs

Drugs with anticholinergic activity are used as adjunctive therapy in all forms of parkinsonism and in the control of drug-induced extrapyramidal disorders. Examples of drugs with anticholinergic activity include benztropine mesylate (Cogentin), biperiden (Akineton), diphenhydramine, procyclidine (Kemadrin), and trihexyphenidyl (Artane). See Summary Drug Table: Antiparkinsonism Drugs for specific uses of these drugs.

Adverse Reactions of Anticholinergic Drugs

Frequently seen adverse reactions to drugs with anticholinergic activity include dry mouth, blurred vision, dizziness, mild nausea, and nervousness. These may become less pronounced as therapy progresses. Other adverse reactions may include skin rash, urticaria (hives), urinary retention, dysuria, tachycardia, muscle weakness, disorientation, and confusion. If any of these reactions are severe, the drug may be discontinued for several days and restarted at a lower dosage, or a different antiparkinsonism drug may be prescribed.

Contraindications, Precautions, and Interactions of Anticholinergic Drugs

These drugs are contraindicated in those with a hypersensitivity to the anticholinergic drugs, those with glaucoma (angle-closure), pyloric or duodenal obstruction, peptic ulcers, prostatic hypertrophy, achalasia (failure of the muscles of the lower esophagus to relax causing difficulty swallowing), myasthenia gravis, and megacolon.

These drugs are used with caution in patients with tachycardia, cardiac arrhythmias, hypertension, hypotension, those with a tendency toward urinary retention, those with decreased liver or kidney function, or those with obstructive disease of the urinary system or gastrointestinal tract. The anticholinergic drugs are given with caution to an older adult.

GERONTOLOGIC ALERT

Anticholinergic Drugs
Individuals older than 60 years frequently have increased sensitivity to anticholinergic drugs and require careful monitoring. Confusion and disorientation may occur. Lower doses may be required.

When the anticholinergic drugs are administered with amantadine, there is an increased anticholinergic effect. When digoxin is administered with an anticholinergic drug, digoxin blood levels may be increased, leading to an increased risk for digitalis toxicity. Haloperidol and anticholinergic co-administration may result in worsening of schizophrenic symptoms, decreased haloperidol blood levels, and development of tardive dyskinesia (see Chapter 5). When the anticholinergic drugs are administered with the phenothiazines, there is a decrease in the therapeutic effects of the phenothiazines and an increase in anticholinergic adverse reactions.

COMT Inhibitors

Actions of COMT Inhibitors

A newer classification of antiparkinsonism drugs is the catechol-O-methyltransferase (COMT) inhibitors. Examples of the COMT inhibitors are entacapone (Comtan) and tolcapone (Tasmar).

These drugs are thought to prolong the effect of levodopa by blocking an enzyme, catechol-O-methyltransferase (COMT), which eliminates dopamine. When given with levodopa, the COMT inhibitors increase the plasma concentrations and duration of action of levodopa.

Uses of COMT Inhibitors

The COMT inhibitors are used as adjuncts to levodopa/carbidopa in Parkinson disease. Tolcapone is a potent COMT inhibitor that easily crosses the blood–brain barrier. However, the drug is associated with liver damage and liver failure. Because of the danger to the liver, tolcapone is reserved for people who are not responding to other therapies. Entacapone is a milder COMT inhibitor and is used to help manage fluctuations in the response to levodopa in individuals with Parkinson disease.

Adverse Reactions of COMT Inhibitors

The adverse reactions most often associated with the administration of the COMT inhibitors include disorientation, confusion, light-headedness, dizziness, dyskinesias, hyperkinesias, nausea, vomiting, hallucinations, and fever. Other adverse reactions are orthostatic hypotension, sleep disorders, excessive dreaming, somnolence, and muscle cramps. A serious and possibly fatal adverse reaction that can occur with the administration of tolcapone is liver failure.

ALERT

Tolcapone
A serious and potentially fatal adverse reaction to tolcapone is hepatic injury. Regular blood testing to monitor liver function is usually prescribed. The health care provider may order testing of serum transaminase levels at frequent intervals (e.g., every 2 weeks for the first year and every 8 weeks thereafter). Treatment is discontinued if the ALT (SGPT) exceeds the upper normal limit or signs or symptoms of liver failure develop. The patient is observed for persistent nausea, fatigue, lethargy, anorexia, jaundice, dark urine, pruritus, and right upper quadrant tenderness.

Contraindications, Precautions, and Interactions of COMT Inhibitors

These drugs are contraindicated in patients with a hypersensitivity to the drugs and during pregnancy (category C) and lactation. Tolcapone is contraindicated in patients with liver dysfunction. The COMT inhibitors are used with caution in patients with hypertension, hypotension, and decreased hepatic or renal function.

The COMT inhibitors should not be administered with the monoamine oxidase inhibitors (see Chapter 5) because there is an increased risk of toxicity. If the COMT inhibitors are administered with norepinephrine, dopamine, dobutamine, methyldopa, or epinephrine, then there is a risk of increased heart rate, arrhythmias, and excessive blood pressure changes.

Dopamine Receptor Agonists

Actions of Dopamine Receptor Agonists

The exact mechanism of action of these drugs is not understood. It is thought that these drugs act directly on postsynaptic dopamine receptors of nerve cells in the brain, mimicking the effects of dopamine in the brain.

Uses of Dopamine Receptor Agonists

The dopamine receptor agonists, such as pramipexole (Mirapex) and ropinirole (Requip), are used for the treatment of the signs and symptoms of Parkinson disease.

Adverse Reactions of Dopamine Receptor Agonists

The most common adverse reactions seen with pramipexole and ropinirole include nausea, dizziness, postural hypotension, hallucinations, somnolence, vomiting, confusion, visual disturbances, abnormal involuntary movements, and headache.

Contraindications, Precautions, and Interactions of Dopamine Receptor Agonists

The dopamine receptor agonists are contraindicated in patients with known hypersensitivity to the drugs, severe ischemic heart disease, or peripheral vascular disease. The dopamine receptor agonists are used with caution in patients with dyskinesia, orthostatic hypotension, or hepatic or renal impairment. The dopamine receptor agonists are used cautiously in patients with a history of hallucinations or psychosis, cardiovascular disease, or renal impairment. Both ropinirole and pramipexole are pregnancy category C drugs, and safety during pregnancy has not been established.

There is an increased risk of central nervous system depression when the dopamine receptor agonists are administered with other central nervous system depressants. When administered with levodopa, the dopamine receptor agonists increase the effects of levodopa (a lower dosage of levodopa may be required). In addition, when the dopamine receptor agonists are administered with levodopa, there is an increased risk of hallucinations. When administered with ciprofloxacin, there is an increased effect of the dopamine receptor agonist.

The phenothiazines may decrease the effectiveness of the dopamine receptor agonists. When pramipexole is administered concurrently with cimetidine, ranitidine, verapamil, and quinidine, there is an increased effect of pramipexole. When ropinirole is administered with the estrogens, particularly estradiol, there may be an increased effect of ropinirole.

Patient Management Issues with Antiparkinsonism Drugs

Because of memory impairment and alterations in thinking in some patients with parkinsonism, a history obtained from the patient may be unreliable. It may be necessary for the health care provider to rely on a family member for information about the symptoms of the disorder, the length of time the symptoms have been present, the ability of the patient to perform on activities of daily living, and the patient's current mental condition (e.g., impairment in memory, signs of depression, or withdrawal).

Before starting the drug therapy, a physical assessment of a patient provides a baseline for future evaluations of drug therapy. It also is important that the patient's neurologic status be evaluated.

A patient's response to drug therapy by neurologic observations can be compared with the data obtained during the initial physical assessment. For example, a patient is assessed for clinical improvement of the symptoms of the disease, such as improvement of tremor of head or hands at rest, muscular rigidity, mask-like facial expression, and ambulation stability. Although the drug response may occur slowly in some patients, these observations aid the health care provider in adjusting the dosage of the drug upward or downward to obtain the desired therapeutic results. The patient is evaluated for imbalanced nutrition related to adverse drug effects (nausea, vomiting); the risk for injury related to parkinsonism or adverse drug reactions (dizziness, light-headedness, orthostatic hypotension, loss of balance); impaired physical mobility related to alterations in balance, unsteady gait, dizziness; and constipation related to adverse drug reactions.

Effective management of a patient with parkinsonism requires that the health care provider carefully monitor the drug therapy, provide psychological support, and place a strong emphasis on patient and family teaching, as detailed later in the chapter.

The drugs used to treat parkinsonism also may be used to treat the symptoms of parkinsonism that occur with the administration of some of the psychotherapeutic drugs (see Chapter 5). When used for this purpose, the antiparkinsonism drugs may exacerbate mental symptoms and precipitate a psychosis. A health care provider must observe the patient's behavior at frequent intervals. If sudden behavioral changes are noted, the next dose of the drug is withheld and the health care provider is notified immediately.

ALERT

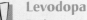 **Levodopa**

Patients receiving levodopa or carbidopa and levodopa must be monitored for the occurrence of choreiform and dystonic movements, such as facial grimacing, protruding tongue, exaggerated chewing motions and head movements, and jerking movements of the arms and legs. If these occur, then the next dose of the drug should be withheld and the health care provider should be notified because it may be necessary to reduce the dosage of levodopa or discontinue use of the drug.

Some patients with parkinsonism communicate poorly and do not tell the health care provider that problems are occurring. A patient with parkinsonism must be observed for outward changes that may indicate one or more adverse reactions. For example, a sudden change in the facial expression or changes in posture may indicate abdominal pain or discomfort, which may be caused by urinary retention, paralytic ileus, or constipation. Sudden changes in behavior may be signs of hallucinations, depression, or other psychotic episodes.

GERONTOLOGIC ALERT

Hallucinations occur more often in older adults receiving the antiparkinsonism drugs, especially when taking the dopamine receptor agonists. Older adults should be assessed for signs of visual, auditory, or tactile hallucinations. The incidence of hallucinations appears to increase with age.

Managing Adverse Reactions of Antiparkinsonism Drugs

Dry Mouth. Some adverse reactions, although not serious, may be uncomfortable. An example of a less serious but uncomfortable adverse reaction is dryness of the mouth. Dry mouth can be relieved by offering frequent sips of water, ice chips, or hard candy (if allowed). If dry mouth is so severe that the patient has difficulty swallowing or speaking, or if loss of appetite and weight loss occurs, then the dosage of the antiparkinsonism drug may be reduced.

Visual Difficulties. Visual difficulties (e.g., adverse reactions of blurred vision and diplopia) may be evidenced by a patient's sudden refusal to read or watch television

or by a patient bumping into objects when walking. Any sudden changes in a patient's behavior or activity must be observed and reported to the health care provider. A patient with visual difficulties may need help walking. The room should be kept well-lighted, scatter and throw rugs should not be used, and any small pieces of furniture or objects that might increase the risk of falling should be removed. The environment must be carefully assessed and necessary adjustments made to ensure a patient's safety.

Gastrointestinal Disturbances. Some patients taking antiparkinsonism drugs experience gastrointestinal disturbances such as nausea, vomiting, or constipation. This can affect a patient's nutritional status. It is a good idea for caregivers to create a calm environment, serve small frequent meals, and serve foods the patient prefers to help improve nutrition. A health care provider may also monitor the patient's weight daily. Gastrointestinal disturbances are sometimes helped by taking the drug with meals. Severe nausea or vomiting may necessitate discontinuing the drug and changing to a different antiparkinsonism drug. With continued use of the drug, nausea usually decreases or is resolved. If constipation is a problem, then the need for a diet high in fiber and increasing fluids in the diet are stressed. A stool softener may be needed to help prevent constipation.

Difficulty Walking. Minimizing the risk for injury is an important aspect in the care of a patient with parkinsonism. These patients may have difficulty walking. Adverse reactions, such as dizziness, muscle weakness, and ataxia (lack of muscular coordination) may further increase difficulty with walking. These individuals are especially prone to falls and other accidents because of their disease process and possible adverse drug reactions. A patient should be helped out of the bed or a chair and with walking and other self-care activities. In addition, assistive devices such as a cane or walker may be helpful. It may be suggested to a patient to wear shoes with rubber soles to minimize the possibility of slipping. Patients are prone to orthostatic hypotension as a result of the drug regimen. These patients are instructed to arise slowly from a sitting or lying position, especially after sitting or lying for a prolonged time.

The On–Off Phenomenon. The **on–off phenomenon** may occur in patients taking levodopa. In this condition, a patient may suddenly alternate between improved clinical status and loss of therapeutic effect. This effect is associated with long-term levodopa treatment. Low doses of the drug, reserving the drug for severe cases, or the use of a "drug holiday" may be prescribed. Should symptoms occur, the health care provider may order a drug holiday that includes complete withdrawal of levodopa for 5 to 14 days, followed by gradually restarting use of the drug at a lower dose.

Educating the Patient and Family About Antiparkinsonism Drugs

The health care provider evaluates a patient's ability to understand the therapeutic drug regimen, to care for himself or herself at home, and to comply with the prescribed drug therapy. If any type of assistance is needed, then the health care provider arranges for a referral to the discharge planning coordinator or social worker.

If a patient requires supervision or help with daily activities and the drug regimen, the family is encouraged to create a home environment that is least likely to result in accidents or falls. Changes such as removing throw rugs, installing a handrail next to the toilet, and moving obstacles that can result in tripping or falling can be made at little or no expense to the family.

Patient Education Box 6-4 includes key points about antiparkinsonism drugs the patient or family should know.

KEY POINTS

● Central nervous system stimulants act in various ways to stimulate different parts of the central nervous system, including actions involving respiration, cardiac and cardiovascular effects, skeletal muscle stimulation, and appetite suppression. Many of these drugs have a potential for dependence.

● Generally, anticonvulsants reduce the excitability of the neurons (nerve cells) of the brain. When neuron excitability is decreased, seizures are theoretically reduced in intensity and frequency of occurrence or, in some instances, are virtually eliminated. For some patients, only partial control of the seizure disorder may be obtained with anticonvulsant drug therapy.

● Parkinsonism is a term that refers to the symptoms of Parkinson disease, as well as the Parkinson-like symptoms that may occur with the use of certain drugs, head injuries, and encephalitis. Drugs used to treat the symptoms associated with parkinsonism are called antiparkinsonism drugs. As with some other types of drugs, it may be necessary to change from one antiparkinsonism drug to another or to increase or decrease the dosage until maximum response is obtained.

● Patient management and teaching for all of these drugs focus on the need for strict dosage control and the management of adverse reactions, many of which are severe.

PATIENT EDUCATION BOX 6-4

Key Points for Patients Taking Antiparkinsonism Drugs

❑ Take this drug as prescribed. Do not increase, decrease, or omit a dose or stop taking the drug unless advised to do so by your health care provider. If you have gastrointestinal upset, take the drug with food.

❑ If you experience dizziness, drowsiness, or blurred vision, avoid driving or performing other tasks that require alertness.

❑ Do not use alcohol unless approved by your health care provider.

❑ Relieve dry mouth by sucking on hard candy (unless you have diabetes) or frequent sips of water. Consult your dentist if dryness of the mouth interferes with wearing, inserting, or removing dentures or causes other dental problems.

❑ Orthostatic hypotension may develop with or without symptoms of dizziness, nausea, fainting, and sweating. Do not rise rapidly after sitting or lying down.

❑ Notify your health care provider if you experience any of these problems: severe dry mouth, inability to chew or swallow food, inability to urinate, feelings of depression, severe dizziness or drowsiness, rapid or irregular heartbeat, abdominal pain, mood changes, and unusual movements of the head, eyes, neck, arms, legs, feet, mouth, or tongue.

❑ Keep all appointments with your health care provider or clinic personnel because close monitoring of therapy is necessary.

❑ When taking levodopa, avoid vitamin B_6 (pyridoxine) because this vitamin may interfere with the action of levodopa (see Patient Education Box 6-5).

❑ If you have diabetes, levodopa may interfere with your urine tests for glucose or ketones. Report any abnormal result to your health care provider before adjusting the dosage of the antidiabetic medication.

❑ If you are taking tolcapone, keep all appointments with your health care provider. Liver function tests are performed periodically and are an important part of therapy. Report any signs of liver failure, such as persistent nausea, fatigue, lethargy, anorexia, jaundice, dark urine, pruritus, and right upper quadrant tenderness.

PATIENT EDUCATION BOX 6-5.

Avoiding Certain Foods While Taking Levodopa

If you are taking levodopa, you must be careful to avoid vitamin B_6 (pyridoxine) because it may interfere with the therapeutic effects of the drug. Most multivitamin supplements contain vitamin B_6. Therefore, be sure to check with your health care provider before taking any vitamin supplements.

Vitamin B_6 is also found in a wide variety of food sources. It may be impossible to avoid these food sources entirely, but you can limit or decrease such intake to enhance or maintain the drug's effectiveness. Following are foods containing vitamin B_6:

Organ meats	Walnuts
Pork	Potatoes
Chicken	Oats
Egg yolk	Bananas
Fish	Yeast
Whole grain cereals	Raisins
Peanuts	Wheat germ
Corn	Molasses

CASE STUDY

Ms. Chang has Parkinson disease. Her personal assistant is responsible for Ms. Chang's home care and needs guidance about the drug amantadine, which has been prescribed for Ms. Chang.

1. The personal assistant needs to be aware of adverse reactions, including:
   a. none when given alone; in combination with levodopa, levodopa side effects
   b. constipation, dry mouth, and depression
   c. blurred vision, increase in hand tremor, and abdominal pain
   d. potential loss of hair and dry skin

2. Ms. Chang is elderly. Both she and her personal assistant request information about amantadine drug therapy. The health care provider may explain that:
   a. individuals older than 60 frequently have increased sensitivity to anticholinergic drugs such as amantadine and require careful monitoring
   b. amantadine may be given alone or in combination with another drug, depending on symptoms and progression of the disease
   c. Ms. Chang is a strong candidate for amantadine use because of her severe heart condition
   d. amantadine was prescribed because it will not interfere with Ms. Chang's alcohol consumption

3. Ms. Chang's personal assistant phones the health care provider 1 month into treatment to report that Ms. Chang seems to be stumbling more frequently, especially when rising. The assistant is instructed to:
   a. contact the health care provider
   b. caution Ms. Chang to rise more slowly, and assist her if necessary
   c. recall whether any dose of the medication was accidentally increased or missed
   d. all of the above

WEBSITE ACTIVITIES

1. Go to the website for the Epilepsy Foundation of America (http://www.efa.org) and conduct a search on the ketogenic diet. Write a brief description of the diet and its use in treating epilepsy in children.

2. Does the website suggest a way for patients and their families to connect with other epilepsy-impacted households? If so, what are they?

REVIEW QUESTIONS

1. The adverse drug reactions of doxapram given for chronic pulmonary disease may include:
   a. headache, dizziness, nausea
   b. diarrhea, drowsiness, hypotension
   c. decreased respiratory rate, weight gain, bradycardia
   d. fever, dysuria, constipation

2. A patient with narcolepsy who is receiving an amphetamine should be instructed to:
   a. record the times of the day the medication is taken
   b. take the medication at bedtime as well as in the morning
   c. take the drug with meals
   d. keep a record of how often periods of sleepiness occur

3. A patient is prescribed phenytoin for a recurrent convulsive disorder. The health care provider informs the patient that the most common adverse reactions are:
   a. related to the gastrointestinal system
   b. associated with the reproductive system
   c. associated with kidney function
   d. related to the central nervous system

4. Which of the following adverse reactions, if observed in a patient prescribed phenytoin, would indicate that the patient may be developing phenytoin toxicity?
   a. severe occipital headache
   b. ataxia
   c. hyperactivity
   d. somnolence

5. The most serious adverse reactions seen with levodopa include:
   a. choreiform and dystonic movements
   b. depression
   c. suicidal tendencies
   d. paranoia

6. Elderly patients prescribed one of the dopamine receptor agonists are monitored closely for which of the following adverse reactions?
   a. occipital headache
   b. hallucinations
   c. paralytic ileus
   d. cardiac arrhythmias

7 Cholinesterase Inhibitors

Actions of Cholinesterase Inhibitors	**Natural Remedies: Ginseng**
Uses of Cholinesterase Inhibitors	**Natural Remedies: Ginkgo Biloba**
Adverse Reactions of Cholinesterase Inhibitors	**Educating the Patient and Family**
Managing Adverse Reactions	**Key Points**
Contraindications, Precautions, and Interactions of Cholinesterase Inhibitors	**Case Study**
	Website Activities
Patient Management Issues with Cholinesterase Inhibitors	**Review Questions**

KEY TERMS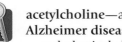

acetylcholine—a natural chemical in the brain that is required for memory and thinking
Alzheimer disease—a disease of the elderly causing progressive deterioration of mental and physical abilities
alanine aminotransferase (ALT)—an enzyme found predominately in the liver; high levels may indicate liver damage
anorexia—a diminished appetite
dementia—decrease in cognitive functioning (memory, decision making, speech, etc.)
ginkgo biloba—an herb that appears to increase blood flow to the brain
ginseng—an herb used to improve energy and mental performance
hepatotoxic—capable of producing liver damage

CHAPTER OBJECTIVES

On completion of this chapter, students will be able to:

1 Define the chapter's key terms.

2 Describe the manifestations of Alzheimer disease.

3 List the uses, general drug actions, general adverse reactions, contraindications, precautions, and interactions of the cholinesterase inhibitors.

4 Discuss important points that patients and family members should know about the use of cholinesterase inhibitors.

FACTS ABOUT ALZHEIMER DISEASE

- Approximately 2 million Americans have Alzheimer disease.
- Almost 50% of individuals in nursing homes and almost half of all people older than 85 years experience the effects of Alzheimer.
- Alzheimer is the fourth leading cause of death in adults.
- The life span of a patient with Alzheimer disease is usually decreased, although a patient may live 3 to 20 years after the diagnosis.

Alzheimer disease is a progressive deterioration of a person's mental and physical abilities from which there is no recovery. Specific pathologic changes occur in the cortex of the brain that are thought to be associated with deficiencies of one or more of the neurohormones, such as acetylcholine or norepinephrine. Alzheimer disease generally occurs in three progressive phases (Box 7-1).

Cholinesterase inhibitors are drugs used to treat Alzheimer disease. They do not cure the disease but help slow its progression. These drugs are used to treat mild to moderate **dementia** (a decrease in cognitive functioning) caused by Alzheimer disease. These patients may also be taking other drugs for symptomatic relief. For example, wandering, irritability, and aggression in people with Alzheimer disease are treated with antipsychotic drugs, such as risperidone and olanzapine (see Chapter 5). Other drugs, such as antidepressants or antianxiety drugs, may be helpful for patients with Alzheimer disease who are experiencing symptoms of depression and anxiety.

Herbal remedies may also be helpful for patients with Alzheimer disease. Ginkgo biloba is a common herb that appears to increase blood flow to the brain and has antioxidant properties. The herb is available over the

Early Phase—Mild Cocgnitive Decline
- Increased forgetfulness
- Decreased social performance
- Some memory deficit
- Mild to moderate anxiety

Early Dementia Phase—Moderately Severe Cognitive Decline
- Needs assistance in activities of daily living
- Unable to recall important aspects of current life
- Difficulty making choices (e.g., what clothes to wear, what to eat)
- Able to recall major facts (e.g., their name and family member's names)

Late Dementia Phase—Severe Cognitive Decline
- Incontinent of urine
- No verbal ability
- No basic psychomotor skills
- Needs help bathing, toileting, and feeding

counter, but there are no standards in the United States to regulate its quality or effectiveness. Patients should not take this or any other herb for Alzheimer disease without first consulting their health care provider. When ginkgo biloba is used with other drugs, such as with warfarin or high doses of vitamin E, the patient has an increased risk for bleeding.

Actions of Cholinesterase Inhibitors

Acetylcholine, a natural chemical in the brain, is required for memory and thinking. Individuals with Alzheimer disease slowly lose this chemical. As their levels of the chemical decrease, these patients experience problems with memory and thinking. The cholinesterase inhibitors act to increase the level of acetylcholine in the central nervous system by inhibiting its breakdown and slowing the destruction of neurons. However, the disease is progressive, and although these drugs alter the progress of the disease, they do not cure the disease.

Uses of Cholinesterase Inhibitors

Cholinesterase inhibitors are used to treat the dementia associated with Alzheimer disease. The effectiveness of these drugs varies from individual to individual. The drugs may noticeably diminish the symptoms of Alzheimer disease, the symptoms may improve only slightly, or the symptoms may continue to progress (only at a slower rate).

Adverse Reactions of Cholinesterase Inhibitors

Adverse reactions of cholinesterase inhibitors include **anorexia** (a diminished appetite), nausea, vomiting, diarrhea, weight loss, abdominal pain, dizziness, and headache. In most situations, these adverse reactions are mild and are usually experienced only early in treatment. When adverse reactions occur, they tend to disappear gradually as the body gets used to the treatment and generally do not last for more than several days.

Tacrine, however, is particularly **hepatotoxic** (capable of producing liver damage). Because tacrine is more likely to cause adverse reactions and drug interactions, it is administered in smaller doses given more frequently; tacrine is rarely used today. Donepezil has fewer and milder side effects and is considered the agent of first choice, although some patients may have a better response with one drug than another. Additional adverse reactions are listed in the Summary Drug Table: Cholinesterase Inhibitors.

Managing Adverse Reactions

When taking the cholinesterase inhibitors, patients may experience nausea and vomiting. Although this can occur with all of the cholinesterase inhibitors, patients taking rivastigmine appear to have more problems with nausea and severe vomiting. Nausea and vomiting should be reported to the health care provider; the drug may be discontinued and then restarted at the lowest dose possible. Restarting therapy at the lower dose helps to reduce the nausea and vomiting.

Weight loss and eating problems related to the inability to swallow are two major problems in the late stage of Alzheimer disease. These problems coupled with the anorexia and nausea associated with use of cholinesterase inhibitors present a challenge for caregivers. The patient should eat a well-balanced diet with foods that are easy to chew and digest. Frequent, small meals may be tolerated better than three regular meals. Offering foods of different consistency and flavor is important in case the patient can handle one form better than another. Fluid intake of 6 to 8 glasses of water daily is encouraged to prevent dehydration.

Physical decline and the adverse reaction of dizziness place the patient at risk for injury. The patient may need help when walking. The use of assistive devices such as walkers or canes may reduce the risk of falls. To minimize the risk of injury, the patient's environment should be controlled and safe.

A patient taking tacrine must be monitored for liver damage. This is usually performed by monitoring **alanine aminotransferase** (ALT) levels. ALT is an enzyme found predominantly in the liver. Disease or injury to

SUMMARY DRUG TABLE   Cholinesterase Inhibitors

Generic Name	Trade Name*	Uses	Adverse Reactions	Dosage Ranges
donepezil HCL *doe-nep'-ah-zill*	Aricept	Mild to moderate dementia of the Alzheimer type	Nausea, vomiting, diarrhea, muscle cramps, fatigue, anorexia, syncope	5–10 mg/d PO
galantamine hydrobromide *ga-lan'-ta-meen*	Reminyl	Mild to moderate dementia of the Alzheimer type	Nausea, vomiting, diarrhea, anorexia, weight loss, abdominal pain, headache, dizziness, lethargy, confusion	4 mg BID PO up to 24 mg/d
rivastigmine tartrate *riv-ah-stig'-meen*	Exelon, Exelon Oral Solution	Mild to moderate dementia of the Alzheimer type	Nausea, vomiting, diarrhea, dyspepsia, anorexia, abdominal pain, insomnia, fatigue, skin rash, dizziness, constipation, somnolence, tremor	1.5–12 mg/d BID PO
tacrine HCL *tay'-krin*	Cognex	Mild to moderate dementia of the Alzheimer type	Diarrhea, loss of appetite, clumsiness, nausea, vomiting, fainting, tachycardia, fever, hypertension or hypotension, skin rash, severe abdominal pain, hepatotoxicity	40–160 mg/d in 4 divided doses PO

*The term *generic* indicates the drug is available in generic form.

the liver causes a release of this enzyme into the bloodstream, resulting in elevated ALT levels.

Contraindications, Precautions, and Interactions of Cholinesterase Inhibitors

The cholinesterase inhibitors are contraindicated in patients with hypersensitivity to the drugs and during pregnancy (pregnancy category B) and lactation.

These drugs are used cautiously in patients with renal or hepatic disease, bladder obstruction, seizure disorders, sick sinus syndrome, gastrointestinal bleeding, and asthma. Individuals with a history of ulcer disease may have a recurrence of bleeding.

When the cholinesterase inhibitors are given to patients using an anticholinergic drug, there is a potential decrease in the activity of the anticholinergic drug. There is a greater risk of theophylline toxicity when

tacrine is administered. There is a synergistic effect when tacrine is administered with succinylcholine, other cholinesterase inhibitors, or cholinergic agonists (e.g., bethanechol).

Patient Management Issues with Cholinesterase Inhibitors

A patient receiving a cholinesterase inhibitor may be treated in a hospital or nursing home or as an outpatient. The patient's cognitive ability and functional ability are assessed before and during therapy. Confusion, agitation, impulsive behavior, speech, ability to perform the activities of daily living, and self-care abilities also are assessed. These assessments will be used to monitor the patient's improvement (if any) after taking a cholinesterase inhibitor. These drugs may slow the progression of the disease but are not a cure for Alzheimer disease.

Physical assessments include obtaining blood pressure measurements on both arms with the patient in a sitting position, pulse, respiratory rate, and body weight. Vital signs are monitored at least daily in hospitalized patients, and any significant change in the vital signs should be reported to the health care provider.

Ongoing assessment of patients taking a cholinesterase inhibitor includes mental and physical assessments. Ongoing assessments will be compared with the initial assessments to monitor the patient's improvement (if any) after taking the cholinesterase inhibitor.

Patients with poor response to drug therapy may require dosage changes, discontinuation of the drug therapy, or the addition of other therapies to the treatment regimen. However, response to these drugs may take several weeks. The symptoms that the patient is experiencing may get better or remain the same, or the patient may experience only a small response to therapy. Any treatment that slows the progression of symptoms in Alzheimer disease is considered successful.

Natural Remedies: Ginseng

Ginseng has been called the "king of herbs" because of its wide use and the benefits attributed to the herb. In early times in China, ginseng was valued as much as gold. Hundreds of ginseng products (e.g., gum, teas, chewing gum, juices) are sold throughout the US. A decade ago, ginseng was the fourth best selling herb in the US, although it has become relatively less popular recently and ranked thirteenth in sales in 2002. The primary use of ginseng is to improve energy and mental performance. The benefits of ginseng are said to include improving endurance during exercise, reducing fatigue, boosting stamina and reaction times, and increasing feelings of well-being.

Additional research is needed before definitive statements can be made about the value of ginseng for improving cognitive performance in Alzheimer patients or others. Some studies have shown improved memory, for example, whereas others have not.

Adverse reactions are rare, but headache, sleeplessness, nervousness, and diarrhea have been reported in individuals taking large amounts of ginseng. The herb should not be taken in combination with stimulants, including substances containing caffeine. Because ginseng can lower blood sugar levels in people with type 2 diabetes, it should not be used by those taking insulin or oral antidiabetic medications without careful glucose monitoring. Ginseng can increase the risk of bleeding problems in patients taking the blood-thinning agent warfarin. Ginseng may also interfere with the heart medication digoxin.

ALERT

Ginseng

Ginseng is contraindicated in individuals with high blood pressure and during pregnancy.

Natural Remedies: Ginkgo Biloba

Ginkgo biloba, one of the oldest known herbs in the world, is used to improve symptoms associated with reduced blood flow to the brain, including short-term memory loss and dizziness. It is also a frequent treatment for ringing in the ears, headache, depression, erectile dysfunction, and anxiety. In the United States, it is classified by the Food and Drug Administration (FDA) as a dietary supplement rather than a drug. It is commercially available over the counter in liquid, capsule, or tablet form.

The leaves of the ginkgo plant contain insufficient quantities of active ingredients for effective use as a medical treatment. Ginkgo extract is most commonly used. Clinical studies of the extract suggest that it is effective in treating established dementia. However, a recent study in the *Journal of the American Medical Association* indicated that for elderly patients with normal memory, gingko did not improve learning, memory, attention, or concentration.

The health improvements associated with ginkgo are not immediate but may begin after 4 to 24 weeks. The potential side effects of regular use of ginkgo include mild gastrointestinal upset, headache, rash, muscle spasms, cramps, and bleeding. Large doses reportedly cause diarrhea, nausea, vomiting, and restlessness.

Patients taking anticlotting medication, including over-the-counter treatments such as aspirin, should avoid taking ginkgo. Taking ginkgo with a thiazide diuretic will increase blood pressure. Patients taking monoamine oxidase inhibitors (MAOIs) should not take ginkgo because of increased risk of toxic reaction.

Educating the Patient and Family

Patients with Alzheimer disease may understand and comprehend the extent and severity of this disease while they are early in the disease process. As their cognitive abilities decrease, however, it is the family who needs to be educated about the disease and the effects of drugs given for treatment. It is often important for family members to assume responsibility for giving drugs to patients at home if they appear unable to manage their own drug therapy.

Patient Education Box 7-1 includes key points about cholinesterase inhibitors the patient or family members should know.

PATIENT EDUCATION BOX 7-1

Key Points for Patients Taking Cholinesterase Inhibitors

❑ Keep all appointments with health care providers because close monitoring of the drug therapy is essential. Dose changes may be needed to achieve the best results.

❑ Take the drug exactly as directed. Do not increase, decrease, or omit a dose or discontinue use of this drug unless directed to do so by your primary health care provider.

❑ Do not drive or perform other hazardous tasks if you feel drowsy. Patients with a diagnosis of Alzheimer disease should not drive.

❑ Do not take any nonprescription drug unless your primary health care provider approves the specific drug.

❑ Keep track of when the drug is taken. Patients in the early stages of forgetfulness can mark their calendar each time they take the medicine or use a pill counter that holds the medicine for each day of the week; such methods can help patients remember to take their medication or know if they have already taken the medication for the day.

❑ Immediately report any of the following adverse reactions: severe vomiting, dehydration, changes in mental functioning, or yellowing of the skin or eyes.

KEY POINTS

● Alzheimer disease is a common progressive deterioration of mental and physical abilities caused by changes in the brain.

● Medications for Alzheimer do not cure the disease but may lessen or delay its symptoms. Cholinesterase inhibitors increase the level of acetylcholine in the central nervous system by inhibiting its breakdown and slowing the destruction of neurons.

● Cholinesterase inhibitors may cause anorexia, nausea, vomiting, diarrhea, weight loss, dizziness, and headache. They are contraindicated during pregnancy and lactation and in patients with a known hypersensitivity, and are used with caution in patients with renal or hepatic disease, bladder obstruction, seizure disorders, sick sinus syndrome, gastrointestinal bleeding, and asthma.

● Patient management issues include physical and cognitive assessments to determine the patient's improvement while on the medication and to monitor and care for adverse reactions.

● Patient and family education issues include monitoring the patient's status for adverse effects and to determine a need for dosage changes.

CASE STUDY

Mr. Alvarez had mild Alzheimer disease diagnosed, and the doctor has prescribed donepezil. Two weeks later, Mr. Alvarez's family is concerned because he does not seem "better" and is experiencing some nausea.

1. His family members need to know that:
   a. It may take a full year before the drug has an effect.
   b. Even if he does not seem to be getting "better," the drug may be helping to keep his symptoms from worsening.
   c. The doctor will double the dosage every week until a positive effect occurs.
   d. He does not need to take the drug on days when he does not feel like it.

2. Mr. Alvarez's symptom of nausea:
   a. is a common adverse effect of donepezil and will likely diminish over time
   b. is probably caused by his Alzheimer disease, not the drug
   c. will become worse the longer he continues to use the drug
   d. is a sign that the drug is improving his cognitive performance

3. Other adverse effects Mr. Alvarez may experience may include:
   a. headache, tingling in his fingers and toes, and a sensation of cold
   b. bleeding, tinnitus, and tachycardia
   c. confusion, insomnia, and frequent brief blackouts
   d. vomiting, weight loss, and headache

WEBSITE ACTIVITIES

1. Go to the website of the U.S. Food and Drug Association (http://www.fda.gov). From the home page, navigate to this agency's information on "recalls and safety alerts." Determine whether any alerts have been issued for either ginseng or ginkgo. (Be sure to check both the current recall list and the archives. Hint: try the Search engine using key terms such as "ginseng safety alert.") If so, read the alert and write a one- or two-sentence summary for your pharmacology instructor.

   1. _____

   2. _____

   3. _____

   4. _____

   5. _____

2. Go to the website of the Alzheimer Disease Education & Referral Center (http://www.alzheimers.org). From the starting page move to the section on treatment, and check whether any new drugs for the treatment of Alzheimer have been added to the four drugs described in this chapter. If so, write a note on any new drug in the same format as in the Summary Drug Table in this chapter, listing the generic and trade names, the uses, and adverse reactions.

   1. _____

   2. _____

   3. _____

   4. _____

   5. _____

REVIEW QUESTIONS

1. Cholinesterase inhibitors are used to treat which of the following conditions associated with Alzheimer disease?
   a. urinary incontinence
   b. dementia
   c. peripheral paralysis
   d. depression

2. Cholinesterase inhibitors act by helping maintain or increase the level of what chemical in the brain?
   a. erythrocytes
   b. gastric acid
   c. cerebrospinal fluid
   d. acetylcholine

3. Adverse reactions that may occur in a patient taking rivastigmine (Exelon) include:
   a. occipital headache
   b. vomiting

c. hyperactivity

d. hypoactivity

4. When a patient with Alzheimer disease is given tacrine (Cognex), which laboratory examination would most likely be prescribed?

a. a complete blood count

b. cholesterol levels

c. alanine aminotransferase (ALT) levels

d. electrolytes

5. A patient taking gingko for Alzheimer may experience:

a. gastrointestinal upset and headache

b. sleepiness and dizziness

c. tremors in the arms and legs

d. an inability to speak normally

8 Antiemetic and Antivertigo Drugs

KEY TERMS

antiemetic—a drug used to treat or prevent nausea or vomiting
antivertigo—a drug used to treat or prevent vertigo
chemoreceptor trigger zone—a group of nerve fibers in the brain that when stimulated by chemicals, such as drugs or toxic substances, sends impulses to the vomiting center of the brain
emesis—the expelled gastric contents; vomitus
nausea—an unpleasant gastric sensation usually preceding vomiting
prophylaxis—a drug or treatment designed for prevention of a condition or symptom
vertigo—an abnormal feeling of spinning or rotation motion that may occur with motion sickness and other disorders
vestibular neuritis—inflammation of the vestibular nerve to the inner ear
vomiting—forceful expulsion of gastric contents through the mouth

CHAPTER OBJECTIVES

On completion of this chapter, students will be able to:

1 Define the chapter's key terms.

2 Discuss the general drug actions, uses, adverse reactions, contraindications, precautions, and interactions of antiemetic and antivertigo drugs.

3 Discuss important points that patients and family members should know about the use of an antiemetic or antivertigo drug.

An **antiemetic** drug is used to treat or prevent **nausea** (unpleasant gastric sensation usually preceding vomiting) or **vomiting** (forceful expulsion of gastric contents through the mouth). An **antivertigo** drug is used to treat or prevent vertigo (a feeling of a spinning or rotation-type motion), which may occur with motion sickness, Ménière's disease of the ear, middle or inner ear surgery, and other disorders.

Vomiting caused by drugs, radiation, and metabolic disorders usually occurs because of stimulation of the **chemoreceptor trigger zone**, a group of nerve fibers in the brain. When these fibers are stimulated by chemicals, such as drugs or toxic substances, impulses are sent to the vomiting center located in the medulla. The vomiting center may also be directly stimulated by disorders such as gastrointestinal irritation, motion sickness, and vestibular neuritis (inflammation of the vestibular nerve in the inner ear).

Actions of Antiemetics and Antivertigo Drugs

These drugs appear to act primarily by inhibiting the chemoreceptor trigger zone or by depressing the sensitivity of the vestibular apparatus of the inner ear. Drugs that act on the chemoreceptor trigger zone are more effective for vomiting caused by stimulation of the chemoreceptor trigger zone, whereas those that act on the vestibular apparatus of the inner ear are more effective for vertigo associated with motion sickness or middle or inner ear surgery.

Uses of Antiemetics and Antivertigo Drugs

Uses of Antiemetic Drugs

An antiemetic is used for **prophylaxis** (prevention) or treatment of nausea and vomiting. An example of prophylactic use is giving an antiemetic before surgery to prevent vomiting during the immediate postoperative period when the patient is recovering from anesthesia. Another example is giving an antiemetic before administration of antineoplastic drugs (drugs used in the treatment of cancer; see Chapter 28), which are likely to cause vomiting.

Antiemetics are also used for other causes of nausea and vomiting such as radiation therapy for a malignancy, bacterial and viral infections, nausea and vomiting caused by drugs, Ménière's disease and other ear disorders, and some neurological diseases and disorders. Some of these drugs also are used to treat the nausea and vomiting that occurs with motion sickness.

Dronabinol is a derivative of the active substance found in marijuana. Dronabinol is a second-line antiemetic and is generally used only after treatment with other antiemetics has failed.

Some antiemetics also are antivertigo drugs (see the Summary Drug Table: Antiemetic and Antivertigo Drugs).

Uses of Antivertigo Drugs

An antivertigo drug is used to treat vertigo, which is usually accompanied by light-headedness, dizziness, and weakness. A person experiencing vertigo often has difficulty walking. Some of the causes of vertigo include inebriation with alcohol, certain drugs, inner ear disease, and postural hypotension. Motion sickness (seasickness, carsickness) has similar symptoms but is caused by repetitive motion (e.g., riding in an airplane, boat, or car). Both vertigo and motion sickness may result in nausea and vomiting.

Antivertigo drugs are essentially antiemetics because many of these drugs, whether used for motion sickness or vertigo, also have direct or indirect antiemetic properties. They prevent the nausea and vomiting that occur because of stimulation of the vestibular apparatus in the ear. Stimulation of this apparatus results in vertigo, which is often followed by nausea and vomiting.

Adverse Reactions of Antiemetics and Antivertigo Drugs

The most common adverse reactions of these drugs are varying degrees of drowsiness. Additional adverse reactions for each drug are listed in the Summary Drug Table: Antiemetic and Antivertigo Drugs.

Managing Adverse Reactions

To prevent accidental falls and other injuries caused by drowsiness, hospitalized patients should be helped out of bed and helped to walk. Patients who experience extreme drowsiness may need to remain in bed and use a call light when assistance is needed.

ALERT

Drowsiness

Many of these drugs cause variable degrees of drowsiness. The patient should avoid activities requiring alertness and may need help when getting out of bed if drowsiness occurs.

Contraindications, Precautions, and Interactions of Antiemetics and Antivertigo Drugs

The antiemetic and antivertigo drugs are contraindicated in patients with known hypersensitivity to these drugs, those in a coma, or those with severe central nervous system depression. In general, these drugs are not recommended during pregnancy or lactation or for uncomplicated vomiting in young children. Metoclopramide is contraindicated in patients with a seizure disorder, breast cancer, pheochromocytoma, or gastrointestinal obstruction. Prochlorperazine is contraindicated in patients with bone marrow depression, blood dyscrasia, Parkinson disease, or severe liver or cardiovascular disease. Thiethylperazine is classified as pregnancy category X and is contraindicated during pregnancy.

Severe nausea and vomiting should not be treated only with antiemetic drugs. The cause of the vomiting must be investigated. Antiemetic drugs may hamper the diagnosis of disorders such as brain tumors, appendicitis, intestinal obstruction, or drug toxicity (e.g., digitalis toxicity). A delayed diagnosis of any of these disorders could have serious consequences for the patient.

Antiemetics and antivertigo drugs are used cautiously in patients with glaucoma or obstructive disease of the gastrointestinal or genitourinary system, in patients with renal or hepatic dysfunction, and in older men with possible prostatic hypertrophy. Promethazine is used cautiously in patients with hypertension, sleep apnea, or epilepsy. Trimethobenzamide is used cautiously in children with a viral illness because it may increase the risk of Reye syndrome.

SUMMARY DRUG TABLE   Antiemetics and Antivertigo Drugs

Generic Name	Trade Name*	Uses	Adverse Reactions	Dosage Ranges
buclizine *byoo'-kli-zeen*	Bucladin-S Softabs	Nausea and vomiting, motion sickness	Drowsiness, confusion, dry mouth, headache, jitteriness, anorexia, nausea, urinary frequency, difficulty urinating	50 mg PO q4–6h; maximum dose, 150 mg/d
chlorpromazine hydrochloride *klor-proe'-ma-zeen*	Thorazine, *generic*	Control of nausea and vomiting, intractable hiccoughs	Drowsiness, hypotension, postural hypotension, hypertension, bradycardia, hypersensitivity reactions, dry mouth, nasal congestion	Nausea and vomiting: 10–25 mg PO q4–6h PRN; 50–100 mg rectal suppository q6–8h PRN; 25–50 mg IM q3–4h PRN; hiccoughs: 25–50 mg PO, IM, slow IV infusion
cyclizine *sye'-kli-zeen*	Marezine	Nausea and vomiting, motion sickness	Same as buclizine	50 mg PO 30 min before exposure to motion, may repeat q4–6h; maximum dose, 200 mg/d
dimenhydrinate *dye-men-hye'-dri-nate*	Dinate, Dramamine, Dramanate, Triptone, *generic*	Prevention and treatment of nausea, vomiting, dizziness, vertigo of motion sickness	Dizziness, confusion, nervousness, restlessness, nausea, vomiting, diarrhea, blurred vision, palpitations	50–100 mg PO q4–6h PRN, maximum dose, 400 mg/d, 50 mg IM as needed, 50 mg IV
diphenhydramine *dye-fen-hye'-dra-meen*	Benadryl, *generic*	Prevention and treatment of motion sickness, antihistamine	Dizziness, sedation, epigastric distress, faintness, allergic reactions, urinary frequency, thickening of bronchial secretions	25–50 mg PO q4–6h, 10–50 mg IM, IV
diphenidol *di-phen'-i-dol*	Vontrol	Vertigo and associated nausea and vomiting, Ménière's disease, middle and inner ear surgery, control of nausea and vomiting in postoperative period, malignancies, inner ear disturbances	Auditory and visual hallucinations, disorientation, drowsiness, dry mouth, nausea, skin rash	25–50 mg PO q4h
dolasetron mesylate *doe-laz-e'-tron*	Anzemet	Prevention of chemotherapy-induced nausea, vomiting, and postoperative nausea and vomiting	Hypotension, hypertension, electrocardiographic changes, headache, dizziness, light-headedness, fatigue, sedation, hunger, constipation	Before chemotherapy: 100 mg within 1 h before chemotherapy; PO nausea and vomiting: 100 mg or 1.8 mg/kg IV

Generic Name	Trade Name*	Uses	Adverse Reactions	Dosage Ranges
dronabinol *droe-nab'-i-nol*	Marinol	Treatment of nausea and vomiting due to antineoplastic drug therapy, appetite stimulant in AIDS patients with weight loss	Palpitations, drowsiness, diarrhea, euphoria, dizziness, paranoid reaction, somnolence, irritability, hallucinations	Antiemetic: 5–15 mg/m^2 1–3 h before chemotherapy, then q2–4h after chemotherapy for a total of 4–6 doses/d; appetite stimulant: 2.5 mg PO BID AC lunch and dinner
granisetron hydrochloride *gran-iz'-e-tron*	Kytril	Prevention and treatment of nausea and vomiting caused by antineoplastic drug therapy	Headache, weakness, somnolence, diarrhea, constipation	10 mg/kg infused IV over 5 min, 30 min before chemotherapy, or 1 mg PO BID
meclizine *mek'-li-zeen*	Antivert, Antivert/25, Antivert/50, *generic*	Vertigo, prevention and treatment of nausea and vomiting caused by motion sickness	Drowsiness, restlessness, rash, urticaria, anorexia, hypotension, dry mouth, nose, and throat	Vertigo: 25–100 mg/d PO in divided doses; nausea and vomiting: 25–50 mg PO 1 h before travel and repeat 24 h PRN
metoclopramide *met-oh-kloe-pra'-mide*	Reglan, generic	Prevention of nausea and vomiting caused by antineoplastic drug therapy	Restlessness, drowsiness, fatigue, lassitude, dizziness, nausea, diarrhea	1–2 mg/kg IV 15–30 min before chemotherapy
ondansetron hydrochloride *on-dan'-sa-tron*	Zofran	Prevention of nausea and vomiting due to antineoplastic drug therapy, prevention of postoperative nausea and vomiting	Diarrhea, headache, fever, weakness, dry mouth, drowsiness, sedation	Chemotherapy: 3 doses of 0.15 mg/kg IV or 32 mg PO 30 min before chemotherapy; postoperative nausea and vomiting; 4 mg IV
perphenazine *per-fen'-a-zeen*	Trilafon, *generic*	Control of nausea and vomiting, intractable hiccoughs	Same as chlorpromazine hydrochloride	8–16 mg/d PO in divided doses, 5–10 mg IM, IV q6h PRN
prochlorperazine hydrochloride *proe-klor-per'-a-zeen*	Compazine, *generic*	Control of nausea and vomiting	Same as chlorpromazine hydrochloride	5–10 mg PO TID, QID; 10–20 mg IM, IV; 25 mg rectal suppository BID; 10–15 mg sustained release
promethazine hydrochloride *proe-meth'-a-zeen*	Phenergan, *generic*	Treatment of motion sickness, prevention of nausea and vomiting associated with anesthesia and surgery	Same as diphenhydramine hydrochloride	Motion sickness: Initial dose 25 mg PO 30 min before travel and repeat in 8–12 h, then 25 mg PO BID, 12.5–25 mg IM, IV; nausea and vomiting: 12.5–25 mg PO, IM, IV
thiethylperazine maleate *thye-eth-il-per'-a-zeen*	Torecan	Nausea and vomiting	Same as chlorpromazine hydrochloride	10 mg PO, IM, PRN 1–3 times per day; maximum dose, 30 mg/d
transdermal scopolamine *skoe-pol'-a-mine*	Transderm-Scop Scopace oral	Prevention of nausea and vomiting due to motion sickness	Drowsiness, dry mouth, blurred vision	One system applied at least 4 h before effect is required, repeat in 3 d scopolamine, if needed; orally, 0.4–0.8 mg PO

Generic Name	Trade Name*	Uses	Adverse Reactions	Dosage Ranges
triflupromazine *trye-flu-proe'-ma-zeen*	Vesprin	Severe nausea and vomiting	Drowsiness, insomnia, vertigo, dry mouth, salivation, nausea, vomiting, anorexia, constipation, urinary retention, extrapyramidal effects (see Chapter 5)	5–15 mg IM q4h, maximum dose, 60 mg/d; 1 mg IV up to 3 mg/d
trimethobenzamide hydrochloride *trye-meth-oh-ben'-za-mide*	Tebamide, T-Gen, Tigan, *generic*	Control of nausea and vomiting	Hypersensitivity reactions, hypotension (IM use), Parkinson-like symptoms, blurred vision, drowsiness, dizziness	250 mg PO TID, QID: 200 mg IM, rectal suppository TID, QID

*The term *generic* indicates that the drug is available in generic form.

Perphenazine, prochlorperazine, promethazine, scopolamine, chlorpromazine, and trimethobenzamide are pregnancy category C drugs. The pregnancy category of diphenidol has not been established. Other antiemetics and antivertigo drugs are classified as pregnancy category B (except for thiethylperazine, which is classified as pregnancy category X).

The antiemetics and antivertigo drugs may have additive effects when used with alcohol and other central nervous system depressants such as sedatives, hypnotics, antianxiety drugs, opiates, and antidepressants. They may cause additive anticholinergic effects (see Chapter 4) when administered with drugs that have anticholinergic activity, such as the antihistamines, antidepressants, phenothiazines, and disopyramide. Antacids decrease the absorption of the antiemetics.

When ondansetron is administered with rifampin, blood levels of ondansetron may be reduced, decreasing the antiemetic effect. Dimenhydrinate may mask the signs and symptoms of ototoxicity when administered with ototoxic drugs, such as the aminoglycosides (see Chapter 25), causing irreversible hearing damage. When lithium is administered with prochlorperazine, the risk of extrapyramidal reactions increases (see Chapter 5).

Patient Management Issues with Antiemetics and Antivertigo Drugs

Patients who have vomited repeatedly are at risk for fluid and electrolyte imbalances. It may be necessary to document the number of times the patient has vomited and the approximate amount of fluid lost. The health care provider should be notified if there is blood in the patient's **emesis** (vomitus) or if the vomiting suddenly becomes more severe.

Before drug therapy begins, vital signs are taken and the patient is assessed for signs of fluid and electrolyte imbalances.

Patients who experience prolonged and repeated episodes of vomiting (e.g., those receiving chemotherapy for malignant disease) may need to be weighed daily or weekly.

If the patient continues vomiting after being given the oral form of an antiemetic drug, then the drug may need to be administered parenterally or as a rectal suppository (if available in these forms) until the risk of vomiting has passed.

A number of different antiemetics are used to prevent nausea in patients being treated for cancer. Most are administered before the chemotherapy is given and for some time afterwards to prevent or relieve nausea and vomiting.

Dehydration is a serious concern in patients experiencing vomiting. If the patient can retain small amounts of oral fluids, then sips of water should be offered at frequent intervals. In addition, the patient is observed for signs of an electrolyte imbalance, particularly sodium and potassium deficits (see Chapter 32); in such cases, parenteral administration of fluids or fluids with electrolytes may be necessary.

GERONTOLOGIC ALERT

Dehydration

An elderly or chronically ill patient experiencing vomiting may have severe dehydration develop in a short time, leading to fluid and electrolyte disturbances. Health care workers should be alert for and immediately report symptoms of dehydration, such as poor skin turgor, dry mucous membranes, decreased urinary output, concentrated urine, increased respiratory rate, irritability, restlessness, or confusion in older adults.

With a hospitalized patient experiencing vomiting, extra care is needed. Soiled bedding or clothing must be changed as needed because the odor of vomitus may only intensify the patient's nausea, vomiting, vertigo, or dizziness. The patient should be given an emesis basin and checked frequently. Patients should have a damp washcloth and towel to wipe their hands and face as needed, as well as mouthwash or frequent oral rinses to remove the disagreeable taste caused by vomiting.

Natural Remedies: Ginger

Ginger, a medicinal herb, is derived from the root of the ginger plant. When dried for consumption, it resembles an ash-colored powder, smells like pepper, and has a spicy taste. Ginger is usually taken to reduce nausea, vomiting, and indigestion. Clinical studies suggest that ginger can be effective in preventing the nausea associated with motion sickness, seasickness, and anesthesia, although results are unclear whether ginger helps people already experiencing the symptoms of seasickness. In the United States, it is classified by the Food and Drug Administration (FDA) as a dietary supplement rather than a drug. It is commercially available over the counter in dried form (chopped, powdered, powdered extract), candied ginger, and tea.

Although conclusive studies have not yet shown that ginger is also effective as a treatment for arthritis pain and inflammation, anecdotal evidence points to that conclusion.

Ginger is not recommended for morning sickness associated with pregnancy and is not advised for patients with gallstones or hypertension. Small amounts present in food preparation are generally regarded as safe. The medicinal use of ginger should cease 2 to 3 weeks before surgery to reduce the risk of bleeding. The only known side effects of ginger are heartburn and heightened taste sensitivity.

Educating the Patient and Family

Patient Education Box 8-1 includes key points about antiemetic and antivertigo drugs that the patient or family members should know.

PATIENT EDUCATION BOX 8-1

Key Points for Patients Taking Antiemetic and Antivertigo Drugs

❑ Avoid driving or performing other hazardous tasks when taking these drugs because drowsiness may occur with use.
❑ Contact the health care provider if nausea, vomiting, or vertigo persists or worsens.
❑ Use these drugs only as directed. Do not increase the dose or frequency of use unless advised by the health care provider.
❑ Do not use alcohol and other drugs with sedative effects except as advised by the health care provider.
❑ Follow the directions for application of transdermal scopolamine that are supplied with the drug.

KEY POINTS

⦿ An antiemetic drug is used to treat or prevent nausea or vomiting. An antivertigo drug is used to treat or prevent vertigo, which may occur with motion sickness, Ménière disease of the ear, middle or inner ear surgery, and other disorders.

⦿ Antiemetics and antivertigo drugs appear to act primarily by inhibiting the chemoreceptor trigger zone, a group of nerve fibers in the brain, or by depressing the sensitivity of the vestibular apparatus of the inner ear.

⦿ The most common adverse reactions of both antiemetics and antivertigo drugs are varying degrees of drowsiness. The patient should avoid activities requiring alertness.

⦿ The antiemetic and antivertigo drugs are contraindicated in patients with known hypersensitivity to these drugs, those in a coma, or those with severe central nervous system depression. In general, these drugs are not recommended during pregnancy or lactation or for uncomplicated vomiting in young children. Specific agents also have specific contraindications and precautions.

⦿ Patients who have vomited repeatedly are at risk for fluid and electrolyte imbalances, especially dehydration.

CASE STUDY

Ms. Davis was prescribed meclizine (Antivert-50) 50 mg for motion sickness. After returning from a long car trip, she tells you that the medicine did not help.

1. When should she have taken the medication to prevent experiencing motion sickness?
   a. the day before the car trip
   b. 1 hour before the car trip began
   c. at the beginning of the car trip
   d. when she first began to feel nauseous

2. Which of the following is *not* a common adverse reaction to meclizine and should therefore be reported to Ms. Davis's health care provider?
   a. bleeding
   b. dry mouth
   c. lack of appetite
   d. drowsiness

3. Before Ms. Davis's next trip, her health care provider prescribes a transdermal scopolamine patch. Ms. Davis needs to remember that:
   a. the patch should be applied at least 4 hours before the trip begins
   b. she may experience drowsiness because of the medication
   c. she should use the patch as directed in the product information sheet
   d. all of the above

WEBSITE ACTIVITIES

1. Go to the Mayo Clinic's public health information website (http://www.mayoclinic.com) and navigate to the "diseases and conditions A–Z" section. Read the information on the treatment of vertigo and write brief answers to these questions:
   a. What is the procedure called BPPV?
   b. What conditions can a physical therapist help with?
   c. When might counseling help a patient?
   d. What other types of drugs might help a patient with Ménière disease?

2. Remaining at the Mayo Clinic's public health information website (http://www.mayoclinic.com), perform a "drug search" on buclizine. Read the provided information and write brief answers to the following questions:
   a. Can children and adolescents take buclizine?
   b. What adverse effects of buclizine may older adults be more susceptible to?
   c. If your health care provider is prescribing buclizine for you, do you need to tell the health care provider if you have glaucoma?

REVIEW QUESTIONS

1. What is the most common adverse reaction in patients receiving an antiemetic?
   a. occipital headache
   b. drowsiness
   c. edema
   d. nausea

2. When an antivertigo drug is prescribed for a patient experiencing motion sickness, the patient should be advised to:
   a. take the drug with food immediately before traveling
   b. administer the drug at least 6 hours before travel
   c. avoid driving or performing hazardous tasks
   d. take the drug at the first sign of motion sickness

3. Which of these drugs is a pregnancy category X drug and should not be taken by a pregnant woman?
   a. dimenhydrinate
   b. scopolamine
   c. promethazine
   d. thiethylperazine

4. Repeated vomiting may lead to what potentially serious condition?
   a. dehydration
   b. stomach ulcers
   c. migraine headache
   d. anaphylaxis

5. The adverse reactions of antiemetics can be completely prevented by:
   a. going to sleep immediately after taking the drug
   b. eating 2 hours before taking the drug
   c. taking twice the prescribed dose of the drug
   d. none of the above

9 Anesthetic Drugs

Local Anesthetics
Uses of Local Anesthetics
Patient Management Issues with Local Anesthetics

Preanesthetic Drugs
Uses of Preanesthetic Drugs
Contraindications, Precautions, and Interactions of Preanesthetic Drugs
Patient Management Issues with Preanesthetic Drugs

General Anesthetics
Uses of General Anesthetics
Administration of General Anesthetics
Patient Management Issues with General Anesthetics

Educating the Patient and Family

Key Points

Case Study

Website Activities

Review Questions

KEY TERMS

analgesia—absence of pain
anesthesia—a loss of feeling or sensation
anesthesiologist— a physician with special training in administering anesthetics
anesthetist—a nurse with special training who is qualified to administer anesthetics
atelectasis—reduction of air in the lung
brachial plexus block—type of regional anesthesia produced by injection of a local anesthetic into the brachial plexus
conduction block—type of regional anesthesia produced by injection of a local anesthetic into or near a nerve trunk
epidural block—type of regional anesthesia produced by injection of a local anesthetic into the space surrounding the dura of the spinal cord
general anesthesia—provision of a pain-free state for the entire body
local anesthesia—provision of a pain-free state in a specific area
local infiltration anesthesia—anesthesia produced by injecting a local anesthetic drug into tissues
neuroleptanalgesia—a state of general quietness achieved through a combination of analgesic and neuroleptic drugs
patency—being open or exposed
preanesthetic drug—a drug given before the administration of anesthesia
regional anesthesia—anesthesia produced by injecting a local anesthetic around nerves to limit the pain signals sent to the brain
spinal anesthesia—a type of regional anesthesia produced by injecting a local anesthetic drug into the subarachnoid space of the spinal cord
transsacral block—type of regional anesthesia produced by injection of a local anesthetic into the epidural space at the level of the sacrococcygeal notch
volatile liquid—a liquid that evaporates on exposure to the air

CHAPTER OBJECTIVES

On completion of this chapter, students will be able to:

1 Define the chapter's key terms.

2 Define the uses and general drug actions of anesthetic drugs.

3 List and briefly describe the four stages of general anesthesia.

This chapter focuses on anesthetic drugs. Because either an anesthesiologist or a nurse anesthetist is responsible for administering this drug group, this chapter's information on dosages, adverse reactions, contraindications, precautions, and interactions will be kept to a minimum.

Anesthesia is a loss of feeling or sensation. Anesthesia may be induced by various drugs that are able to bring about partial or complete loss of sensation. The two types of anesthesia are local anesthesia and general anesthesia.

Local Anesthetics

Local anesthesia, as the term implies, is the condition of a pain-free state in a specific area (or region) of the body. With a local anesthetic, a patient is fully awake but does not feel pain in the area that has been anesthetized. However, some procedures performed under local anesthesia may require a patient to be sedated. Although not fully awake, sedated patients may still hear what is going on around them. A physician or dentist administers a local injectable anesthetic. Table 9-1 lists commonly used local anesthetics.

Uses of Local Anesthetics

Topical Anesthetics

Topical anesthesia involves the application of the anesthetic to the surface of the skin, open area, or mucous membrane. The anesthetic may be applied with a cotton swab or sprayed on the area. This type of anesthesia may be used to desensitize the skin or mucous membrane before the injection of a deeper local anesthetic. In some instances, a topical anesthetic may be applied by a health care provider other than a physician.

Local Infiltration Anesthetics

Local infiltration anesthesia is produced by the injection of a local anesthetic drug into tissues. This type of anesthesia may be used for dental procedures, suturing small wounds, or making an incision into a small area such as that required for removing a superficial tissue sample for biopsy.

Regional Anesthetics

Regional anesthesia is produced by the injection of a local anesthetic around nerves so that the area supplied by these nerves will not send pain signals to the brain. The anesthetized area is usually larger than the area affected by local infiltration anesthesia. Spinal anesthesia and conduction blocks are two types of regional anesthesia.

Spinal Anesthetics. Spinal anesthesia is a type of regional anesthesia resulting from the injection of a local anesthetic drug into the subarachnoid space of the spinal cord, usually at the level of the second lumbar vertebra. There is a loss of feeling (anesthesia) and movement in the lower extremities, lower abdomen, and perineum.

Conduction Block Anesthetics. A **conduction block** is a type of regional anesthesia produced by injection of a local anesthetic drug into or near a nerve trunk. Examples of a conduction block include an **epidural block** (injection of a local anesthetic into the space surrounding the dura of the spinal cord), a **transsacral (caudal) block** (injection of a local anesthetic into the epidural space at the level of the sacrococcygeal notch), and **brachial plexus block** (injection of a local anesthetic into the brachial plexus). Epidural and transsacral blocks are often used in obstetrics. A brachial plexus block may be used for surgery of the arm or hand.

Patient Management Issues with Local Anesthetics

Depending on the procedure performed, preparing a patient for local anesthesia may or may not be similar to preparing the patient for general anesthesia. For example, administering a local anesthetic for dental surgery or for suturing a small wound may require the health care provider to explain to the patient how the anesthetic will be administered. The patient's allergy history may be taken. When applicable, the area of the patient's body to be anesthetized may require preparation, such as cleaning the area with an antiseptic or shaving the area. Other local anesthetic procedures may require the patient to be in a fasting state because a sedative may also be administered. An intravenous sedative such as the antianxiety drug diazepam (Valium) (see Chapter 5)

TABLE 9-1   **Examples of Local Anesthetics**

Generic Name	Trade Name*
ardecaine HCl	Septocaine
bupivacaine HCl	Marcaine HCl, *generic*
chloroprocaine HCl	Nesacaine, Nescaine-MPF
lidocaine HCl	Dilocaine, Xylocaine, *generic*
mepivacaine HCl	Carbocaine, Isocaine HCl
prilocaine HCl	Citanest HCl
procaine HCl, injectable	Novocain, *generic*
ropivacaine	Naropin
tetracaine HCl	Pontocaine HCl

*The term generic indicates the drug is available in generic form.

may also be given during some local anesthetic procedures, such as cataract surgery or surgery performed under spinal anesthesia.

Preanesthetic Drugs

A **preanesthetic drug** is one given before the administration of anesthesia. It is usually used before the administration of general anesthesia but also on occasion before injection of a local anesthetic. The preanesthetic may consist of one drug or a combination of drugs.

Uses of Preanesthetic Drugs

The general purpose of the preanesthetic drug is to prepare the patient for anesthesia.

Narcotic or antianxiety drugs are used to decrease anxiety and apprehension immediately before surgery. The patient who is calm and relaxed can be anesthetized more quickly, usually requires a smaller dose of an induction drug, may require less anesthesia during surgery, and may have a smoother anesthesia recovery period (awakening from anesthesia). Preanesthetic drugs are usually given 30 minutes before surgery.

Cholinergic blocking drugs are used to decrease secretions of the upper respiratory tract. Some anesthetic gases and volatile liquids are irritating to the lining of the respiratory tract and increase mucus secretions. The cough and swallowing reflexes are lost during general anesthesia, and excessive secretions can pool in the lungs, resulting in pneumonia or **atelectasis** (a reduction of air in the lung) after surgery. The cholinergic blocking drug, such as glycopyrrolate (Robinul), dries up secretions of the upper respiratory tract and lessens the possibility of excessive mucus production.

Antiemetics are used to prevent nausea and vomiting during the immediate postoperative recovery period.

GERONTOLOGIC ALERT

Preanesthetic Drugs

Preanesthetic drugs are often not used in patients 60 years or older because many of the medical disorders for which these drugs are contraindicated occur in older individuals. For example, atropine and glycopyrrolate, drugs that can be used to decrease secretions of the upper respiratory tract, are contraindicated in patients with certain medical disorders, such as prostatic hypertrophy, glaucoma, and myocardial ischemia. Other preanesthetic drugs that depress the central nervous system, such as narcotics, barbiturates, and antianxiety drugs with or without antiemetic properties, may also be contraindicated in older individuals.

TABLE 9-2 Examples of Preanesthetic Drugs

Generic Name	Trade Name*
Narcotics	
droperidol	Inapsine
fentanyl	Sublimaze, *generic*
meperidine hydrochloride	Demerol, *generic*
morphine sulfate	Duramorph, *generic*
Barbiturates	
pentobarbital	Nembutal Sodium, *generic*
secobarbital	Generic
Cholinergic-Blocking Drugs	
atropine sulfate	Generic
glycopyrrolate	Robinul, *generic*
scopolamine	Generic
Antianxiety Drugs With Antiemetic Properties	
hydroxyzine	Atarax, Vistaril, *generic*
Antianxiety Drugs	
chlordiazepoxide	Librium, *generic*
diazepam	Valium, *generic*
midazolam	Versed

*The term *generic* indicates the drug is available in generic form.

The preanesthetic drug is usually selected by the anesthesiologist and may consist of one or more drugs (Table 9-2). A narcotic (see Chapter 10), antianxiety drug (see Chapter 5), or barbiturate (see Chapter 5) may be given to relax or sedate a patient. Barbiturates are used only occasionally; narcotics are usually preferred for sedation. A cholinergic blocking drug (see Chapter 4) is given to dry secretions in the upper respiratory tract. Scopolamine and glycopyrrolate also have mild sedative properties, and atropine may or may not produce some sedation. Antianxiety drugs have sedative action; when combined with a narcotic, they allow for a lowering of the narcotic dosage because they potentiate the sedative action of the narcotic. Diazepam (Valium), an antianxiety drug, is one of the more commonly used drugs for preoperative sedation.

Contraindications, Precautions, and Interactions of Preanesthetic Drugs

Preanesthetic drugs must be administered on time to produce their intended effects. Failure to give the preanesthetic drug on time may result in events such as increased respiratory secretions caused by the irritating effect of anesthetic gases and the need for a greater dose of the induction drug because the preanesthetic drug has not had time to sedate a patient.

Patient Management Issues with Preanesthetic Drugs

A health care provider, usually a nurse, evaluates the patient's physical status and explains the anesthesia to the patient. In some situations, an anesthesiologist examines the patient the day or evening before surgery. In some hospitals members of the operating room or postanesthesia recovery room staff visit a patient the night before or the morning of surgery to explain certain facts, such as the time of surgery, the effects of the preanesthetic drug, preparations for surgery, and the postanesthesia recovery room. Proper explanation of anesthesia, the surgery itself, and the events that may occur in preparation for surgery, as well as care after surgery, require a team approach.

Examples of preoperative preparations include fasting from midnight (or the time specified by a health care provider), enemas, shaving of the operative site, use of a hypnotic for sleep the night before, and a preoperative injection approximately 30 minutes before going to surgery.

General Anesthetics

Uses of General Anesthetics

General anesthesia is a condition of a pain-free state for the entire body. When a general anesthetic is given, a patient loses consciousness and feels no pain. Reflexes, such as the swallowing and gag reflexes, are lost during deep general anesthesia (Fig. 9-1). An **anesthesiologist** is a physician with special training in administering anesthesia. A nurse **anesthetist** is a nurse with special training who is qualified to administer anesthetics.

General anesthesia results from the use of one or more drugs. The choice of anesthetic drug depends on many factors, including the patient's general physical condition; the area, organ, or body system undergoing surgery; and the anticipated length of the surgical procedure. An anesthesiologist selects the anesthetic drugs that will produce safe anesthesia, **analgesia** (absence of pain), and, for some surgeries, skeletal muscle relaxation.

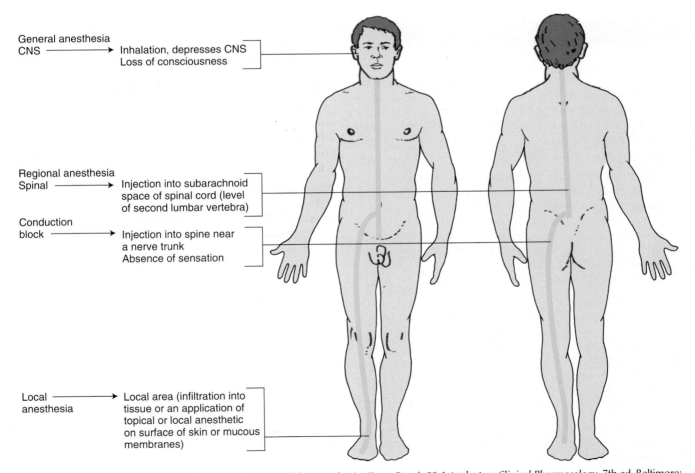

General anesthesia
CNS ⟶ Inhalation, depresses CNS
Loss of consciousness

Regional anesthesia
Spinal ⟶ Injection into subarachnoid space of spinal cord (level of second lumbar vertebra)

Conduction block ⟶ Injection into spine near a nerve trunk
Absence of sensation

Local anesthesia ⟶ Local area (infiltration into tissue or an application of topical or local anesthetic on surface of skin or mucous membranes)

FIGURE 9-1   Sites and mechanisms of action of drugs used for anesthesia. (From Roach SS. *Introductory Clinical Pharmacology*, 7th ed. Baltimore: Lippincott Williams & Wilkins; 2004.)

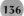

General surgical anesthesia usually has four stages:

- Stage I: analgesia
- Stage II: delirium
- Stage III: surgical analgesia
- Stage IV: respiratory paralysis

Box 9-1 describes the stages of general anesthesia more completely. With newer drugs and techniques, the stages of anesthesia may not be as prominent as those described in Box 9-1. In addition, most patients' movement through the first two stages is very rapid.

Anesthesia begins with a loss of consciousness. This occurs at the end of the induction stage (stage I). The patient relaxes and after becoming unconscious cannot see or hear what is going on. Additional anesthetic drugs are usually administered once the patient is unconscious for deepening anesthesia. Depending on the type of surgery, an endotracheal tube may be inserted into the patient's trachea to ensure an adequate airway and assist in the administration of oxygen and anesthetic drugs. The endotracheal tube is removed during the postanesthesia period when the gag and swallowing reflexes return.

Box 9-1 Stages of General Anesthesia

Stage I
Induction is a part of stage I anesthesia. It begins with the administration of an anesthetic drug and lasts until the patient loses consciousness. With some induction drugs, such as short-acting barbiturates, this stage may last only 5 to 10 seconds.

Stage II
Stage II is a brief stage of delirium and excitement. During this stage, the patient may move about and mumble incoherently, although the patient is unconscious and cannot feel pain. The muscles are somewhat rigid. The patient would have a physical reaction to painful stimuli yet not remember sensing pain. During the first two stages of anesthesia, health care professionals avoid any unnecessary noise or motion around the patient.

Stage III
Stage III is the stage of surgical analgesia, which is usually divided into four planes or substages. The anesthesiologist differentiates these planes by the character of the patient's respirations, eye movements, reflexes, pupil size, and other factors. The level of anesthesia ranges from plane 1 (light) to plane 4 (deep). At plane 2 or 3 the patient is ready for the surgical procedure.

Stage IV
Stage IV is the stage of respiratory paralysis, a rare and dangerous stage of anesthesia. Respiratory arrest may occur.

Administration of General Anesthetics

General anesthetics are most commonly administered by inhalation or intravenously. Volatile liquid anesthetics produce anesthesia when their vapors are inhaled. **Volatile liquids** are liquids that evaporate when exposed to air. Examples of volatile liquids include halothane, desflurane, and enflurane. Gas anesthetics are combined with oxygen and administered by inhalation. Examples of gas anesthetics are nitrous oxide and cyclopropane. Box 9-2 lists commonly used general anesthetics and their uses.

Skeletal Muscle Relaxants

Various skeletal muscle relaxants may be used during general anesthesia (Table 9-3). These drugs are given to produce relaxation of the skeletal muscles during certain types of surgeries, such as those involving the chest or abdomen. They may also be used to facilitate the insertion of an endotracheal tube. Their onset of action is usually rapid (45 seconds to a few minutes), and the duration of action is 30 minutes or more.

Patient Management Issues with General Anesthetics

After surgery a number of patient management issues must be monitored. These include checking the patient's airway for **patency** (being open and clear), assessing the patient's respiratory status and giving oxygen as needed, positioning the patient to prevent aspiration of vomitus and secretions, and checking the patient's blood pressure, pulse, intravenous lines, catheters, drainage tubes, surgical dressings, and casts. The patient's blood pressure, pulse, and respiratory rate may be monitored every 5 to 15 minutes. The patient is checked every 5 to 15 minutes for emergence from anesthesia.

Caution is needed when narcotics are administered after surgery. A patient's respiratory rate, blood pressure, and pulse are taken before these drugs are given and 20 to 30 minutes afterwards (see Chapter 10). The health care provider is contacted if the patient's respiratory rate is below 10 before the drug is given or falls below 10 after the drug is given.

Educating the Patient and Family

Before surgery, the immediate postoperative care is explained to the patient, such as the postanesthesia recovery room or postoperative surgical unit and the activities of physicians, nurses, and other health care workers during this period. The patient is told that his or her vital signs will be monitored frequently and that other equipment, such as intravenous fluids and monitors, may be used.

Box 9-2 **Drugs Used for General Anesthesia**

Methohexital and Thiopental

Methohexital (Brevital) and thiopental (Pentothal), which are ultrashort-acting barbiturates, are used for:

- Induction of anesthesia
- Short surgical procedures with minimal painful stimuli
- In conjunction with or as a supplement to other anesthetics
- Control of convulsive states (thiopental)

These drugs have a rapid onset and a short duration of action. They depress the central nervous system to produce hypnosis and anesthesia but do not produce analgesia. Recovery after a small dose is rapid.

Etomidate

Etomidate (Amidate), a nonbarbiturate, is used for induction of anesthesia. Etomidate also may be used to supplement other anesthetics, such as nitrous oxide, for short surgical procedures. It is a hypnotic without analgesic activity.

Propofol

Propofol (Diprivan) is used for induction and maintenance of anesthesia. It also may be used for sedation during diagnostic procedures and procedures that use a local anesthetic. This drug also is used for continuous sedation of intubated or respiratory-controlled patients in intensive care units.

Midazolam

Midazolam (Versed), a short-acting benzodiazepine central nervous system depressant, is used as a preanesthetic drug to relieve anxiety, for induction of anesthesia, for conscious sedation before minor procedures such as endoscopic procedures, and to supplement nitrous oxide and oxygen for short surgical procedures. When the drug is used for induction anesthesia, the patient gradually loses consciousness during 1 to 2 minutes.

Sevoflurane

Sevoflurane (Ultane) is an inhaled analgesic. It is used for induction and maintenance of general anesthesia in adult and pediatric patients for inpatient and outpatient surgical procedures.

Ketamine

Ketamine (Ketalar) is a rapid-acting general anesthetic. It produces an anesthetic state characterized by profound analgesia, cardiovascular and respiratory stimulation, normal or enhanced skeletal muscle tone, and occasionally mild respiratory depression. Ketamine is used for diagnostic and surgical procedures that do not require relaxation of skeletal muscles, for induction of anesthesia before the administration of other anesthetic drugs, and as a supplement to other anesthetic drugs.

Cyclopropane

An anesthetic gas, cyclopropane has a rapid onset of action and may be used for induction and maintenance of anesthesia. Skeletal muscle relaxation is produced with full anesthetic doses. Disadvantages of cyclopropane are difficulty in detecting the planes of anesthesia, occasional laryngospasm, cardiac arrhythmias, and postanesthesia nausea, vomiting, and headache. Cyclopropane and oxygen mixtures are explosive, which limits the use of this gas anesthetic.

Ethylene

Ethylene is an anesthetic gas with a rapid onset of action and a rapid recovery from its anesthetic effects. It provides adequate analgesia but has poor muscle relaxant properties. The advantages of ethylene include minimal bronchospasm, laryngospasm, and postanesthesia vomiting. A disadvantage of ethylene is hypoxia (low oxygen level in body tissues). Mixtures of ethylene and oxygen are flammable and explosive.

Nitrous Oxide

Nitrous oxide is the most commonly used anesthetic gas. It is a weak anesthetic and is usually used in combination with other anesthetic drugs. It does not cause skeletal muscle relaxation. The chief danger in the use of nitrous oxide is hypoxemia (low arterial oxygen level). Nitrous oxide is nonexplosive.

Enflurane

Enflurane (Ethrane) is a volatile liquid anesthetic that is delivered by inhalation. Induction and recovery from anesthesia are rapid. Muscle relaxation for abdominal surgery is adequate, but greater muscle relaxation may be necessary for other surgeries and may require the use of a skeletal muscle relaxant. Enflurane may produce mild stimulation of respiratory and bronchial secretions when used alone. Hypotension may occur when anesthesia deepens.

Halothane

Halothane (Fluothane) is a volatile liquid given by inhalation for induction and maintenance of anesthesia. Induction and recovery from anesthesia are rapid, and the depth of anesthesia can be rapidly altered. Halothane does not irritate the respiratory tract, and tracheobronchial secretions usually are not increased. Halothane produces moderate muscle relaxation, but skeletal muscle relaxants may be needed for certain types of surgeries. This anesthetic may be given with a mixture of nitrous oxide and oxygen.

Isoflurane

Isoflurane (Forane) is a volatile liquid given by inhalation. It is used for induction and maintenance of anesthesia.

Methoxyflurane

Methoxyflurane (Penthrane), a volatile liquid, provides analgesia and anesthesia. It is usually used in combination with nitrous oxide but may also be used alone. It does not produce good muscle relaxation, and a skeletal muscle relaxant may be required.

Desflurane

Desflurane (Suprane), a volatile liquid, is used for induction and maintenance of anesthesia. A special vaporizer is used to deliver this anesthetic because delivery by mask results in irritation of the respiratory tract.

continues

Box 9-2 **Drugs Used for General Anesthesia**
(continued)

Fentanyl and Droperidol

The narcotic analgesic fentanyl (Sublimaze) and the neuroleptic (major tranquilizer) droperidol (Inapsine) may be used together as a single drug called Innovar. The combination of these two drugs results in **neurolep-tanalgesia**, which is characterized by general quietness, reduced motor activity, and profound analgesia. Complete loss of consciousness may not occur unless other anesthetic drugs are used. A combination of fentanyl and droperidol may be used for the tranquilizing effect and analgesia for surgical and diagnostic procedures. It may also be used as a preanesthetic for the induction of anesthesia and in the maintenance of general anesthesia. Droperidol may be used alone as a tranquilizer, as an antiemetic to prevent nausea and vomiting during the immediate postanesthesia period, as an induction drug, and as an adjunct to general anesthesia. Fentanyl may be used alone as a supplement to general or regional anesthesia. It may also be administered alone or with other drugs as a preoperative drug and as an analgesic during the immediate postoperative (recovery room) period.

Remifentanil Hydrochloride

Remifentanil (Ultiva) is used for induction and maintenance of general anesthesia and for continued analgesia during the immediate postoperative period. This drug is used cautiously in patients with a history of hypersensitivity to fentanyl.

TABLE 9-3 **Examples of Muscle Relaxants Used During General Anesthesia**

Generic Name	Trade Name*
atracurium besylate	Tracrium
cisatracurium besylate	Nimbex
doxacurium chloride	Nuromax
metocurine iodide	Metubine Iodine, *generic*
mivacurium chloride	Mivacron
pancuronium bromide	Pavulon, *generic*
pipecuronium bromide	Arduan
rapacuronium bromide	Raplon
rocuronium bromide	Zemuron
succinylcholine chloride	Anectine, *generic*
tubocurarine chloride	*Generic*
vecuronium bromide	Norcuron, *generic*

*The term *generic* indicates that the drug is available in generic form.

surgery and are referred to as preanesthetic drugs. Cholinergic blocking drugs are used to decrease secretions of the upper respiratory tract. Some anesthetic gases and volatile liquids are irritating to the lining of the respiratory tract and increase mucus secretions. Antiemetics are used to prevent nausea and vomiting during the immediate postoperative recovery period.

◯ Preanesthetic drugs may not be used in patients 60 years or older because many of the medical disorders for which these drugs are contraindicated occur in older individuals.

◯ When a general anesthetic is given, a patient loses consciousness and feels no pain. Reflexes, such as the swallowing and gag reflexes, are lost during deep general anesthesia.

◯ The choice of anesthetic drug depends on many factors, including the patient's general physical condition; the area, organ, or body system being operated on; and the anticipated length of the surgical procedure.

◯ Careful monitoring of a patient is essential after surgery. This usually includes respiratory observation, and checking the patient's pulse, blood pressure, intravenous lines, catheters, drainage tubes, surgical dressings, and casts.

Postoperative patient activities, such as deep breathing, coughing, and leg exercises, are also explained and demonstrated, as appropriate.

KEY POINTS

◯ With a local anesthetic, a patient is fully awake but does not feel pain in the area that has been anesthetized. In some cases the patient may also be sedated.

◯ Local anesthetics may be administered by topical application, local infiltration, or methods to result in regional anesthesia.

◯ Narcotic or antianxiety drugs are used to decrease the patient's anxiety and apprehension immediately before

CASE STUDY

A nurse reports she was reprimanded for not giving a preanesthetic drug on time. She administered the drug 10 minutes before the patient, Sally Smithers, was taken to surgery and placed under general anesthesia. Several hours after the surgery, Ms. Smithers reported that no one told her ahead of time what to expect in the recovery room.

1. How much time should pass between when a preanesthetic drug is administered and surgery commences?
   a. 15 minutes
   b. 30 minutes

c. 45 minutes

    d. 60 minutes

2. What should Ms. Smithers have been informed of before going to surgery?
   a. the physician's and nurse's anticipated activities in the postoperative surgical unit
   b. the weight loss she is anticipated to experience
   c. the necessity of fasting the night before surgery
   d. all of the above

3. If Ms. Smithers had been given ketamine (Ketalar), what type of surgical procedure might she be undergoing?
   a. a procedure in which no relaxation of the skeletal muscles is necessary
   b. a procedure in which relaxation of the skeletal muscles is essential
   c. any outpatient procedure
   d. all of the above

WEBSITE ACTIVITIES

1. Go to the Food and Drug Administration website (www.fda.gov) and conduct a search of the site for nitrous oxide. Write a brief statement about the various uses of nitrous oxide, including any legitimate nonmedical uses.

2. Continuing with the FDA website and nitrous oxide, read any information you uncover about illegal uses of the drug and answer the following questions:
   a. What is the drug's "street name"?
   b. What, if any, recent FDA investigations have taken place regarding nitrous oxide?
   c. Is nitrous oxide as an anesthetic safe for all populations, including children, pregnant and lactating women, etc?

REVIEW QUESTIONS

1. When selecting a drug for general anesthesia, which of the following factors are considered?
   a. the general physical condition of the patient
   b. the time of day the surgery will be conducted
   c. the length of time that has passed since the patient's last general anesthesia
   d. all of the above

2. Which of the following is/are commonly used in obstetrics?
   a. transsacral block
   b. brachial plexus block
   c. epidural block
   d. a and c

3. What is the purpose of cholinergic drugs as preanesthetic drugs?
   a. to decrease secretions of the upper respiratory tract
   b. to decrease anxiety
   c. to prevent postoperative nausea
   d. all of the above

4. Which population is particularly at risk for problems with preanesthetic drugs?
   a. children
   b. patients 60 years or older
   c. pregnant women
   d. anyone weighing less than 100 lbs

KEY TERMS

acute pain—pain that is of short duration and lasts less than 3 to 6 months and can be from mild to severe

agonist–antagonist—a narcotic analgesic that has properties of both the agonist and antagonist

agonist—a category of narcotic analgesic that binds to a receptor and causes a response

analgesic—a drug that alleviates pain

antagonist—a substance that counteracts the action of something else

antipyretic—a drug that reduces elevated body temperature

chronic pain—pain that lasts longer than 6 months and ranges in intensity from mild to severe

epidural—drug administration is performed when a catheter is placed into the epidural space outside of the dura matter of the brain and spinal cord

miosis—pinpoint pupils

opioids—narcotic analgesics obtained from the opium plant

pain—an unpleasant sensory and emotional experience associated with actual or potential tissue damage

partial agonist—a category of narcotic analgesic that binds to a receptor, but the response is limited (i.e., is not as great as with the agonist).

patient-controlled analgesia—a method of pain relief that allows patients to administer their own analgesic by means of an intravenous pump system

Reye syndrome—a life-threatening condition characterized by vomiting and lethargy, progressing to coma

salicylates—drugs that have analgesic, antipyretic, and anti-inflammatory effects

salicylism—a condition produced by salicylate toxicity

tinnitus—ringing sound in the ear

CHAPTER OBJECTIVES

On completion of this chapter, students will be able to:

1 Define the chapter's key terms.

2 Describe the uses, general drug actions, common adverse reactions, contraindications, precautions, and interactions of analgesic and antagonist drugs.

3 Discuss important points to keep in mind when educating the patient and family about the use of analgesic and antagonist drugs.

Pain is an unpleasant sensory and emotional experience that is associated with actual or potential tissue damage. Pain is subjective, and the patient's report of pain should always be taken seriously. Pain management in acute and chronic illness is an important responsibility of health care providers. Many practitioners consider pain as the fifth vital sign and the assessment of pain to be just as important as the assessment of temperature, pulse, respirations, and blood pressure. Accurate assessment of pain is necessary if pain management is to be effective. Patients with pain are often undertreated.

Basically there are three types of pain: acute pain, chronic pain associated with malignant disease, and chronic pain not associated with malignant disease. **Acute pain** is of short duration and lasts less than 3 to 6 months. The intensity of acute pain is from mild to severe. Causes of acute pain include postoperative pain, procedural pain, and traumatic pain. Acute pain usually subsides when the injury heals.

Chronic pain lasts longer than 6 months and ranges in intensity from mild to severe. Chronic pain associated with a malignancy includes the pain of cancer, acquired immunodeficiency syndrome (AIDS), multiple sclerosis, sickle cell disease, and end-stage organ system failure.

A patient's exact cause of chronic pain of a nonmalignant nature may or may not be known. This type of pain includes the pain associated with various neuropathic and musculoskeletal disorders such as headaches, fibromyalgia, rheumatoid arthritis, and osteoarthritis.

This chapter deals with drugs used in the management of pain: nonnarcotic analgesics (salicylates, nonsalicylates, and the nonsteroidal anti-inflammatory drugs [NSAIDs]) and narcotic analgesics. **Analgesics** are drugs that relieve pain. This chapter also includes narcotic antagonists, which are used to counteract the effects of narcotics.

Nonnarcotic analgesics are a group of drugs used to relieve pain without the possibility of causing physical dependency, which can occur with the use of the narcotic analgesics. Nonnarcotic analgesics include salicylates, nonsalicylates (such as acetaminophen), and the NSAIDs. A number of combination nonnarcotic analgesics are available over the counter and by prescription. NSAIDs have emerged as important drugs in the treatment of the chronic pain and inflammation associated with disorders such as rheumatoid arthritis and osteoarthritis. Examples of NSAIDs include celecoxib (Celebrex) and rofecoxib (Vioxx).

Salicylates

Actions of Salicylates

The **salicylates** include aspirin (acetylsalicylic acid) and related drugs, such as magnesium salicylate and sodium salicylate. The salicylates have analgesic (relieves pain), **antipyretic** (reduces elevated body temperature), and anti-inflammatory effects. All the salicylates are similar in pharmacologic activity, but aspirin has a greater anti-inflammatory effect than the other salicylates. Specific salicylates are listed in the Summary Drug Table: Nonnarcotic Analgesics: Salicylates and Nonsalicylates.

The manner in which salicylates relieve pain and reduce inflammation is not fully understood. It is thought that the analgesic action of the salicylates is caused by the inhibition of prostaglandins. Prostaglandins are fatty acid derivatives found in almost every tissue of the body and body fluid. Release of prostaglandin is thought to increase the sensitivity of peripheral pain receptors. The inhibitory action of salicylates on the prostaglandins is also thought to account for the anti-inflammatory activity. Salicylates lower an elevated body temperature by dilating peripheral blood vessels, which in turn cools the body.

Aspirin more potently inhibits prostaglandin synthesis and has greater anti-inflammatory effects than other salicylates. In addition, aspirin also prolongs bleeding time by inhibiting the aggregation (clumping) of platelets. It takes a longer time for the blood to clot after a cut, surgery, or other injury to the skin or mucous membranes. Other salicylates do not have as great an effect on platelets as aspirin. This effect of aspirin on platelets is irreversible and lasts for the life of the platelet (7–10 days).

Uses of Salicylates

The salicylate nonnarcotic analgesics are used for the following purposes:

- Relief of mild to moderate pain
- Reduction of elevated body temperature (except for diflunisal, which is not used as an antipyretic)

- Treatment of inflammatory conditions, such as rheumatoid arthritis, osteoarthritis, and rheumatic fever
- Reduction of the risk of myocardial infarction in those with unstable angina or previous myocardial infarction (aspirin only)
- Reduction of the risk of transient ischemic attacks or strokes in men who have had transient ischemia of the brain caused by fibrin platelet emboli (aspirin only), although this use has not been found effective in women

Adverse Reactions of Salicylates

Gastric upset, heartburn, nausea, vomiting, anorexia, and gastrointestinal bleeding may occur with salicylate use. Although these drugs are relatively safe when taken as recommended, their use can occasionally result in more serious reactions. Some individuals are allergic to aspirin and other salicylates. Salicylate allergy causes hives, rash, angioedema, bronchospasm with asthma-like symptoms, and anaphylactoid reactions.

Loss of blood through the gastrointestinal tract occurs with salicylate use. The amount of blood lost is insignificant with one normal dose. However, use of these drugs over a long period, even in normal doses, can result in a significant blood loss.

Salicylate toxicity produces a condition called **salicylism**. The symptoms of this condition are listed in Box 10-1. Mild salicylism usually occurs with repeated administration of large doses of a salicylate. This condition is reversible with reduction of the drug dosage.

Managing Adverse Reactions of Salicylates

When high doses of salicylates are administered (such as for severe arthritic disorders), the patient should be observed for signs of salicylism. If signs of salicylism occur,

Box 10-1 **Symptoms of Salicylism**
• Dizziness • Tinnitus (a ringing sound in the ear) • Impaired hearing • Nausea • Vomiting • Flushing • Sweating • Rapid deep breathing • Tachycardia • Diarrhea • Mental confusion • Lassitude • Drowsiness • Respiratory depression and coma (large doses)

SUMMARY DRUG TABLE   Nonnarcotic Analgesics: Salicylates and Nonsalicylates

Generic Name	Trade Name	Uses	Adverse Reactions	Dosage Ranges
Salicylates aspirin (acetylsalicylic acid) *ass'-purr-in*	Bayer, Ecotrin, Empirin, *generic*	Analgesic, antipyretic, anti-inflammatory	Nausea, vomiting, epigastric distress, gastrointestinal bleeding, tinnitus, allergic and anaphylactic reactions; salicylism with overuse	325–650 mg PO with up to 8 g/d PO in divided doses; 325–650 mg rectally
buffered aspirin *ass'-purr-in*	Ascriptin, Asprimox, Buffered Aspirin, Buffex, *generic*	Same as aspirin	Same as aspirin	Same as aspirin
choline salicylate *co-leen'-sal-ih'-sah-late*	Arthropan	Same as aspirin	Same as aspirin	870 mg q3–4h (maximum 6 times/d)
diflunisal *dye-floo-'ni-sal*	Dolobid, *generic*	Same as aspirin	Same as aspirin	500–1000 mg/d in 2 divided doses (maximum dose, 1.5 g/d)
magnesium salicylate *mag-nee'-see-um-sal-ih'-sah-late*	Extra Strength Doan's, Magan, Mobidin	Same as aspirin	Same as aspirin	600 mg PO q4h or 1160 mg TID PRN
salsalate *sal-sa'-late*	Amigesic, Disalcid, Salflex, Salsitab, *generic*	Same as aspirin	Same as aspirin	3000 mg/d PO in divided doses
sodium salicylate *soe-de-yum-sal-ih'-sah-late*	*Generic*	Same as aspirin	Same as aspirin	325–650 mg PO q4h
sodium thiosalicylate *soe-de-yum-thi-oh-sal-ih'-sah-late*	Rexolate, *generic*	Same as aspirin	Same as aspirin	50–150 mg IM q4–6h
Nonsalicylate acetaminophen *a-sea-tah-min'-oh-fen*	Temptra, Tylenol, *generic*	Analgesic, antipyretic	Rare when used as directed; skin eruptions, urticaria, hemolytic anemia, pancytopenia, jaundice, hepatotoxicity	325–650 mg/d PO q4–6h or 1 g PO 3–4 times daily; maximum dose, 4 g/d

* The term *generic* indicates the drug is available in generic form.

then the health care provider should be notified before the next dose is given because a reduction in dose or determination of the plasma salicylate level may be necessary. Therapeutic salicylate levels are between 100 and 300 mcg/mL. Symptoms associated with different salicylate levels are as follows:

- Levels greater than 150 mcg/mL may result in symptoms of mild salicylism, such as **tinnitus** (ringing in the ears), difficulty in hearing, dizziness, nausea, vomiting, diarrhea, mental confusion, central nervous system depression, headache, sweating, and hyperventilation (rapid, deep breathing).
- Levels greater than 250 mcg/mL may result in symptoms of mild salicylism plus headache, diarrhea, thirst, and flushing.
- Levels greater than 400 mcg/mL may result in respiratory alkalosis, hemorrhage, excitement, confusion, asterixis (involuntary jerking movements especially of the hands), pulmonary edema, convulsions, tetany (muscle spasms), fever, coma, shock, and renal and respiratory failure.

ALERT

Salicylate Gastrointestinal Toxicity

Serious gastrointestinal toxicity can cause bleeding, ulceration, and perforation that may occur at any time during therapy, with or without symptoms. Although minor gastrointestinal problems are common, patients receiving long-term therapy may experience ulceration and bleeding, even if they experienced no previous gastric symptoms.

The color of the patient's stools must be checked. Black or dark stools or bright red blood in the stool may indicate gastrointestinal bleeding. Any change in the color of the stool should be reported to the health care provider.

A patient given salicylates must be monitored for signs and symptoms of acute salicylate toxicity or salicylism (see Box 10-1). The initial treatment includes inducing emesis (vomiting) or gastric lavage to remove any unabsorbed drug from the stomach. Activated charcoal diminishes salicylate absorption if given within 2 hours of ingestion. Further therapy is supportive. Hemodialysis is effective in removing the salicylate but is used only in patients with severe salicylism.

The patient also should be assessed for tinnitus or impaired hearing. Tinnitus or impaired hearing probably indicates high blood salicylate levels. If this is suspected, then the drug should be withheld and any sensory alterations reported immediately. It should be explained to the patient that any hearing loss will disappear after the drug therapy is discontinued.

GERONTOLOGIC ALERT

Salicylates

Salicylates are often prescribed for the pain and inflammation of arthritis. Because older adults have a higher incidence of both rheumatoid arthritis and osteoarthritis and may use nonnarcotic analgesics on a long-term basis, they are particularly vulnerable to gastrointestinal bleeding. Patients should be encouraged to take the drug with a full glass of water or with food because this may decrease the gastrointestinal effects.

ALERT

Salicylates in Children

Studies suggest that the use of salicylates (especially aspirin) may be involved in the development of **Reye syndrome** in children with chickenpox or influenza. This rare but life-threatening disorder is characterized by vomiting and lethargy, progressing to coma. Therefore, use of salicylates is not recommended for children with chickenpox, fever, or flu-like symptoms. Acetaminophen is recommended instead.

Contraindications, Precautions, and Interactions of Salicylates

The salicylates are contraindicated in patients with known hypersensitivity and in pregnant women. Aspirin is a pregnancy category D drug and may produce adverse maternal effects (such as anemia, postpartum hemorrhage, and prolonged gestation or labor). Aspirin used in pregnancy may also cause adverse fetal effects, such as low birth weight, intracranial hemorrhage in premature infants, stillbirth, or neonatal death. Other salicylates (salsalate and magnesium salicylate) are pregnancy category C drugs.

Because the salicylates prolong bleeding time, they are contraindicated in those with bleeding disorders or bleeding tendencies. These include patients with gastrointestinal bleeding (attributed to any cause), blood dyscrasias, and those receiving anticoagulant or antineoplastic drugs. Children or teenagers with influenza or chickenpox should not take the salicylates, particularly aspirin.

The salicylates are used cautiously in patients with hepatic or renal disease, preexisting hypoprothrombinemia, or vitamin K deficiency and during lactation. The drugs are also used with caution in patients with gastrointestinal irritation such as peptic ulcers, mild diabetes, or gout.

Food containing salicylate (curry powder, paprika, licorice, prunes, raisins, and tea) may increase the risk of adverse reactions. Coadministration of a salicylate with activated charcoal decreases the absorption of the salicylate. Antacids may decrease the effects of the salicylate. Coadministration with a carbonic anhydrase inhibitor increases the risk of salicylism. Aspirin may increase the risk of bleeding during heparin administration. Coadministration with a nonsteroidal anti-inflammatory drug (NSAID) may increase the blood levels.

Natural Remedies: Willow Bark

Willow bark has a long history of use as an analgesic, dating back to the time of Hippocrates, when it was common for patients to chew on the bark to reduce fever or inflammation. Its other important medicinal quality is to relieve pain. When used as a medicinal herb, willow bark is collected in early spring from young willow branches, when the bark is most tender. White willow in particular is used medicinally.

Salicylate was originally isolated from willow bark and identified as the most likely source of the bark's anti-inflammatory effects. Its chemical structure was replicated in the laboratory and mass-produced as synthetic salicylic acid. Years later, a modified version (acetylsalicylic acid) was first sold as aspirin. Aspirin became the most widely used pain reliever, fever reducer, and anti-inflammatory agent, and willow bark lost popularity. Synthetic anti-inflammatory drugs work quickly and have a higher potency than willow bark. Willow bark takes longer to work and may have to be taken in fairly high doses to achieve a noticeable effect. However, willow bark has fewer adverse reactions than salicylates. Although adverse reactions are rare with willow bark, it should be used with caution in patients with peptic ulcers and medical conditions in which aspirin is contraindicated, including patients taking blood-thinning medications such as warfarin. Patients taking anticoagulant or antiplatelet medications should avoid the use of willow bark altogether.

Willow bark is also purported to help with sexual dysfunction, diarrhea, tendonitis, bursitis, and some forms of arthritis. Scientific study has been insufficient to verify the accuracy of these claims.

In the United States, the Food and Drug Administration classifies willow bark as an herb. It is available as an over-the-counter (OTC) drug and is commonly consumed in tea and tincture form.

Nonsalicylate Analgesics

The major drug classified as a nonsalicylate analgesic is acetaminophen (Tylenol, Datril, Panadol). Acetaminophen is the only drug of this kind available in the United States at this time. It is the most widely used aspirin substitute for patients who are allergic to aspirin or who experience extreme gastric upset when taking aspirin. Acetaminophen is also the drug of choice for treating children with fever and flu-like symptoms.

Actions of Nonsalicylate Analgesics

The mechanism of action of acetaminophen is unknown. Like the salicylates, acetaminophen has both analgesic and antipyretic activity. However, acetaminophen does not have an anti-inflammatory action and is of no value in the treatment of inflammation or inflammatory disorders.

Uses of Nonsalicylate Analgesics

Acetaminophen is used to relieve mild to moderate pain and to reduce elevated body temperature (fever). This drug is particularly useful for those with aspirin allergy and bleeding disorders, such as bleeding ulcer or hemophilia, those receiving anticoagulant therapy, and those who have recently had minor surgical procedures. Although acetaminophen has no anti-inflammatory action, it may be used to relieve the pain and discomfort associated with arthritic disorders.

Adverse Reactions of Nonsalicylate Analgesics

Acetaminophen causes few adverse reactions when used as recommended. Adverse reactions associated with the use of acetaminophen usually occur with long-term use or when the recommended dosage is exceeded. Adverse reactions include skin eruptions, urticaria (hives), hemolytic anemia, pancytopenia (a reduction in all cellular components of the blood), hypoglycemia, jaundice (yellow discoloration of the skin), hepatotoxicity (damage to the liver), and hepatic failure (seen in chronic alcoholics taking the drug).

Acute acetaminophen poisoning or toxicity can occur after a single 10- to 15-g dose of acetaminophen. Dosages of 20 to 25 g may be fatal. With excessive dosages the liver cells necrose (die). Death can occur because of liver failure. The risk of liver failure is higher in chronic alcoholics.

Signs of acute acetaminophen toxicity include the following:

- nausea
- vomiting
- confusion
- liver tenderness
- hypotension
- arrhythmias
- jaundice
- acute hepatic and renal failure

Managing Adverse Reactions to Nonsalicylate Analgesics

Acetaminophen is usually well-tolerated, and few adverse reactions are seen if the drug is given in recommended amounts. It is important not to exceed the recommended dosage. If a patient is an alcoholic or chronic user of alcohol, then acetaminophen intake is limited to no more than 2 g/d.

ALERT

Acetaminophen Toxicity

Any signs of acetaminophen toxicity, such as nausea, vomiting, anorexia, malaise, diaphoresis, abdominal pain, confusion, liver tenderness, hypotension, arrhythmias, jaundice, and acute hepatic and renal failure, must be reported immediately to the health care provider. Early diagnosis is important because liver failure may be reversible.

Toxicity is treated with gastric lavage, preferably within 4 hours of ingestion of the acetaminophen. Liver function studies are performed frequently. Acetylcysteine (Mucomyst) is an antidote to acetaminophen toxicity, protecting liver cells and destroying acetaminophen metabolites. It is administered by nebulization within 24 hours after ingestion of the drug and after the gastric lavage. In lieu of gastric lavage, the health care provider may prescribe syrup of ipecac to induce vomiting.

Contraindications, Precautions, and Interactions of Nonsalicylate Analgesics

Hypersensitivity to acetaminophen is a contraindication.

Hepatotoxicity has occurred in chronic alcoholics after therapeutic dosages. Patients taking acetaminophen should avoid alcohol if taking more than an occasional dose of acetaminophen and should avoid taking acetaminophen concurrently with a salicylate or NSAID. Acetaminophen is classified as pregnancy category B and can be used cautiously during pregnancy and lactation. If an analgesic is necessary, then it appears safe for short-term use. The drug is used cautiously in patients with severe or recurrent pain or high or continued fever, which may indicate the presence of a serious illness. If pain persists for more than 5 days or if redness or swelling is present, then the health care provider should be consulted.

GERONTOLOGIC ALERT

Acetaminophen

An older adult with liver damage should use acetaminophen only with caution.

Acetaminophen may alter blood glucose test results, causing falsely lower blood glucose values. Use with barbiturates, hydantoins, isoniazid, or rifampin may increase the toxic effects and possibly decrease the therapeutic effects of acetaminophen. The effects of loop diuretics may be decreased when administered with acetaminophen. Hepatotoxicity has occurred in chronic alcoholics taking moderate doses of acetaminophen.

Patient Management Issues with Salicylates and Nonsalicylates

The patient should be monitored for relief of pain. If pain recurs, then its severity, location, and intensity should be assessed. In inpatients, the vital signs are monitored every 4 hours or more frequently if necessary. Hot, dry, flushed skin and decreased urinary output may develop with prolonged fever, and dehydration may occur. The patient's joints are assessed for reduced inflammation and greater mobility.

Any adverse reactions, such as unusual or prolonged bleeding or dark stools, must be reported to the health care provider.

ALERT

Acetaminophen Use

The patient's overall health and alcohol usage must be assessed before acetaminophen is prescribed. Patients who are malnourished or abuse alcohol are at risk for hepatotoxicity (damage to the liver) with the use of acetaminophen.

Some health care providers may not prescribe an antipyretic for patients with an elevated temperature because of evidence suggesting that fever activates the immune system to produce disease-fighting antibodies. The decision to treat an elevated temperature with an antipyretic depends in part on the cause of the fever and the patient's physical condition.

A patient receiving these drugs may have an acute or chronic disorder with varying degrees of mobility. The patient may be in acute pain or have longstanding mild to moderate pain. These patients may need help walking or with other activities.

Salicylates are given with food, milk, or a full glass of water to prevent gastric upset. If gastric distress occurs, then the health care provider is notified because other drug therapy may be necessary. An antacid may be prescribed to minimize gastrointestinal distress.

Patients should not take salicylates for at least 1 week before any type of major or minor surgery, including dental surgery, because of the possibility of postoperative bleeding. In addition, patients should not use salicylates after any type of surgery until complete healing has occurred. A patient may use acetaminophen or an

NSAID after surgery or a dental procedure when relief of mild pain is necessary.

Acetaminophen is taken with a full glass of water. A patient may take this drug with meals or on an empty stomach.

Nonsteroidal Anti-inflammatory Drugs (NSAIDs)

The nonsteroidal anti-inflammatory drug (NSAID) group contains more than 70 drugs, with new drugs frequently becoming available. Some texts include the salicylates within the NSAID group, whereas others do not. Their chemical and physiologic effects are similar. The NSAIDs are also nonnarcotic analgesics. This section covers the NSAID group generally and describes four commonly used NSAIDs in more specifics: celecoxib (Celebrex), ibuprofen (Advil), naproxen (Naprosyn), and rofecoxib (Vioxx). Other NSAIDs are listed in the Summary Drug Table: Nonsteroidal Anti-inflammatory Drugs. Like salicylates, NSAIDs have anti-inflammatory, antipyretic, and analgesic effects.

Actions of NSAIDs

NSAIDs are so named because they are not steroids and thus do not cause the adverse reactions associated with steroids (see Chapter 23), yet they have anti-inflammatory effects along with their analgesic and antipyretic properties. Although their exact mechanisms of actions are not known, NSAIDs are thought to act by inhibiting prostaglandin synthesis by inhibiting the action of the enzyme cyclooxygenase, which is responsible for prostaglandin synthesis. The anti-inflammatory effects of the NSAIDs result from inhibition of cyclooxygenase-2 (COX-2). The gastrointestinal adverse reactions are caused by inhibition of cyclooxygenase-1 (COX-1).

The newer NSAIDs (celecoxib and rofecoxib) appear to work by specifically inhibiting the COX-2 enzyme without inhibiting the COX-1 enzyme. Celecoxib and rofecoxib relieve pain and inflammation with less potential for gastrointestinal adverse reactions. Traditional NSAIDs, such as ibuprofen and naproxen, are thought to reduce pain and inflammation by blocking COX-2. Unlike celecoxib and rofecoxib, these drugs also inhibit COX-1, the enzyme that helps maintain the lining of the stomach. This inhibition of COX-1 causes the unwanted gastrointestinal reactions, such as stomach irritation and ulcers.

Uses of NSAIDs

The individual NSAIDs have a variety of uses, including the following conditions:

- relief of signs and symptoms of osteoarthritis, rheumatoid arthritis, and other musculoskeletal disorders

- mild to moderate pain relief
- primary dysmenorrhea (painful menstruation)
- fever reduction

Other uses of individual NSAIDs are given in the Summary Drug Table: Nonsteroidal Anti-inflammatory Drugs.

General Adverse Reactions of NSAIDs

Many adverse reactions are associated with the use of NSAIDs, although many patients take these drugs and experience few, if any, of these effects. Adverse reactions include the following:

- Gastrointestinal: nausea, vomiting, diarrhea, constipation, epigastric pain, indigestion, abdominal distress or discomfort, intestinal ulceration, stomatitis, jaundice, bloating, anorexia, and dry mouth
- Central nervous system: dizziness, anxiety, lightheadedness, vertigo, headache, drowsiness, insomnia, confusion, depression, and psychic disturbances
- Cardiovascular: congestive heart failure, decreased or increased blood pressure, and cardiac arrhythmias
- Renal: hematuria, cystitis, elevated blood urea nitrogen, polyuria, dysuria, oliguria, and acute renal failure in those with impaired renal function
- The senses: visual disturbances, blurred or diminished vision, diplopia, swollen or irritated eyes, photophobia, reversible loss of color vision, tinnitus, taste change, and rhinitis
- Hematologic: neutropenia, eosinophilia, leukopenia, pancytopenia, thrombocytopenia, agranulocytosis, and aplastic anemia
- Skin: rash, erythema, irritation, skin eruptions, exfoliative dermatitis, Stevens-Johnson syndrome, ecchymosis (bruising), and purpura
- Metabolic/endocrinologic: decreased appetite, weight increase or decrease, hyperglycemia, hypoglycemia, flushing, sweating, menstrual disorders, and vaginal bleeding
- Other: thirst, fever, chills, and vaginitis

Common Adverse Reactions of Specific NSAIDs

Celecoxib

The most common adverse reactions of celecoxib include dyspepsia (upset stomach), abdominal pain, diarrhea, nausea, and headache. Like other NSAIDs, celecoxib may compromise renal function. Aminotransferase levels may be elevated.

Ibuprofen

This drug is available over the counter without a prescription. The drug is used in children with juvenile arthritis and for fever reduction in children 6 months to

SUMMARY DRUG TABLE   Nonsteroidal Anti-Inflammatory Drugs

Generic Name	Trade Name*	Uses	Adverse Reactions	Dosage Ranges
celecoxib *sell-ah-cocx'-ib*	Celebrex	Acute and long-term treatment of the signs and symptoms of rheumatoid arthritis and osteoarthritis; reduction of the number of colorectal polyps in familial adenomatous polyposis	Headache, dizziness, somnolence, insomnia, dyspepsia, rash, fatigue, ophthalmic changes	100–200 mg PO BID as needed.
diclofenac sodium *dye-kloe'-fen-ak*	Voltaren, *generic*	Signs and symptoms of rheumatoid arthritis and osteoarthritis, ankylosing spondylitis	Nausea, gastric or duodenal ulcer formation, gastrointestinal (GI) bleeding	Osteoarthritis: 100–150 mg/d PO in divided doses; rheumatoid arthritis: 150–200 mg/d PO in divided doses; ankylosing spondylitis: 100–125 mg/d PO in divided doses
diclofenac potassium	Cataflam, *generic*	Signs and symptoms of rheumatoid arthritis and osteoarthritis, ankylosing spondylitis	Nausea, gastric or duodenal ulcer formation, gastrointestinal (GI) bleeding	Osteoarthritis: 50 mg PO BID–TID Rheumatoid arthritis: 50 mg PO BID–TID Ankylosing spondylitis: 25 mg PO QID with 25 mg hs PRN
etodolac *ee-toe-doe'-lak*	Lodine, Lodine XL, *generic*	Osteoarthritis, mild to moderate pain, rheumatoid arthritis	Dizziness, tiredness, nausea, dyspepsia, rash, constipation, bleeding, diarrhea	Osteoarthritis, rheumatoid arthritis: Maintenance, 600–1200 mg/d in divided doses. Maximum dose 1200 mg/d
fenoprofen calcium *fen-oh-proe'-fen*	Nalfon, *generic*	Signs and symptoms of rheumatoid arthritis and osteoarthritis, long-term management of mild to moderate pain	Dizziness, visual disturbances, jaundice, nausea, vomiting, peptic ulcer	Rheumatoid arthritis and osteoarthritis: 300–600 mg PO TID, QID: pain: 200 mg PO q4–8h
flurbiprofen *flure-bi'-proe-fen*	Ansaid, *generic*	Signs and symptoms of rheumatoid arthritis and osteoarthritis	Nausea, vomiting, diarrhea, constipation, gastric or duodenal ulcer formation, GI bleeding, headache	Up to 300 mg/d PO in divided doses
ibuprofen *eye-byoo'-proe-fen*	Advil, Genpril, Nuprin, Motrin, *generic*	Mild to moderate pain, rheumatoid disorders, painful dysmenorrhea	Nausea, dizziness, somnolence, dyspepsia, gastric or duodenal ulcer formation, GI bleeding, headache	Arthritis disorders: 1.2–3.2 g/d PO in divided doses; pain: 400 mg PO q4–6h; dysmenorrhea: 400 mg PO q4h

Generic Name	Trade Name*	Uses	Adverse Reactions	Dosage Ranges
indomethacin *in-doe-meth'-a-sin*	Indocin, *generic*	Rheumatoid arthritis, ankylosing spondylitis, moderate to severe osteoarthritis, acute painful shoulder, acute gouty arthritis	Nausea, constipation, gastric or duodenal ulcer formation, GI bleeding, hematologic changes	Anti-inflammatory and analgesic: 25–50 mg PO BID–TID not to exceed 200 mg/d Acute painful shoulder: 75–150 mg/d PO in 3–4 divided doses
ketoprofen *kee-toe-proe'-fen*	Orudis, Oruvail, *generic*	Mild to moderate pain, rheumatoid disorders, painful dysmenorrhea	Dizziness, visual disturbances, nausea, constipation, vomiting, diarrhea, gastric or duodenal ulcer formation, GI bleeding	Arthritis: 150–300 mg/d in divided doses; Primary dysmenorrhea: 25–50 mg q6–8h PRN
ketorolac *kee'-toe-role-ak*	Toradol, *generic*	Short-term management of pain; osteoarthritis, rheumatoid arthritis	Dyspepsia, nausea, GI pain, pain at injection site, drowsiness	30–60 mg IM initially, followed by half the initial dose q6h PRN; 10 mg q4–6h PO, PRN; maximum dose, 40 mg/d
meclofenamate *me-kloe-fen-am'-ate*	*Generic*	Rheumatoid arthritis; mild to moderate pain; dysmenorrhea	Headache, dizziness, tiredness, insomnia, nausea, dyspepsia, constipation, rash, bleeding	Rheumatoid arthritis: 200–400 mg/d PO in 3–4 doses; pain: 50 mg q4–6h, maximum dose, 400 mg/d; dysmenorrhea: 100 mg PO TID
mefenamic acid *me-fe-nam'-ik*	Ponstel	Moderate pain that does not exceed 1 wk	Dizziness, tiredness, nausea, dyspepsia, rash, constipation, bleeding, diarrhea	500 mg followed by 250 mg q6h PO PRN, maximum dose, 1 wk of therapy
meloxicam *mel-ox'-i-kam*	Mobic	Osteoarthritis	Nausea, dyspepsia, GI pain, headache, dizziness, somnolence, insomnia, rash	7.5–15 mg PO QD
nabumetone *nah-byew'-meh-tone*	Relafen	Rheumatoid arthritis and osteoarthritis	Dizziness, tiredness, nausea, dyspepsia, rash, constipation, bleeding, diarrhea	1000–2000 mg/d PO
naproxen *na-prox'-en*	Aleve, Anaprox, Naprosyn, Naprelan, *generic*	Management of inflammatory disorders including rheumatoid arthritis and osteoarthritis, management of mild to moderate pain, treatment of dysmenorrhea	Dizziness, visual disturbances, headache, nausea, vomiting, gastric or duodenal ulcer formation, GI bleeding	Pain, primary dysmenorrhea: 500 mg initially then 250 mg q6–8h; arthritic disorders: 250–500 mg PO BID
oxaprozin *oks-a-pro'-zin*	Daypro	Rheumatoid arthritis and osteoarthritis	Dizziness, tiredness, nausea, dyspepsia, rash, constipation, bleeding, diarrhea	1200 mg PO QD

Generic Name	Trade Name*	Uses	Adverse Reactions	Dosage Ranges
piroxicam *peer-ox'-i-kam*	Feldene, *generic*	Mild to moderate pain, rheumatoid arthritis and osteoarthritis	Nausea, vomiting, diarrhea, drowsiness, gastric or duodenal ulcer formation, GI bleeding	20 mg/d PO as a single dose or 10 mg PO BID
rofecoxib *roh-fah-cox'-ib*	Vioxx	Signs and symptoms of osteoarthritis, management of acute pain, primary dysmenorrhea	Same as celecoxib	Osteoarthritis: 12.5 mg or 25 mg/d PO Dysmenorrhea and acute pain: 50 mg PO QD for no more than 5 days
sulindac *sul-in'-dak*	Clinoril, *generic*	Mild to moderate pain, rheumatoid arthritis, ankylosing spondylitis, osteoarthritis, gouty arthritis	Nausea, vomiting, diarrhea, constipation, gastric or duodenal ulcer formation, GI bleeding	150–200 mg PO BID for 1–2 wk, then reduce dose (not to exceed 400 mg/d)
tolmetin sodium *tole'-met-in*	Tolectin	Mild to moderate pain, rheumatoid arthritis and osteoarthritis	Nausea, vomiting, diarrhea, constipation, gastric or duodenal ulcer formation, GI bleeding	400 mg PO TID or BID, not to exceed 2 g/d
valdecoxib *val-dah-cox'-hib*	Bextra	Osteoarthritis, rheumatoid arthritis, primary dysmenorrhea	Headache, nausea, dyspepsia, abdominal pain, anemia	Arthritis 10 mg/d PO; primary dysmenorrhea, 20 mg BID PRN

*The term *generic* indicates the drug is available in generic form.

12 years. Common adverse reactions of ibuprofen include headache, dizziness, drowsiness, nausea, dyspepsia, gastrointestinal pain, and rash.

Naproxen

Common adverse reactions of naproxen include headache, vertigo (dizziness), drowsiness, insomnia, nausea, dyspepsia, gastrointestinal pain, and rash.

Rofecoxib

Common adverse reactions of rofecoxib include headache, dizziness, drowsiness, insomnia, dyspnea (shortness of breath), hemoptysis (pulmonary or bronchial bleeding), and rash.

Managing Adverse Reactions of NSAIDs

A patient receiving an NSAID must be monitored for adverse drug reactions throughout therapy. Because these drugs can cause many adverse reactions, the health care provider must be notified of any symptoms of the patient. Gastrointestinal reactions are the most common and can be severe and sometimes fatal, especially in those prone to upper gastrointestinal disease.

ALERT

NSAIDs

The health care provider should be notified immediately, and the next dosage of the NSAID withheld, if any gastric symptoms occur, especially nausea, vomiting, diarrhea, evidence of bleeding (blood in stool, tarry stools), or abdominal pain.

NSAIDs may cause visual disturbances. Any symptoms of blurred or diminished vision or changes in color vision should be reported to the health care provider. Corneal deposits and retinal disturbances may also occur. Therapy may be discontinued if ocular changes are noted. Because some patients do not notice visual changes, patients on long-term therapy require periodic eye examinations.

General Contraindications, Precautions, and Interactions of NSAIDs

NSAIDs are contraindicated in patients with known hypersensitivity to any NSAID, because these drugs have a cross-sensitivity. Hypersensitivity to aspirin is a contraindication for all NSAIDs. NSAIDs are contraindicated during the third trimester of pregnancy and during lactation.

NSAIDs are used cautiously in the elderly and in patients with bleeding disorders, renal disease, cardiovascular disease, or hepatic impairment. Patients older than 65 years taking NSAIDs have an increased risk of ulcer formation. Most NSAIDs are classified as pregnancy category B. In general, NSAIDs are used with extreme caution during early pregnancy, especially in large doses.

NSAIDs prolong bleeding time and increase the effects of anticoagulants, lithium, cyclosporine, and the hydantoins. These drugs may decrease the effects of diuretics or antihypertensive drugs. Long-term use of NSAIDs with acetaminophen may increase the risk of renal impairment.

Contraindications, Precautions, and Interactions of Specific NSAIDs

Celecoxib

Celecoxib is contraindicated in patients who are allergic to the drug or to sulfonamides, other NSAIDs, or aspirin. It also is contraindicated during pregnancy (category C) and lactation.

The drug is used cautiously in patients with a history of peptic ulcer, patients older than 60 years, and patients taking an anticoagulant or steroids. In rare instances, serious stomach problems such as bleeding can occur without warning. When celecoxib is given with an anticoagulant, the patient has an increased risk for bleeding.

Ibuprofen

Ibuprofen is contraindicated in individuals who are allergic to the drug or other NSAIDs; in patients with hypertension, peptic ulceration, or gastrointestinal bleeding; and during pregnancy (category B) and lactation. The drug is used cautiously in patients with renal or liver dysfunction.

When ibuprofen is taken with lithium, the patient has an increased risk of lithium toxicity. Ibuprofen may cause a diuretic to have a decreased effect when they are taken together. Ibuprofen may cause a decreased antihypertensive effect of beta-adrenergic blocking drugs.

Naproxen

Naproxen is contraindicated in patients who are allergic to the drug or to other NSAIDs. It is also contraindicated during pregnancy (category B) and lactation. The drug is used cautiously in patients with asthma, hypertension, cardiac problems, peptic ulcer disease, or impaired liver or kidney function.

Like ibuprofen, naproxen increases the risk of lithium toxicity when a patient is taking both drugs. When naproxen is administered with an anticoagulant, the patient has an increased risk for bleeding. When naproxen is administered with an antihypertensive, the antihypertensive's effect is diminished. Naproxen decreases the diuretic effect of diuretics.

Rofecoxib

Rofecoxib is contraindicated in patients who are allergic to the drug or to any of the NSAIDs or sulfonamides. The drug is not used during pregnancy (category C) or lactation. Rofecoxib is used cautiously in patients with impaired renal or hepatic function, in patients with a history of gastrointestinal bleeding or peptic ulcer disease, and in patients with congestive heart failure, asthma, or hypertension.

Drug interactions with rofecoxib are similar to those with the other NSAIDs, such as an increased risk of bleeding when taken with anticoagulants and a possible risk of lithium toxicity when taken with lithium.

Patient Management Issues with Nonsteroidal Anti-inflammatory Drugs (NSAIDs)

The patient is monitored for relief of pain. If pain recurs, then its severity, location, and intensity are assessed. An inpatient's vital signs are monitored every 4 hours or more frequently if necessary. Hot, dry, flushed skin and decreased urinary output may develop with prolonged fever and dehydration. The patient's joints are assessed for reduced inflammation and greater mobility. Any adverse reactions, such as unusual or prolonged bleeding or dark stools, should be reported to the health care provider. Patients who do not experience a therapeutic response to one NSAID may respond to another NSAID. However, several weeks of treatment may be necessary for a full therapeutic response to develop.

NSAIDs are prescribed for the pain and inflammation of arthritis. Because older adults more commonly have rheumatoid arthritis and osteoarthritis and may use the NSAID for a long-term, they are particularly vulnerable to gastrointestinal bleeding. The patient should take the drug with a full glass of water or with food because this may decrease the gastrointestinal effects.

GERONTOLOGIC ALERT

Adverse Reactions to NSAIDs

Age appears to increase the possibility of adverse reactions to NSAIDs. The risk of serious ulcer disease in adults older than 65 years is increased with higher doses of NSAIDs. Therapy often begins with reduced dosages, which are increased slowly.

Patients with pain in their the limbs or joints may need additional comfort measures. Therapy may include the use of heat or cold along with joint rest. Various orthodontic devices, such as splints and braces, may be used to support inflamed joints. Braces, splints, and assistive mobility devices such as canes, crutches, and walkers help ease pain.

Educating the Patient and Family About Salicylates, Nonsalicylates, and Nonsteroidal Anti-inflammatory Drugs (NSAIDs)

A nonnarcotic analgesic or an NSAID may be prescribed for a patient for a prolonged period, such as for arthritis. Some patients may discontinue their use of the drug, fail to take the drug at the prescribed or recommended intervals, increase their dose, or decrease the time interval between doses, especially if their symptoms change. The patient and family must understand that the drug should be taken even when symptoms are relieved. Patient Education Boxes 10-1 and 10-2 include key points about nonnarcotic analgesics the patient or family members should know. Patient Education Box 10-3 include key points about NSAIDs for the patient or family.

Many NSAIDs are available as OTC products. OTC formulations such as ibuprofen (Advil, Motrin, and Nuprin), ketoprofen (Orudis), and naproxen sodium (Aleve) are available to any consumer. The potential for misuse and abuse is high, especially because frequent advertisements on television and in print herald the wonderful benefits of these products. Therefore, patients need to be educated about these products, emphasizing the following points:

- Indications for using the drug (the reason the patient might take it)
- Dosage information, including frequency and maximum daily amounts
- Possible drug–drug and drug–food interactions
- Possible adverse effects, including life-threatening ones such as bleeding

---

PATIENT EDUCATION BOX 10-1

Key Points for Patients Taking Nonnarcotic Analgesics

❑ Take the drug exactly as prescribed by the health care provider. Do not increase or decrease the dosage, and do not take any over-the-counter (OTC) drugs without first consulting your health care provider. Notify your health care provider or dentist if the pain is not relieved.

❑ Take the drug with food or a full glass of water unless told otherwise by your health care provider. If you experience gastric upset, then take the drug with food or milk. If the problem persists, then contact your health care provider.

❑ Inform all health care providers, including your dentist, when you take these drugs regularly or occasionally.

❑ If you use the drug to reduce fever, then contact your health care provider if your temperature continues elevated for more than 24 hours.

❑ Do not consistently use an OTC nonnarcotic analgesic to treat chronic pain without first consulting your health care provider.

❑ Severe or recurrent pain or high or continued fever may indicate a serious illness. If your pain persists more than 10 days (in an adult), or if your fever persists more than 3 days, then consult your health care provider.

SALICYLATES

❑ If taking a salicylate, then notify your health care provider if you have any of the following symptoms: ringing in the ears, gastrointestinal pain, nausea, vomiting, flushing, sweating, thirst, headache, diarrhea, episodes of unusual bleeding or bruising, or dark stools. (See Patient Education Box 10-2 on detecting gastrointestinal bleeding.)

❑ All drugs deteriorate with age. Salicylates often deteriorate more rapidly than many other drugs. If there is a vinegar odor to the salicylate, then discard the entire contents of the container. Purchase salicylates in small amounts when used only occasionally. Keep the container tightly closed at all times because salicylates deteriorate rapidly when exposed to air, moisture, or heat.

❑ The ingredients of some OTC drugs contain aspirin. The name of the salicylate may not appear in the name of the drug but is listed on the label. Do not use these products while taking a salicylate, especially during high-dose or long-term salicylate therapy. Consult the pharmacist about the product's ingredients if you are in doubt.

❑ If you are to have surgery or a dental procedure, such as tooth extraction or gum surgery, then notify your health care provider or dentist. Salicylates may be discontinued 1 week before the procedure because of the possibility of postoperative bleeding.

ACETAMINOPHEN

❑ If you have arthritis, then do not change from aspirin to acetaminophen without consulting your health care provider. Acetaminophen lacks the anti-inflammatory properties of aspirin.

❑ Notify your health care provider if you have any of the following adverse reactions: dyspnea, weakness, dizziness, blue discoloration of the nailbeds, unexplained bleeding, bruising, or sore throat.

❑ Do not drink alcoholic beverages.

PATIENT EDUCATION BOX 10-2

Detecting Gastrointestinal Bleeding

Patients with a musculoskeletal disorder commonly receive salicylates or NSAIDs to help control inflammation and pain. In addition, these drugs are readily available over the counter. A patient who is prescribed one drug, such as NSAIDs, may also take an OTC salicylate, such as aspirin, for headaches or additional pain relief. When taken alone, these drugs may cause gastrointestinal irritation, possibly leading to gastrointestinal bleeding. If taken in combination or in high doses, or for long periods of time, the patient's risk for gastrointestinal bleeding increases dramatically. Therefore, the patient may be taught how to look for signs and symptoms of gastrointestinal bleeding. Patients should be instructed to report any of the following:

❑ Abdominal pain or distention, especially any sudden increases
❑ Vomiting that appears bright red or blood streaked (indicates fresh or recent bleeding) dark red, brown, or black, similar to the consistency of coffee grounds (indicates partial digestion of retained blood)
❑ Stools that appear black, loose and tarry, or bright red, red streaked, maroon, or dark mahogany

Patients should check their stools for occult blood (guaiac) by doing the following:

1. Gather the necessary supplies, including chemical testing solution, testing card, applicator, and a watch with a second hand.
2. After passing stool and opening the flap of the testing card, obtain a sample of stool and place a thin smear on the first window or slot marked as "1" or "A."
3. Obtain a second sample from another area of the same stool and place a thin smear on the second window or slot marked as "2" or "B."
4. Close the flap of the test card.
5. If your health care provider or laboratory will be checking the test results, then return the test card to them. If you are checking the sample, then proceed as follows:
6. Turn the test card over and open the flap.
7. Open the bottle of chemical testing solution.
8. Place two drops of the solution onto each sample area of the paper.
9. Wait 30 to 60 seconds.
10. Observe the paper for a color change. If there is no color change, then the results are negative. If either area of the paper turns blue, then the results are positive for blood and you should contact your health care provider as soon as possible.

PATIENT EDUCATION BOX 10-3

Key Points for Patients Taking NSAIDs

❑ Take the drug exactly as prescribed by your health care provider. Do not increase or decrease the dosage, and do not take any over-the-counter (OTC) drugs without first consulting your health care provider. Notify your health care provider or dentist if the pain is not relieved.
❑ Take the drug with food or a full glass of water unless indicated otherwise by your health care provider. If you experience gastric upset, then take the drug with food or milk. If the problem persists, then contact your health care provider.
❑ Inform all health care providers, including dentists, if you take these drugs regularly or occasionally.
❑ If you use the drug to reduce fever, then contact your health care provider if your temperature continues elevated for more than 24 hours.
❑ Do not consistently use an OTC nonnarcotic analgesic to treat chronic pain without first consulting your health care provider.

❑ Severe or recurrent pain or high or continued fever may indicate a serious illness. If your pain persists more than 10 days (in an adult), or if your fever persists more than 3 days, then consult your health care provider.
❑ Do not use aspirin or other salicylates when taking an NSAID.
❑ The drug may take several days to take effect (relief of pain and tenderness). If some or all of your symptoms are not relieved after 2 weeks of therapy, then continue taking the drug, but notify your health care provider.
❑ These drugs may cause drowsiness, dizziness, or blurred vision. Use caution while driving or performing tasks that require alertness.
❑ Notify your health care provider if you have any of the following adverse reactions: skin rash, itching, visual disturbances, weight gain, edema, diarrhea, black stools, nausea, vomiting, or persistent headache.

- The need to read and heed all manufacturer's instructions, including the maximum number of days one should use the drug and when to notify the health care provider (e.g., if fever is not resolved within 3 days or pain persists)

Although this patient education is not a fool-proof remedy for preventing possible misuse and abuse, it can help minimize the risk of problems associated with over-the-counter NSAIDs.

Narcotic Analgesics

Narcotic analgesics are controlled substances (see Chapter 1) used to treat moderate to severe pain. Narcotic antagonists, which are drugs that counteract the effects of narcotic analgesics by competing with narcotic at receptor sites, are used to reverse the depressant effects of narcotic analgesics.

Actions of Narcotic Analgesics

Opioid analgesics are narcotic drugs derived from the opium plant. More than 20 different alkaloids are present in the unripe seed of the opium poppy plant. The analgesic properties of opium have been known for hundreds of years. Narcotics obtained from raw opium (also called opiates, opioids, or opiate narcotics) include morphine, codeine, hydrochlorides of opium alkaloids, and camphorated tincture of opium.

Morphine is extracted from raw opium and treated chemically to produce the semisynthetic narcotics hydromorphone, oxymorphone, oxycodone, and heroin. Heroin is an illegal narcotic in the United States and is not used in medicine. Synthetic narcotics are laboratory-made analgesics with properties and actions similar to the natural opioids. Examples of synthetic narcotic analgesics are methadone, levorphanol, remifentanil, and meperidine. Additional narcotics are listed in the Summary Drug Table: Narcotic Analgesics.

Narcotic analgesics are classified as agonists, partial agonists, and mixed agonists–antagonists. An **agonist** binds to a receptor and causes a response. A **partial agonist** binds to a receptor but has only a limited response. Antagonists bind to a receptor and cause no response of their own, but an antagonist can reverse the effects of an agonist. This reversal occurs possibly because the antagonist competes with the agonist for the receptor site. (Narcotic antagonists are discussed later in this chapter.) An **agonist–antagonist** drug has properties of both the agonist and antagonist.

Narcotic analgesics are categorized based on the opioid receptor sites where they are active. Five categories of opioid receptors have been identified, three of which are

TABLE 10-1 Activities Within the Body Associated With Receptor Sites

Receptor	Bodily Response
Mu	Morphine-like supraspinal analgesia, respiratory and physical depression, miosis, reduced G motility
Delta	Dysphoria, psychotomimetic effects (e.g., hallucinations), respiratory and vasomotor stimulations caused by drugs with antagonist activity
Kappa	Sedation and miosis

involved in the actions of narcotic analgesics; these are called the mu, kappa, and delta receptors. Table 10-1 identifies the responses in the body associated with each of these receptors.

Remifentanil is a very short-acting agonist with potent analgesic activity. It is a mu opioid agonist with rapid onset and peak effect, and short duration of action. The mixed agonist–antagonist drugs act on the mu receptors by competing with other substances at the mu receptor (antagonist activity) and are agonists at other receptors. Partial agonists have limited agonist activity at the mu receptor. The actions of the narcotic analgesics on the various organs and structures of the body (also called secondary pharmacological effects) are shown in Box 10-2.

Uses of Narcotic Analgesics

The major use of narcotic analgesics is to manage moderate to severe acute and chronic pain. The ability of a narcotic analgesic to relieve pain depends on several factors, such as the drug, the dose, the route of administration, the type of pain, the patient, and the length of time the drug has been administered. Morphine is the most widely used opioid and is an effective drug for moderately severe to severe pain. Morphine is considered the prototype or "model narcotic." Morphine's actions, uses, and ability to relieve pain are standards to which other narcotic analgesics are often compared. Other narcotics, such as meperidine and levorphanol, are effective for the treatment of moderate to severe pain. For mild to moderate pain, the health care provider may order a narcotic such as codeine or pentazocine.

In addition to the management of moderate to severe acute and chronic pain, narcotic analgesics may be used for the following reasons:

- To lessen anxiety and sedate a patient before surgery. Patients who are relaxed and sedated when anesthesia is given are easier to anesthetize (requiring a smaller dose of an induction anesthetic), as well as easier to maintain under anesthesia.

SUMMARY DRUG TABLE   Narcotic Analgesics

Generic Name	Trade Name*	Uses	Adverse Reactions**	Dosage Ranges
Agonist alfentanil HCL *al-fen'-ta-nil*	Alfenta	Analgesic, anesthetic	Respiratory depression, skeletal muscle rigidity, light-headedness, sedation, constipation, dizziness, nausea, vomiting	Individualize dosage and titrate to obtain desired effect
codeine *koe'-deen*	*Generic*	Analgesic, antitussive	Sedation, sweating, headache, dizziness, lethargy, confusion, light-headedness	Analgesic: 15–60 mg q4–6h PRN PO, IV, SC, IM; antitussive: 10–20 mg PO q4–6h; maximum dose, 120 mg/24 h
fentanyl *fen'-ta-nil*	Sublimaze, *generic*	Analgesic, anesthesia before, during, and after surgery	Sedation, sweating, headache, vertigo, lethargy, confusion, light-headedness, nausea, vomiting, respiratory depression	Preanesthesia: 0.05–0.1 mg IM; postoperative: 0.05–0.1 mg IM; anesthesia: administered by anesthesiologist
fentanyl *fen'-ta-nil* transmucosal system	Actiq, Fentanyl Oralet	Fentanyl Oralet: only as anesthetic premedication Actiq: only as management of breakthrough cancer pain	Sedation, sweating, headache, vertigo, lethargy, confusion, light-headedness, nausea, vomiting, respiratory depression	Individualize dosage: Oralet up to 5 mcg/kg/dose (lozenges) Actiq: 200 mcg/dose (lozenge on a stick)
fentanyl *fen'-ta-nil* transdermal system	Duragesic	Chronic pain	Sedation, sweating, headache, vertigo, lethargy, confusion, light-headedness, nausea, vomiting, respiratory depression	Individualized dosage: 25–100 mcg/h as a transdermal patch
hydromorphone *hy-droe-mor'-fone*	Dilaudid	Analgesic	Sedation, vertigo, lethargy, confusion, light-headedness, nausea, vomiting, respiratory depression	2–4 mg PO, IM, SC q4–6h; 3 mg q6–8h rectally
levomethadyl acetate *lev-oh-meth'-a-dil*	ORLAAM	Opioid dependence	Sedation, lethargy, nausea, vomiting, clamminess, sweating, vertigo, unusual dreams, respiratory depression	Individualized dosage of 60–90 mg PO 3 times/wk
levorphanol tartrate *lee-vor'-fa nole*	Levo-Dromoran	Analgesic, preoperative medication	Dizziness, sedation, nausea, vomiting, dry mouth, sweating, respiratory depression	2–3 mg PO, SC, IM q4h PRN; 1 mg IV q3–8 h PRN

Generic Name	Trade Name*	Uses	Adverse Reactions**	Dosage Ranges
meperidine *me-per'-i-deen*	Demerol	Analgesic, preoperative medication, support of anesthesia	Light-headedness, sedation, constipation, dizziness, nausea, vomiting, respiratory depression	50–150 mg PO, IM, SC, q3–4h PRN
methadone *meth'-a-doan*	Dolophine	Analgesic, detoxification and temporary maintenance treatment of narcotic abstinence syndrome	Light-headedness, dizziness, sedation, nausea, vomiting, constipation, respiratory depression	Analgesic: 2.5–10 mg PO, IM, SC q4h PRN; detoxification: 10–40 mg PO, IV
morphine sulfate *mor'-feen*	MS Contin, Roxanol	Analgesic, preoperative sedation, adjunct to anesthesia, dyspnea due to pulmonary edema, pain associated with MI	Sedation, hypotension, increased sweating, constipation, dizziness, drowsiness, nausea, vomiting, dry mouth, somnolence, respiratory depression	10–30 mg PO q4h PRN; 10–20 mg rectally q4h; 5–20 mg IM SC q4h PRN; 2.5–15mg/70 kg IV
opium *oh'-pee-um*	Camphorated tincture of opium, Paregoric	Analgesic, anti-diarrheal	Light-headedness, dizziness, sedation, nausea, vomiting, constipation, suppression of cough reflex, dry mouth	Paregoric: 5–10 mL PO QID; 10% liquid: 0.6 mL PO QID
oxycodone *ox-ee-koe'-done*	OxyContin, OxyIR, Roxicodone	Analgesic	Light-headedness, sedation, constipation, dizziness, nausea, vomiting, sweating, respiratory depression	OxyContin: 10–20 mg PO q12h; OxyIR: 5 mg for breakthrough pain
oxymorphone *ox-ee-mor'-fone*	Numorphan	Analgesic, preoperative sedation, obstetric analgesia	Light-headedness, sedation, constipation, dizziness, nausea, vomiting, respiratory depression	1–1.5 mg SC or IM q4–6h PRN; 0.5 mg IV; 5 mg rectally q4–6h
propoxyphene *proe-pox'-i-feen*	Darvon, Darvocet-N, Darvon-N	Analgesic	Light-headedness, sedation, constipation, dizziness, nausea, vomiting, respiratory depression	Darvon: 65 mg PO q4h PRN Darvocet-N and Darvon-N: 100 mg PO q4h, maximum dose, 600 mg/d
remifentanil HCL *reh-mih-fen'-tah-nill*	Ultiva	anesthesia	Light-headedness, sedation, skeletal muscle rigidity, nausea, vomiting, respiratory depression, sweating	0.5–1 mcg/kg/min

Generic Name	Trade Name*	Uses	Adverse Reactions**	Dosage Ranges
Partial Agonist buprenorphine *byoo-pre-nor'-feen*	Buprenex	Analgesia	Light-headedness, sedation, constipation, dizziness, nausea, vomiting, respiratory depression	0.03 mg q6h PRN IV or IM
butorphanol *byoo-tor'fa-nole*	Stadol, Stadol NS	Analgesia, preoperative to support anesthesia	Light-headedness, sedation, constipation, dizziness, nausea, vomiting, respiratory depression	1–4 mg IM; 0.5–2 mg IV; nasal spray (NS): 1 mg (spray) repeat in 60–90 min. May repeat q3–4h
Agonist Antagonist nalbuphine *nal'-byoo-feen*	Nubain, generic	Analgesia	Light-headedness, sedation, constipation, dizziness, nausea, vomiting, respiratory depression	10 mg/70 kg SC, IM, IV q3–6h PRN
pentazocine *pen-taz'-oh-seen*	Talwin, Talwin NX	Analgesia	Light-headedness, sedation, constipation, dizziness, nausea, vomiting, respiratory depression	50–100 mg PO q3–4h PRN; up to 30 mg IM, SC, IV q3–4h PRN
pentazocine combination	Talacen (pentazocine) and acetaminophen	Analgesia	Light-headedness, sedation, constipation, dizziness, nausea, vomiting, respiratory depression	1 tablet q4h

*The term *generic* indicates the drug is available in generic form.
**The adverse reactions of the narcotic analgesics are discussed extensively in the chapter. Some of the reactions may be less severe or intense than others.

- To support anesthesia (as an adjunct during anesthesia)
- For obstetrical analgesia
- To relieve anxiety in patients with dyspnea associated with pulmonary edema
- Intrathecally or epidurally to relieve pain for extended periods without apparent loss of motor, sensory, or sympathetic function
- To relieve pain associated with heart attack (morphine)
- To manage opiate dependence (levomethadyl)
- For detoxification of and temporary maintenance of narcotic addiction (methadone)
- To induce conscious sedation before a diagnostic or therapeutic procedure
- To treat severe diarrhea and intestinal cramping (camphorated tincture of opium)
- To relieve severe, persistent cough (codeine, although the drug's use has declined)

Narcotic Analgesic Use in Management of Opioid Dependence

Two opioids are used in the treatment and management of opiate dependence: levomethadyl and methadone. Levomethadyl is given in opiate dependency clinics where control can be maintained over delivery of the drug. Because of its potential for serious and life-threatening proarrhythmic effects, levomethadyl is used only to treat addicted patients who do not respond to other treatments. Levomethadyl is administered three times per week (Monday/Wednesday/Thursday or Tuesday/Thursday/Saturday). Daily use of the usual dose would cause serious overdose.

Methadone, a synthetic narcotic, may be used for the relief of pain, but it also is used in the detoxification and maintenance treatment of those addicted to narcotics. Detoxification involves withdrawing the patient from the narcotic while preventing withdrawal symptoms.

Box 10-2 Secondary Pharmacological Effects of Narcotic Analgesics

- **Cardiovascular:** peripheral vasodilation, decreased peripheral resistance, inhibition of baroreceptors (pressure receptors located in the aortic arch and carotid sinus that regulate blood pressure), orthostatic hypotension, and fainting
- **Central nervous system:** euphoria, drowsiness, apathy, mental confusion, alterations in mood, reduction in body temperature, feelings of relaxation, dysphoria (depression accompanied by anxiety), nausea, and vomiting are caused by direct stimulation of the emetic chemoreceptors located in the medulla. The degree to which these occur usually depends on the drug and the dose.
- **Dermatologic:** histamine release, pruritus, flushing, and red eyes
- **Gastrointestinal:** decrease in gastric motility (prolonged emptying time); decrease in biliary, pancreatic, and intestinal secretions; delay in digestion of food in the small intestine; and increase in resting tone, with the potential for spasms, epigastric distress, or biliary colic (caused by constriction of the sphincter of Oddi). These drugs can cause constipation and anorexia.
- **Genitourinary:** urinary urgency and difficulty with urination, caused by spasms of the ureter. Urinary urgency also may occur because of the action of the drugs on the detrusor muscle of the bladder. Some patients may have difficulty urinating because of contraction of the bladder sphincter.
- **Respiratory:** depressant effects on respiratory rate (caused by a reduced sensitivity of the respiratory center to carbon dioxide)
- **Cough:** suppression of the cough reflex by exerting a direct effect on the cough center in the medulla. Codeine has the most noticeable effect on the cough reflex.
- **Medulla:** Nausea and vomiting can occur when the chemoreceptor trigger zone located in the medulla is stimulated. To a varying degree, narcotic analgesics also depress the chemoreceptor trigger zone. Therefore, nausea and vomiting may or may not occur when these drugs are given.

Maintenance therapy is designed to reduce the patient's desire to return to the drug that caused addiction and to prevent withdrawal symptoms. The dosages used vary with the patient, the length of time the individual has been addicted, and the average daily amount of the addictive drug that had been used. Patients enrolled in an outpatient methadone program for detoxification or maintenance therapy on methadone must continue to receive methadone when hospitalized.

Adverse Reactions of Narcotic Analgesics

The adverse reactions differ according to whether the narcotic analgesic acts as an agonist or as an agonist–antagonist.

Adverse Reactions of Agonists

One of the major hazards of narcotic administration is respiratory depression, in which the respiratory rate and depth decrease. The most common adverse reactions include light-headedness, dizziness, sedation, constipation, anorexia, nausea, vomiting, and sweating. When these effects occur, the health care provider may lower the dose in an effort to eliminate or decrease their intensity. Other adverse reactions that may occur with the administration of an agonist narcotic analgesic include:

- Central nervous system: euphoria, weakness, headache, pinpoint pupils, insomnia, agitation, tremor, and impairment of mental and physical tasks
- Gastrointestinal: dry mouth and biliary tract spasms
- Cardiovascular: flushing of the face, peripheral circulatory collapse, tachycardia, bradycardia, and palpitations
- Genitourinary: spasms of the ureters and bladder sphincter, urinary retention or hesitancy
- Allergic: pruritus, rash, and urticaria
- Other: physical dependence, pain at injection site, and local tissue irritation

Adverse Reactions of Agonist–Antagonists

Administration of a narcotic agonist–antagonist may result in symptoms of narcotic withdrawal in those addicted to narcotics. Other adverse reactions include sedation, nausea, vomiting, sweating, headache, vertigo, dry mouth, euphoria, and dizziness.

Managing Adverse Drug Reactions

Any significant change in a patient's vital signs should immediately be reported to the health care provider. Narcotic analgesics can cause hypotension. Particularly vulnerable are postoperative patients and individuals whose ability to maintain blood pressure has been compromised.

ALERT

Narcotic Analgesics

The narcotic analgesic should be withheld and the health care provider contacted immediately if any of the following are present:

- a significant decrease in the respiratory rate or a respiratory rate of 10/min or below
- a significant increase or decrease in the pulse rate or a change in the pulse quality
- a significant decrease in blood pressure (systolic or diastolic) or a systolic pressure below 100 mm Hg

Patients receiving long-term opioid therapy rarely have problems with respiratory depression. In instances in which respiratory depression occurs, a narcotic antagonist may be ordered by the health care provider if the respiratory rate continues to fall.

GERONTOLOGIC ALERT
Narcotic Analgesics

 Older adults are especially prone to adverse reactions of narcotic analgesics, particularly respiratory depression, somnolence (sedation), and confusion. The health care provider may order a lower dosage of the narcotic for an older adult.

Narcotics may depress the patient's cough reflex. Patients regularly receiving a narcotic, even for a few days, should be encouraged to cough and breathe deeply every 2 hours. This prevents the pooling of secretions in the lungs, which can lead to hypostatic pneumonia and other lung problems. If a patient experiences nausea and vomiting, then the health care provider should be notified. A different analgesic or an antiemetic may be necessary.

Risk for Injury. Narcotics may produce orthostatic hypotension, which causes dizziness. The patient may need help walking and rising slowly from a sitting or lying position. **Miosis** (pinpoint pupils) may occur with some narcotics and is most pronounced with morphine, hydromorphone, and hydrochlorides of opium alkaloids. Miosis decreases the ability to see in dim light. The room should be well lit during daytime hours, and the patient should ask for help when getting out of bed at night.

Constipation. Constipation can occur with repeated doses of a narcotic. A daily record of bowel movements is kept and the health care provider is informed if constipation appears to be a problem. Most patients should begin taking a stool softener or laxative with the initial dose of a narcotic analgesic. Many patients need to continue taking a laxative as long as they take the narcotic analgesic. If a patient is constipated despite the use of a stool softener, then the health care provider may prescribe an enema or another means of relieving constipation.

Imbalanced Nutrition. When a narcotic is prescribed for a prolonged time, anorexia (loss of appetite) may occur. Those receiving a narcotic for the relief of pain caused by terminal cancer often have severe anorexia from both the disease and the narcotic. Food intake is assessed after each meal. When anorexia is prolonged, the patient is weighed weekly or as ordered by the health care provider. It is important to notify the health care provider of continued weight loss and anorexia.

Narcotic Drug Dependence. Most patients receiving a narcotic analgesic for medical purposes do not develop dependence. However, drug dependence can occur when a narcotic is administered over a long period. For some patients, such as those who are terminally ill and in severe pain, drug dependence is not considered a problem because the most important task is to keep patients as comfortable as possible for the time they have remaining (see the section on "Relieving Chronic Severe Pain").

When a patient does not have a painful terminal illness, drug dependence must be avoided. Signs of drug dependence include the appearance of withdrawal symptoms (acute abstinence syndrome) when the narcotic is discontinued, requests for the narcotic at frequent intervals around the clock, personality changes if the narcotic is not given immediately, and constant reports of pain and failure of the narcotic to relieve pain. Although these behaviors can have other causes, drug dependence should be considered. Specific symptoms of the abstinence syndrome are listed in Box 10-3.

Drug dependence can also occur in a newborn whose mother was dependent on opiates during pregnancy. Withdrawal symptoms in the newborn usually appear during the first few days of life. Symptoms include irritability, excessive crying, yawning, sneezing, increased respiratory rate, tremors, fever, vomiting, and diarrhea.

Contraindications, Precautions, and Interactions of Narcotic Analgesics

All narcotic analgesics are contraindicated in patients with known hypersensitivity. These drugs are contraindicated in patients with acute bronchial asthma, emphysema, or upper airway obstruction and

---

Box 10-3 Symptoms of the Abstinence Syndrome

Early Symptoms	Late Symptoms
Yawning	Muscle spasm
Lacrimation	Fever
Rhinorrhea	Nausea
Sweating	Vomiting
	Kicking movements
Intermediate Symptoms	Weakness
	Depression
Mydriasis	Body aches
Tachycardia	Weight loss
Twitching	Severe backache
Tremor	Abdominal and leg pains
Restlessness	Hot and cold flashes
Irritability	Insomnia
Anxiety	Repetitive sneezing
Anorexia	Increased blood pressure, respiratory rate, and heart rate

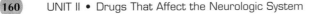

in patients with head injury or increased intracranial pressure. The drugs are also contraindicated in patients with convulsive disorders, severe renal or hepatic dysfunction, or acute ulcerative colitis. Narcotic analgesics are pregnancy category C drugs (oxycodone is category B) and are not recommended for use during pregnancy or labor because they may prolong labor or cause respiration depression of the neonate. The use of narcotic analgesics is recommended during pregnancy only if the benefit to the mother outweighs the potential harm to the fetus.

These drugs are used cautiously in the elderly and in patients with undiagnosed abdominal pain, liver disease, a history of addiction to the opioids, hypoxia, supraventricular tachycardia, prostatic hypertrophy, or renal or hepatic impairment. Obese patients must be monitored closely for respiratory depression while taking a narcotic analgesic. The drug is used cautiously during lactation, and the mother is advised to wait at least 4 to 6 hours after taking the drug before breastfeeding the infant. Narcotics are used cautiously in patients undergoing biliary surgery because these drugs may cause spasm of the sphincter of Oddi.

Narcotic analgesics potentiate the central nervous system depressant properties of other central nervous system depressants, such as alcohol, antihistamines, antidepressants, sedatives, phenothiazines, and monoamine oxidase inhibitors. Use of a narcotic analgesic within 14 days of a MAO inhibitors (see Chapter 4) may potentiate the effect of either drug. Patients taking an agonist–antagonist narcotic analgesic may experience withdrawal symptoms if they have been abusing or using narcotics.

The agonist–antagonists drugs can cause opioid withdrawal symptoms in those who are physically dependent on an opioid. The patient has an increased risk of respiratory depression, hypotension, and sedation when narcotic analgesics are administered too soon after barbiturate general anesthesia.

Patient Management Issues with Narcotic Analgesics

When a narcotic is given for the first time, certain questions are considered by the health care provider. The answers may influence the choice of a specific narcotic. The patient is asked the following:

- Does the pain keep you awake at night? Prevent you from falling asleep or staying asleep?
- What makes your pain worse?
- Does the pain affect your mood? Are you depressed? Irritable? Anxious?
- What over-the-counter or herbal remedies have you used for the pain?
- Does the pain affect your activity level? Are you able to walk? Perform self-care activities?

Other factors to consider are:

- A patient's subjective description of the pain (What does the pain feel like?)
- Location(s) of the pain
- Intensity, severity, and duration of the pain
- Any factors that influence the pain
- Quality of the pain
- Patterns of coping
- Effects of previous therapy (if applicable)
- The health care provider's observations of a patient's behavior

The health care provider may request that a patient evaluate the pain using a standardized pain scale measurement tool. The pain is usually rated on a scale of 1 to 10, with 10 being the most severe pain and 1 being the least discomfort. Failure to adequately assess pain is a major factor in the common undertreatment of pain.

When these drugs are administered, the health care provider should regularly ask about the pain and believe the patient's and family's reports of pain. The exact location of the pain, a description of the pain (e.g., sharp, dull, or stabbing), and an estimate of when the pain began are assessed each time the patient requests a narcotic analgesic. Further questioning and more detailed information about the pain are necessary if the pain is different from that experienced previously or if it is in a different area. Not all instances of a change in pain type, location, or intensity require notifying the health care provider. For example, if a patient recovering from recent abdominal surgery experiences pain in the leg, then the health care provider should be notified immediately. However, it may not be necessary to contact the health care provider for pain that is slightly worse because the patient has been moving in bed.

In addition, if any controllable factors (e.g., uncomfortable position, cold room, drafts, bright lights, noise, thirst) may decrease the patient's tolerance to pain, then the adjustment should be made as soon as possible.

Narcotic analgesics can produce serious or potentially fatal respiratory depression if given too frequently or in excessive doses. Respiratory depression may occur in patients receiving a normal dose if the patient is vulnerable, such as in weakened state or debilitated state. Elderly, cachectic, or debilitated patients may receive a reduced initial dose until their response to the drug is known. If the respiratory rate drops to 10/min or below, then the patient must be monitored frequently and the health care provider notified immediately.

Relieving Acute Pain

The health care provider should be notified if the analgesic is ineffective because a higher dose or a different narcotic analgesic may be required.

During the time when the drug is producing its greatest analgesic effect, usually 1 to 2 hours after being administered, the patient may need help getting out of bed and performing therapeutic activities, such as deep breathing, coughing, and leg exercises (when ordered).

Patient-controlled analgesia (PCA) allows patients to administer their own analgesic by means of an intravenous pump system (Fig. 10-1). The dose and the time interval permitted between doses is programmed into the device to prevent accidental overdosage.

Many postoperative patients require narcotics less often when they are able to self-administer a narcotic for pain. Because the self-administration system is under the control of a nurse or health care provider, who adds the drug to the infusion pump and sets the time interval (or lockout interval) between doses, the patient cannot receive an overdose of the drug.

Relieving Chronic Severe Pain

Morphine is the most widely used drug for chronic severe pain, such as pain associated with cancer. The fact that this drug can be given orally, subcutaneously, intramuscularly, intravenous, and rectally in the form of a suppository allows tremendous versatility. Medication for chronic pain should be scheduled around the clock and not given on a PRN (as needed) basis. Most patients with cancer can be treated with oral morphine. The oral route is preferred as long as a patient is able to swallow or can tolerate sublingual administration. Respiratory depression is less likely to occur when the drug is given orally.

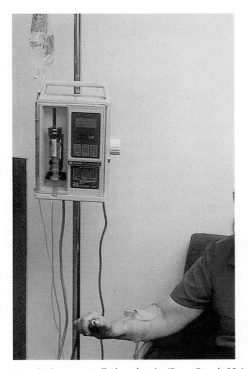

FIGURE 10-1   Patient-controlled analgesia. (From Roach SS. Introductory Clinical Pharmacology, 7th ed. Baltimore: Lippincott Williams & Wilkins; 2004.)

OxyContin is a controlled-released form of oxycodone for moderate to severe pain when a continuous, around-the-clock analgesic is needed for an extended period of time. OxyContin is not intended for use as a PRN analgesic. A patient may experience fewer adverse reactions with oxycodone than morphine, and the drug is effective and generally considered safe for the elderly. The tablets are to be swallowed whole and should not be broken, chewed, or crushed.

Fentanyl transdermal is a transdermal system that is effective for the severe pain associated with cancer. The transdermal system allows for a timed-release patch containing the drug fentanyl used over a 72-hour period. A small number of patients may require systems applied every 48 hours. Adverse effects are monitored in the same manner as for other narcotic analgesics (e.g., the health care provider is notified if the respiratory rate is 10/min or less).

GERONTOLOGIC ALERT

Transdermal Drug Administration

The use of the transdermal route in the elderly is questionable because the amount of subcutaneous tissue is reduced by the aging process.

On rare occasions when pain is not relieved by the narcotic analgesic alone, a mixture of an oral narcotic and other drugs may be used to obtain relief. Brompton's mixture is commonly used in these situations. In addition to a narcotic, such as morphine or methadone, other drugs may be used in the solution, including antidepressants, stimulants, aspirin, acetaminophen, and tranquilizers. The pharmacist prepares the solution according to the health care provider's instructions. The patient should be monitored for the adverse reactions of each drug in the solution. The time interval for administration varies. Some health care providers may order the mixture on an as-needed basis; others may order it given at regular intervals.

When narcotics are administered for severe pain, the goal is to prevent or control the patient's pain, not to prevent addiction. Patients taking a narcotic for severe pain rarely become addicted. Although some dependence may occur in rare instances, a patient who recovers from the illness may be gradually weaned from the drug.

When long-acting forms of a narcotic are used, a fast-acting form may be given for breakthrough pain. Patients should be given the drug as ordered and on time. Oral transmucosal fentanyl (Actiq) is used to treat breakthrough pain. Making a patient wait for the effect of a long-acting drug may result in withdrawal symptoms, which will only add to the pain of the illness.

Tolerance results over a period of time in the patient taking a narcotic analgesic. The rate at which a patient develops tolerance varies according to the dosage, the route or administration, and the individual. Patients taking oral or transdermal morphine develop tolerance more slowly than those taking the drug parenterally. Some patients develop tolerance quickly and need larger doses every few weeks, whereas others are maintained on the same dosage schedule throughout the course of their illness.

The risk of respiratory depression is a concern for health care professionals who administer narcotics and may cause some to hesitate to administer the drug. However, respiratory depression rarely occurs in patients using a narcotic for pain because these patients usually very quickly develop tolerance to the respiratory depressant effects of the drug. Naloxone can be administered to reverse the narcotic effects if absolutely necessary.

ALERT

Naloxone

Naloxone should be administered with great caution and only when necessary in patients receiving a narcotic for severe pain. Naloxone cancels out all of the pain-relieving effects of the narcotic and may lead to withdrawal symptoms or the return of pain.

Epidural Pain Management

Epidural administration of certain narcotic analgesics, specifically morphine and fentanyl, is an alternative to the intramuscular or oral route. **Epidural** administration is performed when a catheter is placed into the epidural space outside the dura matter of the brain and spinal cord. The analgesic effect is produced by the direct effect on the opiate receptors in the dorsal horn of the spinal cord. Epidural administration offers several advantages over other routes. Lower total dosages of the drug are used, fewer adverse reactions occur, and the patient has greater comfort with epidural administration.

Access to the epidural route is made through the use of a percutaneous epidural catheter. The epidural catheter is placed into the space between the dura mater and the vertebral column (Fig. 10-2). The drug injected through the catheter spreads freely throughout all the tissues in the space, interrupting pain conduction at the points where sensory fibers exit from the spinal cord. The narcotic is administered either by bolus or by continuous infusion pump.

This type of pain management is used for postoperative pain, labor pain, and cancer pain. The most serious adverse reaction associated with the administration of narcotics by the epidural route is respiratory depression. A patient may also experience sedation, confusion, nausea, pruritus, or urinary retention. Fentanyl is increas-

ingly used as an alternative to morphine sulfate because patients experience fewer adverse reactions.

Educating the Patient and Family About Narcotic Analgesics

The health care provider explains to the patient that the drug he or she is receiving is for pain. Additional information is also often included, such as how often the drug can be taken. Patient Education Box 10-4 explains the process of receiving drugs through a PCA infusion pump.

Narcotics for outpatient use may be prescribed in the oral form or as a timed-release transdermal patch. In certain cases, such as when terminally ill patients are being cared for at home, the health care provider may instruct the family in the parenteral administration of the drug or use of PCA. Patient Education Box 10-5 explains key points a patient or family member need to know about narcotics.

Herbal Remedies: Passion Flower

The term "passion flower" denotes many of the approximately 400 species of the herb. Long thought to be an herb with calming qualities, passion flower was banned by the United States Food and Drug Administration (FDA) in 1978 for a lack of proven effectiveness as a sedative and sleep aid. Passion flower has been used in medicine to treat pain, anxiety, and insomnia. Some herbalists use the herb to treat symptoms of parkinsonism. In Germany, passion flower is available as an over-the-counter (OTC) sedative in combination with other herbs, such a valerian, chamomile, and hops, for promoting relaxation, rest, and sleep. Although no adverse reactions have been reported, large doses may cause central nervous system depression. The use of passion flower is contraindicated in pregnancy and in patients taking a monoamine oxidase inhibitor (MAOI). Passion flower contains coumarin, and the risk of bleeding may be increased in patients taking warfarin and passion flower.

Narcotic Antagonists

An **antagonist** is a substance that counteracts the action of something else. An antagonist drug has an affinity for a cell receptor and by binding to it prevents the cell from responding to another drug. Thus, a narcotic antagonist reverses the actions of a narcotic. Specific antagonists have been developed to reverse the respiratory depression associated with the opiates. Two narcotic antagonists in use today are naloxone (Narcan) and naltrexone (ReVia); see the Summary Drug Table: Narcotic Antagonists. Naloxone can restore respiratory function within 1 to 2 minutes after administration. Naltrexone

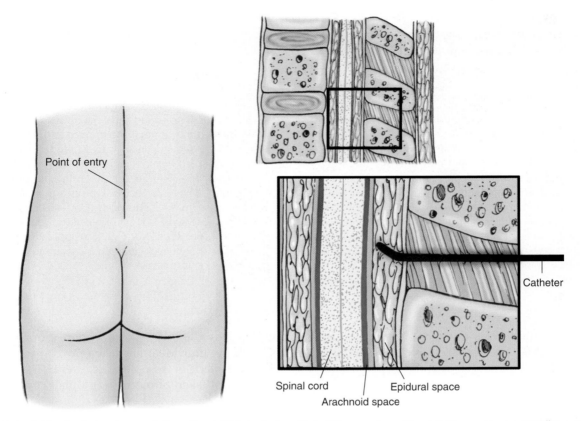

FIGURE 10-2 Epidural catheter placement. (From Roach SS. Introductory Clinical Pharmacology, 7th ed. Baltimore: Lippincott Williams & Wilkins; 2004.)

PATIENT EDUCATION BOX 10-4

Key Points for Receiving Drugs through A PCA Infusion Pump

Patients using a PCA system need to be taught and/or shown:

❏ The location of the control button that activates the administration of the drug
❏ The difference between the control button and the button to call the health care provider (when both are similar in appearance and feel)
❏ The machine regulates the dose of the drug as well as the time interval between doses
❏ If the control button is used too soon after the last dose, then the machine will not deliver the drug until the correct time
❏ Pain relief should occur soon after pushing the button
❏ Call the health care provider if pain relief does not occur after two successive doses

In some situations, narcotic analgesics may be ordered for pain relief using patient-controlled analgesia (PCA). If the patient will be receiving PCA at home, then the following steps are reviewed with the patient and the caregiver:

❏ How the pump works
❏ What drug is being given

❏ When to administer a dose
❏ What the power source is (battery or electricity)
❏ What to do if the battery fails or a power failure occurs
❏ How to check the insertion site
❏ How to change the cartridge or syringe

If the patient or caregiver will be responsible for changing the drug cartridge or syringe, then the following steps are taught:

1. Obtain the new syringe with the drug (if refrigerated, remove it at least 30 minutes before using).
2. Attach the pump-specific tubing to the drug.
3. Prime the tubing.
4. Turn off the pump and clamp the infusion tubing.
5. Remove the tubing from the infusion site.
6. Flush the site (if ordered).
7. Remove the used cartridge or syringe from the pump.
8. Insert the new cartridge or syringe into the pump.
9. Connect the new infusion tubing to the infusion site.
10. Turn on the pump and allow the patient to obtain a drug dose when needed.

PATIENT EDUCATION BOX 10-5

Key Points for Patients Taking Narcotics

❑ This drug may cause drowsiness, dizziness, and blurring of vision. Be cautious when driving or performing tasks requiring alertness.

❑ Do not drink alcoholic beverages unless your health care provider approves. Alcohol may intensify the action of the drug and cause extreme drowsiness or dizziness. In some instances, drinking while taking a narcotic can have extremely serious and even life-threatening consequences that may require emergency medical treatment.

❑ Take the drug as directed by the container label and do not exceed the prescribed dose. Contact your health care provider if the drug is not effective.

❑ If you experience gastrointestinal upset, take the drug with food.

❑ Notify your health care provider if you experience severe nausea, vomiting, or/and constipation.

❑ To put on a transdermal patch, remove the patch from the package and immediately apply it to the skin of your upper torso. To ensure complete contact with the skin, press on it for 10 to 20 seconds with your palm. After 72 hours, remove the patch. Put on a new one if prescribed. Use only water to cleanse the site before putting it on because soaps, oils, and other substances may irritate the skin. Rotate your sites of application. Fold the used patch carefully so that it adheres to itself, and dispose of it appropriately.

---

is used primarily for the treatment of narcotic dependence to block the effects of the opiates, especially the euphoric effects experienced in opiate dependence.

Naloxone

Actions of Naloxone

Administration of naloxone prevents or reverses the effects of the opiates. The exact mechanism of action is not fully understood, but it is believed that naloxone re-

verses opioid effects by competing for opiate receptor sites. If the individual has taken or received an opiate, then the effects of the opiate are reversed. If the individual has not taken or received an opiate, then naloxone has no drug activity.

Uses of Naloxone

This drug is used for complete or partial reversal of narcotic depression, including respiratory depression. Narcotic depression may be caused by intentional or acci-

SUMMARY DRUG TABLE   Narcotic Antagonists

Generic Name	Trade Name*	Uses	Adverse Reactions	Dosage Ranges
nalmefene *nal'-me-feen*	Revex	Complete or partial reversal of opioid effects	Nausea, vomiting, tachycardia, hypertension, return of postoperative pain, fever, dizziness	Initial dose: 0.5 mg/70 kg IV PRN, second dose of 1 mg/70 kg 2–5 min later; maximum dose, 1.5 mg/70 kg
naloxone hydrochloride *nal-ox'-ohn*	Narcan	Narcotic overdose, postoperative narcotic depression	Abrupt reversal of narcotic depression may result in nausea, vomiting, sweating, increased blood pressure, tachycardia	0.4–2 mg IV initially with additional doses repeated at 2–3 min intervals; smaller doses used for postoperative narcotic depression
naltrexone hydrochloride *nal-trex'-ohn*	ReVia, Depade	Narcotic addiction, alcohol dependence	Anxiety, difficulty sleeping, abdominal cramps, nasal congestion, joint and muscle pain, nausea, vomiting, dizziness, irritability	Maintenance treatment: 50 mg PO daily or 100 mg every other day, or 150 mg PO every third day; 2 mL IV, SC

* The term generic *indicates the drug is available in generic form.*

dental overdose (self-administration by an individual), accidental overdose by medical personnel, or a drug idiosyncratic reaction. Naloxone also may be used to diagnose a suspected acute opioid overdosage.

Adverse Reactions of Naloxone

Although not a true adverse reaction of naloxone, the abrupt reversal of narcotic depression may result in nausea, vomiting, sweating, tachycardia, increased blood pressure, and tremors.

Contraindications, Precautions, and Interactions of Naloxone

Naloxone is contraindicated in those with a hypersensitivity to narcotic antagonists. Naloxone is used cautiously in those with a narcotic addiction. Naloxone is used cautiously in patients with cardiovascular disease, pregnant women (pregnancy category B), and infants of opioid-dependent mothers.

These drugs may produce withdrawal symptoms in those physically dependent on a narcotic drug. These patients must not have taken any opiate for the last 7 to 10 days. Naloxone may prevent the action of opioid antidiarrheals, antitussives, and analgesics. This drug is used cautiously during lactation.

Naltrexone

Actions of Naltrexone

Naltrexone completely blocks the effects of intravenous opiates, as well as drugs with agonist–antagonist actions (butorphanol, nalbuphine, and pentazocine). The mechanism of action appears to be the same as that for naloxone.

Uses of Naltrexone

Naltrexone is used to treat persons dependent on opioids. Patients receiving naltrexone have been detoxified and are enrolled in a program for treatment of narcotic addiction. Naltrexone, along with other methods of treatment, such as counseling or psychotherapy, is used to maintain an opioid-free state. Patients taking naltrexone on a scheduled basis will not experience any narcotic effects if they use an opioid.

Adverse Reactions of Naltrexone

Administration of naltrexone may result in anxiety, difficulty sleeping, abdominal cramps, nasal congestion, joint and muscle pain, nausea, vomiting, dizziness, irritability, depression, fatigue, and drowsiness.

Contraindications, Precautions, and Interactions of Naltrexone

Naltrexone is contraindicated in those with a hypersensitivity to narcotic antagonists. Naltrexone is contraindicated during pregnancy (category C). Naltrexone is used cautiously in those with a narcotic addiction; in patients with cardiovascular disease, acute hepatitis, liver failure, or depression; and in patients who are suicidal. Naltrexone is used cautiously during lactation.

Naltrexone may produce withdrawal symptoms in those physically dependent on narcotics. These patients must not have taken any opiate for the last 7 to 10 days. Concurrent use of naltrexone with thioridazine may cause increased drowsiness and lethargy. Naltrexone may prevent the action of opioid antidiarrheals, antitussives, and analgesics.

Patient Management Issues with Narcotic Antagonists

Narcotic Antagonists for Respiratory Depression

As part of the ongoing assessment during the administration of naloxone, the patient's blood pressure, pulse, and respiratory rate are monitored frequently, usually every 5 minutes, until the patient responds. After the patient has shown response to the drug, vital signs are monitored every 5 to 15 minutes. The health care provider should be notified if any adverse drug reactions occur because additional medical treatment may be needed. The patient's respiratory rate, rhythm, and depth; pulse; blood pressure; and level of consciousness are monitored until the effects of the narcotic wear off.

ALERT

Naloxone

The effects of some narcotics may last longer than the effects of naloxone. A repeat dose of naloxone may be ordered by the health care provider if results obtained from the initial dose are unsatisfactory. How long the patient is closely observed depends on the patient's response to the narcotic antagonist.

Narcotic Antagonists for Treatment of Opioid Dependency

Each time a patient visits the outpatient clinic, the patient's response to therapy is evaluated and the health care provider looks for any signs that drug dependency might again be a problem. These signs might include ineffective coping related to difficulty staying drug-free, anxiety, or other factors, including an indifference to the requirements of the treatment program.

Entering a program for drug dependency may cause great anxiety. Possible causes of anxiety include the socioeconomic impact of drug dependency, questions about the effectiveness of the treatment program, and concern over remaining drug free. Individuals vary in their ability to communicate their fears and concerns. At times, the health care provider may be able to identify situations causing anxiety and explore possible solutions to the many problems faced by these patients.

One of the greatest problems experienced by those with former drug dependency is remaining drug-free. Some people find it difficult to break away from situations, individuals, or pressures that promote drug use. Because of this, some opioid users entering a drug rehabilitation program may eventually not report to the program or agency to receive their drug and thus become more likely to return to using an opiate.

All staff members in a rehabilitation program should work to encourage the patient to stick with the regimen and to identify situations in which the patient is encouraged to return to drug use.

Educating the Patient and Family About Narcotic Antagonists

Patients under treatment for narcotic addiction should be instructed to wear or carry identification indicating that they are receiving naltrexone. If a patient taking naltrexone requires hospitalization, then medical personnel must be aware of therapy with this drug. Narcotics administered to these patients have no effect and cannot relieve pain. The health care provider must decide what methods must be used to control pain in patients receiving naltrexone.

Patients taking naltrexone should be made aware of the impact of therapy. While they are taking the drug, any use of heroin or another opiate generally will have no effect. Large doses of heroin or other opiates, however, can overcome the drug's effect and result in coma or death.

KEY POINTS

● Nonnarcotic analgesics are drugs used to relieve pain without the possibility of causing physical dependency, such as can occur with the use of the narcotic analgesics. Nonnarcotic analgesics include the salicylates, nonsalicylates (acetaminophen), and nonsteroidal anti-inflammatory drugs (NSAIDs).

● Adverse reactions of salicylate drugs include gastric upset, heartburn, nausea, vomiting, anorexia, and gastrointestinal bleeding. Adverse reactions of acetaminophen usually occur with chronic use or when the recommended dosage is exceeded, and are otherwise uncommon.

● Many adverse reactions may occur with NSAIDs. However, many patients take these drugs and experience few if any side effects.

● Narcotic analgesics are controlled substances used to treat moderate to severe pain. Narcotic analgesics are classified as agonists, partial agonists, and mixed agonists–antagonists. Drugs that counteract the effects of the narcotic analgesics are narcotic antagonists.

● One of the major hazards of agonist narcotic administration is respiratory depression. The most common adverse reactions to agonists include light-headedness, dizziness, sedation, constipation, anorexia, nausea, vomiting, and sweating. Administration of a narcotic agonist–antagonist may result in symptoms of narcotic withdrawal in those addicted to narcotics.

● Morphine is the most widely used drug in the management of chronic severe pain, such as pain associated with cancer. This drug can be given orally, subcutaneously, intramuscularly, intravenous, and rectally in the form of a suppository and has tremendous versatility.

CASE STUDY

Mr. Nunn, age 68 years, has been prescribed an NSAID for the treatment of arthritis and has been taking the drug for 2 weeks. During an outpatient appointment, Mr. Nunn says that he has noticed very little improvement in his arthritis and complains of nausea, difficulty hearing, constipation, and bloating.

1. When he finishes describing his ailments, it is important to:
   a. stress the importance of informing the health care provider of his ailments before taking the next dose of the NSAID
   b. make a mental note of his concerns but realize they pose no immediate threat to his health
   c. tell him NSAIDs often create these conditions at the onset; patients find that the reactions tend to subside over time
   d. none of the above

2. As you are speaking with Mr. Nunn, he compliments on your red shoes. Your shoes are white. What is the most likely explanation?
   a. Mr. Nunn is color blind.
   b. Mr. Nunn's entire color spectrum may be off, because visual disturbances can be an adverse reaction to NSAIDs
   c. This is an adverse reaction created by the combination of medication for hypertension and the NSAID
   d. Mr. Nunn's vision changes are an indication of life-threatening adverse reaction.

3. Mr. Nunn's age is:
   a. irrelevant to his condition because NSAIDs do not require special considerations for geriatric patients
   b. a consideration because the likelihood of visual disturbances increases with advanced age
   c. a consideration because of gastrointestinal symptoms
   d. a factor that should result in beginning treatment with a larger dosage

WEBSITE ACTIVITIES

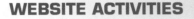

1. Go to the Mayo Clinic website (www.mayoclinic.org) and search for information about the use of an epidural for labor pain management. Write a brief statement about what an expectant mother might learn from the site.

2. Continuing on the Mayo Clinic website, search for the most current information on cancer pain management. Write a brief statement outlining what you learn.

REVIEW QUESTIONS

1. Which of the following symptoms would you expect in a patient experiencing salicylism?
   a. dizziness, tinnitus, mental confusion
   b. diarrhea, nausea, weight loss
   c. constipation, anorexia, rash
   d. weight gain, hyperglycemia, urinary frequency

2. Patients taking aspirin are instructed to avoid foods containing salicylates because this increases the risk of adverse reactions. Which foods should patients avoid?
   a. salt, soft drinks
   b. broccoli, milk
   c. prunes, tea
   d. liver, pepper

3. The health care provider observes a patient for which of these common adverse reactions when administering naproxen?
   a. headache, dyspepsia
   b. blurred vision, constipation
   c. anorexia, tinnitus
   d. stomatitis, confusion

4. It is explained to patients that some narcotics may be used as part of the preoperative medication regimen to:
   a. increase their intestinal motility
   b. facilitate passage of an endotracheal tube
   c. enhance the effects of a skeletal muscle relaxant
   d. lessen their anxiety and provide sedation

5. Which narcotic antagonist is most likely prescribed for treatment of a patient experiencing an overdose of a narcotic?
   a. naltrexone
   b. naloxone
   c. naproxen
   d. nifedipine

Unit III • Drugs That Affect the Respiratory System

11 Antihistamines and Decongestants

KEY TERMS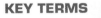
antihistamine—a drug used to counteract the effects of histamine on body organs and structures
decongestant—a drug that reduces the swelling of nasal passages
epigastric distress—discomfort in the abdomen
expectoration—the elimination of thick, tenacious mucus from the respiratory tract by spitting it up
histamine—a substance in various body tissues, such as the heart, lungs, gastric mucosa, and skin, that is produced in response to injury
photosensitivity—exaggerated response to brief exposure to the sun, resulting in moderate to severe sunburn
rebound—causing the opposite of the desired effect
vasoconstriction—a narrowing of the blood vessel

CHAPTER OBJECTIVES

On completion of this chapter, students will be able to:

1 Define the chapter's key terms.

2 Understand disorders involving the respiratory system and how antihistamines and decongestants are used to treat these disorders.

3 Describe the uses, general drug actions, general adverse reactions, contraindications, precautions, and interactions of antihistamines and decongestants.

4 Discuss important points a patient or family member should know about using an antihistamine or decongestant.

The respiratory system consists of the upper and lower airways, the lungs, and the thoracic cavity. The function of the respiratory system is to exchange oxygen and carbon dioxide from the blood in the lungs. Any change in a patient's respiratory status has the potential to affect every other body system because all cells need an adequate supply of oxygen for optimal functioning. This chapter focuses on drugs used to treat some of the more common disorders affecting the respiratory system, particularly allergies and the congestion associated with certain respiratory disorders.

Histamine is a substance present in various tissues of the body, such as the heart, lungs, gastric mucosa, and

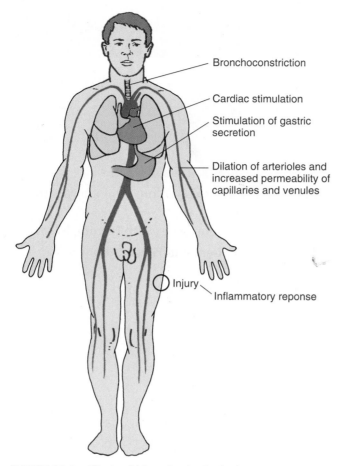

Bronchoconstriction

Cardiac stimulation

Stimulation of gastric secretion

Dilation of arterioles and increased permeability of capillaries and venules

Injury

Inflammatory reponse

FIGURE 11-1 Effects of histamine in the body. (From Roach SS. *Introductory Clinical Pharmacology,* 7th ed. Baltimore: Lippincott Williams & Wilkins; 2004.) (Adapted from Reiss & Evans. *Pharmacological Aspects of Nursing Care,* 3rd ed.)

skin (Fig. 11-1). The highest concentration of histamine is found in basophils (a type of white blood cell) and mast cells that are found near capillaries. Histamine is released in response to injury. It acts on areas such as the vascular system and smooth muscle, producing dilation of arterioles and an increased permeability of capillaries and venules. Dilation of the arterioles results in localized redness. An increase in the permeability of small blood vessels allows fluid to escape from these blood vessels into the surrounding tissues, which produces localized swelling. Thus, the release of histamine produces an inflammatory response. Histamine is also released in allergic reactions or hypersensitivity reactions, such as anaphylactic shock.

Antihistamines are drugs used to counteract the effects of histamine on body organs and structures.

A **decongestant** is a drug that reduces swelling of the nasal passages, which in turn opens clogged nasal passages and enhances drainage of the sinuses. These drugs are used for the temporary relief of nasal congestion caused by the common cold, hay fever, sinusitis, and other respiratory allergies.

Actions of Antihistamines

Antihistamines block most, but not all, of the effects of histamine. They do this by competing for histamine at histamine receptor sites, thereby preventing histamine from entering these receptor sites and producing its effect on body tissues. Some antihistamines have additional effects, such as antipruritic (prevents itching), antiemetic (prevents vomiting), and sedative effects.

Uses of Antihistamines

The general uses of the antihistamines include relief of the symptoms of seasonal and perennial allergies, allergic and vasomotor rhinitis, allergic conjunctivitis, mild and uncomplicated angioneurotic edema and urticaria, relief of allergic reactions to drugs, blood, or plasma, relief of coughs caused by colds or allergy, adjunctive therapy in anaphylactic shock, treatment of parkinsonism, relief of nausea and vomiting, relief of motion sickness, sedation, and as adjuncts to analgesics. Each antihistamine may be used for one or more of these reasons.

Examples of antihistamines include diphenhydramine (Benadryl), loratadine (Claritin), fexofenadine (Allegra), and cetirizine (Zyrtec). A new antihistamine, desloratadine (Clarinex), is the active metabolite of loratadine and is intended to eventually replace loratadine (Claritin). Topical corticosteroid nasal sprays such as fluticasone propionate (Flonase) or triamcinolone acetonide (Nasacort AQ) are also used for nasal allergy symptoms. See Chapter 30 for more information about topical corticosteroids. Additional antihistamines are listed in the Summary Drug Table: Antihistamines.

Examples of nasal decongestants include phenylephrine (Neo-Synephrine) and oxymetazoline (Afrin), which are available as nasal sprays or drops, and pseudoephedrine (Sudafed), which is taken orally. Additional nasal decongestants are listed in the Summary Drug Table: Systemic and Topical Nasal Decongestants.

Adverse Reactions of Antihistamines

Drowsiness and sedation are common adverse reactions of many of the antihistamines. Some antihistamines appear to cause more drowsiness and sedation than others. These drugs may also have varying degrees of anticholinergic (cholinergic blocking) effects, which may result in dryness of the mouth, nose, and throat and a thickening of bronchial secretions. Several newer preparations (e.g., loratadine) cause little, if any, drowsiness and fewer anticholinergic effects than other antihistamines. Some antihistamines may cause dizziness, disturbed coordination, fatigue, hypotension, headache,

SUMMARY DRUG TABLE   Antihistamines

Generic Name	Trade Name*	Uses	Adverse Reactions	Dosage Ranges
brompheniramine maleate *brome-fen-ir'-a-meen*	Bromphen, Dimetane, *generic*	Allergic symptoms; allergic reactions to blood or plasma; adjunctive therapy in anaphylactic reactions	Drowsiness, sedation, dizziness, disturbed coordination, hypotension, headache, blurred vision, thickening of bronchial secretions	4 mg PO q4–6h; 8–12 mg PO of sustained-release form q12h; maximum dosage, 40 mg/d IM, SC, IV in divided doses
cetirizine HCl *se-tear'-i-zeen*	Zyrtec	Seasonal rhinitis, chronic urticaria	Sedation, diarrhea, somnolence	5–10 mg daily PO; maximum dosage, 20 mg/d
chlorpheniramine maleate *klor-fen-eer'-a-meen*	Aller-Chlor, Chlor-Trimeton, *generic*	Allergic symptoms, hypersensitivity reactions, including anaphylaxis and transfusion reactions	Drowsiness, sedation, hypotension, palpitations, blurred vision, dry mouth, urinary hesitancy	4 mg PO q4–6h; sustained-release form: 8–12 mg PO q8–12h; 5–20 mg IM, SC, IV
clemastine fumarate *klem'-as-teen*	Tavist	Allergic rhinitis, urticaria	Drowsiness, sedation, hypotension, palpitations, blurred vision, dry mouth, urinary hesitancy	1.34 mg PO BID to 8.04 mg/d
desloratadine *des-low-rah'-tah-deen*	Clarinex	Seasonal or perennial allergic rhinitis	Headache, fatigue, drowsiness, dry mouth, nose, and throat	Adults and children 12 years and older: 5 mg once daily PO
diphenhydramine hydrochloride *edye-fen-hye'-dra-meen*	Benadryl, Hyrexin, Tusstat, *generic*	Allergic symptoms, hypersensitivity reactions, including anaphylaxis and transfusion reactions, motion sickness, sleep aid, antitussive, parkinsonism	Drowsiness, dry mouth, anorexia, blurred vision, urinary frequency	25–50 mg PO q4–6h; 10–400 mg IM, IV
fexofenadine *fecks-oh-fen'-a-deen*	Allegra	Seasonal rhinitis, urticaria	Drowsiness, nausea, headache, back pain, upper respiratory infection	30–60 mg PO BID; maximum dosage, 180 mg/d
hydroxyzine *hye-drox'-i-zeen*	Atarax, Vistaril, *generic*	Pruritus, sedation (oral only), adjunctive therapy for analgesia (parenteral only), antiemetic (parenteral)	Drowsiness, dry mouth, dizziness, wheezing, chest tightness	25 mg 3–4 times per day PO; 25–100 mg IM; sedation, 50–100 mg PO
loratadine *lor-a'-ta-dine*	Claritin, Claritia, Reditabs	Allergic rhinitis	Dizziness, migraine headache, tremors, conjunctivitis, blurred vision, altered salivation	PO 10 mg/d
promethazine HCl *proe-meth'-a-zeen*	Anergan, Phenergan, *generic*	Allergic symptoms, motion sickness, nausea and vomiting associated with anesthesia and surgery, adjunct to analgesics, sedation and apprehension, preoperative and postoperative sedation	Excessive sedation, confusion, disorientation, dizziness, fatigue, blurred vision, dry mouth	Allergy: 12.5–25 mg PO, 25 mg IM, IV; motion sickness, 25 mg BID; nausea, vomiting: 12.5–25 mg PO, IM, IV; preoperative: 50 mg IM or PO the night before surgery
tripelennamine HCl *trip-el-en'-a-meen*	PBZ, PBZ-SR	Seasonal allergic rhinitis	Moderate sedation, mild gastrointestinal distress, paradoxical excitation	PO 25–50 mg q4–6h; SR: 1 (100-mg) tablet in am and 1 tablet in pm

SUMMARY DRUG TABLE   Systemic and Topical Nasal Decongestants

Generic Name	Trade Name*	Uses	Adverse Reactions	Dosage Ranges
ephedrine *e-fed'-rin*	Pertz-D	Nasal congestion	Nasal burning, stinging, dryness, rebound nasal congestion	2–3 drops or small amount of jelly in each nostril q4h; maximum use, 3–4 d
epinephrine HCl *ep-i-nef'-rin*	Adrenalin Chloride	Nasal congestion	Same as ephedrine	2–3 drops or spray in each nostril q4–6h
naphazoline HCl *na-faz'-o-line*	Privine	Nasal congestion	Same as ephedrine	1–2 drops in each nostril PRN maximum dosage, q3h for drops and q4–h for spray
oxymetazoline HCl *oxy-met-az'-oh-leen*	Afrin, Dristan 12-hour Nasal, *generic*	Nasal congestion	Same as ephedrine	2–3 drops or sprays q10–12h
phenylephrine HCl *fen-ill-ef'-rin*	Alconefrin, Neo-Synephrine	Nasal congestion	Same as ephedrine	1–2 sprays of 0–25% solution q3–4h
phenylpropanolamine HCl *fen-ill-proe-pan-ole'-a-meen*	Propagest, *generic*	Nasal congestion	Anxiety, restlessness, anorexia, arrhythmias, nervousness, nausea, vomiting, blurred vision	25 mg PO q4h; maximum dosage, 150 mg/d; discontinued in US
pseudoephedrine HCl *soo-dow-e-fed'-rin*	Sudafed, *generic*	Nasal congestion	Same as phenyl-propanolamine HCl	60 mg PO q4–6h
tetrahydrozoline HCl *tet-rah-hi-draz'-oh-leen*	Tyzine	Nasal congestion	Same as phenyl-propanolamine HCl	2–4 drops in each nostril 3–4 times/d
xylometazoline HCl *zye-low-met-az'-oh-leen*	Otrivin	Nasal congestion	Same as ephedrine	2– drops or sprays in each nostril q8–10h

*The term *generic* indicates the drug is available in generic form.

epigastric distress, and **photosensitivity** (exaggerated response to brief exposure to the sun, resulting in moderate to severe sunburn). Although these drugs are sometimes used to treat allergies, a drug allergy can occur with the use of an antihistamine. Symptoms that may indicate an allergy to these drugs include skin rash, urticaria, and anaphylactic shock.

Contraindications, Precautions, and Interactions of Antihistamines

Antihistamines are contraindicated in patients with a known hypersensitivity and during pregnancy. Although the antihistamines are classified in pregnancy category B (chlorpheniramine, dexchlorpheniramine, clemastine, diphenhydramine, and loratadine) or category C (fexofenadine, hydroxyzine, and prome-

thazine), they are generally contraindicated during pregnancy. Several possible associations with congenital malformations have been reported along with jaundice, hyperreflexia, and prolonged extrapyramidal symptoms in infants whose mothers have received antihistamines (particularly promethazine) during pregnancy. Use of antihistamines during the third trimester of pregnancy has been associated with severe reactions (convulsions) in the infant. The antihistamines are also contraindicated in lactating women; these drugs pass readily into breast milk and may adversely affect newborns.

Antihistamines are used cautiously in patients with bronchial asthma, cardiovascular disease, narrow-angle glaucoma, symptomatic prostatic hypertrophy, hypertension, impaired kidney function, peptic ulcer, urinary retention, pyloroduodenal obstruction, or hyperthyroidism.

Anticholinergic effects are likely to increase when antihistamines are administered with a monamine oxidase inhibitor (MAOI), and additive sedative effects occur if they are administered with central nervous system depressants (e.g., narcotic analgesics or alcohol). When cimetidine and loratadine are administered together, the patient has a risk of increased loratadine levels.

Patient Management Issues with Antihistamines

Most antihistamines are given orally with food to prevent gastrointestinal upset. The patient's risk of injury is greater when adverse drug reactions such as drowsiness, dizziness, or disturbed coordination are experienced. If drowsiness is severe or if other problems such as dizziness or a disturbance in muscle coordination occur, then the patient may require assistance with walking or with other activities.

ALERT

Antihistamines and Lower Respiratory Tract Diseases

Antihistamines should not be taken by patients with lower respiratory tract diseases, including asthma. The drying effect of the antihistamine may cause thickening of respiratory secretions and make **expectoration** more difficult.

GERONTOLOGIC ALERT

Antihistamines

Older adults are more likely to experience anticholinergic effects (e.g., dryness of the mouth, nose, and throat), dizziness, sedation, hypotension, and confusion from antihistamines. Any unusual adverse effects should be reported to the health care provider.

Educating the Patient and Family About Antihistamines

Patient Education Box 11-1 includes key points about antihistamines that the patient or family members should know.

Actions of Decongestants

Nasal decongestants are sympathomimetic drugs, which produce localized **vasoconstriction** of the small blood vessels of the nasal membranes. Vasoconstriction re-

duces swelling in nasal passages (decongestive activity). Nasal decongestants may be applied topically by drops or spray, and some are available in oral form.

Uses of Decongestants

Decongestants are used to treat the congestion associated with rhinitis, hay fever, allergic rhinitis, sinusitis, and the common cold. In addition, they are adjunctive therapy for middle ear infections to decrease congestion around the eustachian tube. Nasal inhalers may relieve ear block and pressure pain during air travel. Many have oral as well as topical forms, but topical application is more effective than the oral route.

Adverse Reactions of Decongestants

When used topically in prescribed doses, decongestants usually have minimal systemic effects in most individuals. Nasal burning, stinging, and dryness may sometimes occur. Oral decongestants may cause tachycardia and other cardiac arrhythmias, nervousness, restlessness, insomnia, blurred vision, nausea, and vomiting. When the topical form is used frequently, or if the liquid is swallowed, the same adverse reactions of oral decongestants may occur.

Contraindications, Precautions, Interactions of Decongestants

Decongestants are contraindicated in patients with known hypersensitivity, hypertension, or severe coronary artery disease. These drugs are also contraindicated in patients taking monoamine oxidase inhibitors (MAOIs). Naphazoline is contraindicated in patients with glaucoma.

Decongestants are used cautiously in patients with hyperthyroidism, diabetes mellitus, prostatic hypertrophy, ischemic heart disease, and glaucoma. Safe use of decongestants during pregnancy (pregnancy category C) and lactation has not been established. Pregnant women should consult with their health care provider before using these drugs.

Additive sympathomimetic effects may develop when decongestants are administered with other sympathomimetic drugs (see Chapter 4). Use of a nasal decongestant along with a MAOI may cause hypertensive crisis. Use of a decongestant with a beta-adrenergic blocking drug may cause hypertension or bradycardia. When ephedrine is administered with theophylline, the patient is at increased risk for theophylline toxicity.

Patient Management Issues with Decongestants

Overuse of the topical form of these drugs can cause **rebound** nasal congestion. This means that the congestion becomes worse with continued use of the drug. Although congestion may be relieved for a brief time after the drug is used, it recurs within a short time, which prompts the patient to use the drug at more frequent intervals, perpetuating the rebound congestion. To minimize the occurrence of rebound nasal congestion, drug therapy should be discontinued gradually by initially discontinuing the medication first in one nostril, then in the other.

After using a topical nasal decongestant, some patients may experience a mild, transient stinging sensation. This usually disappears with continued use.

⚠ ALERT

Nasal Decongestants and Hypertension or Heart Disease

Nonprescription nasal decongestants should not be used by patients with hypertension or heart disease unless approved by their health care provider.

GERONTOLOGIC ALERT

Decongestants

Patients older than 60 years are at greater risk for experiencing adverse reactions to decongestants. Too large of a dose may cause hallucinations, convulsion, and central nervous system depression.

Educating the Patient and Family About Decongestants

Patient Education Box 11-2 includes key points about decongestants that the patient or family members should know.

KEY POINTS

⬤ Any change in a patient's respiratory status has the potential to affect every other body system because all cells need an adequate supply of oxygen for optimal functioning.

PATIENT EDUCATION BOX 11-2

Key Points for Patients Taking or Using Decongestants

Some outpatients may not use decongestants as prescribed. Family members may need to monitor the patient's use and report any adverse reactions that occur.

❑ Remember that overuse of topical nasal decongestants can make the symptoms worse.

❑ Nasal burning and stinging may occur with the topical decongestants. This effect usually disappears with use. If burning or stinging becomes severe, then stop using the drug and discuss this problem with your health care provider, who may prescribe or recommend another drug.

❑ When using a spray, do not allow the tip of the container to touch the nasal mucosa. Do not share the container with anyone.

❑ To use the spray, sit upright and sniff hard for a few minutes after spraying.

❑ To use nose drops, lie on your bed and hang your head over the edge (Fig. 11-2). After using the drops, remain with your head down a few moments and turn your head from side to side.

❑ If using an inhaler, then warm the inhaler in your hand first; wipe the inhaler after each use.

❑ If your symptoms do not improve in 7 days or if you have a high fever, then consult your health care provider before continuing use.

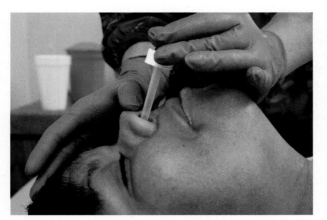

FIGURE 11-2 Position for administering decongestant nose drops. Photo credit: Rick Brady

⊙ Antihistamines are used to counteract the effects of histamine on body organs and structures, a substance present in various tissues of the body produced in response to injury.

⊙ Antihistamines may cause dizziness, disturbed coordination, fatigue, hypotension, headache, epigastric distress, and photosensitivity. Drowsiness and sedation are also common adverse reactions of many of the antihistamines. Symptoms that may indicate an allergy to these drugs include skin rash, urticaria, and anaphylactic shock.

⊙ A decongestant reduces swelling of the nasal passages, which in turn opens clogged nasal passages and enhances drainage of the sinuses.

⊙ Oral decongestants may cause tachycardia and other cardiac arrhythmias, nervousness, restlessness, insomnia, blurred vision, nausea, and vomiting. Decongestants are contraindicated in patients with known hypersensitivity, hypertension, and severe coronary artery disease. These drugs are also contraindicated in patients taking monoamine oxidase inhibitors (MAOIs). Naphazoline is contraindicated in patients with glaucoma.

CASE STUDY

Mrs. Martin, 76, has experienced repeated common colds and as a result, for the past 4 months, she has relied on a topical nasal decongestant to relieve her symptoms. She reports that her other cold symptoms have subsided but that her congestion seems worse, and at times she experiences blurred vision.

1. Which of the following is the likely culprit for Mrs. Martin's exacerbated congestion?
    a. she is experiencing rebound congestion
    b. her cold symptoms may be caused instead by an allergy
    c. she may be experiencing anticholinergic effects
    d. she may need to increase the dosage of the topical nasal decongestant

2. Mrs. Martin's blurred vision may be caused by:
    a. a drug interaction if she is using a drug to treat hypertension
    b. her gender, because women are more likely to have an adverse reaction to topical nasal decongestants
    c. overuse of the topical nasal decongestant
    d. using the nasal decongestant too soon after meals

3. On examination, Mrs. Martin is discovered to have glaucoma. Her doctor asks her whether she is currently taking any medication, and Mrs. Martin explains about the topical nasal decongestant. What drug will the physician avoid prescribing Mrs. Martin, given her current decongestant use?
    a. a monoamine oxidase inhibitor (MAOI)
    b. aspirin
    c. ephedrine
    d. neophylline

WEBSITE ACTIVITIES

1. Go to the website of the U.S. Food and Drug Administration (www.fda.gov). From this page, conduct a search for the criteria the FDA considered in their decision to approve Claritin or any other antihistamine that has been approved as an OTC drug. For example, type "Claritin" into the search box on the FDA home page.

2. On the website of the American Academy of Allergy, Asthma, and Immunology is an article about asthma that defines a "second-generation antihistamine" (www.aaaai.org/patients/seniorsandasthma/medications_and_dosage.stm). Write a brief summary of the definition.

REVIEW QUESTIONS

1. Which of the following is a common adverse reaction of antihistamines?
   a. sedation
   b. blurred vision
   c. headache
   d. hypertension

2. When antihistamines are given to patients receiving central nervous system depressants, a potential adverse effect may be:
   a. an increase in anticholinergic effects
   b. excessive sedation
   c. seizure activity
   d. loss of hearing

3. A patient receives a prescription for phenylephrine (Neo-Synephrine). Overuse of this drug may:
   a. result in hypotensive episodes
   b. decrease sinus drainage
   c. cause rebound nasal congestion
   d. dilate capillaries in the nasal mucosa

4. Antihistamines are not routinely given to patients with lower respiratory disorders because:
   a. the depressant effects may cause a hypotensive crisis
   b. stimulation of the central nervous system may occur, resulting in paradoxical excitement
   c. the effects of these drugs on the respiratory tract may cause secretions to thicken
   d. antihistamines may irritate the bronchi, causing bronchospasm

12 Bronchodilators and Antiasthma Drugs

KEY TERMS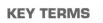

asthma—a reversible obstructive disease of the lower airway

sympathomimetics—drugs that mimic the activities or actions of the sympathetic nervous system

bronchodilator—a drug used to relieve bronchospasm associated with respiratory disorders

theophyllinization—process of giving the patient a higher initial dose, called a loading dose, of a prescription drug to bring blood levels of theophylline to a therapeutic range more quickly

leukotrienes—substances that are released by the body during the inflammatory process and constrict the bronchia

xanthine derivatives—drugs that stimulate the central nervous system and result in bronchodilation

CHAPTER OBJECTIVES

On completion of this chapter, students will be able to:

1 Define the chapter's key terms.

2 Describe common disorders of the respiratory system and the drugs used to treat them.

3 List the uses, general drug actions, general adverse reactions, contraindications, precautions, and interactions of the bronchodilators and antiasthma drugs.

4 Discuss important points to keep in mind when speaking to patients and family members about the use of a bronchodilator or an antiasthma drug.

FACTS ABOUT ASTHMA

- In the United States, the number of new cases of asthma is increasing at a rate faster than any other chronic disease.
- The number of Americans with asthma diagnosed doubled between 1980 and 1998 to approximately 17.3 million.
- 33% of newly diagnosed cases are in children.
- The number of deaths attributed to asthma has tripled in the past 20 years to more than 5500 in the United States per year.

Within recent years, a number of new drugs have been introduced to treat respiratory disorders, such as bronchial **asthma** and disorders that produce chronic airway obstruction. This chapter discusses the **bronchodilators**, drugs that have been around for a long time but are still effective in specific instances, and newer antiasthma drugs that have proven to be highly effective in the prophylaxis (prevention) of breathing difficulty.

Asthma is a respiratory condition characterized by recurrent attacks of dyspnea (difficulty breathing) and wheezing caused by spasmodic constriction of the bronchi. With asthma, the body responds with a massive inflammatory response. During the inflammatory process, large amounts of histamine are released from the mast cells of the respiratory tract, causing symptoms such as increased mucus production and edema of the airway and resulting in bronchospasm and inflammation. With asthma, the airways become narrow, the muscles around the airway tighten, the inner lining of the bronchi swell, and extra mucus clogs the smaller airways.

Asthma is a reversible obstructive disease of the lower airway. Patients with asthma experience airway obstruction caused by bronchospasm and bronchoconstriction, inflammation and edema of the lining of the bronchioles, and the production of thick mucus that can plug the airway (Fig. 12-1).

There are three types of asthma:

- Extrinsic (also referred to as allergic asthma), resulting from response to an allergen such as pollen, dust, and animal dander

- Intrinsic asthma (also called nonallergic asthma), caused by chronic or recurrent respiratory infections, emotional upset, and exercise
- Mixed asthma, caused by both intrinsic and extrinsic factors

Extrinsic or allergic asthma causes the immunoglobin (IgE) inflammatory response. With exposure, the IgE antibodies are produced and attach to mast cells in the lungs. Re-exposure to the antigen causes them to bind to the IgE antibody, releasing histamine and other mast cell products. The release of these products causes bronchospasm, mucous membrane swelling, and excessive mucus production. Gas exchange is impaired, causing carbon dioxide to be trapped in the alveoli so that oxygen is unable to enter. Figure 12-2 identifies the asthmatic pathway from both the intrinsic and extrinsic stimulus.

Other disorders of the lower respiratory tract include emphysema (a lung disorder in which the terminal

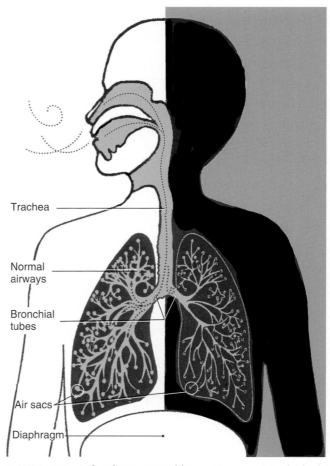

Trachea

Normal airways

Bronchial tubes

Air sacs

Diaphragm

FIGURE 12-1   Left column. Normal lungs: Air comes into the body through the nose and mouth. Air then goes through the trachea pipe into all the airways. The air reaches the tiny air sacs deep in the lungs, where gas exchanges takes place. **Right column.** Lungs in asthma: In asthma, the patient has trouble moving air through the lungs because airways become narrow as the muscles in their walls tighten and the airway walls swell up. The swollen walls give off extra mucus, which clogs the narrowed airways. (From Roach SS. *Introductory Clinical Pharmacology*, 7th ed. Baltimore: Lippincott Williams & Wilkins; 2004.)

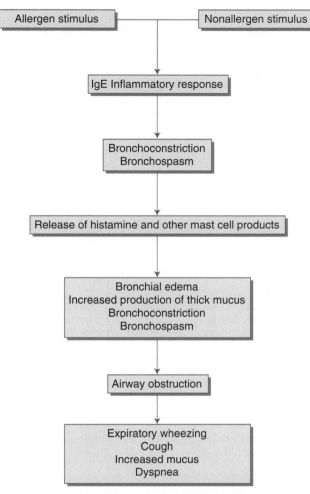

FIGURE 12–2 Asthmatic pathway from intrinsic and extrinsic stimulus. (From Timby B, Scherer J, Smith N. *Introductory Medical-Surgical Nursing*, 7th ed. Philadelphia: Lippincott Williams & Wilkins; 1999.)

bronchioles or alveoli become enlarged and plugged with mucus) and chronic bronchitis (chronic inflammation and possibly infection of the bronchi). Chronic obstructive pulmonary disease (COPD) is the name given collectively to emphysema and chronic bronchitis because the airflow is limited most of the time. Asthma that is persistent and present most of the time may also be referred to as COPD.

ALERT

Bronchospasm

Acute bronchospasm causes severe respiratory distress and a wheezing sound from the forceful expiration of air. It is considered a medical emergency. It is characterized by severe respiratory distress, dyspnea, forceful expiration, and wheezing. These symptoms should be reported to the health care provider immediately.

Bronchodilators

A bronchodilator is a drug used to relieve bronchospasm associated with respiratory disorders, such as bronchial asthma, chronic bronchitis, and emphysema. These conditions are progressive disorders characterized by a decrease in the inspiratory and expiratory capacity of the lung. Collectively, they are often referred to as COPD. A patient with COPD experiences dyspnea (difficulty breathing) with physical exertion, has difficulty inhaling and exhaling, and may have a chronic cough.

The two major types of bronchodilators are the **sympathomimetics** and the xanthine derivatives. The anticholinergic drug ipratropium bromide (Atrovent) is used for bronchospasm associated with COPD, chronic bronchitis, and emphysema. Ipratropium is included in the Summary Drug Table: Bronchodilators. Chapter 4 describes the anticholinergic drugs (cholinergic blocking drugs).

Bronchodilators: Sympathomimetics

Examples of sympathomimetic bronchodilators include albuterol (Ventolin), epinephrine (Adrenalin), salmeterol (Serevent), and terbutaline (Brethine). Many of the sympathomimetics used as bronchodilators are beta-2 receptor agonists (e.g., albuterol, salmeterol, and terbutaline). Additional information concerning the various sympathomimetic drugs is given in the Summary Drug Table: Bronchodilators.

Actions of Sympathomimetics

When bronchospasm occurs, there is a decrease in the lumen (or inside diameter) of the bronchi, which decreases the amount of air taken into the lungs with each breath. This decreased amount of air taken into the lungs results in respiratory distress. Use of a bronchodilating drug opens the bronchi and allows more air to enter the lungs, which in turn completely or partially relieves respiratory distress.

Uses of Sympathomimetics

Sympathomimetics (drugs that mimic the sympathetic nervous system) are used primarily to treat reversible airway obstruction caused by bronchospasm associated with acute and chronic bronchial asthma, exercise-induced bronchospasm, bronchitis, emphysema, bronchiectasis (abnormal condition of the bronchial tree), or other obstructive pulmonary diseases.

Adverse Reactions of Sympathomimetics

A sympathomimetic bronchodilator may result in restlessness, anxiety, increased blood pressure, palpitations,

SUMMARY DRUG TABLE Bronchodilators

Generic Name	Trade Name*	Uses	Adverse Reactions	Dosage Ranges
Sympathomimetics albuterol sulfate *al-byoo'-ter-ole*	Proventil, Ventolin, Volmax, *generic*	Bronchospasm, prevention of exercise-induced bronchospasm (EIB)	Palpitations, tachycardia, hypertension, tremor, dizziness, shakiness, nervousness, nausea, vomiting	2–4 mg TID, QID PO; 1–2 inhalations q4–6h; 2 inhalations before exercise; may also be given by nebulization; Volmax: 4–8 mg q12h PO, up to 32 mg/d
bitolterol mesylate *bye-tole'-ter-ole*	Tornalate	Asthma, bronchospasm	Palpitations, hypertension, dizziness, vertigo, tremor, nervousness, headache, throat irritation	2 inhalations q8h; inhalation solution; 2.5 mg over 10–15 min with continuous flow system or 1 mg with intermittent flow system
ephedrine sulfate *e-fed'-rin*	*Generic*	Asthma, bronchospasm	Palpitations, tachycardia, hypertension, arrhythmias, dizziness, vertigo, shakiness, nervousness, headache, insomnia, nausea, vomiting	25–50 mg PO q3–4h PRN; 25–50 mg IM, SC, IV
epinephrine *ep-i-nef'-rin*	Adrenalin, Epinephrine Mist, Primatene Mist, *generic*	Asthma, bronchospasm	Palpitations, tachycardia, hypertension, arrhythmias, dizziness, vertigo, shakiness, nervousness, headache, insomnia, nausea, vomiting, anxiety, fear, pallor	Inhalation aerosol: individualize dose; injection: solution 1:1000, 0.3–0.5 mL SC, IM; Suspension (1:200): 0.1–0.3 mL SC only
formoterol fumarate *for-moh'-te-rol*	Foradil Aerolizer	Maintenance treatment of asthma, prevention of EIB	Palpitations, tachycardia, dizziness, nervousness	One 12-mg capsule q12h using Aerolizer Inhaler; EIB one 12-mcg capsule 15 min before exercise using the Aerolizer Inhaler
isoetharine *eye-soe-eth'-a-reen*	*Generic*	Asthma, bronchospasm	Palpitations, tachycardia, hypertension, tremor, dizziness, nervousness, weakness, restlessness, hyperactivity, headache, insomnia, nausea, vomiting	Hand-held nebulizer: 3–7 inhalations 1:3 dilution or 4 inhalations undiluted
isoproterenol HCl *eye-soe-proe- ter'-a-nole*	Isuprel, *generic*	Bronchospasm during anesthesia, vasopressor during shock	Palpitations, tachycardia, chest tightness, angina, shakiness, nervousness, weakness, hyperactivity, headache, nausea, vomiting, flushing, sweating	0.01–0.02 mg IV, repeat if necessary; dilute 1 mL of a 1:5000 solution to 10 mL with sodium chloride injections of 5% dextrose IV

Generic Name	Trade Name*	Uses	Adverse Reactions	Dosage Ranges
levalbuterol HCl *lev-al-byoo'-ter-ole*	Xopenex	Bronchospasm	Tachycardia, nervousness, anxiety, pain, dizziness, rhinitis, cough, cardiac arrhythmias	0.63 mg TID, every 6–8h by nebulization; if no response, dose may be increased to 1.25 mg TID by nebulization
metaproterenol sulfate *met-a-proe- ter'-e-nole*	Alupent, *generic*	Asthma, bronchospasm	Tachycardia, tremor, nervousness, shakiness, nausea, vomiting	Aerosol 2–3 inhalations q3–4h; do not exceed 12 inhalations
pirbuterol acetate *peer-byoo'-ter-ole*	Maxair Autohaler, Maxair Inhaler	Asthma, bronchospasm	Shakiness, nervousness, nausea, tachycardia	2 inhalations q4–6h; do not exceed 12 inhalations
salmeterol *sal-mee'-ter-ol*	Serevent	Asthma, bronchospasm	Palpitations, tachycardia, tremor, nervousness, headache, nausea, vomiting, heartburn, GI distress, diarrhea, cough, rhinitis	Asthma/bronchospasm: aerosol, 2 inhalations BID morning and evening; inhalation powder, 1 (50 mcg) inhalation BID
terbutaline sulfate *ter-byoo'-ta-leen*	Brethine, *generic*	Asthma, bronchospasm	Palpitations, tremor, dizziness, vertigo, shakiness, nervousness, drowsiness, headache, nausea, vomiting, GI upset	2.5–5 mg q6h PO TID during waking hours; 0.25 mg SC (may repeat one time if needed)
aminophylline *am-in-off'-i-lin*	***Xanthine Derivatives*** Phyllocontin, Truphylline, *generic*	Symptomatic relief or prevention of bronchial asthma and reversible bronchospasm of chronic bronchitis and emphysema	Nausea, vomiting, diarrhea, headache, insomnia, irritability, hyperglycemia, hypotension, cardiac arrhythmias, tachycardia, tachypnea, seizures	Individualize dosage: base adjustments on clinical responses, monitor serum theophylline levels, maintain therapeutic range of 10–20 mcg/mL; base dosage on lean body mass
dyphylline *dye'-fi-lin*	Lufyllin	Same as aminophylline	Same as aminophylline	Up to 15 mg/kg PO QID; 250–500 mg IM
oxtriphylline *ox-trye'-fi-lin*	Choledyl, *generic*	Same as aminophylline	Same as aminophylline	4.7 mg/kg q8h PO; sustained action: 1 tablet q12h PO
theophylline *thee-off'-i-lin*	Theo-24, Theo-dur, Theolair, Slo-bid, Uniphyl, *generic*	Same as aminophylline	Same as aminophylline	Long-term therapy: 16 mg/kg/24h or 400 mg/24h in divided doses; monitor serum theophylline levels
Anticholinergic ipratropium bromide *ih-prah-trow'-pea- um*	Atrovent, *generic*	Bronchospasm associated with chronic obstructive pulmonary disease, chronic bronchitis and emphysema, rhinorrhea	Dryness of the oropharynx, nervousness, irritation from aerosol, dizziness, headache, GI distress, dry mouth, exacerbation of symptoms, nausea, palpitations	Aerosol: 2 inhalations (36 µg) QID, not to exceed 12 inhalations; solution: 500 mg (1 unit dose vial) TID, QID by oral nebulization; nasal spray: 2 sprays per nostril BID, TID of 0.03% or 2 sprays per nostril TID, QID of 0.06%

*The term *generic* indicates the drug is available in generic form.

cardiac arrhythmias, and insomnia. When these drugs are used by inhalation, excessive use (more often than recommended) may result in paradoxical bronchospasm.

Managing Adverse Reactions

Patients who have difficulty breathing and are receiving a sympathomimetic drug may experience extreme anxiety, nervousness, and restlessness, which may be caused by their breathing difficulty or the action of the sympathomimetic drug. In these patients, it may be difficult to determine if the patient is having an adverse drug reaction or if the problem is related to the respiratory disorder. Patients who are extremely apprehensive are observed more frequently until their respirations are near normal, and the health care provider is notified. The patient's blood pressure and pulse should be closely monitored during therapy and any significant changes reported. Health care workers should speak and act in a calm manner, being careful not to increase the patient's anxiety or nervousness caused by the sympathomimetic drug. Explaining the effects of the drug may help the patient to tolerate these uncomfortable adverse reactions.

GERONTOLOGIC ALERT

Sympathomimetic Bronchodilators in Older Adults

Older adults taking sympathomimetic bronchodilators are at increased risk for adverse reactions related to the cardiovascular system (tachycardia, arrhythmias, palpitations, and hypertension) as well as adverse reactions related to the central nervous system (restlessness, agitation, insomnia).

Contraindications, Precautions, and Interactions of Sympathomimetics

Sympathomimetic bronchodilators are contraindicated in patients with known hypersensitivity, cardiac arrhythmias associated with tachycardia, organic brain damage, cerebral arteriosclerosis, or narrow-angle glaucoma. Salmeterol is contraindicated during acute bronchospasm. Sympathomimetics are used cautiously in patients with hypertension, cardiac dysfunction, hyperthyroidism, glaucoma, diabetes, prostatic hypertrophy, or a history of seizures.

Sympathomimetic drugs are used cautiously during pregnancy (all are pregnancy category C, except terbutaline, which is pregnancy category B) and lactation.

When the sympathomimetics are used concurrently with another sympathomimetic drug (see Chapter 4), additive adrenergic effects can occur. When used with a monoamine oxidase inhibitor (see Chapter 6), the patient is at increased risk for a hypertensive crisis. When a

sympathomimetic is administered with a β-adrenergic blocker, the drugs may inhibit the cardiac, bronchodilating, and vasodilating effects of the sympathomimetic. When a β-blocker such as propranolol is administered with a sympathomimetic such as epinephrine, an initial hypertensive episode may occur, followed by bradycardia. Concurrent use of a sympathomimetic with an oxytocic drug may result in severe hypotension. When a sympathomimetic is administered with theophylline, the patient has an increased risk for cardiotoxicity. When epinephrine is administered with insulin or an oral hypoglycemic drug, the patient may require an increased dose of the hypoglycemic drug.

Bronchodilators: Xanthine Derivatives

Xanthine derivatives, also called methylxanthines, are drugs that stimulate the central nervous system and result in bronchodilation. Examples are theophylline and aminophylline. Additional information concerning the xanthine derivatives is found in the Summary Drug Table: Bronchodilators.

Actions of Xanthine Derivatives

Xanthine derivatives, although a different class of drugs, also have bronchodilating activity by means of their direct relaxation of the smooth muscles of the bronchi.

Uses of Xanthine Derivatives

Xanthine derivatives are used for symptomatic relief or prevention of bronchial asthma and reversible bronchospasm associated with chronic bronchitis and emphysema.

For acute respiratory symptoms, rapid theophyllinization using one of the xanthine derivatives may be required. **Theophyllinization** is accomplished by giving the patient a higher initial dose, called a loading dose, to bring blood levels to therapeutic range more quickly than waiting several days for the drug to exert a therapeutic effect.

Adverse Reactions of Xanthine Derivatives

Adverse reactions of xanthine derivatives include nausea, vomiting, restlessness, nervousness, tachycardia, tremors, headache, palpitations, increased respirations, fever, hyperglycemia, and electrocardiographic changes.

Managing Adverse Reactions

Patients taking theophylline may report heartburn because the drug relaxes the lower esophageal sphincter, allowing gastroesophageal reflux. Heartburn is minimized if the patient remains in an upright position and sleeps with the head of the bed elevated. A patient taking theophylline must be frequently monitored for signs of toxicity. A daily plasma theophylline level is useful in monitoring for toxicity. Obtaining serum blood samples to measure theophylline levels at the time of peak absorption, 1 or 2 hours after administration for immediate-release products or 5 to 9 hours after the morning dose for most sustained-released preparations, is advised. The patient should not have missed any doses during the previous 48 hours. The patient should be discouraged from drinking coffee before blood is drawn to determine the blood theophylline level because coffee can cause a false elevation of drug concentration levels. Toxicity is more likely to occur in patients requiring high doses or during prolonged therapy. Any symptoms associated with toxicity should be reported.

Contraindications, Precautions, and Interactions of Xanthine Inhibitors

Xanthine derivatives are contraindicated in those with known hypersensitivity, peptic ulcers, seizure disorders (unless well-controlled with appropriate anticonvulsant medication), serious uncontrolled arrhythmias, or hyperthyroidism.

Xanthine derivatives are used cautiously in patients older than 60 years and in patients with cardiac disease, hypoxemia, hypertension, congestive heart failure, or liver disease. Aminophylline, dyphylline, oxtriphylline, and theophylline are pregnancy category C drugs and are used cautiously during pregnancy and lactation.

When a xanthine bronchodilator is administered with a sympathomimetic drug (see Chapter 4), additive central nervous system and cardiovascular effects may occur.

If a patient eats large amounts of charcoal-broiled foods while taking a xanthine, then the therapeutic effect of the xanthine may be diminished. Certain foods contain xanthine (e.g., coffee, colas, or chocolate) and may increase the risk of cardiac and central nervous system adverse reactions. Cigarettes, nicotine gum and patches, barbiturates, phenytoin, loop diuretics, isoniazid, and rifampin may decrease the effectiveness of the xanthines. There is an increased risk of xanthine toxicity when the drugs are administered with influenza vaccination, oral contraceptives, glucocorticoids, β-adrenergic blockers, cimetidine, macrolides, thyroid hormones, or allopurinol.

A L E R T

Theophylline Toxicity
Notify the health care provider immediately if any of the following signs of theophylline toxicity develop: anorexia, nausea, vomiting, diarrhea, confusion, abdominal cramping, headache, restlessness, insomnia, tachycardia, arrhythmias, or seizures.

Antiasthma Drugs: Corticosteroids

Along with the bronchodilators, several types of drugs are effective in the treatment of asthma, including corticosteroids.

Actions of Corticosteroids

Corticosteroids, such as beclomethasone (Beclovent), flunisolide (AeroBid), and triamcinolone (Azmacort), are given by inhalation and act to decrease the inflammatory process in the airways of patients with asthma. In addition, corticosteroids increase the sensitivity of the β2-receptors. With increased sensitivity of the β2-receptors, the β2-receptor agonist drugs are more effective.

Uses of Corticosteroids

The corticosteroids are used in the management and prophylactic treatment of the inflammation associated with chronic asthma or allergic rhinitis.

Adverse Reactions of Corticosteroids

When used to manage chronic asthma, corticosteroids are most often given by inhalation. Adverse reactions to corticosteroids are less likely to occur when the drugs are given by inhalation rather than taken orally. Occasionally, patients may experience throat irritation causing hoarseness, cough, or fungal infection of the mouth and throat. Vertigo or headache also may occur. See Chapter 23 for adverse reactions after oral administration of corticosteroids. A more complete listing of the adverse reactions associated with corticosteroids is given in the Summary Drug Table: Antiasthma Drugs.

A L E R T

Inhaled Corticosteroids
Bronchospasm may occur after administration of an inhaled corticosteroid. If an immediate increase in wheezing indicating bronchospasm occurs after administration of a corticosteroid inhalant, then the health care provider immediately administers a short-acting inhaled bronchodilator. The inhaled corticosteroid is discontinued and an alternate treatment started.

Managing Adverse Reactions

Some antiasthma drugs may cause an unpleasant taste in the mouth. Having the patient take frequent sips of water, suck on sugarless candy, or chew gum helps to alleviate the problem. If dizziness occurs, then the patient may need help walking. For nausea, frequent small meals are recommended rather than three larger meals.

SUMMARY DRUG TABLE   Antiasthma Drugs

Generic Name	Trade Name	Uses	Adverse Reactions	Dosage Ranges
Corticosteroids beclomethasone dipropionate *be-kloe-meth'-a-sone*	Beconase AQ, QVAR, Vanceril, Vanceril Double Strength	Respiratory inhalant use: asthma Intranasal use: seasonal or perennial rhinitis, prevention of recurrence of nasal polyps after surgical removal	Oral, laryngeal, pharyngeal irritation, fungal infections, suppression of hypothalamic-pituitary-adrenal function	Respiratory inhalation use: 2 inhalations (84–168 mg) TID, QID; maximum dosage, 20 inhalations (840 mcg/d). Intranasal therapy: 1 inhalation (42–84 mcg) in each nostril BID, QID (168–336 mcg/d)
budesonide *bue-des'-oh-nide*	Pulmicort Respules, Pulmicort Turbuhaler	Turbuhaler: management of chronic asthma in adults and children older than age 6 yr; Respules: maintenance treatment of asthma and as prophylactic therapy in children 12 mo to 8 yr; Additional indication: improvement of symptoms of mild to moderate acute laryngotracheal-bronchitis (croup), seasonal or perennial rhinitis (nasal spray)	Oral, laryngeal, pharyngeal irritation, fungal infections, suppression of HPA function	Individualized dosage by oral inhalation Adults: 200–800 mcg BID; children 6 years and older: 200–400 mcg BID; children 12 mo to 8 yr: 0.5–1 mcg total daily dose administered once or twice daily in divided doses
flunisolide *floo-niss'-oh-lide*	AeroBid, AeroBid-M	Chronic asthma Respiratory inhalant: asthma Intranasal: rhinitis	Oral, laryngeal, pharyngeal irritation, fungal infections, suppression of HPA function	Adults: 2 inhalations BID; maximum dose, 4 inhalations BID; Intranasal: 2 sprays each nostril BID (maximum dosage, 8 sprays/d)
fluticasone propionate *flew-tick'-ah-sone pro'-pee-oh-nate*	Flovent, Flovent Rotadisk	Prophylactic maintenance and treatment of asthma	Oral, laryngeal, pharyngeal irritation, fungal infections, suppression of HPA function	Aerosol: 88–880 mcg BID; powder: adults and adolescents 100–1000 mcg BID; children 4–11 yr, 500–600 mcg BID
triamcinolone acetonide *trye-am-sin'-oh-lone*	Azmacort	Maintenance and prophylactic treatment of asthma; for asthma patients who require systemic corticosteroid administration when adding an inhaled corticosteroid may reduce or eliminate the need for systemic corticosteroids	Oral, laryngeal, pharyngeal irritation, fungal infections, suppression of HPA function	Adults: 2 inhalations TID, QID; maximum daily dosage 16 inhalations; children 6–12 yr: 1–2 inhalations TID, QID; maximum daily dosage, 12 inhalations

Generic Name	Trade Name	Uses	Adverse Reactions	Dosage Ranges
Leukotriene Receptor Antagonists				
montelukast sodium *mon-tell-oo'-kast*	Singulair	Prophylaxis and treatment of chronic asthma in adults and children older than 2 yr	Headache, dizziness, dyspepsia, gastroenteritis, influenza symptoms, cough, abdominal pain, fatigue	Adults and children older than 15 yr: 10 mg PO in the evening; children 6–14 years: 1 5-mg chewable tablet daily, in the evening; children 2–5 years: 1 4-mg chewable tablet daily, in the evening
zafirlukast *zah-fir'-luh-kast*	Accolate	Prophylaxis and treatment of chronic asthma in adults and children 12 yr or older	Headache, dizziness, nausea, diarrhea, abdominal pain, vomiting, infection, pain, asthenia, accidental injury, myalgia, fever, ALT elevation	20 mg BID PO
Leukotriene Formation Inhibitors				
zileuton *zye-loot'-on*	Zyflo	Prophylaxis and treatment of chronic asthma in adults and children 12 yr or older	Dyspepsia, nausea, headache, pain, abdominal pain, asthenia, myalgia, accidental injury, ALT elevation	600 mg QID PO
Mast Cell Stabilizers				
cromolyn *kroe'-moe-lin*	Intal, Nasalcrom	Prophylaxis of severe bronchial asthma; prevention of exercise-induced asthma (EIA) Nasal preparations: prevention and treatment of allergic rhinitis	Dizziness, headache, nausea, dry and irritated throat, rash, joint swelling and pain	Nebulizer solution: 20 mg (1 capsule) inhaled QID Aerosol: adults and children aged 5 yr and older, 2 metered sprays QID Nasal solution: 1 spray each nostril 3–6 times/d Oral: adults and children aged 13 yr and older: 2 ampules QID 30 min before meals and at bedtime; children 2–12 yr, 1 ampule QID before meals and at bedtime; do not exceed 40 mg/kg/d
nedocromil *nee-doc'-ro-mill*	Tilade	Maintenance therapy in mild to moderate bronchial asthma Treatment of itching caused by allergic conjunctivitis (ophthalmic)	Cough, nausea, pharyngitis, rhinitis, vomiting, dyspepsia, chest pain, headache, bronchospasm	2 inhalations QID Eyedrops 1–2 g HS each eye BID

*The term *generic* indicates the drug is available in generic form.

The inhalers, particularly the corticosteroid or mast cell aerosols, may cause throat irritation and infection with *Candida albicans*. The patient is instructed to use strict oral hygiene, cleanse the inhaler as directed in the package directions, and use the proper technique when taking an inhalation. These measures decrease the incidence of candidiasis and help soothe the throat. Occasionally an antifungal drug may be prescribed to manage the candidiasis.

Contraindications, Precautions, and Interactions of Corticosteroids

Corticosteroids are contraindicated in patients with hypersensitivity and patients with acute bronchospasm, status asthmaticus, or other acute episodes of asthma. Vanceril is contraindicated for the relief of symptoms that can be controlled by a bronchodilator and other nonsteroidal medications and in the treatment of nonasthmatic bronchitis.

Corticosteroids are used cautiously in patients with compromised immune systems, glaucoma, kidney or liver disease, convulsive disorders, or diabetes; those taking systemic corticosteroids; and during pregnancy (pregnancy category C) and lactation.

Ketoconazole may increase plasma levels of budesonide and fluticasone.

Antiasthma Drugs: Leukotriene Receptor Antagonists and Leukotriene Formation Inhibitors

Leukotriene receptor antagonists include montelukast sodium (Singulair) and zafirlukast (Accolate). Zileuton (Zyflo) is classified as a leukotriene formation inhibitor. Additional information concerning these drugs is found in the Summary Drug Table: Antiasthma Drugs.

Actions of Leukotriene Receptor Antagonists and Leukotriene Formation Inhibitors

Leukotrienes are bronchoconstrictive substances released by the body during inflammation. When leukotriene production is inhibited, bronchodilation is facilitated. Zileuton acts by decreasing the formation of leukotrienes. Although the result is the same, montelukast and zafirlukast work in a slightly different manner. Montelukast and zafirlukast are considered leukotriene receptor antagonists because they inhibit leukotriene receptor sites in the respiratory tract, preventing airway edema and facilitating bronchodilation.

Uses of Leukotriene Receptor Antagonists and Leukotriene Formation Inhibitors

Zafirlukast and zileuton are used in the prophylaxis and treatment of chronic asthma in adults and children older than 12 years. Montelukast is used in the prophylaxis and treatment of chronic asthma in adults and in children older than 2 years. Leukotriene receptor antagonists and leukotriene formation inhibitors should never be administered during an acute asthma attack. These agents are used for the management of chronic asthma and are not bronchodilators.

Adverse Reactions of Leukotriene Receptor Antagonists and Leukotriene Formation Inhibitors

Adverse reactions of zafirlukast (Accolate) include headache, dizziness, myalgia, pain, nausea, diarrhea, abdominal pain, vomiting, and fever. Montelukast (Singulair) may cause headache, dizziness, dyspepsia, flu-like symptoms, cough, abdominal pain, and fatigue. Adverse reactions of zileuton (Zyflo) include dyspepsia, nausea, abdominal pain, and headache. Liver enzyme elevations may occur with the administration of zileuton; these elevations may continue to rise, remain unchanged, or resolve with continued therapy. Alanine aminotransferase (ALT) is an enzyme produced by the liver that acts as a catalyst in the transamination reaction necessary for amino acid production. ALT is found in liver cells in high concentrations. When liver damage occurs, ALT levels increase, which makes ALT testing a valuable test for monitoring liver function.

Managing Adverse Reactions

The patient is carefully monitored for hepatic transaminase levels at the beginning of treatment and during therapy with zileuton. ALT levels are measured before treatment begins, once per month for the first 3 months, then every 2 to 3 months for the remainder of the first year. After the first year, ALT levels are measured periodically. If symptoms of liver impairment (such as right upper quadrant pain, nausea, fatigue, lethargy, pruritus, jaundice, or flu-like symptoms) occur or if the ALT elevation is greater than five times the upper limits of normal, then the drug is discontinued. Transaminase levels are monitored until they return to normal.

Contraindications, Precautions, and Interactions of Leukotriene Receptor Antagonists and Leukotriene Formation Inhibitors

These drugs are contraindicated in patients with a known hypersensitivity. Montelukast, zafirlukast, and zileuton are not used in the reversal of bronchospasm in acute asthma attacks. Zileuton is contraindicated in patients with active liver disease.

The drugs are used cautiously in patients with hepatic dysfunction and during pregnancy (zafirlukast and montelukast are pregnancy category B drugs, and zileuton is pregnancy category C) and lactation.

Administration of zafirlukast and aspirin increases plasma levels of zafirlukast. When zafirlukast is administered with warfarin, there is an increased effect of the anticoagulant. Administration of zafirlukast and theophylline or erythromycin may result in a decreased level of zafirlukast. Administration of montelukast with aspirin or NSAIDs is avoided in patients with known aspirin sensitivity. Administration of zileuton with propranolol increases the activity of the propranolol; with theophylline increases serum theophylline levels; and with warfarin may increase prothrombin time. A prothrombin blood test should be performed regularly in the event that dosages of warfarin need to be decreased.

Antiasthma Drugs: Mast Cell Stabilizers

Mast cell stabilizers include cromolyn sodium (Intal) and nedocromil sodium (Tilade).

Actions of Mast Cell Stabilizers

These drugs inhibit the release of substances that cause bronchoconstriction and inflammation from the mast cells in the respiratory tract.

Uses of Mast Cell Stabilizers

Mast cell stabilizers are used in combination with other drugs in the treatment of asthma and other allergic disorders, including allergic rhinitis (using a nasal solution), and in the prevention of exercise-induced bronchospasm. When a mast cell stabilizer is used along with another antiasthma drug, a reduction in dosage of the drugs may be possible after using the mast cell stabilizer for 3 to 4 weeks. These drugs may be given by nebulization, as an aerosol spray, or as an oral concentrate.

When added to an existing treatment regimen, other medications such as corticosteroids are decreased gradu-ally when the patient experiences a therapeutic response to cromolyn in 2 to 4 weeks and the asthma is under good control. The corticosteroid or other antiasthma drug may be reinstituted based on the patient's symptoms. If use of the mast cell stabilizers must be discontinued for any reason, then the dosage is gradually tapered.

Adverse Reactions of Mast Cell Stabilizers

The more common adverse reactions associated with mast cell stabilizers include headache, dizziness, nausea, fatigue, hypotension, and an unpleasant taste in the mouth. These drugs may cause nasal or throat irritation when given intranasally or by inhalation. A more complete listing of the adverse reactions of mast cell stabilizers is given in the Summary Drug Table: Antiasthma Drugs.

Contraindications, Precautions, and Interactions of Mast Cell Stabilizers

Mast cell stabilizers are contraindicated in patients with a known hypersensitivity and in patients during attacks of acute asthma because they may worsen bronchospasm during the acute asthma attack.

Mast cell stabilizers are used cautiously in patients with impaired renal or hepatic function and during pregnancy (pregnancy category B) and lactation. No significant drug interactions have been reported.

Educating the Patient and Family about Bronchodilators and Antiasthma Drugs

Patient Education Box 12-1 includes key points about bronchodilators and antiasthma drugs that the patient and family members should know.

PATIENT EDUCATION BOX 12-1

Key points for Patients about Bronchodilators and Antiasthma Drugs

If the patient is to use an aerosol inhaler for administration of the bronchodilator, then follow these general guidelines:

❏ Drink 6 to 8 glasses of water each day to decrease the thickness of secretions.
❏ Do not use nonprescription drugs (some may contain sympathomimetic drugs) unless your health care provider approves them.
❏ Stop smoking. Smoking may make it difficult to adjust the dosage and may worsen breathing problems.

❏ Do not puncture metered dose inhalers or store them near heat or open flame; the contents of such inhalers are under pressure. Never throw the container into a fire or incinerator. If you notice an unusual smell or taste with use of the inhaler, then stop using it and contact your health care provider.

For treatment with sympathomimetics, follow these guidelines:

❏ Do not exceed the recommended dosage.

continues

PATIENT EDUCATION BOX 12-1 *(continued)*

Key points for Patients about Bronchodilators and Antiasthma Drugs

❏ These drugs may cause nervousness, insomnia, and restlessness (especially the sympathomimetics). Contact your health care provider if your symptoms become severe.

❏ Contact your health care provider if you experience palpitations, tachycardia, chest pain, muscle tremors, dizziness, headache, flushing, or difficulty with urination or breathing.

❏ Salmeterol is not meant to relieve acute asthmatic symptoms. Notify your health care provider immediately if salmeterol becomes less effective for relief of your symptoms, if you need more inhalations than usual, or if you need more than the maximum number of inhalations of short-acting bronchodilators.

❏ Formoterol fumarate (Foradil Aerolizer) is administered only by oral inhalation using the Aerolizer inhaler. When using the Aerolizer inhaler, do not exhale into the device. Always store formoterol capsules in the blister pack and remove them immediately before use. Always discard the capsule and Aerolizer inhaler by the expiration date included in the manufacturer's instructions. When treatment with formoterol begins, discontinue the regular use of the short-acting β2-agonist and use it only for relief of acute asthma symptoms. Do not substitute formoterol for inhaled oral corticosteroids and do not reduce your use of the corticosteroids.

For treatment with xanthine derivatives, follow these guidelines:

❏ Avoid foods that contain xanthine, such as colas, coffee, and chocolate, as well as charcoal-grilled foods.

❏ If you experience gastrointestinal upset, then take the drug with food. Do not chew or crush coated or sustained-release tablets.

❏ Do not change from one brand to another without consulting your health care provider.

For treatment with corticosteroid inhalants, follow these guidelines:

❏ Rinse your mouth with water without swallowing after each dose to reduce the risk of oral candidiasis.

❏ Carry a warning card indicating the need for supplemental systemic steroids in the event of stress or severe asthmatic attack that is unresponsive to bronchodilators.

❏ Do not stop the drug therapy abruptly.

❏ These drugs are not bronchodilators and do not contain medication to provide rapid relief of breathing difficulties during an asthma attack.

❏ If taking bronchodilators by inhalation, then use the bronchodilator several minutes before the corticosteroid to enhance application of the steroid into the bronchial tract.

For treatment with leukotriene receptor agonists and leukotriene formation inhibitors, follow these guidelines:

❏ Zafirlukast: Take this drug regularly as prescribed, even during symptom-free times. Do not use it to treat acute episodes of asthma.

❏ Montelukast: Take once daily in the evening, even when free of symptoms. Contact your health care provider if your asthma is not well controlled. This drug is not for the treatment of an acute attack. Avoid taking aspirin and or NSAIDs while taking montelukast.

❏ Zileuton: This drug is not a bronchodilator, so do not use it for an acute episode of asthma. Contact your health care provider if you need a bronchodilator more often than usual or more than the maximum number of inhalations in a 24-hour period. This drug can interact with other drugs; consult your health care provider before starting or stopping any prescription or nonprescription drug. Have liver enzyme tests performed on a regular basis. Immediately report any symptoms of liver dysfunction, such as upper right quadrant pain, nausea, fatigue, lethargy, pruritus, and jaundice.

For treatment with mast cell stabilizers, follow these guidelines:

❏ Inform your health care provider if your asthma symptoms do not improve within 4 weeks after starting treatment. Your health care provider may discontinue the drug therapy.

❏ Cromolyn: To prevent exercise-induced asthma, this drug should be taken approximately 15 minutes before activity but no earlier than 1 hour before the expected activity. The oral form should be taken at least 30 minutes before meals and at bedtime. Do not mix the drug with any other food or beverage.

KEY POINTS

⬤ Asthma is a respiratory condition characterized by recurrent attacks of dyspnea (difficulty breathing) and wheezing caused by spasmodic constriction of the bronchi. Asthma is a reversible obstructive disease of the lower airway. Airway obstruction is caused by bronchospasm and bronchoconstriction, inflammation and edema of the lining of the bronchioles, and the production of thick mucus that can plug the airway.

⬤ Antiasthma drugs are used in various combinations to treat and manage asthma. Using several drugs may be more beneficial than using a single drug.

⬤ A bronchodilator is a drug used to relieve bronchospasm associated with respiratory disorders, such as bronchial asthma, chronic bronchitis, and emphysema.

⬤ Patients who have difficulty breathing and are receiving a sympathomimetic drug may experience extreme anxiety, nervousness, and restlessness, which may be caused by their breathing difficulty or the action of the sympathomimetic drug.

⚪ Xanthine derivatives relax the smooth muscles of the bronchia and are used for symptomatic relief or prevention of bronchial asthma and reversible bronchospasm associated with chronic bronchitis and emphysema.

⚪ Adverse reactions of xanthine derivatives include nausea, vomiting, restlessness, nervousness, tachycardia, tremors, headache, palpitations, increased respirations, fever, hyperglycemia, and electrocardiographic changes.

⚪ Corticosteroids are given by inhalation and act to decrease the inflammatory process in the airways of patients with asthma.

⚪ Adverse reactions of corticosteroids are less likely to occur when the drugs are given by inhalation rather than taken orally. Occasionally, patients may experience throat irritation causing hoarseness, cough, or fungal infection of the mouth and throat. Vertigo or headache also may occur.

⚪ Leukotrienes are bronchoconstrictive substances released by the body during the inflammatory process; when leukotriene production is inhibited, bronchodilation is facilitated.

⚪ Adverse reactions of leukotriene receptor antagonists and leukotriene formation inhibitors are specific to each drug. Zafirlukast (Accolate) may cause headache, dizziness, myalgia, pain, nausea, diarrhea, abdominal pain, vomiting, and fever. Montelukast (Singulair) may cause headache, dizziness, dyspepsia, flu-like symptoms, cough, abdominal pain, and fatigue. Zileuton (Zyflo) may cause dyspepsia, nausea, abdominal pain, headache, and liver enzyme elevations.

⚪ Mast cell stabilizers inhibit the release of substances that cause bronchoconstriction and inflammation from the mast cells in the respiratory tract.

⚪ The more common adverse reactions associated with the mast cell stabilizers include headache, dizziness, nausea, fatigue, hypotension, and an unpleasant taste in the mouth. These drugs may cause nasal or throat irritation when given intranasally or by inhalation.

CASE STUDY

Ms. Sinclair, who lives alone, says that the montelukast (Singulair) her physician prescribed is not having the desired effect. She broke her reading glasses and admits she does not remember how often she is supposed to take it.

1. How often and at what time of day should Ms. Sinclair take montelukast (Sinclair)?
   a. once daily in the evening
   b. twice daily in the morning and evening
   c. every 8 hours
   d. once daily in the morning

2. Which of the following *is not* a common adverse reaction of montelukast (Sinclair) and should be reported to Ms. Sinclair's health care provider?
   a. headache
   b. dizziness
   c. cough
   d. red, itchy rash

3. Ms. Sinclair's granddaughter, who is 1 year old, has chronic asthma, also. Ms. Sinclair mentions that the child had an attack while visiting, and Ms. Sinclair wondered whether giving her montelukast (Sinclair) might have helped. The correct response would be:
   a. the drug is not recommended for anyone younger than age 2 years
   b. the drug is not used in the reversal of bronchospasm in acute asthma attacks
   c. montelukast (Sinclair) is intended to prevent airway edema
   d. all of the above

WEBSITE ACTIVITIES

1. Go to the website for the National Institutes of Health (http://health.nih.gov) and perform a search for the health topic "asthma." Look in the section of articles from the National Institute of Allergy and Infectious Diseases for the page "Asthma: A Concern for Minority Populations." Write brief answers to the following questions:
   a. What population groups are more susceptible to asthma than others and why?

b. Name two environmental factors that may be causing an increase in the number of new cases of asthma reported each year.

1. _____

2. _____

2. Go to the NIH home page (http://www.nih.gov) and perform a general search for "cromolyn" (search box at top of screen). Scan the listings of "MEDLINEplus Drug Information" for Cromolyn (Inhalation). Read the provided information and answer the following questions.

a. What case studies have been conducted on the use of cromolyn by pregnant women?
b. What does the NIH advise for women who are breast-feeding with regard to cromolyn use?
c. What reason is given for advising patients with irregular heartbeats to avoid cromolyn use?

REVIEW QUESTIONS

1. When the sympathomimetics are administered to older adults there is an increased risk of:
a. gastrointestinal effects
b. nephrotoxic effects
c. neurotoxic effects
d. cardiovascular effects

2. Zafirlukast (Accolate) has what primary treatment function?
a. anti-inflammatory
b. symptomatic relief
c. prophylactic
d. mast cell stabilizer

3. A common adverse reaction that may occur with xanthine derivatives is:
a. hyperglycemia
b. hypoglycemia
c. gastric acid
d. sleepiness

4. Which food(s) should be avoided when taking a xanthine derivative?
a. shellfish
b. products containing nuts
c. cola and coffee
d. dairy products

5. To reduce the likelihood of exercise-induced asthma, cromolyn should be taken:
a. 2 hours before exertion
b. 15 minutes to 1 hour before exertion
c. as needed to control symptoms while exercising
d. 30 minutes before a meal and at bedtime

13 Antitussives, Mucolytics, and Expectorants

KEY TERMS   **antitussive**—a drug used to relieve coughing
auscultating—listening to sounds within the body
coughing—the forceful expulsion of air from the lungs
dyspnea—shortness of breath
expectorant—a drug that aids in raising thick, tenacious mucus from the respiratory passages
mucolytic—a drug that loosens respiratory secretions
nebulization—the dispersing of liquid medication in a mist of extremely fine particles to be inhaled into the deeper parts of the respiratory tract
nonproductive cough—a dry, hacking cough that produces no secretions
productive cough—a cough that expels secretions from the lower respiratory tract

CHAPTER OBJECTIVES

On completion of this chapter, students will be able to:

1 Define the chapter's key terms.

2 Describe the uses, general drug actions, adverse reactions, contraindications, precautions, and interactions of antitussive, mucolytic, and expectorant drugs.

3 Discuss important points to keep in mind when educating the patient or family members about the use of an antitussive, mucolytic, or expectorant drug.

Upper respiratory infections are among the most common afflictions of humans. The drugs used to treat the discomfort associated with an upper respiratory infec-

tion include antitussives, mucolytics, and expectorants. Many of these drugs are available as nonprescription (over-the-counter) drugs, whereas others are available only by prescription.

Actions of Antitussives

Some antitussives depress the cough center located in the medulla and are called centrally acting drugs. Codeine and dextromethorphan are examples of centrally acting antitussives. Other antitussives are peripherally acting drugs, which act by anesthetizing stretch receptors in the respiratory passages, thereby decreasing coughing. An example of a peripherally acting antitussive is benzonatate (Tessalon).

Coughing is the forceful expulsion of air from the lungs. A cough may be productive or nonproductive. With a **productive cough**, secretions from the lower respiratory tract are expelled. A **nonproductive cough** is a dry, hacking one that produces no secretions. An **antitussive** is a drug used to relieve coughing. Many antitussive drugs are combined with another drug, such as an antihistamine or expectorant, and sold as nonprescription cough medicine. Other antitussives, either alone or in combination with other drugs, are available by prescription only.

Uses of Antitussives

Antitussives are used to relieve a nonproductive cough. When the cough is productive of sputum, it should be treated by the health care provider who, based on a physical examination, may or may not prescribe or recommend an antitussive. The color and amount of any sputum present may indicate an infection, particularly in patients with a productive cough.

If the patient's sleep is frequently interrupted by coughing, then the problem should be discussed with the health care provider.

Adverse Reactions of Antitussives

Use of codeine may result in respiratory depression, euphoria, light-headedness, sedation, nausea, vomiting, and hypersensitivity reactions. The more common adverse reactions of antitussives are listed in the Summary Drug Table: Antitussive, Mucolytic, and Expectorant Drugs. When used as directed, nonprescription cough medicines containing two or more ingredients have few adverse reactions. However, those that contain an antihistamine may cause drowsiness.

ALERT

Extended Use of Nonprescription Cough Medicine

If the patient is taking a nonprescription cough medicine for a cough that has lasted for more than 10 days or is accompanied by fever, chest pain, severe headache, or skin rash, then the patient should be advised to consult with the health care provider.

Contraindications, Precautions, and Interactions of Antitussives

Antitussives are contraindicated in patients with a known hypersensitivity. Narcotic antitussives (those with codeine) are contraindicated in premature infants

or during labor when delivery of a premature infant is anticipated. Codeine is a pregnancy category C drug, except in a pregnant woman at term or when taken for extended periods, when it is considered a pregnancy category D drug.

All antitussives are given with caution to patients with a persistent or chronic cough or when the cough is accompanied by excessive secretion. Individuals with a high fever, rash, persistent headache, nausea, or vomiting should take antitussives only when advised by their health care provider. Antitussives containing codeine are used with caution in patients having an acute asthmatic attack, those with congestive obstructive pulmonary disease (COPD), and those with pre-existing respiratory disorders. Administration of codeine may obscure the diagnosis in patients with acute abdominal conditions.

Antitussives containing codeine are classified as pregnancy category C (during pregnancy) and pregnancy category D (during labor) drugs. Safe use of non-narcotic antitussives during pregnancy has not been established. They are used with caution and only when clearly needed during pregnancy and lactation.

Narcotic antitussives are used cautiously in patients with head injury and increased intracranial pressure, acute abdominal disorders, convulsive disorders, hepatic or renal impairment, prostatic hypertrophy, or asthma or other respiratory conditions.

Other central nervous system depressants and alcohol may cause additive depressant effects when administered with antitussives containing codeine. When dextromethorphan is administered with the monoamine oxidase inhibitors (see Chapter 5), patients may experience hypotension, fever, nausea, jerking motions of the leg, and coma.

One problem associated with the use of antitussives is related to its drug action. Although not an adverse reaction, depression of the cough reflex can cause a pooling of secretions in the lungs. A pooling of secretions that are normally removed by coughing may result in more serious problems, such as pneumonia and atelectasis. For this reason, using an antitussive for a productive cough is often contraindicated.

Another problem can arise from the use of nonprescription cough medicine for self-treatment of a chronic cough. Indiscriminate use of antitussives by the general public may prevent early diagnosis and treatment of serious disorders, such as lung cancer and emphysema.

Patient Management Issues with Antitussives

Periodically taking and recording vital signs and **auscultating** the lungs helps establish a baseline for patient's condition. When a patient has a cough, the frequency of

SUMMARY DRUG TABLE Antitussive, Mucolytic, and Expectorant Drugs

Generic Name	Trade Name*	Uses	Adverse Reactions	Dosage Ranges
Antitussives Narcotic codeine sulfate *koe'-deen*	*Generic*	Suppression of non-productive cough, relief of mild to moderate pain	Sedation, nausea, vomiting, dizziness, constipation, CNS depression	10–20 mg PO q4–6h; maximum dosage 120 mg/d
Nonnarcotic benzonatate *ben-zoe'-naa-tate*	Tessalon Perles, *generic*	Symptomatic relief of cough	Sedation, headache, mild dizziness, constipation, nausea, GI upset, skin eruptions, nasal congestion	Adults and children older than 10 yr: 100 mg TID (up to 600 mg/d)
dextromethorphan HBr *dex-troe-meth-or'-fan*	Drixoral Cough Liquid Caps, Robitussin Pediatric, Sucrets, Suppress, Trocal	Symptomatic relief of cough	Sedation, headache, mild dizziness, constipation, nausea, GI upset, skin eruptions, nasal congestion	Adults and children older than 12 yr: 10–30 mg q4–8h, sustained release (SR) 60 mg q12h PO; children 6–12 yr: 5–10 mg q4h or 15 mg q6–8h, SR 30 mg q12h PO; children 2–6 years: 2.5–7.5 mg q4–8h, SR 15 mg q12h PO
dextromethorphan HBr and benzocaine	Spec-T, Tetra-Formula, Cough X, Vicks Formula 44 Cough	Symptomatic relief of cough	Same as dextromethorphan HBr	Varies, depending on formulation; take as directed on package
diphenhydramine HCI *dye-fen-hye'-dra-meen*	Benadryl, *generic*	Symptomatic relief of cough, allergies, sleep aid, motion sickness, Parkinson's disease	Sedation, headache, mild dizziness, constipation, nausea, GI upset, skin eruptions, postural hypotension	Adults: 25 mg q4h PO not to exceed 150 mg/d; children (6–12 yr): 25 mg PO q4h (not to exceed 75 mg/d); children 2–6 yr, 6.25 mg q4h (not to exceed 25 mg/d)
Mucolytic acetylcysteine *a-se-teel-sis'-tay-een*	Mucomyst, *generic*	Reduction of viscosity of mucus in acute and chronic bronchopulmonary disease, tracheostomy care, atelectasis due to mucus obstruction	Stomatitis, nausea, vomiting, fever, drowsiness, bronchospasm, irritation of the trachea and bronchi	10 mL of 20% solution or 2–20 mL of 10% solution q2–6h
Expectorants guaifenesin (glyceryl guaiacolate) *gwye-fen'-e-sin*	Fenesin, Humibid LA, Liquibid Muco-Fen-LA, Tussin, *generic*	Relief of dry, nonproductive cough, and in the presence of mucus in the respiratory tract	Nausea, vomiting, dizziness, headache, rash	Adults and children 12 yr and older: 100–400 mg PO q4h; children 6–12 yr: 100–200 mg q4h PO; children 2–6 yr: 50–100 mg q4h

Generic Name	Trade Name*	Uses	Adverse Reactions	Dosage Ranges
potassium iodide *poe-tass'-ee-um-eye-o-dide*	Pima, SSKI, *generic*	Symptomatic relief of chronic pulmonary diseases for which tenacious mucus complicates the problem	Iodine sensitivity or iodinism (sore mouth, metallic taste, increased salivation, nausea, vomiting, epigastric pain, parotid swelling, and pain)	300–1000 mg PO after meals BID or TID, up to 1.5 g PO TID
terpin hydrate *ter'-pin-high'-drate*	*generic*	Symptomatic relief of dry, nonproductive cough	Drowsiness, nausea, vomiting or abdominal pain	85–170 mg TID or QID PO

*The term *generic* indicates the drug is available in generic form.

coughing, whether the cough is productive or nonproductive, and whether the cough interrupts sleep or causes pain in the chest or other parts of the body should be noted.

Actions of Mucolytics and Expectorants

A **mucolytic** is a drug that loosens respiratory secretions. An **expectorant** is a drug that aids in raising thick, tenacious mucus from the respiratory passages to be coughed out.

A drug with mucolytic activity appears to reduce the viscosity (thickness) of respiratory secretions by direct action on the mucus. An example of a mucolytic drug is acetylcysteine (Mucomyst).

Expectorants increase the production of respiratory secretions, which in turn appears to decrease the viscosity of the mucus. This helps to raise secretions from the respiratory passages. An example of an expectorant is guaifenesin.

Uses of Mucolytics and Expectorants

Uses of Mucolytics

The mucolytic acetylcysteine may be used as part of the treatment of bronchopulmonary diseases such as emphysema. It is primarily given by **nebulization** (liquid medication in a mist form inhaled into respiratory tract) but also may be directly instilled into a tracheostomy to liquefy (thin) secretions. Mucolytic drugs are effective as adjunctive therapy in patients with chronic bronchopulmonary diseases, such as chronic emphysema, emphysema with bronchitis, chronic asthma, tuberculosis, and bronchiectasis, and acute bronchopulmonary diseases, such as pneumonia and tracheobronchitis. It is also used for pulmonary conditions of cystic fibrosis and in

tracheostomy care. Acetylcysteine has an additional use in preventing liver damage caused by acetaminophen overdosage.

Uses of Expectorants

Expectorants are used to help raise respiratory secretions. An expectorant may also be included along with one or more additional drugs, such as an antihistamine, decongestant, or antitussive, in some prescription and nonprescription cough medicines.

Adverse Reactions of Mucolytics and Expectorants

Common adverse reactions of mucolytic and expectorant drugs include nausea, vomiting, and drowsiness. Other adverse reactions are listed in the Summary Drug Table: Antitussive, Mucolytic, and Expectorant Drugs.

Contraindications, Precautions, and Interactions of Mucolytics and Expectorants

Expectorants and mucolytics are contraindicated in patients with a known hypersensitivity. The expectorant potassium iodide is contraindicated during pregnancy (pregnancy category D).

Expectorants are used cautiously in patients with persistent cough that may be caused by a serious condition needing medical evaluation. Acetylcysteine is used cautiously in those with severe respiratory insufficiency or asthma and in older adults or debilitated patients. Expectorants are used cautiously during pregnancy and lactation. Acetylcysteine is a pregnancy category B drug; guaifenesin is a pregnancy category C drug.

No significant interactions have been reported when the expectorants are used as directed. The exception is iodine products. Lithium and other antithyroid drugs may potentiate the hypothyroid effects of these drugs if used concurrently with iodine products. When potassium-containing medications and potassium-sparing diuretics are administered with iodine products, the patient may experience hypokalemia, cardiac arrhythmias, or cardiac arrest. Thyroid function tests may also be altered by iodine.

Patient Management Issues with Mucolytics and Expectorants

The respiratory status of the patient is assessed before a drug is administered. Lung sounds, amount of dyspnea (if any), and consistency of sputum (if present) are documented. A description of the sputum is important as a baseline for future comparison.

Any increase in sputum or change in its consistency is assessed after a drug has been administered as well. Patients with thick, tenacious mucus may have difficulty breathing. The health care provider should be notified if the patient has difficulty breathing because of an inability to raise sputum and clear the respiratory passages.

If any problem occurs during or after treatment, or if the patient is uncooperative, then the problem should be discussed with the health care provider.

Educating the Patient and Family About Antitussives, Mucolytics, and Expectorants

Patient Education Box 13-1 includes key points about antitussives, mucolytics, and expectorants that the patient or family members should know.

KEY POINTS

◉ Drugs used to treat the discomfort associated with an upper respiratory infection include nonprescription and prescription antitussives, mucolytics, and expectorants.

◉ Some centrally acting antitussives depress the cough center located in the medulla. Peripherally acting antitussives act by anesthetizing stretch receptors in the respiratory passages, thereby decreasing coughing.

◉ A drug with mucolytic activity appears to reduce the viscosity (thickness) of respiratory secretions by direct action on the mucus.

◉ Expectorants increase the production of respiratory secretions, which in turn appears to decrease the viscosity of the mucus. This helps to raise secretions from the respiratory passages.

◉ When used as directed, nonprescription cough medicines containing two or more ingredients have few adverse reactions. However, those that contain an antihistamine may cause drowsiness.

◉ Narcotic antitussives are used cautiously in patients with head injury and increased intracranial pressure,

PATIENT EDUCATION BOX 13-1

Key Points for Patients Taking Antitussives, Mucolytics, and Expectorants

ANTITUSSIVES

❑ Indiscriminate use of nonprescription cough medicines, especially when coughing produces sputum, is not advised.

❑ Read the label carefully, follow the dosage recommendations, and consult your health care provider if your cough persists for more than 10 days or if you experience fever or chest pain.

❑ If an antitussive is prescribed for use at home, then the following information is important:
   ❑ Do not exceed the recommended dose.
   ❑ If you experience chills, fever, chest pain, or sputum production, contact your health care provider as soon as possible.
   ❑ Drink plenty of fluids.
   ❑ If taking oral capsules, then do not chew or break open the capsules; swallow them whole.
   ❑ If your cough is not relieved or becomes worse, then contact your health care provider.
   ❑ Avoid irritants such as cigarette smoke, dust, or fumes to decrease throat irritation. Take frequent sips of water, suck on sugarless hard candy, or chew gum to diminish coughing.
   ❑ Codeine may impair mental or physical abilities required for potentially hazardous tasks. Be cautious when driving or performing tasks requiring alertness, coordination, or physical dexterity. Do not use with alcohol or other central nervous system depressants (e.g., antidepressants, hypnotics, sedatives, tranquilizers). Codeine may cause orthostatic hypotension (reduced blood pressure and dizziness) when rising too quickly from a sitting or lying position. Do not take it for persistent or chronic cough, such as occurs with smoking, asthma, or emphysema, or when the cough is accompanied by excessive secretions, except when prescribed by your health care provider.
   ❑ Notify your health care provider if you have difficulty breathing because of an inability to raise sputum and clear the respiratory passages.

MUCOLYTICS AND EXPECTORANTS

❑ For mucolytics and expectorants, the signs and symptoms of possible adverse reactions and impaired respiratory function include changes in cough, the color or amount of sputum, shortness of breath, or difficulty breathing. Notify your health care provider immediately if you experience any of these.

acute abdominal disorders, convulsive disorders, hepatic or renal impairment, prostatic hypertrophy, asthma, or other respiratory conditions. All antitussives are given with caution to patients with a persistent or chronic cough or when the cough is accompanied by excessive secretion. Individuals with a high fever, rash, persistent headache, nausea, or vomiting should take antitussives only when advised by their health care provider.

● Expectorants are used cautiously in patients with persistent cough that may be caused by a serious condition needing medical evaluation. Acetylcysteine is used cautiously in those with severe respiratory insufficiency or asthma and in older adults or debilitated patients. Expectorants are used cautiously during pregnancy and lactation. Adverse reactions include nausea, vomiting, and drowsiness.

CASE STUDY

Ms. Tollster, a teacher, has had a cough for 2 weeks. She is finding it difficult to teach because her lung congestion is interfering with her ability to speak loudly and for prolonged periods. She has elected to take an over-the-counter (OTC) cough suppressant/decongestant but is dissatisfied with the results.

1. What action is best for her to take?
   a. visit her health care provider, given that her congestion has lasted more than 10 days
   b. drink more water to help raise sputum
   c. consider whether her cough is productive
   d. all of the above

2. Ms. Tollster's health care provider prescribes guaifenesin (Tussin). She later mentions that although her congestion has improved, she believes she is experiencing an adverse reaction to Tussin. Which of the following is *not* a common adverse reaction and should be reported to Ms. Tollster's health care provider?
   a. dry mouth
   b. nausea
   c. headache
   d. rash

3. Ms. Tollster says that she is taking Tussin every 2 hours. What is the proper interval between dosages?
   a. every 2 hours
   b. every 4 hours
   c. twice daily
   d. at bedtime with a glass of water

WEBSITE ACTIVITIES

1. Go to the Cystic Fibrosis Foundation website (http://www.cff.org) and navigate to their Publications page, then to the "Patient and Family Education" section. Read the article on glutathione, a new drug being investigated for cystic fibrosis patients. Write a brief statement about the status of this research.

2. Go to the National Institute of Health website Medlineplus website (http://medlineplus.gov) and click on the heading for Drug Information. Use the A–Z drug list to search for acetylcysteine, and read the "Before Using this Medicine" section. What two medical conditions should patients tell their health care providers about before using acetylcysteine?

REVIEW QUESTIONS

1. What symptom is an antitussive used to relieve?
   a. productive cough
   b. nonproductive cough
   c. lung congestion
   d. nasal congestion

2. Dextromethorphan has which of the following as a potential adverse reaction?
   a. constipation
   b. gastrointestinal upset
   c. skin eruptions
   d. all of the above

3. Emphysema can best be treated by which class of drugs?
   a. antitussives
   b. mucolytics
   c. expectorants
   d. none of the above

4. Auscultating the lungs is an important diagnostic tool because it:
   a. allows a baseline to be determined
   b. determines the color of sputum
   c. helps to determine how the patient's vocal chords are affected by congestion
   d. may indicate whether an allergen is present

5. Narcotic antitussives are used cautiously when the following condition is present:
   a. head injury
   b. glaucoma
   c. arthritis
   d. gastrointestinal disorders

14 | Drugs for Heart Conditions: Cardiotonic, Miscellaneous Inotropic, and Antiarrhythmic Drugs

KEY TERMS

action potential—an electrical impulse that passes from cell to cell in the myocardium, stimulating fibers to shorten and causing muscular contraction (systole)

atrial fibrillation—a cardiac arrhythmia characterized by rapid contractions of the atrial myocardium, resulting in an irregular and often rapid ventricular rate

arrhythmia—a disturbance or irregularity in the heart rate or rhythm, or both

blockade effect—the action of antiarrhythmic drugs blocking stimulation of beta receptors of the heart by adrenergic neurohormones

cardiac output—the amount of blood leaving the left ventricle with each contraction

cinchonism—a term for quinidine toxicity

depolarization—the movement of a stimulus passing along the nerve; the positive ions move from outside the cell into the cell, and the negative ions move from inside the cell to outside the cell

digitalization—a series of digitalis doses given until the drug begins to exert a full therapeutic effect

ejection fraction—the amount of blood that the ventricle ejects per beat in relationship to the amount of blood available to eject

heart failure—denoted by the area of the initial ventricle dysfunction: left-side (left-ventricular) dysfunction and right-side (right ventricular) dysfunction; because both sides work together, both sides are affected in heart failure

ischemic—marked by reduced blood flow caused by arterial narrowing or blockage or other causes

left ventricular dysfunction—also called left ventricular systolic dysfunction, the most common form of heart failure

polarization—the point at which positive ions on the outside and negative ions on the inside of the cell membrane are in equilibrium

positive inotropic action—the increased force of the contraction of the muscle (myocardium) of the heart through the use of cardiotonic drugs

proarrhythmic effect—the development of a new arrhythmia or the worsening of an existing arrhythmia caused by an antiarrhythmic drug

refractory period—the period between transmissions of nerve impulses along a nerve fiber

repolarization—the movement back to the original state of positive and negative ions after a stimulus passes along the nerve fiber; the positive ions are on the outside and the negative ions on the inside of the nerve cell

---

CHAPTER OBJECTIVES

On completion of this chapter, students will be able to:

1 Define the chapter's key terms.

2 Describe the uses, general drug actions, adverse reactions, contraindications, precautions and interactions of cardiotonic, miscellaneous inotropic, and antiarrhythmic drugs.

3 Discuss important points to keep in mind when educating the patient or family members about the use of a cardiotonic, miscellaneous inotropic, or antiarrhythmic drug.

This chapter considers two kinds of drugs prescribed for heart disorders: cardiotonics and antiarrhythmics.

Cardiotonics are drugs used to improve the efficiency and contraction of the heart muscle (myocardium), leading to improved blood flow to all tissues of the body. These drugs have long been used to treat congestive heart failure (CHF), a condition in which the heart cannot pump enough blood to meet the tissue needs of the body. Although the term "congestive heart failure" continues to be used by some, a more accurate term is simply "heart failure."

Approximately 4.5 million Americans have heart failure. It is the most frequent cause of hospitalization for individuals older than 65 years. With treatment, some patients may lead nearly normal lives, but more than 50% of individuals with severe heart failure die each year. Heart failure is a complex clinical syndrome that can result from any number of cardiac or metabolic disorders such as **ischemic** heart disease, hypertension, or hyperthyroidism (Fig. 14-1). Any condition that impairs the ability of the ventricles to pump blood can lead to heart failure.

Antiarrhythmic drugs are primarily used to treat cardiac arrhythmias. A cardiac **arrhythmia** is a disturbance or irregularity in the heart rate or rhythm, or both, which may require use of one of the antiarrhythmic drugs. Examples of cardiac arrhythmias are listed in Table 14-1.

An arrhythmia may occur as a result of heart disease or from a disorder that affects cardiovascular function. Conditions such as emotional stress, hypoxia, and electrolyte imbalance also may trigger an arrhythmia. An electrocardiogram (ECG) provides a record of the electrical activity of the heart. Careful interpretation of the ECG along with a thorough physical assessment is necessary to determine the cause and type of arrhythmia. The goal of antiarrhythmic drug therapy is to restore normal cardiac function and to prevent life-threatening arrhythmias.

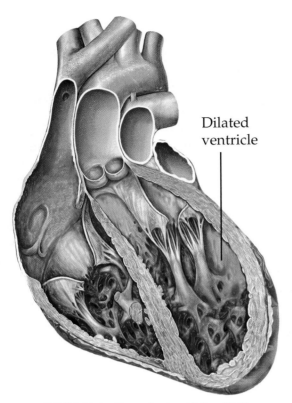

Dilated ventricle

FIGURE 14-1   Congestive heart failure (CHF).

Cardiotonics and Miscellaneous Inotropic Drugs

Heart failure causes a number of neurohormonal changes as the body tries to compensate for the increased workload of the heart. Box 14-1 describes this neurohormonal response.

The sympathetic nervous system increases the secretions of catecholamines (the neurohormones epinephrine and norepinephrine), which results in increased heart rate and vasoconstriction. The activation of the renin-angiotensin-aldosterone (RAA) system occurs because of decreased perfusion to the kidneys. As

> ### Box 14-1 Neurohormonal Responses Related to Heart Failure
>
> In heart failure, the body activates neurohormonal compensatory mechanisms, which result in:
> - Increased secretion of neurohormones by the sympathetic nervous system
> - Activation of the renin-angiotensin-aldosterone (RAA) system
> - Remodeling of the cardiac tissue

the RAA system is activated, levels of angiotensin II and aldosterone rise, which increases the blood pressure, adding to the workload of the heart. These increases in neurohormonal activity cause a remodeling of cardiac muscle cells, leading to hypertrophy of the heart, an increased need for oxygen, and cardiac necrosis, which worsens the heart failure. Heart tissue changes increase the cellular mass of cardiac tissue, change the shape of the ventricle(s), and reduce the heart's ability to contract effectively.

Heart failure is usually described in terms of the area of initial ventricle dysfunction: left-side (left ventricular) dysfunction or right-side (right ventricular) dysfunction. Left ventricular dysfunction leads to pulmonary symptoms such as dyspnea and moist cough. Right ventricular dysfunction leads to neck vein distention, peripheral edema, weight gain, and hepatic engorgement. Because both sides of the heart work together, ultimately both sides are affected in heart failure. Typically the left side of the heart is affected first, followed by right ventricular involvement. Box 14-2 lists the most common symptoms of heart failure.

Left ventricular dysfunction, also called left ventricular systolic dysfunction, is the most common form of heart failure and results in decreased cardiac output and decreased **ejection fraction** (the amount of blood that the ventricle ejects per beat in relationship to the amount of blood available to eject). Normally the ejection fraction is greater than 60%. With left ventricular systolic

TABLE 14-1   Common Types of Arrhythmias

Arrhythmia	Description
Atrial flutter	Rapid contraction of the atria (up to 300 bpm) at a rate too rapid for the ventricles to pump efficiently
Atrial fibrillation	Irregular and rapid atrial contraction, resulting in a quivering of the atria and causing an irregular and inefficient ventricular contraction
Premature ventricular contractions	Beats originating in the ventricles instead of the sinoatrial node in the atria, causing the ventricles to contract before the atria and resulting in a decrease in the amount of blood pumped to the body
Ventricular tachycardia	A rapid heartbeat with a rate of more than 100 bpm, usually originating in the ventricles
Ventricular fibrillation	Rapid disorganized contractions of the ventricles resulting in the inability of the heart to pump any blood to the body, which will result in death unless treated immediately

Box 14-2 Common Symptoms of Heart Failure

Left Ventricular Dysfunction:
- Shortness of breath with exercise
- Dry, hacking cough or wheezing
- Orthopnea (difficulty breathing while lying flat)
- Restlessness and anxiety

Right Ventricular Dysfunction:
- Swollen ankles, legs, or abdomen, leading to pitting edema
- Anorexia
- Nausea
- Nocturia (the need to urinate frequently at night)
- Weakness
- Weight gain as the result of fluid retention

Other symptoms include:
- Palpitations, fatigue, or pain when performing normal activities
- Tachycardia or irregular heart rate
- Dizziness or confusion

dysfunction, the ejection fraction in less than 40%, and the heart is enlarged and dilated.

Until recently, a cardiotonic and a diuretic were the treatment of choice for heart failure. Drugs such as angiotensin-converting enzyme (ACE) inhibitors and beta blockers have now become the treatment of choice. See Chapters 4, 16, and 19 for more information on the beta blockers, ACE inhibitors, and diuretics, respectively.

Digoxin (Lanoxin) is the most commonly used cardiotonic drug. Other terms for cardiotonics are cardiac glycosides or digitalis glycosides.

Miscellaneous drugs with positive inotropic action such as inamrinone and milrinone (Primacor) are nonglycosides used in the short-term management of heart failure. Although in the past the cardiotonics were a mainstay of treatment for heart failure, currently they are used as the fourth line of treatment for patients who continue to experience symptoms after using ACE inhibitors, diuretics, and beta blockers. See the Summary Drug Table: Cardiotonics and Miscellaneous Inotropic Drugs for information concerning these drugs.

SUMMARY DRUG TABLE Cardiotonics and Miscellaneous Inotropic Drugs

Generic Name	Trade Name*	Uses	Adverse Reactions	Dosage Ranges
Cardiotonics digoxin *di-jox'-in*	Digitek, Lanoxicaps, Lanoxin, *generic*	Heart failure (HF), atrial fibrillation, atrial flutter, paroxysmal atrial tachycardia	Headache, weakness, drowsiness, visual disturbances, nausea, vomiting, anorexia, arrhythmias	Loading dose: 0.75–1.25 mg or 0.125–0.25 mg IV; maintenance: 0.125–0.25 mg/d PO
Miscellaneous Inotropic Drugs inamrinone lactate *in-am'-ri-none*	Inocor, *generic*	Short-term management of HF in patients with no response to digitalis, diuretics, or vasodilators	Arrhythmia, hypotension, nausea, vomiting, abdominal pain, anorexia, hepatotoxicity	IV: 0.75 mg/kg bolus, may repeat in 30 min; maintenance: IV 5–10 μg/kg/min, not to exceed 10 mg/kg/d
milrinone lactate *mill'-ri-none*	Primacor	HF	Ventricular arrhythmias, hypotension, angina/chest pain, headaches, hypokalemia	IV: up tp 1.13 mg/kg/d
Antidote Digoxin Specific digoxin immune fab (ovine)	Digibind	Antidote for digoxin toxicity	Hypokalemia, re-emergence of atrial fibrillation or CHF	IV: dosage depends on serum digoxin level or estimate of the amount of digoxin ingested; average dose up to 800 mg (20 vials)

*The term *generic* indicates the drug is available in generic form.

Actions of Cardiotonic Drugs

Cardiotonics act in two ways:

- Increase cardiac output through positive inotropic activity
- Decrease the conduction velocity through the atrioventricular (AV) and sinoatrial (SA) nodes in the heart

These are described in the following sections.

Increased Cardiac Output

Cardiotonic drugs increase the force of the contraction of the muscle (myocardium) of the heart. This is called a **positive inotropic action**. When the force of contraction of the myocardium is increased, the amount of blood leaving the left ventricle with each contraction, called **cardiac output**, is increased.

The most profound effect of a cardiotonic drug occurs in patients with heart failure. In heart failure, the heart, weakened by disease or age, cannot pump a sufficient amount of blood to meet the demands of the body. A decreased amount of oxygenated blood leaves the left ventricle during each myocardial contraction (decreased cardiac output). A marked decrease in cardiac output deprives the kidneys, brain, and other vital organs of an adequate blood supply. The weakened heart also cannot pump enough circulated blood back into the heart. The blood accumulates or congests in the body's tissues. With congestion, legs and ankles swell. Fluid collects in the lungs, and the individual finds it increasingly difficult to breathe, especially when lying down. When the kidneys are deprived of an adequate blood supply, they cannot effectively remove water, electrolytes, and waste products from the bloodstream. Excess fluid (edema) may occur in the lungs or tissues, increasing the congestion. The body attempts to make up for this cardiac output deficit by increasing the heart rate, which in turn circulates more blood through the kidneys, brain, and other vital organs. Often, however, this increased heart rate ultimately fails to deliver an adequate amount of blood to the kidneys and other vital organs. The increased heart rate also places added strain on the heart's muscle, which may further weaken the heart. Untreated, congestion worsens and may prevent the heart from pumping enough blood to keep the individual alive.

When a cardiotonic drug is administered, the positive inotropic action increases the force of the contraction, resulting in an increased cardiac output. When cardiac output is increased, the blood supply to the kidneys and other vital organs is increased. Water, electrolytes, and waste products are removed in adequate amounts, and the symptoms of inadequate heart action or heart failure are relieved. In most instances, the heart rate also decreases. This occurs because vital organs are now receiving an adequate blood supply because of the increased force of myocardial contraction.

Depression of the Sinoatrial (SA) and Atrioventricular (AV) Nodes

Cardiotonics also affect the transmission of electrical impulses in the conduction system of the heart. The conduction system of the heart involves a group of specialized nerve fibers consisting of the SA node, the AV node, the bundle of His, and the branches of Purkinje (Fig. 14-2). Each heartbeat (contraction of the ventricles) results from an electrical impulse that normally starts in the SA node, is then received by the AV node, and travels down the bundle of His and through the Purkinje fibers. When the electrical impulse reaches the Purkinje fibers, the ventricles contract. Normally, once the ventricles contract, another electrical impulse is generated by the SA node, and the cycle begins again. Cardiotonic drugs depress the SA node and slow conduction of the electrical impulse to and through the AV node. Slowing this part of the transmission of nerve impulses decreases the number of impulses and the

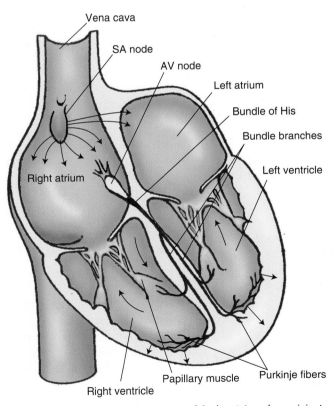

FIGURE 14-2   The conducting system of the heart. Impulses originating in the SA node are transmitted through the atria to the AV node down the bundle of His and the bundle branches through the Purkinje fibers to the ventricles. (From Roach SS. *Introductory Clinical Pharmacology*, 7th ed. Baltimore: Lippincott Williams & Wilkins; 2004.)

number of ventricular contractions per minute, thereby decreasing the heart rate and allowing the heart to function more normally. The therapeutic effects of cardiotonics on atrial arrhythmias are thought to be related to the depressive action on the SA and AV nodes and baroreceptor sensitization.

Uses of Cardiotonic Drugs

The cardiotonics are used to treat heart failure and atrial fibrillation. **Atrial fibrillation** is a cardiac arrhythmia characterized by rapid contractions of the atrial myocardium, resulting in an irregular and often rapid ventricular rate. Arrhythmias are discussed later in this chapter.

Adverse Reactions of Cardiotonic Drugs

Adverse reactions are dose dependent. Dosages are individualized based on several factors, including the following:

- the patient's ideal body weight
- the patient's renal function, evaluated by creatinine clearance
- the patient's age (infants and children require lower dosages, and the elderly may have decreased renal function, requiring a lower dosage)
- the patient's other medications, other medical problems, or other factors affecting the activity of digoxin

Because some patients are more sensitive to the adverse reactions of digoxin, the dosage is selected carefully and adjusted as the clinical condition indicates. Adverse reactions were more common and severe in past years before careful attention was given to weight, renal function, and the concurrent administration of certain medications.

There is a narrow margin of safety between the full therapeutic effects and the toxic effects of cardiotonic drugs. Even normal doses of a cardiotonic drug can cause toxic drug effects. Because substantial individual variations may occur, the dosage must be individualized. The term digitalis toxicity (or digitalis intoxication) is used when toxic drug effects occur when digoxin is administered. The signs of digitalis toxicity are listed in Box 14-3.

Digoxin has a rapid onset and a short duration of action. If the drug is withheld, then the toxic effects of digoxin will disappear rapidly. At times, the health care provider may deem it necessary to administer digoxin immune fab if a life-threatening digoxin overdosage occurs.

Box 14-3 Signs of Digitalis Toxicity

- Gastrointestinal: anorexia (usually the first sign), nausea, vomiting, diarrhea
- Muscular: weakness
- Central nervous system: headache, apathy, drowsiness, visual disturbances (blurred vision, disturbance in yellow/green vision, halo effect around dark objects), mental depression, confusion, disorientation, delirium
- Cardiac: changes in pulse rate or rhythm; electrocardiographic changes, such as bradycardia, tachycardia, premature ventricular contractions, bigeminal (two beats followed by a pause), or trigeminal (three beats followed by a pause) pulse. Other arrhythmias (abnormal heart rhythms) also may be seen.

Managing Adverse Reactions of Cardiotonic Drugs

Digitalis toxicity can occur even when normal doses are being administered or when a patient has been receiving a maintenance dose. Many symptoms of toxicity are similar to the symptoms of the heart conditions for which a patient is receiving the cardiotonic. This makes careful assessment of a patient a critical aspect of care.

ALERT

Digitalis Toxicity

The drug should be withheld and the health care provider informed immediately if the patient shows any signs of digitalis toxicity, if the patient has any change in pulse rhythm or a marked increase or decrease in the pulse rate since the last time it was taken, or if the patient's general condition appears to have worsened.

GERONTOLOGIC ALERT

Digitalis Toxicity

Older adults are particularly prone to digitalis toxicity. All older adults must be carefully monitored for signs of digitalis toxicity.

The patient is also closely observed for other adverse drug reactions, such as anorexia, nausea, vomiting, and diarrhea. Some adverse drug reactions are also signs of digitalis toxicity, which can be serious. Any patient symptom or comment should be carefully considered, recorded on the patient's chart, and brought to the attention of the health care provider.

Usually digoxin toxicity can be successfully treated by simply withdrawing the drug. However, life-threatening toxicity is treated with digoxin immune fab (Digibind). Digoxin immune fab, composed of digoxin-specific antigen-binding fragments (fab), is used as an antidote in the treatment of digoxin overdosage. The dosage depends on the amount of digoxin the patient was given. Digoxin immune fab is administered by the intravenous route during a 30-minute period. Few adverse reactions have been observed with the use of immune fab, but there is a possibility of a worsening of the heart failure, low cardiac output, hypokalemia, or atrial fibrillation. Hypokalemia is of particular concern in patients taking digoxin immune fab, particularly because hypokalemia usually coexists with toxicity.

Contraindications, Precautions, and Interactions of Cardiotonics

Cardiotonics are contraindicated in patients with known hypersensitivity, ventricular failure, ventricular tachycardia, or AV block, and in the presence of digitalis toxicity.

Cardiotonics are given cautiously in patients with an electrolyte imbalance (especially hypokalemia, hypocalcemia, and hypomagnesemia), severe carditis, heart block, myocardial infarction, severe pulmonary disease, acute glomerulonephritis, or impaired renal or hepatic function. Digoxin and digoxin immune fab are classified as pregnancy category C drugs. Fetal toxicity and neonatal death have been reported from maternal digoxin overdosage. These drugs are used only when the potential benefit outweighs the potential harm to the fetus.

When a cardiotonic is taken with food, absorption is slowed, but the amount absorbed is the same. However, if taken with high-fiber meals, absorption of the cardiotonic may be decreased. Cardiotonics react with many different drugs. Drugs that may increase plasma digitalis levels leading to toxicity include amiodarone, benzodiazepines, cyclosporine, diphenoxylate, indomethacin, itraconazole, macrolides (erythromycin, clarithromycin), propafenone, quinidine, quinine, spironolactone, tetracyclines, and verapamil. Drugs that may decrease plasma digitalis levels include the oral aminoglycosides, antacids, antineoplastics (bleomycin, carmustine, cyclophosphamide, methotrexate, and vicristine), activated charcoal, cholestyramine, colestipol, kaolin/pectin, neomycin, penicillamine, rifampin, St. John's wort, and sulfasalazine. Thyroid hormones may decrease the effectiveness of digoxin, requiring a larger dosage of digoxin. Thiazide and loop diuretics may increase diuretic-induced electrolyte disturbances, predisposing the patient to digitalis-induced arrhythmias.

Patients taking a diuretic and a digitalis glycoside must be monitored closely. Thiazide and loop diuretics (see Chapter 19) may increase the risk and effects of toxicity.

Miscellaneous Inotropic Drugs

Inamrinone and milrinone have inotropic actions and are used in the short-term management of severe heart failure that is not controlled by digitalis. Milrinone is used more often than inamrinone, appears to be more effective, and has fewer adverse reactions. Both drugs are given intravenously (IV), and close monitoring is required during therapy. The patient's heart rate and blood pressure must be continuously monitored with either drug. If hypotension occurs, then the drug is discontinued or the rate of administration reduced. Continuous cardiac monitoring is necessary because life-threatening arrhythmias may occur. These drugs do not cure, but rather control, the signs and symptoms of heart failure.

Patient Management Issues with Cardiotonic and Miscellaneous Inotropic Drugs

Cardiotonics are potentially toxic drugs. Therefore, the patient must be observed closely, especially during initial therapy. Before therapy is started, the patient is assessed to establish a database for comparison during therapy. The physical assessment should include:

- taking blood pressure, apical–radial pulse rate, respiratory rate
- auscultating the lungs, noting any unusual sounds during inspiration and expiration
- examining the extremities for edema
- checking the jugular veins for distention
- measuring weight
- inspecting sputum raised (if any), and noting the appearance (e.g., frothy, pink-tinged, clear, yellow)
- looking for evidence of other problems, such as cyanosis, shortness of breath on exertion (if the patient is allowed out of bed) or when lying flat, and mental changes

The health care provider also may order laboratory and diagnostic tests, such as an electrocardiogram, renal and hepatic function tests, complete blood count, serum enzymes, and serum electrolytes. These tests are reviewed before the first dose of the drug is given. Renal function is particularly important because diminished renal function could affect the dosage of digoxin. Because digoxin reacts with many medications, a careful drug history must also be taken.

Patients being started on therapy with a cardiotonic are said to be "digitalized." Digitalization may be accomplished by two general methods:

- rapid digitalization (accomplished by administering a loading dose)
- gradual digitalization (giving a maintenance dose allowing the body to gradually accumulate therapeutic blood levels)

Digitalization involves a series of doses given until the drug begins to exert a full therapeutic effect. The digitalizing, or loading, dose is administered in several doses, with approximately half the total digitalization dose administered in the first dose. Additional fractions of the digitalis dose are administered at 6- to 8-hour intervals. Once a full therapeutic effect is achieved, a patient is usually prescribed a maintenance dose schedule. Digoxin injections are usually used for rapid digitalization; digoxin tablets or capsules are used for maintenance therapy.

Digitalizing doses vary, and the health care provider may decide to achieve full digitalization rapidly or slowly, depending on a patient's diagnosis, age, current condition, and other factors.

During digitalization, the patient's blood pressure, pulse, and respiratory rate are taken every 2 to 4 hours or as ordered by the health care provider. This time interval may be increased or decreased, depending on the patient's condition and the route of drug administration.

Serum levels (digoxin) may be ordered daily during the period of digitalization and periodically during maintenance therapy. Periodic electrocardiograms, serum electrolytes, hepatic and renal function tests, and other laboratory studies also may be ordered.

The patient is observed for signs of digitalis toxicity every 2 to 4 hours during digitalization and 1 or 2 times per day when a maintenance dose is being given. If digitalis toxicity develops, then the health care provider may discontinue digitalis use until all signs of toxicity are gone. If severe bradycardia occurs, then atropine (see Chapter 4) may be ordered. If digoxin has been given, then the health care provider may order blood tests to determine drug serum levels.

Diuretics (see Chapter 19) may be ordered for some patients receiving a cardiotonic drug. Diuretics and other conditions or factors, such as gastrointestinal suction, diarrhea, and old age, may produce low serum potassium levels (hypokalemia). The health care provider may order a potassium salt to be given orally or IV.

ALERT

Hypokalemia and Digitalis Toxicity

Hypokalemia makes the heart muscle more sensitive to digitalis, thereby increasing the possibility of developing digitalis toxicity. The patient must be closely and frequently observed for signs of digitalis toxicity.

Patients with hypomagnesemia (low magnesium plasma levels) are at increased risk for digitalis toxicity. If low magnesium levels are detected, then the health care provider may prescribe magnesium replacement therapy.

Educating the Patient and Family About Cardiotonic Drugs

In some instances, a cardiotonic may be prescribed for a prolonged period. Some patients may discontinue use of the drug, especially if they feel better and their original symptoms have been relieved. The patient and family members must understand that the prescribed drug must be taken exactly as directed by the health care provider.

The health care provider may want the patient to monitor his or her pulse rate daily during cardiotonic therapy. The patient or family member is shown the correct technique for taking the pulse (see Patient Education Box 14-1: Monitoring Pulse Rate). The health care provider may also want a patient to omit the next dose of the drug and call him or her if the pulse rate falls below a certain level (usually 60 bpm in an adult, 70 bpm in a child, and 90 bpm in an infant). These instructions should be emphasized as part of patient teaching. Patient Education Box 14-2 includes key points about taking a cardiotonic drug that the patient or family member should know.

Antiarrhythmic Drugs

Actions of Antiarrhythmic Drugs

Cardiac muscle (myocardium) has properties of both nerve and muscle. Some cardiac arrhythmias are caused by the generation of an abnormal number of electrical impulses (stimuli). Table 14.1 describes common types of arrhythmias. These abnormal impulses may come

---

PATIENT EDUCATION BOX 14-1

Monitoring Pulse Rate

When patients go home with digoxin, they need to monitor the pulse rate to prevent possible adverse reactions. They should be taught to perform the following steps:

❑ Use a watch with a second hand.
❑ Sit down and rest your nondominant arm on a table or chair armrest.
❑ Place the index and third fingers of your dominant hand just below the wrist bone on the thumb side of your nondominant arm.
❑ Feel for a beating or pulsing sensation. This is your pulse.
❑ Count the number of beats for 30 seconds (if the pulse is regular) and multiply by 2. If the pulse is irregular, then count the number of beats for 60 seconds.
❑ Record the number of beats of your pulse and keep a log of your reading.
❑ If you notice the pulse rate is more than 100 bpm or less than 60 bpm, then call your health care provider immediately.

Key Points for Taking a Cardiotonic Drug

- ❑ Do not discontinue use of this drug without first checking with your health care provider (unless instructed to do otherwise). Do not miss a dose and do not take an extra dose.
- ❑ Take this drug at the same time each day.
- ❑ Take your pulse before taking the drug, and withhold the drug and notify your health care provider if your pulse rate is less than 60 bpm or more than 100 bpm.
- ❑ Do not take antacids or nonprescription cough, cold, allergy, antidiarrheal, and diet (weight-reducing) drugs unless their use has been approved by your health care provider. Some of these drugs interfere with the action of the cardiotonic drug or cause other, potentially serious, problems.
- ❑ Contact your health care provider if you experience nausea, vomiting, diarrhea, unusual fatigue, weakness, vision change (such as blurred vision, changes in colors of objects, or halos around dark objects), or mental depression.
- ❑ Carry an identification card describing the disease process and your medication regimen.
- ❑ Keep the drug in its original container.
- ❑ Follow the dietary recommendations (if any) made by your health care provider.
- ❑ Your health care provider will closely monitor your drug therapy. Keep all appointments for visits or laboratory or diagnostic tests.

from the sinoatrial node or may be generated in other areas of the myocardium.

Antiarrhythmic drugs are classified according to their effects on the action potential of cardiac cells and their presumed mechanism of action. There are four basic classifications of antiarrhythmic drugs, and several subclasses. Drugs in each class have certain similarities, yet each drug has subtle differences that make it unique.

Class I Antiarrhythmic Drugs

Class I antiarrhythmic drugs, such as moricizine, have a membrane-stabilizing or anesthetic effect on the cells of the myocardium. Class I antiarrhythmic drugs contain the largest number of drugs of the four classifications. Because the actions differ slightly, they are subdivided into classes I-A, I-B, and I-C.

Class I-A Drugs

The drugs quinidine, procainamide, and disopyramide are examples of class I-A drugs. Quinidine depresses myocardial excitability, which is the ability of the my-

ocardium to respond to an electrical stimulus. Because the ability of the myocardium to respond to some but not all electrical stimuli is depressed, the pulse rate decreases and the arrhythmia is corrected. Quinidine also prolongs the refractory (resting) period and decreases the height and rate of the action potential of the impulses traveling through the myocardium.

All cells are electrically polarized, with the inside of the cell more negatively charged than the outside. The difference in electrical charge is called the resting membrane potential. Nerve and muscle cells are excitable, and the resting membrane potential can change in response to electrochemical stimuli. The **action potential** is an electrical impulse that passes from cell to cell in the myocardium, stimulating the fibers to shorten, causing muscular contraction (systole). After the action potential passes, the fibers relax and return to their resting length (diastole). An action potential generated in one part of the myocardium passes almost simultaneously through all of the fibers, causing rapid contraction.

Only one impulse can pass along a nerve fiber at any given time. After the passage of an impulse, there is a brief pause, or interval, before the next impulse can pass along the nerve fiber. This pause is called the **refractory period**, which is the period between the transmission of nerve impulses along a nerve fiber. When the refractory period is lengthened, the number of impulses traveling along a nerve fiber within a given time is decreased. For example, a patient has a pulse rate of 120 bpm. If the refractory period between each impulse is lengthened and the height and rate of the rise of action potential are decreased, then fewer impulses would be generated each minute, and the pulse rate would decrease. Procainamide is thought to act by decreasing the rate of diastolic depolarization in the ventricles, decreasing the rate and height of the action potential and increasing the fibrillation threshold. Disopyramide (Norpace) decreases the rate of depolarization of myocardial fibers during the diastolic phase of the cardiac cycle, prolongs the refractory period, and decreases the rate of rise of the action potential.

Nerve cells have positive ions on the outside and negative ions on the inside of the cell membrane when they are at rest (Fig. 14-3). This is called **polarization**. When a stimulus passes along the nerve, the positive ions move from outside the cell into the cell, and the negative ions move from inside the cell to outside the cell. This movement of ions is called **depolarization**. Unless positive ions move into and negative ions move out of a nerve cell, a stimulus (or impulse) cannot pass along the nerve fiber. Once the stimulus has passed along the nerve fiber, the positive and negative ions move back to their original place. This movement is called **repolarization**. When the rate of depolarization is decreased, the stimulus must literally wait for this process before it can pass along the nerve fiber. Decreasing the rate of depolarization there-

Polarization

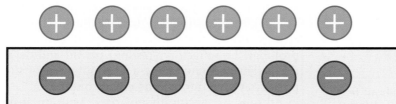

When the nerve cell is polarized positive, ions (⊕) are on the outside of the cell membrane and the negative ions (⊖) are on the inside of the cell membrane.

Depolarization

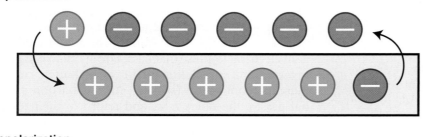

In response to a stimulus, the positive ions move from the outside to the inside of the cell membrane, while the negative ions move to the outside.

Repolarization

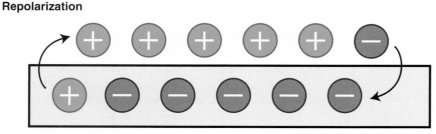

After the stimulus has passed along the nerve fiber, the ions move back to their original place until another stimulus occurs.

FIGURE 14-3 Polarization, depolarization, and repolarization. (From Roach SS. *Introductory Clinical Pharmacology*, 7th ed. Baltimore: Lippincott Williams & Wilkins; 2004.)

fore decreases the number of impulses that can pass along a nerve fiber during a specific time period.

Class I-B Drugs

Lidocaine (Xylocaine), the representative class I-B drug, raises the threshold in the ventricular myocardium. The threshold is the lowest intensity stimulus that will cause a response in a nerve fiber. A stimulus must be of a specific intensity (strength, amplitude) to pass along a given nerve fiber (Fig. 14-4).

For example, let us say a certain nerve fiber has a threshold of 10. If a stimulus rated as 9 reaches the fiber, then it will not pass along the fiber because its intensity is lower than the fiber's threshold of 10. If a stimulus of 14 reaches the fiber, however, then it will pass along the fiber because its intensity is greater than the fiber's threshold of 10. If the threshold of a fiber is raised from 10 to 15, then only those stimuli greater than 15 can pass along the nerve fiber.

Some cardiac arrhythmias result from too many stimuli present in the myocardium. Some of these are weak or of low intensity but are still able to excite myocardial tissue. Lidocaine, by raising the threshold of myocardial fibers, reduces the number of stimuli that can pass along these fibers and therefore decreases the pulse rate and corrects the arrhythmia. Mexiletine (Mexitil) and tocainide (Tonocard) are also antiarrhythmic drugs with actions similar to those of lidocaine.

Class 1-C Drugs

Flecainide (Tambocor) and propafenone (Rythmol) are examples of class I-C drugs. These drugs have a direct stabilizing action on the myocardium, decreasing the height and rate of rise of cardiac action potentials, thus slowing conduction in all parts of the heart.

Class II Antiarrhythmic Drugs

Class II antiarrhythmic drugs include beta-adrenergic blocking drugs, such as acebutolol (Sectral), esmolol (Brevibloc), and propranolol (Inderal). These drugs also decrease myocardial response to epinephrine and norepinephrine (adrenergic neurohormones) because of their ability to block stimulation of beta receptors of the heart (see Chapter 4). Adrenergic neurohormones stimulate the beta receptors of the myocardium and therefore increase the heart rate. Blocking the effect of these neurohormones decreases the heart rate. This is called a **blockade effect**.

Class III Antiarrhythmic Drugs

Bretylium (Bretylol) prolongs repolarization, prolongs refractory period, and increases the ventricular fibrillation threshold. Amiodarone (Cordarone) appears to act directly on the cardiac cell membrane, prolonging the

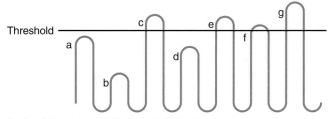

A stimulus must reach the threshold to cause a response in a nerve fiber. Note that stimuli **a**, **b**, and **d** do *not* reach the threshold; therefore, they do *not* cause a response in a nerve fiber. Stimuli **c**, **e**, **f**, and **g** do reach and surpass the threshold, resulting in stimulation of nerve fiber.

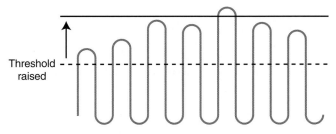

After receiving lidocaine hydrochloride (Xylocaine HCl), the threshold is raised to a higher level, allowing fewer stimuli to reach the threshold. This results in decreased stimulation of the nerve fiber and prevents conduction of the nerve impulses causing the arrhythmia.

FIGURE 14-4   The threshold phenomenon. (From Roach SS. *Introductory Clinical Pharmacology*, 7th ed. Baltimore: Lippincott Williams & Wilkins; 2004.)

refractory period and repolarization and increasing the ventricular fibrillation threshold. Newer class III antiarrhythmic drugs include ibutilide (Corvert) and dofetilide (Tikosyn). These two drugs are used to convert atrial fibrillation or flutter to a normal sinus rhythm. Ibutilide acts by prolonging the action potential, producing a mild slowing of the sinus rate and atrioventricular conduction. Dofetilide selectively blocks potassium channels, widens the QRS complex, and prolongs the action potential. The drug has no effect on calcium channels or cardiac contraction.

Class IV Antiarrhythmic Drugs

Class IV antiarrhythmic drugs include verapamil (Calan) and the other calcium channel blockers. Calcium channel blockers produce their antiarrhythmic action by inhibiting the movement of calcium through channels across the myocardial cell membranes and vascular smooth muscle. Contraction of cardiac and vascular smooth muscle depends on the movement of calcium ions into these cells through specific ion channels. By reducing the calcium flow, conduction through the sinoatrial (SA) and atrioventricular (AV) nodes is slowed and the refractory period is prolonged, resulting in suppression of the arrhythmia. The calcium channel blockers are also called slow channel blockers or calcium antagonists. Two calcium channel blockers used as

antiarrhythmics are verapamil and diltiazem. Dosage ranges for the antiarrhythmic drugs are given in the Summary Drug Table: Antiarrhythmic Drugs.

Uses of Antiarrhythmic Drugs

Specific uses of the antiarrhythmic drugs are given in the Summary Drug Table: Antiarrhythmic Drugs. In general, these drugs are used to prevent and treat cardiac arrhythmias, such as premature ventricular contractions (PVCs), ventricular tachycardia (VT), premature atrial contractions (PACs), paroxysmal atrial tachycardia (PAT), atrial fibrillation, and atrial flutter. Some of the antiarrhythmic drugs are also used for other conditions. For example, propranolol may also be used for patients with myocardial infarction. This drug has reduced the risk of death and repeated myocardial infarctions in those surviving the acute phase of a myocardial infarction. Additional uses include control of tachycardia in those with pheochromocytoma (a tumor of the adrenal gland that secretes excessive amounts of norepinephrine), migraine headaches, angina pectoris caused by atherosclerosis, and hypertrophic subaortic stenosis.

Adverse Reactions of Antiarrhythmic Drugs

General adverse reactions common to most antiarrhythmic drugs include light-headedness, weakness, hypotension, bradycardia, and drowsiness. Adverse reactions of specific antiarrhythmic drugs are given in the Summary Drug Table: Antiarrhythmic Drugs. All antiarrhythmic drugs may cause new arrhythmias or worsen existing arrhythmias, even though they are administered to resolve an existing arrhythmia. This phenomenon is called the **proarrhythmic effect**. This effect ranges from an increase in frequency of premature ventricular contractions (PVCs), to the development of more severe ventricular tachycardia, to ventricular fibrillation, and may lead to death. Proarrhythmic effects may occur at any time but occur more often if an excessive dosage is given, if the preexisting arrhythmia is life threatening, or if the drug is given IV.

Managing Adverse Reactions of Antiarrhythmic Drugs

Adverse reactions must be reported to the health care provider either routinely or urgently. A patient with a dry mouth is not in danger, for example, even though the condition is uncomfortable. Although this reaction is reported to the health care provider, it is not an emergency. In some instances patients must tolerate minor adverse reactions. A patient with severe bradycardia or prolonged nausea and vomiting, however, is in a potentially dangerous situation. The health care provider is

SUMMARY DRUG TABLE   Antiarrhythmic Drugs

Generic Name	Trade Name*	Uses	Adverse Reactions	Dosage Ranges
Class I disopyramide *dye-soe-peer'-a-mide*	Norpace, Norpace CR, *generic*	Suppression and treatment of sustained ventricular tachycardia	Dry mouth, constipation, urinary hesitancy, blurred vision, nausea, fatigue, dizziness, headache, rash, hypotension, CHF	Ventricular arrhythmias: dosage individualized, 400–800 mg/d PO in divided doses
flecainide *fle-kay'-nide*	Tambocor	Paroxysmal atrial fibrillation/flutter and superventricular tachycardia	Dizziness, headache, faintness, unsteadiness, blurred vision, headache, nausea, dyspnea, CHF, fatigue, palpitations, chest pain	Initial dose: 50 mg PO q12h; maximum dosage, 300 mg/d
lidocaine HCl *lye'-doe-kane*	Xylocaine, *generic*	Ventricular arrhythmias	Light-headedness, nervousness, bradycardia, hypotension, drowsiness, apprehension	50–100 mg IV bolus; 1–4 mg/min IV infusion 20–50 mg/kg/min; 300 mg IM
mexiletine HCl *Max-ill'-i-teen*	Mexitil	Ventricular arrhythmias	Palpitations, nausea, vomiting, chest pain, heartburn, dizziness, light-headedness, rash	Initial dose: 200 mg PO q8h; maximum dosage, 1200 mg/d PO
moricizine *Mor-i'-siz-een*	Ethmozine	Life-threatening ventricular arrhythmias	Cardiac rhythm disturbances, existing arrhythmias worsened, palpitations, dizziness, headache, nausea, anxiety	600–900 mg/d PO in 3 equally divided doses
procainamide HCl *Proe-kane-a'-mide*	Pronestyl, Pronestyl SR, Procanbid	Life-threatening ventricular arrhythmias	Hypotension, disturbances of cardiac rhythm, urticaria, fever, chills, nausea, vomiting, rash, confusion, dizziness, weakness, anorexia	Oral: 50 mg/kg/d PO in divided doses q3h; IM: 0.5–1.0 g q4–8h; IV: 500–600 mg over 25–30 min then 2–6 mg/min
propafenone HCl *Proe-paf'-a-non*	Rythmol	Life-threatening ventricular arrhythmias	Dizziness, nausea, vomiting, constipation, unusual taste, first-degree AV block	Initial dose: 150 mg PO q8h; may be increased to 300 mg PO q8h
quinidine gluconate	Quinaglute, *generic*	Premature atrial and ventricular contractions, atrial tachycardia and flutter, paroxysmal atrial fibrillation, chronic atrial fibrillation	Ringing in the ears, hearing loss, nausea, vomiting, dizziness, headache, rash, disturbed vision, proarrhythmia	Administer test dose of 1 tablet PO or 200 mg IM to test for idiosyncratic reaction; 200–300 mg TID, QID or 300–600 mg q8h or q/12h for SR; IM 600 mg quinidine gluconate, then 400 mg q2h; IV 300 mg quinidine gluconate slow IV at 1 mL/min of diluted solution

Generic Name	Trade Name*	Uses	Adverse Reactions	Dosage Ranges
quinidine sulfate quinidine poly galacturonate *kwin'-i-deen*	Quinidex Cardio-quin			
tocainide HCl *to-kay'-nide*	Tonocard	Life-threatening ventricular arrhythmias	Light-headedness, nausea, vomiting, tremor, vertigo, paresthesia, numbness, hallucinations, restlessness, sedation, blurred vision, cardiac arrhythmias	Initial dose: 400 mg PO q8h; may be increased to 1800 mg/d PO in divided doses
Class II acebutolol *ah-see-byoo'-toe-lol*	Sectral, *generic*	Ventricular arrhythmias, hypertension	Hypotension, nausea, diaphoresis, headache, fatigue, weakness, dizziness, impotence, CHF	Arrhythmias: initially 200 mg q12h PO; may increase to 1200 mg/d in 2 divided doses; hypertension: 400 mg/d in 1 or 2 doses PO; maintenance, 200–1200 mg in divided doses
esmolol HCl *ez'-moe-lol*	Brevibloc	Rapid, short-term treatment of ventricular rate in superventricular arrhythmia, sinus tachycardia	Dizziness, headache, hypotension, nausea, cold extremities, bradycardia	Loading dose: 500 µg/kg/min IV for 1 minute, followed by infusion of 50 µg/kg/min IV for 4 min; maintenance dose, 25 µg/kg/min IV

*The term *generic* indicates the drug is available in generic form.

contacted immediately because additional treatment may be necessary.

Proarrhythmic effects (worsening of the existing arrhythmia or development of a new arrhythmia) may occur, such as severe ventricular tachycardia or ventricular fibrillation. It is often difficult to distinguish proarrhythmic effects from a patient's preexisting arrhythmia.

ALERT

Antiarrhythmic Drugs and New Arrhythmias

Antiarrhythmic drugs are capable of causing new arrhythmias, as well as an exacerbation of existing arrhythmias. Any new arrhythmia or exacerbation of an existing arrhythmia must be reported to the health care provider immediately.

Some antiarrhythmic drugs may cause dizziness and light-headedness, especially during early therapy. The patient may need help walking or with other activities until these symptoms are no longer present.

GERONTOLOGIC ALERT

Adverse Reactions to Antiarrhythmic Drugs

When older adults take the antiarrhythmic drugs, they are at greater risk for adverse reactions such as the development of additional arrhythmias or aggravation of existing arrhythmias, hypotension, and congestive heart failure (CHF). A dosage reduction may be indicated. Careful monitoring is necessary for early identification and management of adverse reactions. The health care provider monitors the intake and output and reports any signs of CHF, such as increase in weight, decrease in urinary output, or shortness of breath.

Some antiarrhythmic drugs such as quinidine, procainamide, mexiletine, tocainide, or verapamil may cause agranulocytosis. Any signs of agranulocytosis such as fever, chills, sore throat, or unusual bleeding or bruising should be reported.

The management of adverse reactions of specific antiarrhythmic drugs is described in the following sections.

Managing Adverse Reactions of Quinidine

The most common adverse reactions of quinidine include nausea, vomiting, abdominal pain, diarrhea, or anorexia. **Cinchonism** is the term used to describe quinidine toxicity, which occurs with high blood levels of quinidine. The occurrence of any of the following signs or symptoms of cinchonism must be reported: ringing in the ears (tinnitus), hearing loss, headache, nausea, dizziness, vertigo, and light-headedness. These symptoms may appear after a single dose of quinidine has been administered. The patient is kept in a supine position throughout IV administration to minimize hypotension.

Managing Adverse Reactions of Procainamide

Adverse reactions of procainamide therapy include nausea, loss of appetite, and vomiting. Small meals eaten frequently may be better-tolerated than three full meals. Administering the drug with meals may decrease gastrointestinal effects.

Managing Adverse Reactions of Dipopyramide

Because of the cholinergic blocking effects of disopyramide (see Chapter 4), urinary retention may occur. Urinary output is monitored closely, especially during the initial period of therapy. If a patient's fluid intake is sufficient but the output is low, then the lower abdomen is palpated for bladder distention. If urinary retention occurs, then catheterization may be necessary.

Dryness of the mouth and throat caused by the cholinergic blocking action of this drug also may occur. The patient is urged to take frequent sips of water to relieve this problem. In addition, postural hypotension may occur during the first few weeks of disopyramide therapy. The patient is advised to make position changes slowly. In some instances, a patient may require assistance in getting out of the bed or chair.

Managing Adverse Reactions of Lidocaine

Lidocaine is an emergency drug used in the treatment of life-threatening ventricular arrhythmias. Constant cardiac monitoring is essential when this drug is administered by the IV or intramuscular (IM) route. The patient must be observed closely for signs of respiratory depression, bradycardia, change in mental status, respiratory arrest, convulsions, and hypotension. An oropharyngeal airway and suction equipment are kept at the bedside in case the patient has convulsions.

If pronounced bradycardia occurs, then the health care provider may order emergency measures, such as the administration of IV atropine or isoproterenol (see Chapter 4). Any sudden change in the patient's mental state should be reported to the health care provider immediately because a decrease in the dosage may be necessary.

Managing Adverse Reactions of Tocainide and Mexiletine

Tremors indicate that the maximum dosage of tocainide or mexiletine has been reached. Adverse effects related to the central nervous system or gastrointestinal tract may occur during initial therapy and must be reported to the health care provider.

Managing Adverse Reactions of Flecainide and Propafenone

When flecainide is administered, the patient must be carefully monitored for cardiac arrhythmias. Life support equipment, including a pacemaker, should be kept on stand-by during administration.

To minimize adverse reactions, dosage is increased slowly at a minimum of 3- to 4-day intervals.

Managing Adverse Reactions of Propranolol

Patients receiving IV propranolol require continuous cardiac monitoring. The blood pressure and pulse are monitored frequently during the dosage adjustment period and periodically throughout therapy.

Managing Adverse Reactions of Bretylium

Hypotension or postural hypotension occurs in approximately 50% of the patients receiving bretylium. Therefore, patients need to be carefully monitored for these conditions. The patient is instructed to change position slowly. Most individuals adjust to blood pressure changes within a few days.

Contraindications, Precautions, and Interactions of Antiarrhythmic Drugs

The antiarrhythmic drugs are contraindicated in patients with a known hypersensitivity, and during pregnancy and lactation. Most antiarrhythmic drugs are pregnancy category B or C drugs, indicating that safe use of these drugs during pregnancy, lactation, or in children has not been established. The antiarrhythmic drug amiodarone is a pregnancy category D drug, indicating that fetal harm can occur when the agent is administered to a pregnant woman. It is used only if the potential benefits outweigh the potential hazards to the fetus. Antiarrhythmic drugs are contraindicated in patients with second- or third-degree AV block (if the patient has no artificial pacemaker), severe congestive heart failure (CHF), aortic stenosis, hypotension, or cardiogenic shock. Quinidine and procainamide are contraindicated in patients with myasthenia gravis (see Chapter 4).

All antiarrhythmic drugs are used cautiously in patients with renal or hepatic disease. When renal or hepatic dysfunction is present, a dosage reduction may be necessary. All patients should be observed for renal and hepatic dysfunction. Quinidine and procainamide are used cautiously in patients with CHF. Disopyramide is used cautiously in patients with CHF, myasthenia gravis, or glaucoma, and in men with prostate enlargement. Bretylium is used cautiously in patients with digitalis toxicity because the initial release of norepinephrine with digitalis toxicity may exacerbate arrhythmias and symptoms of toxicity. Verapamil is used cautiously in patients with a history of serious ventricular arrhythmias or CHF. Electrolyte disturbances such as hypokalemia, hyperkalemia, or hypomagnesemia may alter the effects of the antiarrhythmic drugs. The patient's electrolytes are monitored frequently and imbalances corrected as soon as possible.

When two antiarrhythmic drugs are administered concurrently, the patient may experience additive effects and is at increased risk for drug toxicity. When quinidine and procainamide are administered with digitalis, the risk of digitalis toxicity is increased. The pharmacologic effects of procainamide may be increased when procainamide is administered with quinidine. When quinidine is administered with the barbiturates or cimetidine, quinidine serum levels may be increased. When quinidine is administered with verapamil, the patient has an increased risk of hypotensive effects. When quinidine is administered with disopyramide, the patient has an increased risk of increased disopyramide blood levels and/or decreased serum quinidine levels.

Propranolol may increase procainamide plasma levels. Additive cholinergic effects may occur when procainamide is administered with other drugs with anticholinergic effects. There is the potential for additive cardiodepressant effects when procainamide is administered with lidocaine. When a beta blocker, such as Inderal, is administered with lidocaine, the patient has an increased risk of lidocaine toxicity.

Propranolol may alter the effectiveness of insulin or oral hypoglycemic drugs. Dosage adjustments may be necessary.

Dofetilide is not administered with cimetidine because dofetilide plasma levels may be increased by as much as 50%. When treatment for gastric disorders is necessary, patients receiving dofetilide should take omeprazole, ranitidine, or antacids as an alternative to cimetidine.

Verapamil may cause an additive hypotensive effect when administered with other antihypertensives, alcohol, or nitrates. Verapamil increases plasma digoxin levels and may cause bradycardia or CHF.

Patient Management Issues with Antiarrhythmic Drugs

The health care provider performs initial preadministration assessments before starting therapy with any of the antiarrhythmic drugs. These assessments include taking blood pressure, pulse, and respiratory rates, and assessing the patient's general condition.

Because all antiarrhythmic drugs may produce proarrhythmic effects, a careful preadministration assessment is essential. It is often difficult to distinguish a proarrhythmic effect from the patient's underlying rhythm disorder, so it is important that each patient taking an antiarrhythmic drug be assessed with cardiac monitoring before therapy begins and thereafter to determine if the patient is experiencing a therapeutic response to the drug, developing another arrhythmia, or experiencing worsening of the original arrhythmia.

The health care provider may also order laboratory and diagnostic tests, renal and hepatic function tests, a complete blood count, serum enzymes, and serum electrolytes. An electrocardiogram (ECG) may be performed to provide baseline data for comparison during therapy.

When interacting with a patient being treated for an arrhythmia, any significant changes should be reported immediately to the health care provider, including a change in blood pressure, pulse rate, or rhythm; respiratory difficulty; a change in respiratory rate or rhythm; or a change in the patient's general condition.

Educating the Patient and Family About Antiarrhythmic Drugs

The adverse drug effects that may occur with use of the antiarrhythmic drug are explained to the patient and family. To ensure compliance with the prescribed drug regimen, the importance of taking these drugs exactly as prescribed is emphasized. It may be necessary to teach patients or their family members how to take their pulse rate. The patient is advised to report any changes in the pulse rate or rhythm to the health care provider. Patient Education Box 14-3 reviews self-monitoring of the pulse rate with antiarrhythmic therapy.

Patient Education Box 14-4 includes key points about antiarrhythmic drugs that the patient and family should know.

KEY POINTS

⬤ The cardiotonics are used to increase the efficiency and improve the contraction of the heart muscle, which leads to improved blood flow to all tissues of the body.
⬤ The antiarrhythmic drugs are primarily used to treat cardiac arrhythmias. An arrhythmia may occur as a result of heart disease or from a disorder that affects cardiovascular function. Conditions such as emotional stress, hypoxia, and electrolyte imbalance also may trigger an arrhythmia.

PATIENT EDUCATION BOX 14-3

Self-monitoring Pulse Rate With Antiarrhythmic Therapy

The health care provider:

❑ Explains the purpose of self-monitoring of pulse rate when receiving antiarrhythmic therapy.

❑ Instructs the patient about the importance of drug therapy and taking drug exactly as prescribed.

❑ Provides written instruction for monitoring pulse rate (see Patient Education Box 14-1: Monitoring Pulse Rate).

❑ Encourages self-monitoring before each dose.

❑ Reviews acceptable pulse rate ranges for taking the drug, both verbally and in writing.

❑ Encourages recording of pulse rates in a log.

❑ Emphasizes need to notify the health care provider should the pulse rate fall outside acceptable range or the rhythm changes.

❑ Reassures the patient that results of therapy will be monitored by periodic laboratory and diagnostic tests and follow-up visits with the health care provider.

❑ Assists with arrangements for follow-up as necessary.

● Digitalis increases cardiac output through positive inotropic activity and decreases the conduction velocity through the atrioventricular (AV) and sinoatrial (SA) nodes in the heart.

● There is a narrow margin of safety between the full therapeutic effects and the toxic effects of cardiotonic drugs. Even normal doses of a cardiotonic drug can cause toxic drug effects.

● Inamrinone and milrinone have inotropic actions and are used in the short-term management of severe heart failure that is not controlled by the digitalis preparations.

● Class I antiarrhythmic drugs, such as moricizine, have a membrane-stabilizing or anesthetic effect on the cells of the myocardium, making them valuable in treating cardiac arrhythmias. Class II antiarrhythmic drugs include beta-adrenergic blocking drugs, such as acebutolol (Sectral), esmolol (Brevibloc), and propranolol (Inderal), which also decrease myocardial response to epinephrine and norepinephrine (adrenergic neurohormones) by their ability to block stimulation of beta receptors of the heart

● General adverse reactions common to most antiarrhythmic drugs include light-headedness, weakness, hypotension, bradycardia, and drowsiness. Antiarrhythmic drugs are contraindicated in patients with a known hypersensitivity and during pregnancy and lactation.

PATIENT EDUCATION BOX 14-4

Key Points for Taking Antiarrhythmic Drugs

❑ Take the drug at the prescribed intervals. Do not omit a dose or increase or decrease the dose unless advised to do so by your health care provider. Do not stop taking the drug unless advised to do so by your health care provider.

❑ Do not take any nonprescription drug unless your health care provider has approved it.

❑ Do not drink alcoholic beverages or smoke unless these have been approved by your health care provider.

❑ Follow the directions on the drug label, such as taking the drug with food.

❑ Do not chew tablets or capsules; instead, swallow them whole.

❑ Do not attempt to drive or perform hazardous tasks if you feel light-headed or dizzy.

❑ Notify your health care provider as soon as possible if you have any adverse effects.

❑ If you experience dry mouth, then take frequent sips of water, allow ice chips to dissolve in your mouth, or chew (sugar-free) gum.

❑ Remember that the wax matrix of sustained-release tablets of procainamide (Procan SR only) is not absorbed by the body and may be seen in the stool. This is normal.

❑ Keep all appointments with your health care provider, clinic, or laboratory because your therapy needs to be closely monitored.

❑ If you have diabetes and are taking propranolol, then adhere to your prescribed diet and check your blood glucose levels one to two times per day (or as recommended by you health care provider). Report elevated glucose levels to your health care provider as soon as possible because an adjustment in the dosage of insulin or oral hypoglycemic drugs may be necessary.

❑ Keep all follow-up visits with your health care provider to monitor progress.

CASE STUDY

Mr. Brannen has been taking digoxin for 4 weeks and is in for a follow-up visit.

1. Which of the following questions should Mr. Brannen be asked to determine whether potentially serious side effects are occurring?
   a. whether his appetite has changed
   b. whether he is experiencing numbness in his limbs
   c. whether he is dizzy when rising
   d. all of the above

2. Mr. Brannen says that he thinks the digoxin is causing heartburn. When questioned, he admits that he is frequently consuming antacids to combat the heartburn. The correct response is:
   a. antacids are fine; there is no cause for concern
   b. antacids should be avoided while on digoxin because they may interfere with the action of the digoxin
   c. excess stomach acid is a common side effect of digoxin use and may have to be tolerated; he should check with his health care provider
   d. ignore the symptom

3. Which of the following drugs would be prescribed if digoxin toxicity develops?
   a. digoxin immune fab
   b. milrinone
   c. inamrinone lactate
   d. any inotropic drug

4. During rapid digitalization, the first dose will be:
   a. the smallest dose in case the patient is allergic to digoxin
   b. given orally, with succeeding doses given intravenously
   c. approximately half of the total digitalization dose
   d. approximately three quarters of the total digitalization dose

WEBSITE ACTIVITIES

1. Go to the American Heart Association (AHA) website (www.americanheart.org) and click on "Children: Heart Disease and Health." Then select "Children and Exercise." Write a brief statement about the significance of cholesterol in children.

2. Return to the AHA home page and click on the general topic of "News." Write a brief statement summarizing any new information on the topic of "Heart News."

REVIEW QUESTIONS

1. Which of the following is commonly associated with left ventricular systolic dysfunction?
   a. ejection fraction of 60% or more
   b. ejection fraction less than 40%
   c. increased cardiac output
   d. normal cardiac output

2. Which of the following statements would be included in a teaching plan for a patient taking an antiarrhythmic drug as an outpatient?
   a. take the drug without regard to meals
   b. limit fluid intake during the evening hours

c. avoid drinking alcoholic beverages unless their consumption has been approved by the health care provider

d. eat a diet high in potassium

3. Which of the following adverse reactions of lidocaine (Xylocaine) should be reported immediately to the health care provider?

a. sudden change in mental status

b. dry mouth

c. occipital headache

d. light-headedness

4. Which of the following drugs, when given with quinidine (Quinidex), would increase the patient's risk for hypotension?

a. verapamil (Calan)

b. propranolol (Inderal)

c. encainide (Enkaid)

d. disopyramide (Norpace)

15 Antianginal and Peripheral Vasodilating Drugs

KEY TERMS

angina—a disorder often caused by atherosclerotic plaque formation in the coronary arteries, which causes decreased oxygen supply to the heart muscle and results in chest pain or pressure

atherosclerosis—a disease characterized by deposits of fatty plaques on the inner wall of arteries

intermittent claudication—a group of symptoms characterized by pain in the calf muscle of one or both legs, caused by walking and relieved by rest

lumen—the inside diameter of a vessel such as an artery

prophylaxis—prevention

transdermal system—a convenient form of drug administration in which the drug is impregnated in a pad and absorbed through the skin

vasodilation—an increase in the size of blood vessels, primarily small arteries and arterioles

CHAPTER OBJECTIVES

On completion of this chapter, students will be able to:

1 Define the chapter's key terms.

2 Describe the uses, general drug actions, adverse reactions, contraindications, precautions, and interactions of antianginal and peripheral vasodilating drugs.

3 Discuss important points to keep in mind when educating patients and their families about the use of antianginal and peripheral vasodilating drugs.

Diseases of the arteries can cause serious problems such as coronary artery disease, cerebral vascular disease, and peripheral vascular disease. Drug therapy for vascular diseases may include drugs that dilate blood vessels and thereby increase blood supply to an area.

Atherosclerosis is a disease characterized by deposits of fatty plaques on the inner wall of arteries. These deposits result in a narrowing of the **lumen** (inside diameter) of the artery and a decrease in blood supply to the area served by the artery (Fig. 15-1).

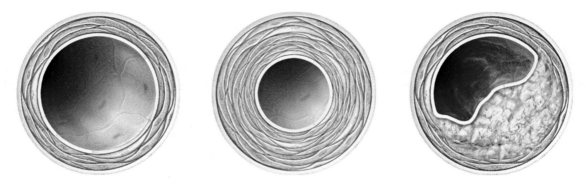

FIGURE 15-1 Schematic illustration of a plague in atherosclerosis. (From Bullock BL. *Focus on Pathophysiology*. Baltimore: Lippincott Williams & Wilkins; 2000.) (Image provided by Anatomical Chart Co.)

This chapter discusses two different types of drugs whose primary purpose is to increase blood supply to an area by dilating blood vessels: the antianginal and peripheral vasodilating drugs. Vasodilating drugs relax the smooth muscle layer of arterial blood vessels, which results in **vasodilation**, an increase in the size of blood vessels, primarily small arteries, and arterioles. Because peripheral, cerebral, or coronary artery disease usually results in decreased blood flow to an area, drugs that dilate narrowed arterial blood vessels will increase the blood flow to the affected area. Increasing the blood flow to an area may result in complete or partial relief of symptoms. Vasodilating drugs sometimes relieve the symptoms of vascular disease, but in some cases drug therapy provides only minimal and temporary relief. Many vasodilating drugs are also used to treat hypertension. Their use as antihypertensives is discussed in Chapter 16.

Antianginal Drugs

Angina is a disorder often caused by atherosclerotic plaque formation in the coronary arteries, which causes a decrease in the oxygen supply to the heart muscle and results in chest pain or pressure. Any activity that increases the workload of the heart, such as exercise or simply climbing stairs, can precipitate an angina attack. Antianginal drugs relieve chest pain or pressure by dilating the coronary arteries and increasing the blood supply to the myocardium.

Antianginal drugs include the nitrates and calcium channel blockers. Chapter 4 discusses adrenergic blocking drugs, which are also used to treat angina and other disorders.

Nitrates

Actions of Nitrates

The nitrates, such as isosorbide (Isordil) and nitroglycerin have a direct relaxing effect on the smooth muscle layer of blood vessels. This increases the lumen of the artery or arteriole and increases the amount of blood flowing through these vessels. An increased blood flow results in an increased oxygen supply.

Uses of Nitrates

The nitrates are used to treat angina pectoris. Some of these drugs, such as isosorbide dinitrate (Isordil), are used for **prophylaxis** (prevention) and long-term treatment of angina, whereas others, such as sublingual nitroglycerin (Nitrostat), are used to relieve the pain of acute anginal attacks when they occur. See the Summary Drug Table: Antianginal Drugs for additional uses of the nitrates. Intravenous nitroglycerin is also used to control perioperative hypertension associated with surgical procedures.

Adverse Reactions of Nitrates

The nitrate antianginal drugs all have the same adverse reactions, although the intensity of some reactions may vary with the drug and the dose. A common adverse reaction is headache, especially early in therapy. Hypotension, dizziness, vertigo, and weakness may also occur. Flushing caused by dilation of small capillaries near the surface of the skin may also occur.

The nitrates are available in various forms, including sublingual and translingual forms. Some adverse reactions result from the method of administration. For example, sublingual nitroglycerin may cause a local burning or tingling in the mouth. However, a patient must be aware that an absence of this effect does not indicate a decrease in the drug's potency. Contact dermatitis may occur from use of the transdermal delivery system.

In many instances, the adverse reactions associated with the nitrates lessen and often disappear with continued use of the drug. However, for some patients, these adverse reactions become severe, and the health care provider may lower the dose until symptoms

SUMMARY DRUG TABLE   Antianginal Drugs

Generic Name	Trade Name*	Uses	Adverse Reactions	Dosage Ranges
Nitrates amyl nitrite *am-il-nye-trite*	*Generic*	Relief of angina pectoris	Headache, hypotension, dizziness, vertigo, weakness, flushing	Crush capsule and wave under nose, taking 1–6 inhalations; may repeat in 3–5 min
isosorbide mononitrate, oral *eye-soe-sor'-bide*	ISMO, Imdur, Monoket, *generic*	Prevention of angina pectoris	Headache, hypotension, dizziness, vertigo, weakness, flushing	20 mg BID PO with the two doses given 7h apart; extended-release tablets: 30–60 mg once daily may be increased to 240 mg/d PO
isosorbide dinitrate sublingual and chewable *eye-soe-sor'-bide*	Isordil, Sorbitrate, *generic*	Treatment and prevention of angina pectoris	Headache, hypotension, dizziness, vertigo, weakness, flushing	Treatment: 2.5–5 mg sublingual; prevention: 2.5–5 mg SL, 5 mg chewable
isosorbide Dinitrate, oral *eye-soe-sor'-bide*	Dilatrate SR, Isordil Tembids, Isordil Titradose, Sorbitrate, *generic*	Treatment and prevention of angina pectoris	Headache, hypotension, dizziness, vertigo, weakness, flushing	Initial dose 5–20 mg PO; maintenance dose 10–40 mg BID, TID; sustained release: 40 mg/d; daily maximum dose, 160 mg/d PO
nitroglycerin, Intravenous *Nye-troe-gli'-ser-in*	Nitro-Bid IV, Tridil, *generic*	Control of blood pressure in perioperative hypertension and in immediate postoperative period, CHF associated with acute MI, angina pectoris unresponsive to recommended doses of nitrates or beta blockers	Headache, hypotension, dizziness, vertigo, weakness, flushing	Initially 5 mcg/min via IV infusion pump; may increase to 20 mcg/min
nitroglycerin, sublingual *Nye-troe-gli'-ser-in*	NitroQuick, Nitrostat	Acute relief of an attack of angina pectoris or prophylaxis of angina pectoris	Headache, hypotension, dizziness, vertigo, weakness, flushing	1 tablet under tongue or in buccal pouch at first sign of an acute anginal attack; may repeat q5 min until relief or 3 tablets have been taken
nitroglycerin, translingual *Nye-troe-gli'-ser-in*	Nitrolingual	Acute relief of an attack or prophylaxis of angina pectoris	Headache, hypotension, dizziness, vertigo, weakness, flushing	1–2 metered dose sprays onto or under the tongue; maximum of 3 metered doses in 15 min

Generic Name	Trade Name*	Uses	Adverse Reactions	Dosage Ranges
nitroglycerin, transmucosal *Nye-troe-gli'-ser-in*	Nitrogard	Prevention of angina pectoris	Headache, hypotension, dizziness, vertigo, weakness, flushing	1 tablet q3–5h between lip and gum or between cheek and gum
nitroglycerin, sustained release *Nye-troe-gli'-ser-in*	Nitroglyn, Nitrong, Nitro-Time, *generic*	Prevention of angina pectoris	Headache, hypotension, dizziness, vertigo, weakness, flushing	2.5–2.6 mg TID, QID PO up to 26 mg QID
nitroglycerin transdermal systems *Nye-troe-gli'-ser-in*	Deponit, Minitran, Nitro-Dur, Transderm-Nitro, *generic*	Prevention of angina pectoris	Headache, hypotension, dizziness, vertigo, weakness, flushing	One system daily 0.2–0.8 mg/h
Nitroglycerin, topical *Nye-troe-gli'-ser in*	Nitro-Bid, Nitrol, *generic*	Prevention and treatment of angina pectoris	Headache, hypotension, dizziness, vertigo, weakness, flushing	1–5 inches q4–8h
Calcium Channel Blocking Drugs nmlodipine *am-low'-dih-peen*	Norvasc	Hypertension, chronic stable angina, vasospastic angina (Prinzmetal's angina)	Dizziness, light-headedness, headache, nervousness, nausea, diarrhea, constipation peripheral edema, angina, bradycardia, AV block, flushing, rash, nasal congestion, cough	Individualize dosage; 5–10 mg PO once daily
bepridil HCl *be'-pri-dil*	Vascor	Chronic stable angina	Dizziness, light-headedness, headache, nervousness, nausea, diarrhea, constipation, peripheral edema, angina, bradycardia, AV block, flushing, rash, nasal congestion, cough	Individualize dosage; 200–400 mg/d PO
diltiazem HCl *dil-tye'-a-zem*	Cardizem, Cardizem CD, Dilacor XR, Tiamate, Tiazac, *generic*	Oral: Angina pectoris, chronic stable angina, essential hypertension Parenteral: atrial fibrillation or flutter, paroxysmal supraventricular tachycardia	Dizziness, light-headedness, headache, nervousness, nausea, diarrhea, constipation, peripheral edema, angina, bradycardia, AV block, flushing, rash, nasal congestion, cough	Tablets: 30–360 mg/d in divided doses; sustained-release: Cardizem SR 120–360 mg/d; Cardizem CD angina 120–240 mg once daily; Dilacor XR, 180–480 mg once daily PO; Tiazac, 120–240 mg/d for hypertension Parenteral: 0.25 mg/kg IV bolus; 5–15 mg/h IV

Generic Name	Trade Name*	Uses	Adverse Reactions	Dosage Ranges
nicardipine HCl *nye-kar'-de-peen*	Cardene, Cardene IV, Cardene SR, *generic*	Chronic stable angina, hypertension, short-term treatment of hypertension when oral therapy is not desirable	Dizziness, light-headedness, headache, nervousness, nausea, diarrhea, constipation, peripheral edema, angina, bradycardia, AV block, flushing, rash, nasal congestion, cough	Angina: individualize dosage; immediate release only, 20–40 mg TID PO Hypertension: individualize dosage; immediate release, 20–40 mg/d TID PO; sustained release, 30–60 mg BID PO; 0.5–2.2 mg/h IV by infusion
nifedipine *nye-fed'-i-peen*	Adalat, Procardia, Procardia XL, *generic*	Vasospastic angina (Prinzmetal's angina), chronic stable angina, hypertension (sustained-release only)	Dizziness, light-headedness, headache, nervousness, nausea, diarrhea, constipation, peripheral edema, angina, bradycardia, AV block, flushing, rash, nasal congestion, cough	10–20 mg TID PO; may increase to 120 mg/d; sustained release: 30–60 mg/d PO; may increase to 120 mg/d
verapamil HCl *ver-ap'-a-mil*	Calan, Calan SR, Isoptin, Isoptin SR, Verelan, *generic*	Angina, arrhythmias, essential hypertension, supraventricular tachycardia (parenteral only), atrial flutter/fibrillation (parenteral only)	Dizziness, light-headedness, headache, nervousness, nausea, diarrhea, constipation, peripheral edema, angina, bradycardia, AV block, flushing, rash, nasal congestion, cough	Individualize dosage; do not exceed 480 mg/d; essential hypertension: 240 mg/d, sustained release 80 mg TID; ER capsules, 100–300 mg HS

*The term *generic* indicates the drug is available in generic form.

subside. The dose may then be slowly increased if the lower dosage does not provide relief from the symptoms of angina.

Contraindications, Precautions, and Interactions of Nitrates

The nitrates are contraindicated in patients with a known hypersensitivity, severe anemia, closed-angle glaucoma, postural hypertension, cerebral hemorrhage, allergy to adhesive (transdermal system), or constrictive pericarditis. Amyl nitrate is contraindicated during pregnancy (pregnancy category X).

The nitrates are used cautiously in patients with severe hepatic or renal disease, severe head trauma, acute myocardial infarction, or hypothyroidism, and during pregnancy (pregnancy category C, except for amyl nitrate) or lactation.

If the nitrates are administered with the antihypertensives, alcohol, calcium channel blockers, or the phenothiazines, then there may be an increased hypotensive effect. When nitroglycerin is administered intravenously, the effects of heparin may be decreased. Increased nitrate serum concentrations may occur when the nitrates are administered with aspirin.

Patient Management Issues with Nitrates

Patients using nitrates are monitored for the frequency and severity of any episodes of angina pain. With treatment, episodes of angina should be eliminated or decrease in frequency and severity. Any chest pain that does not respond to three doses of nitroglycerin given every 5 minutes for 15 minutes should be reported to the health care provider.

The nitrates may be administered by the sublingual (under the tongue), buccal (between the cheek and gum), oral, intravenous (IV), or transdermal route. Nitroglycerin may be administered by the sublingual, buccal, topical, transdermal, oral, or IV route. If the buccal form of nitroglycerin is prescribed, then the patient is instructed to place the buccal tablet between the cheek and gum or between the upper lip and gum above the incisors and allow it to dissolve. Patients can be shown how and where to place the tablet in the mouth. Absorption of sublingual and buccal forms depends on saliva. Dry mouth decreases absorption.

Nitroglycerin may also be administered by a metered spray canister that is used to abort an acute anginal attack. The spray is directed from the canister onto or under the tongue. The canister meters each dose, delivering the same dose each time the canister top is depressed. The patient is instructed not to inhale the spray. For some individuals, the spray is more convenient than the small tablets placed under the tongue.

ALERT

 Sublingual Nitroglycerine Doses

The dose of sublingual nitroglycerin may be repeated every 5 minutes until pain is relieved or until the patient has received three doses in a 15-minute period. One or two sprays of translingual nitroglycerin may be used to relieve angina, but no more than three metered doses are recommended within a 15-minute period.

The health care provider should be notified if a patient frequently has anginal pain, if the pain worsens, or if the pain is not relieved after three doses within a 15-minute period. A change in the dosage of the drug or other treatment may be necessary.

Nitroglycerin may also be administered in topical (ointment) form. The ointment is usually applied to the chest or back. Application sites are rotated to prevent inflammation of the skin. Areas that may be used for application include the chest (front and back), abdomen, and upper arms and legs.

ALERT

Application of Nitroglycerine Ointment

Nitroglycerin ointment *must not* be rubbed into a patient's skin because this will immediately deliver a large amount of the drug through the skin. Care must be exercised in applying topical nitroglycerin. The ointment must not come in contact with the fingers or hands of the person applying the ointment, because the drug will be absorbed through his or her skin.

For many patients, nitroglycerin **transdermal systems** are convenient and easier to use because the drug is absorbed through the skin. In transdermal systems,

the drug is impregnated in a pad. The pad is applied to the skin once per day for 10 to 12 hours.

Tolerance to the vascular and anginal effects of nitrates may develop, particularly in patients taking high dosages, those prescribed longer-acting products, and those on frequent dosing schedules. Patients using transdermal nitroglycerin patches are particularly prone to tolerance because the nitroglycerin is released at a constant rate, maintaining steady plasma concentrations. Research has shown that applying the patch in the morning and leaving it in place for 10 to 12 hours, followed by removing it for the next 10 to 12 hours, yields better results and delays tolerance to the drug.

Nitroglycerin is also available as oral tablets to be swallowed. The patient should take it on an empty stomach unless the health care provider orders otherwise. If the patient experiences nausea, then the health care provider should be notified. Taking the tablet or capsule with food may be ordered to relieve nausea. The sustained-released preparation must be swallowed, not crushed or chewed.

Because of the risk of tolerance to oral nitrates developing, the health care provider may prescribe a short-acting preparation 2 or 3 times daily, or a sustained-release preparations once or twice daily.

Nitroglycerin is also available in IV form, administered by a health care provider.

Educating the Patient and Family About Nitrates

The patient and family must have a thorough understanding of the treatment of chest pain with an antianginal drug. These drugs are used either to prevent angina from occurring or to relieve the pain of angina. The therapeutic regimen (dose, time of day the drug is taken, how often to take the drug, how to take or apply the drug) is explained to the patient. Patient Education Box 15-1 includes key points about nitrates that the patient or family should know.

Calcium Channel Blockers

Actions of Calcium Channel Blockers

Systemic and coronary arteries are influenced by the movement of calcium across cell membranes of vascular smooth muscle. The contractions of cardiac and vascular smooth muscle depend on the movement of extracellular calcium ions through specific ion channels. Calcium channel blockers, such as amlodipine (Norvasc), diltiazem (Cardizem), nicardipine (Cardene), nifedipine (Procardia), and verapamil (Calan), inhibit the movement of calcium ions across cell membranes. This results in less calcium available for the transmission of nerve impulses (Fig. 15-2). This drug action of the calcium chan-

PATIENT EDUCATION BOX 15-1

Key Points for Patients Taking Nitrates

- ❑ Do not drink alcohol unless it is permitted by your health care provider.
- ❑ Notify your health care provider if the drug does not relieve pain or if pain becomes more intense despite use of this drug.
- ❑ Follow the recommendations of your health care provider regarding frequency of use.
- ❑ Take oral capsules or tablets (except sublingual) on an empty stomach unless your health care provider directs otherwise.
- ❑ Keep an adequate supply of the drug on hand for situations such as vacations, bad weather conditions, and holidays.
- ❑ Keep a record of the frequency of acute anginal attacks (date, time of the attack, drug, and dose used to relieve the acute pain), and bring this record to each health care provider visit.

NITRATES

- ❑ Headache is a common adverse reaction but should decrease with continued therapy. If headache persists or becomes severe, then notify your health care provider because a change in dosage may be needed. Headache may be a marker of the drug's effectiveness. Do not try to avoid headaches by altering your treatment schedule because loss of headache may be associated with simultaneous loss of drug effectiveness. You may use aspirin or acetaminophen for headache relief.
- ❑ Do not change from one brand of nitrates to another without consulting your pharmacist or health care provider. Products manufactured by different companies may not be equally effective.

ORAL NITRATES

- ❑ When taking nitroglycerin for an acute attack of angina, sit or lie down. To relieve severe light-headedness or dizziness, lie down, elevate and move your extremities, and breathe deeply.
- ❑ Keep capsules and tablets in their original containers because nitroglycerin must be kept in a dark container and protected from exposure to light. Never mix this drug with any other drug in a container. Nitroglycerin will lose its potency in containers made of plastic or if mixed with other drugs.
- ❑ Always replace the cover or cap of the container as soon as the oral drug or ointment is removed from the container or tube. Replace caps or covers tightly because the drug deteriorates on contact with air.
- ❑ If your chest pain persists, changes character, increases in severity, or is not relieved by following the recommended dosing regimen, then seek prompt medical attention.

SUBLINGUAL OR BUCCAL ADMINISTRATION

- ❑ Do not handle sublingual tablets any more than necessary.
- ❑ Check the expiration date on the container of sublingual tablets. If the expiration date has passed, then do not use the tablets. Instead, purchase a new supply. Unused tablets should be discarded 6 months after the original bottle is opened.
- ❑ Do not swallow or chew sublingual or transmucosal tablets; allow them to dissolve slowly. The tablet may cause a burning or tingling in your mouth, but the absence of this effect does not indicate a decrease in potency. Older adults are less likely to have this burning or tingling sensation.

TRANSLINGUAL/TRANSMUCOSAL

- ❑ The directions for use of translingual nitroglycerin are supplied with the product. Follow the instructions regarding using and cleaning the canister.
- ❑ This drug may be used prophylactically 5 to 10 minutes before engaging in activities that precipitate an attack.
- ❑ At the onset of an anginal attack, spray one or two metered doses onto or under the tongue. Do not use more than three metered doses within 15 minutes.
- ❑ When using the transmucosal form, insert the tablet between the lip and gum above the incisors or between the cheek and gum.

TOPICAL OINTMENT OR TRANSDERMAL SYSTEM

- ❑ Instructions for application of the topical ointment or transdermal system are provided with the product. Read these instructions carefully.
- ❑ Apply the topical ointment or transdermal system at approximately the same time each day.
- ❑ Be sure the area is clean and thoroughly dry before applying the topical ointment or transdermal system, and rotate the application sites. Apply the transdermal system to the chest (front and back), abdomen, and upper or lower arms and legs. Firmly press the patch to ensure contact with the skin. If the transdermal system comes off or becomes loose, then apply a new system. Apply the topical ointment to the front or the back of the chest. If applying to the back, then another person should apply the ointment.
- ❑ When using the topical ointment form or transdermal system, cleanse old application sites with soap and warm water as soon as the ointment or transdermal system is removed.
- ❑ To use the topical ointment, apply a thin layer on the skin using the paper applicator (you may need instructions regarding this technique). Do not touch the ointment with your fingers.
- ❑ Wash your hands before and after applying the ointment.

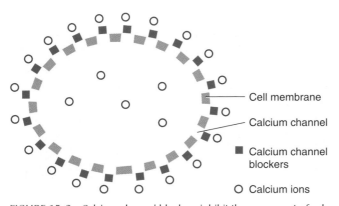

FIGURE 15-2 Calcium channel blockers inhibit the movement of calcium ions across the cell membrane. When calcium channels are blocked by drug molecules, muscle contraction is decreased, causing the smooth muscles of the arteries and arterioles to dilate. (From Roach SS. *Introductory Clinical Pharmacology*, 7th ed. Baltimore: Lippincott Williams & Wilkins; 2004.)

nel blockers (also known as slow channel blockers) has several effects on the heart, including an effect on the smooth muscle of arteries and arterioles. These drugs dilate coronary arteries and arterioles, which in turn deliver more oxygen to cardiac muscle. Dilation of peripheral arteries reduces the workload of the heart. The end effect of these actions drugs is the same as that of the nitrates.

Uses of Calcium Channel Blockers

Calcium channel blockers are primarily used to prevent anginal pain associated with certain forms of angina, such as vasospastic (Prinzmetal's variant) angina and chronic stable angina. They are not used to stop anginal pain once it has occurred. When angina is caused by coronary artery spasm, these drugs are recommended when the patient cannot tolerate therapy with beta-adrenergic blocking drugs (see Chapter 4) or the nitrates. Calcium channel blockers used as antianginals are listed in the Summary Drug Table: Antianginal Drugs. Some calcium channel blocking drugs have additional uses. Verapamil affects the conduction system of the heart and may be used to treat cardiac arrhythmias. Diltiazem, nicardipine, nifedipine, and verapamil also are used in the treatment of essential hypertension (see Chapter 16).

Adverse Reactions of Calcium Channel Blockers

Adverse reactions to the calcium channel blocking drugs usually are not serious and rarely require discontinuation of the drug therapy. The more common adverse reactions include dizziness, light-headedness, nausea, diarrhea, constipation, peripheral edema, headache, bradycardia, flushing, dermatitis, skin rash, and nervousness. See the Summary Drug Table: Antianginal Drugs for a more complete listing of the adverse reactions of specific calcium channel blockers.

Managing Adverse Drug Reactions of All Antianginal Drugs

Patients receiving these drugs must be carefully monitored for adverse reactions. During initial therapy, headache and postural hypotension may occur, and if so the health care provider must be notified because a dose change may be necessary. Patients having episodes of postural hypotension need help walking and with other activities. Patients experiencing episodes of postural hypotension are instructed to take the drug in a sitting or supine position and to remain in that position until symptoms disappear. Hypotension may be accompanied by paradoxical bradycardia and increased angina pectoris. Adverse reactions such as headache, flushing, and postural hypotension often become less severe or even disappear after a period of time.

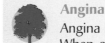

GERONTOLOGIC ALERT

Severity of Hypotensive Effects

Older adults may have a greater hypotensive effect after taking an antianginal drug than do younger adults. An older adult must be closely monitored during dosage adjustments.

If a patient has frequent chest pain or reports dizziness or light-headedness, then blood pressure is monitored frequently. A patient may need help walking if dizziness occurs. In addition, the patient should be asked about the anginal pain. In some patients, the pain may be entirely relieved, whereas in others it may be less intense or less frequent or may occur only with prolonged exercise. All information should be recorded in the patient's chart because this helps the health care provider plan future therapy and make dosage adjustments if required.

GERONTOLOGIC ALERT

Angina

Angina is a common problem in older adults. When an older adult requires an antianginal drug, the dosage may be reduced to compensate for impaired renal function or heart disease. Older patients are at increased risk for postural hypotension. Their blood pressure and ability to walk should be monitored closely.

When the drug regimen for angina pectoris is terminated, the drug dosage is gradually reduced to prevent withdrawal reactions. Abrupt withdrawal of a calcium channel blocker may cause an increase in chest pain. This phenomenon is called rebound angina and is most likely the result of the increased flow of calcium into cells, causing the coronary arteries to spasm. Therefore, calcium channel blockers are gradually withdrawn rather than discontinued abruptly.

Contraindications, Precautions, and Interactions of Calcium Channel Blockers

Calcium channel blockers are contraindicated in patients who are hypersensitive to them and in those with sick sinus syndrome, second-degree or third-degree AV block (except with a functioning pacemaker), hypotension (systolic pressure less than 90 mm Hg), ventricular dysfunction, or cardiogenic shock. Calcium channel blockers are used cautiously during pregnancy (pregnancy category C) and lactation and in patients with congestive heart failure (CHF), hypotension, or renal or hepatic impairment.

The effects of the calcium channel blockers are increased when administered with cimetidine or ranitidine. A decrease in effectiveness of the calcium channel blockers may occur when the agents are administered with phenobarbital or phenytoin. Calcium channel blockers have an antiplatelet effect (inhibition of platelet function) when administered with aspirin, causing easy bruising, petechiae (pinpoint purple–red spot caused by intradermal hemorrhage), and bleeding. An additive depressive effect on the myocardium occurs when a calcium channel blocker is administered with a beta-adrenergic blocking drug. When a calcium channel blocker is administered with digoxin, the patient has an increased risk for digitalis toxicity.

Patient Management Issues with Calcium Channel Blockers

Patients receiving calcium channel blockers should be monitored for signs of CHF, such as dyspnea, weight gain, peripheral edema, abnormal lung sounds (crackles or rales), and jugular vein distention. Any symptoms of CHF should be reported immediately to the health care provider.

With a few exceptions, calcium channel blockers may be taken without regard to meals. If gastrointestinal upset occurs, then the drug may be taken with meals. Verapamil and bepridil frequently cause gastric upset and are routinely given with meals. Verapamil capsules may be opened and sprinkled on foods or mixed in liquids. Sometimes the tablet coverings of verapamil are expelled in the stool. This causes no change in the effect of the drug and should be of no concern to a patient.

For patients who have difficulty swallowing diltiazem, the tablets can be crushed and mixed with food or liquids. However, a patient should swallow the sustained-released tablets whole and not chew or divide them. When nifedipine is ordered sublingually, the capsule is punctured with a sterile needle and the liquid squeezed under the tongue or in the buccal pouch.

Educating the Patient and Family About Calcium Channel Blockers

The patient and family members need a thorough understanding of how chest pain is treated with an antianginal drug. These drugs are used either to prevent angina from occurring or to relieve the pain of angina. The therapeutic regimen (dose, time of day the drug is taken, how often to take the drug, how to take or apply the drug) is explained to the patient. Patient Education Box 15-2 includes key points about calcium channel blockers that the patient or family members should know.

Peripheral Vasodilating Drugs

In contrast to antianginal drugs, which are used primarily for angina, the peripheral vasodilating drugs are given for disorders that affect blood vessels of the extremities. Unfortunately, although these drugs increase blood flow to nonischemic areas (areas with adequate blood flow), there is no conclusive evidence that blood flow is increased in ischemic areas (areas that lack adequate blood flow) that are in critical need of improved perfusion. Because of the lack of evidence of the effectiveness of the peripheral vasodilating drugs, most are labeled as "possibly effective" in the treatment of peripheral vascular disorders. These drugs are not as widely used now as they were in the past. Many peripheral dilating drugs are used for hypertension and are discussed in Chapter 14.

PATIENT EDUCATION BOX 15-2

Key Points for Patients Taking Calcium Channel Blockers

❑ Do not chew or divide sustained-released tablets. Swallow them whole.

❑ Notify your health care provider if you experience any of the following: increased severity of chest pain or discomfort, irregular heartbeat, palpitations, nausea, shortness of breath, swelling of your hands or feet, or severe and prolonged episodes of light-headedness and dizziness.

❑ If your health care provider prescribes one of these drugs plus a nitrate, then take both drugs exactly as directed to obtain the best results of the combined drug therapy.

❑ Make position changes slowly to minimize hypotensive effects.

❑ These drugs can cause dizziness or drowsiness. Do not drive or engage in hazardous activities until you know how you will respond to the drug.

Actions of Peripheral Vasodilating Drugs

Peripheral vasodilating drugs, such as isoxsuprine (Vasodilan), act on the smooth muscle layers of peripheral blood vessels, primarily by blocking alpha-adrenergic nerves and stimulating beta-adrenergic nerves. For a review of the effect of stimulation and blocking effects on adrenergic nerve fibers, see Chapter 4. Cilostazol (Pletal) inhibits platelet aggregation and dilates vascular beds, particularly in the femoral area. The exact mechanism of action is unknown.

Uses of Peripheral Vasodilating Drugs

Peripheral vasodilating drugs are chiefly used in the treatment of peripheral vascular diseases, such as arteriosclerosis obliterans, Raynaud phenomenon, and spastic peripheral vascular disorders. Short-term use is rarely beneficial or permanent. Improvement, if it occurs, takes place gradually during weeks of therapy.

The peripheral vasodilating drugs also have other uses, such as the relief of symptoms associated with cerebral vascular insufficiency and circulatory disturbances of the inner ear. More specific uses of individual peripheral vasodilating drugs are given in the Summary Drug Table: Peripheral Vasodilators and Miscellaneous Vasodilating Drugs.

Intermittent claudication is a group of symptoms characterized by pain in the calf muscle of one or both legs, caused by walking and relieved by rest. It is a manifestation of peripheral vascular disease, in which atherosclerotic lesions develop in the femoral artery, diminishing blood supply to the lower leg. Cilostazol (Pletal) is a phosphodiesterase II inhibitor (a drug that inhibits platelet aggregation and dilates vascular beds,

particularly in the femoral area) used for the symptoms of intermittent claudication. This drug increases the walking distance possible in those with intermittent claudication. This drug is listed under Miscellaneous Drugs in the Summary Drug Table: Peripheral Vasodilators and Miscellaneous Vasodilating Drugs.

Adverse Reactions of Peripheral Vasodilating Drugs

Adverse reactions associated with these drugs are variable. Some of the more common adverse reactions are listed in the Summary Drug Table: Peripheral Vasodilators and Miscellaneous Vasodilating Drugs. Because these drugs dilate peripheral arteries, they may cause some degree of hypotension. They also cause a physiologic increase in the pulse rate (tachycardia). Some of these drugs also cause flushing of the skin, which can range from mild to moderately severe. Nausea, vomiting, flushing, headache, and dizziness may also occur with the use of these drugs. Adverse effects of cilostazol include headache, diarrhea, palpitations, dizziness, pharyngitis, hypotension, and cardiac arrhythmias.

Monitoring Adverse Drug Reactions of Peripheral Vasodilating Drugs

If the patient experiences adverse reactions, then the health care provider should be notified. It is important to note the severity of the adverse reactions on a patient's record. In some instances, adverse reactions are mild and a patient may need to tolerate them.

Some patients may experience dizziness and lightheadedness, especially during early therapy. If these effects should occur, then the patient should be helped

SUMMARY DRUG TABLE   Peripheral Vasodilators and Miscellaneous Vasodilating Drugs

Generic Name	Trade Name*	Uses	Adverse Reactions	Dosage Ranges
isoxsuprine HCl *eye-soks-u'-preen*	Vasodilan, Voxsuprine, *generic*	Peripheral vascular disease (PVD), Raynaud's disease	Hypotension, tachycardia, chest pain, nausea, vomiting, abdominal distress, rash, weakness, palpitations	10–20 mg PO TID, QID
papaverine HCL *pa-pav'-er-reen*	Pavabid Plateau, Pavagen, *generic*	Relief of cerebral and peripheral ischemia associated with arterial spasm, myocardial ischemia complicated by arrhythmias	Nausea, abdominal distress, vertigo, sweating, flushing, rash, excessive sedation	150–300 mg PO q12h
Miscellaneous Drugs cilostazol *sill-oh-stay'-zole*	Pletal	Reduction of symptoms of intermittent claudication	Headache, diarrhea, palpitations, dizziness, nausea, rhinitis, abdominal pain, tachycardia	100 mg BID PO

*The term *generic* indicates the drug is available in generic form.

with walking and other activities and is instructed to ask for help when getting out of bed.

Contraindications, Precautions, and Interactions of Peripheral Vasodilating Drugs

The peripheral vasodilating drugs are contraindicated in patients with a known hypersensitivity, in women in the immediate postpartum period (isoxsuprine causes uterine relaxation), and in patients with arterial bleeding. Safe use during pregnancy has not been established (pregnancy category C). Cilostazol is contraindicated in patients with CHF and during pregnancy (pregnancy category C). These drugs are used cautiously in patients with bleeding tendencies, severe cerebrovascular or cardiovascular disease, or recent myocardial infarction. There are no significant drug–drug interactions.

Patient Management Issues with Peripheral Vasodilating Drugs

Therapeutic results may not occur immediately from the peripheral vasodilating drug. In some instances, results are minimal. The patient's involved extremities are assessed daily for changes in color and temperature and the patient's comments regarding relief from pain or discomfort are recorded. Blood pressure and pulse should be monitored once or twice per day because these drugs may cause a decrease in blood pressure. The anticipated result of therapy for cerebral vascular disease is an improvement in the patient's mental status. When the drug is taken for intermittent claudication, a patient is assessed for increased walking distance without pain.

These drugs are often prescribed for outpatients. Positive results of therapy for a peripheral vascular disorder may include a decrease in pain, discomfort, and cramping; increased warmth in the extremities; and stronger peripheral pulses. Patients taking these drugs for relief of symptoms of peripheral vascular disorders often become discouraged about the lack of effectiveness of drug therapy. A patient may need to be encouraged to continue with the prescribed drug regimen and to follow the health care provider's recommendations regarding additional methods of treating the disorder. The patient is reminded that although signs of improvement may be rapid, improvement usually occurs slowly over many weeks. A patient's affected areas are examined at each visit to the health care provider's office and the findings are recorded in a patient's record.

Educating the Patient and Family About Peripheral Vasodilating Drugs

To ensure compliance to the drug regimen, the patient and family members must understand that improvement will likely be gradual, although some improvement may be noted in a few days. The patient is encouraged to continue with drug therapy and to follow the health care provider's recommendations regarding care of the affected extremities even if improvement is slow. Patient Education Box 15-3 includes key information about peripheral vasodilating drugs that patients and family members should know.

Natural Remedies: L-Arginine

L-arginine is an amino acid found in various foods that is commonly sold in health food specialty shops as a supplement capable of improving vascular health and sexual function in men. It is currently promoted in "medical food" form, as a soy-based candy bar. As a supplement, L-arginine is marketed as a way to prevent heart disease, boost muscle growth, improve wound healing, and combat fatigue.

L-arginine may be beneficial in improving health in individuals with congestive heart failure, peripheral artery disease, angina, hypertension, hyperlipidemia, and type 2 diabetes. It appears to increase nitric oxide concentrations. Abnormalities of the vascular endothelial cells may cause vasoconstriction, inflammation, and

PATIENT EDUCATION BOX 15-3

Key Points for Patients Taking Peripheral Vasodilating Drugs

- ❑ If you experience nausea, vomiting, or diarrhea, then contact your health care provider. These drugs may also cause flushing, sweating, headache, tiredness, jaundice, skin rash, anorexia, and abdominal distress. Notify your health care provider if these effects become pronounced.
- ❑ Dizziness may occur. Avoid driving and other potentially dangerous tasks, as well as making sudden position changes. Dangle your legs over the side of the bed for a few minutes when getting up in the morning or after lying down. If dizziness persists, then contact your health care provider.
- ❑ Be careful when walking up or down stairs or when walking on ice, snow, a slick pavement, or slippery floors.
- ❑ Stop smoking.
- ❑ For peripheral vascular disease, follow your health care provider's recommendations regarding exercise, avoiding exposure to cold, keeping the extremities warm, and avoiding injury to the extremities.
- ❑ The therapeutic effects of drugs for peripheral vascular disease may not occur for 2 weeks and may take up to 12 weeks.
- ❑ Take cilostazol (Pletal) 30 minutes before or 2 hours after meals. Do not take the drug with grapefruit juice.

thrombolytic activity. These abnormalities are partially attributable to degradation of nitric oxide. L-arginine's ability to increase nitric oxide is the basis for its effectiveness in improving some vascular disease states.

Oral doses of 9 to 30 g per day are well-tolerated. No adverse reactions were reported in those taking 9 g per day. Higher doses may cause nausea and mild diarrhea. L-arginine may exacerbate sickle cell crisis and should be used with caution in those with sickle cell anemia.

KEY POINTS

◉ Antianginal drugs relieve chest pain or pressure by dilating coronary arteries, increasing the blood supply to the myocardium.

◉ The nitrates are used to treat angina pectoris. Some of these drugs are used for prophylaxis (prevention) and long-term treatment of angina, whereas others are used to relieve the pain of acute anginal attacks when they occur. A common adverse reaction of these drugs is headache, especially early in therapy. Hypotension, dizziness, vertigo, and weakness may also occur.

◉ Calcium channel blockers are primarily used to prevent anginal pain associated with certain forms of angina. They are not used to stop anginal pain once it has occurred. The more common adverse reactions include dizziness, light-headedness, nausea, diarrhea, constipation, peripheral edema, headache, bradycardia, flushing, dermatitis, skin rash, and nervousness.

◉ Peripheral vasodilating drugs are given for disorders that affect blood vessels of the extremities and are chiefly used in the treatment of peripheral vascular diseases, such as arteriosclerosis obliterans, Raynaud phenomenon, and spastic peripheral vascular disorders. Short-term use is rarely beneficial or permanent. Adverse reactions associated with these drugs are variable.

CASE STUDY

Mr. Braden has peripheral vascular disease and is prescribed isoxsuprine hydrochloride (Vasodilan). He has many questions about his drug treatment.

1. In the past 30 days, Mr. Braden has experienced abdominal distress. What potential side effects are associated with isoxsuprine hydrochloride?
   a. vertigo, excessive sedation, and sweating
   b. double vision, stiff limbs, and insomnia
   c. chest pain, abdominal distress, and nausea
   d. none of the above

2. Mr. Braden did a little research on his own and asks about intermittent claudation. What definition best describes this term?
   a. lower back pain
   b. pain when walking
   c. pain in legs from overexertion
   d. blood flow restrictions to the extremities

3. Mr. Braden also asks about the use of natural remedies for his condition. He read recently that L-arginine may be helpful for him, and he wants to know more about it. He can be told that:
   a. L-arginine's ability to increase nitric oxide supports its use for vascular health
   b. it is generally included in the list of treatments for angina, but not for peripheral vascular disease
   c. it is available in tea form and is recommended only in this form because of potency concerns
   d. none of the above

WEBSITE ACTIVITIES

1. Go to the Food and Drug Administration website page (www.fda.gov). Using the general site search box, search for information about heart disease in women by entering the keywords "women heart disease" to find the 1994 article entitled "Women and Heart Disease." Read the section of this article that discusses angina as a diagnostic sign for heart disease. What is a key difference between men and women in terms of the value of chest pain as a diagnostic clue to heart disease?

2. Go to the website of the American Heart Association (www.americanheart.org). From the opening page go to the Diseases and Conditions page, then to the "Other Conditions" section to find the article on Angina Pectoris. Skim this article to find the sections on stable and unstable angina. Write a brief paragraph summarizing the difference and the importance of treating unstable angina.

REVIEW QUESTIONS

1. What condition(s) may exist in older adults and require a reduction in dosage of antianginal drugs?
   a. impaired renal function or heart disease
   b. glaucoma
   c. diabetes or hypoglycemia
   d. rheumatoid arthritis

2. Which of the following is the most common adverse reaction of nitrates?
   a. hyperglycemia
   b. headache
   c. fever
   d. anorexia

3. Nitroglycerin ointment is administered by:
   a. rubbing the ointment into the scalp
   b. applying the ointment every hour or until the angina is relieved
   c. applying the ointment to a clean, dry area of skin
   d. spreading it under the tongue

4. If a patient taking a calcium channel blocker experiences orthostatic hypotension, then the patient is instructed to:
   a. remain in a supine position until the effects subside
   b. make position changes slowly to minimize hypotensive effects
   c. increase the dosage of the calcium channel blocker
   d. discontinue use of the calcium channel blocker until the hypotensive effects diminish

Actions of Antihypertensive Drugs

Uses of Antihypertensive Drugs

Adverse Reactions to Antihypertensive Drugs
Monitoring Adverse Reactions

Contraindications, Precautions, and Interactions of Antihypertensives

Herbal Remedies

Patient Management Issues with Antihypertensives

Educating the Patient and Family

Key Points

Case Study

Website Activities

Review Questions

KEY TERMS

aldosterone—a hormone that promotes the retention of sodium and water, which may contribute to a rise in blood pressure

angiotensin-converting enzyme—a naturally occurring enzyme that converts angiotensin I to angiotensin II, which is a powerful vasoconstrictor

blood pressure—the force of the blood against the walls of the arteries

endogenous—substances normally manufactured by the body

essential hypertension—hypertension without a known cause

hypertension—usually defined as a systolic pressure more than 140 mm Hg or a diastolic pressure more than 90 mm Hg

hypokalemia—low blood potassium

hyponatremia—low blood sodium

isolated systolic hypertension—a condition of only an elevated systolic pressure

malignant hypertension—hypertension in which the diastolic pressure usually exceeds 130 mm Hg

secondary hypertension—hypertension in which a direct cause can be identified

CHAPTER OBJECTIVES

On completion of this chapter, students will be able to:

1 Define the chapter's key terms.

2 Describe the general drug actions, uses, adverse reactions, contraindications, precautions, and interactions of antihypertensive drugs.

3 Explain why blood pressure determinations are important during therapy with an antihypertensive drug.

4 Discuss important points to keep in mind when educating the patient and family members about the use of antihypertensive drugs.

Blood pressure is the force of the blood against the walls of the arteries. Blood pressure rises and falls throughout the day. When the blood pressure stays elevated over time, the person is said to have hypertension. A systolic pressure less than 120 mm Hg and a diastolic blood pressure less than 80 mm Hg (120/80) are considered normal. **Hypertension**, often called high blood pressure, is usually defined as a systolic pressure more than 140 mm Hg and a diastolic pressure more than 90 mm Hg. Table 16-1 identifies normal blood pressure levels for adults and the different levels of hypertension. Patients in the prehypertension range require frequent blood pressure monitoring; patients with stage 1 or 2 hypertension should be under the care of a physician. Hypertension is serious because it causes the heart to work harder and contributes to atherosclerosis. It increases the risk of heart disease, congestive heart failure, kidney disease, blindness, and stroke.

FACTS ABOUT HYPERTENSION

- 50 million Americans have hypertension
- More than 90% of cases of hypertension have no known cause
- You are more likely to have hypertension if your parents have it
- Hypertension is called "the silent killer" because it has no warning symptoms but increases one's risk of dying from cardiovascular disease
- Because most people with hypertension do not know they have the condition, only one fourth of hypertensive people are being treated.

Source: American Society of Hypertension

Box 16-1 Risk Factors for Hypertension

- Smoking
- Age (women older than 65 years and men older than 55 years of age)
- Obesity
- Diabetes
- Lack of physical activity
- Chronic alcohol consumption
- Family history of cardiovascular disease
- Sex (men and postmenopausal women)

Most cases of hypertension have no known cause. When there is no known cause, the term **essential hypertension** is used. Essential hypertension has been linked to certain risk factors, such as diet and lifestyle. Box 16-1 identifies the risk factors associated with hypertension.

In the United States, blacks are twice as likely as whites to have hypertension. After age 65 years, black women have the highest incidence of hypertension. Essential hypertension cannot be cured but can be controlled. Many individuals experience hypertension as they grow older. For many older individuals, the systolic pressure gives the most accurate diagnosis of hypertension. Box 16-2 discusses the importance of systolic pressure.

Once essential hypertension develops, management of this disorder becomes a lifetime task. When a direct cause of the hypertension can be identified, the condition is described as **secondary hypertension**. Among the known causes of secondary hypertension, kidney disease ranks first, with tumors or other abnormalities of the adrenal glands following. In **malignant hypertension**, the diastolic pressure usually exceeds 130 mm

Hg. Managing the medical condition causing secondary hypertension results in the patient regaining a normal blood pressure.

Malignant hypertension is a dangerous condition that develops rapidly and requires immediate medical attention. Patients with malignant hypertension experience organ damage as the result of hypertension. Target organs of hypertension include the heart, kidney, and eyes (retinopathy).

Most health care providers prescribe lifestyle changes for patients to reduce risk factors before prescribing drugs. The health care provider may recommend measures, such as weight loss (if the patient is overweight), reduction of stress, regular aerobic exercise, quitting smoking (if applicable), and dietary changes, such as a decrease in sodium (salt) intake. Most people with hypertension are "salt-sensitive," which means that any salt or sodium more than the minimal bodily need is too much for them and leads to an increase in blood pressure. Dietitians usually recommend the Dietary Approaches to Stop Hypertension (DASH) diet. Studies indicate that blood pressure can be reduced by eating a diet low in saturated fat, total fat, and cholesterol and rich in fruits, vegetables, and low-fat dairy foods. The DASH diet includes whole grains, poultry, fish, and nuts and has reduced amounts of fats, red meats,

TABLE 16-1 Blood Pressure Levels for Adults

Category	Systolic* (in mm Hg)		Diastolic* (in mm Hg)
Normal	<120	and	<80
Prehypertension	120–139	or	80–89
Stage 1 hypertension	140–159	or	90–99
Stage 2 hypertension	≥160	or	≥100

*If systolic and diastolic pressures fall into different categories, then the patient's treatment status is the higher category.
From the Seventh Report of the Joint National Committee on Prevention, Detection, Evaluation and Treatment of High Blood Pressure, U.S. Department of Health and Human Services, May 2003. http://www.nhlbi.nih.gov/guidelines/hypertension/index.htm.

Box 16-2 Importance of Systolic Blood Pressure

In most individuals, the systolic pressure increases sharply with age, whereas the diastolic pressure increases until approximately age 55 years and then declines. Older individuals with only an elevated systolic pressure have a condition known as **isolated systolic hypertension** (ISH). When the systolic pressure is high, blood vessels become less flexible and stiffen, leading to cardiovascular disease and kidney damage. Research indicates that treating ISH saves lives and reduces illness. The treatment is the same for ISH as for other forms of hypertension.

sweets, and sugared beverages. The diet is rich in potassium, calcium, magnesium, protein, and fiber. Stress-reducing techniques, such as relaxation techniques, meditation, and yoga, may also be a part of the treatment regimen.

When drug therapy is begun, the health care provider may first prescribe a diuretic (Chapter 19) or beta blocker (Chapter 4) because these drugs have been shown to be highly effective. However, as in many other diseases and conditions, there is no "best" single drug, drug combination, or medical regimen for treatment of hypertension. After examination and evaluation of the patient, the health care provider selects the antihypertensive drug and therapeutic regimen that will probably be most effective. Figure 16-1 shows an algorithm for the treatment of hypertension. In some instances, it may be necessary to change to another antihypertensive drug or add a second antihypertensive drug if the patient does not experience a response to therapy. The health care provider also recommends that a patient continue with stress reduction, dietary modification, and other lifestyle modifications important in the control of hypertension.

The types of drugs used for the treatment of hypertension include:

- Vasodilating drugs: for example, hydralazine (Apresoline) and minoxidil (Loniten)
- β-adrenergic blocking drugs: for example, atenolol (Tenormin), metoprolol (Lopressor), and propranolol (Inderal)
- Antiadrenergic drugs (centrally acting): for example, guanabenz (Wytensin) and guanfacine (Tenex)
- Antiadrenergic drugs (peripherally acting): for example, guanadrel (Hylorel) and guanethidine (Ismelin)
- Alpha (α)-adrenergic blocking drugs: for example, doxazosin (Cardura) and prazosin (Minipress)
- Calcium channel blocking drugs: for example, amlodipine (Norvasc) and diltiazem (Cardizem)
- Angiotensin-converting enzyme (ACE) inhibitors: for example, captopril (Capoten), enalapril (Vasotec), and lisinopril (Prinivil)
- Angiotensin II receptor antagonists: for example, irbesartan (Avapro), losartan (Cozaar), and valsartan (Diovan)
- Diuretics: for example, furosemide (Lasix) and hydrochlorothiazide (HydroDIURIL)

For additional information concerning the antiadrenergic drugs (both centrally and peripherally acting) and the α-adrenergic and β-adrenergic blocking drugs, see Chapter 4. For more information on the calcium channel blockers, see Chapter 15. Information on the vasodilating drugs and the diuretics can be found in Chapters 15 and 19, respectively. The angiotensin-converting enzyme

(ACE) inhibitors and the angiotensin II receptor antagonists are discussed in this chapter.

In addition to these antihypertensive drugs, many antihypertensive combinations are available, such as Ser-Ap-Es, Timolide 10-25, Aldoril, and Lopressor (Table 16-2). Most combination antihypertensive drugs combine an antihypertensive and a diuretic.

Actions of Antihypertensive Drugs

Many antihypertensive drugs lower the blood pressure by dilating or increasing the size of the arterial blood vessels (vasodilation). Vasodilation creates an increase in the lumen (the space or opening within an artery) of the arterial blood vessels, which in turn increases the amount of space available for the blood to circulate. Because blood volume (the amount of blood) remains relatively constant, an increase in the space in which the blood circulates (the blood vessels) lowers the pressure of the fluid (measured as blood pressure) in the blood vessels. Although the method by which antihypertensive drugs dilate blood vessels varies, the result remains basically the same. Antihypertensive drugs with vasodilating activity include:

- Adrenergic blocking drugs
- Antiadrenergic blocking drugs
- Calcium channel blocking drugs
- Vasodilating drugs

Another type of antihypertensive drug is the diuretic. The mechanism by which the diuretics reduce elevated blood pressure is unknown, but it is thought to be based, in part, on their ability to increase the excretion of sodium from the body. The actions and uses of diuretics are discussed in Chapter 19.

The mechanism of action of the **angiotensin-converting enzyme** (ACE) inhibitors is not fully understood. It is believed that these drugs may prevent (or inhibit) the activity of angiotensin-converting enzyme, which converts angiotensin I to angiotensin II, a powerful vasoconstrictor. Both angiotensin I and ACE are normally manufactured by the body and are therefore called **endogenous** substances. The vasoconstricting activity of angiotensin II stimulates the secretion of the endogenous hormone aldosterone by the adrenal cortex. **Aldosterone** promotes the retention of sodium and water, which may contribute to a rise in blood pressure. By preventing the conversion of angiotensin I to angiotensin II, this chain of events is interrupted, sodium and water are not retained, and the blood pressure decreases. The angiotensin II receptor antagonists act to block the vasoconstrictor and aldosterone effects of angiotensin II at various receptor sites, resulting in a lowering of the blood pressure.

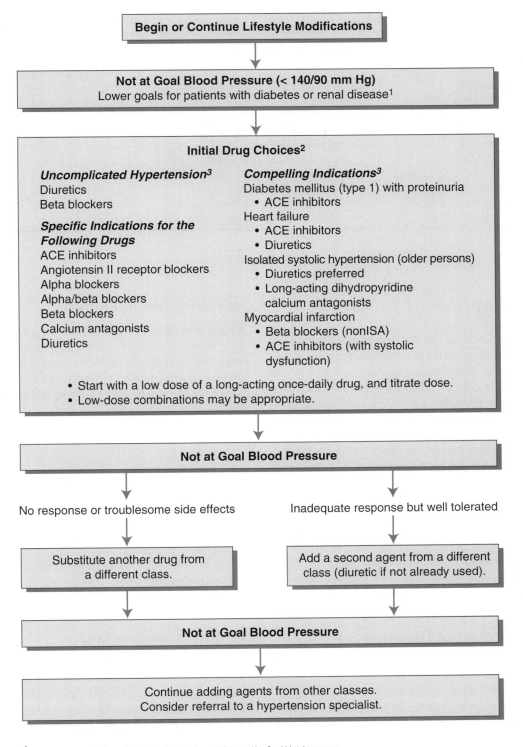

FIGURE 16-1 Algorithm for the treatment of hypertension. (From Roach SS. *Introductory Clinical Pharmacology,* 7th ed. Baltimore: Lippincott Williams & Wilkins; 2004.)

TABLE 16-2   Examples of Selected Antihypertensive Combinations

Trade Name	Diuretic Constituent	Antihypertensive
Aldoril-15	hydrochlorothiazide (15 mg)	methyldopa (250 mg)
Apresazide	hydrochlorothiazide (50 mg)	hydralazine (50 mg)
Combipres	chlorthalidone (15 mg)	clonidine (0.1 mg)
Hydropres-50	hydrochlorothiazide (50 mg)	reserpine (0.125 mg)
Lopressor 100/50	hydrochlorothiazide (50 mg)	metoprolol (100 mg)
Minizide 5	polythiazide (0.5 mg)	prazosin (5 mg)
Ser-Ap-Es	hydrochlorothiazide (15 mg) hydralazine (25 mg)	reserpine (0.1 mg)
Tenoretic 100	chlorthalidone (25 mg)	atenolol (100 mg)
Timolide 10–25	hydrochlorothiazide (25 mg)	timolol maleate (10 mg)
Zestoretic	hydrochlorothiazide (12.5 mg)	lisinopril (20 mg)

Uses of Antihypertensive Drugs

Antihypertensives are used in the treatment of hypertension. Although many antihypertensive drugs are available, not all drugs may work equally well in a given patient. In some instances, the health care provider may find it necessary to prescribe a different antihypertensive drug when a patient experiences no response to therapy. Some antihypertensive drugs are used only in severe cases of hypertension and when other less potent drugs have failed to lower the blood pressure. At times, two antihypertensive drugs may be given together to achieve a better response (see Figure 16-1).

Diazoxide (Hyperstat IV) and nitroprusside (Nitropress) are examples of intravenous (IV) drugs that may be used to treat hypertensive emergencies. A hypertensive emergency is a case of extremely high blood pressure that does not respond to conventional antihypertensive drug therapy.

Adverse Reactions of Hypertensive Drugs

When any antihypertensive drug is given, postural or orthostatic hypotension may occur in some patients, especially early in therapy. Postural hypotension is the occurrence of dizziness and light-headedness when the individual rises suddenly from a lying or sitting position. Orthostatic hypotension occurs when the individual has been standing in one place for a long time. These reactions can be prevented or minimized by having a patient rise slowly from a lying or sitting position and by avoiding standing in one place for a prolonged period.

Additional adverse reactions to antihypertensive drugs are listed in the Summary Drug Table: Antihypertensive Drugs. For the adverse reactions of diuretics, see the Summary Drug Table: Diuretics in Chapter 19.

Monitoring Adverse Reactions

A patient is observed for adverse drug reactions because their occurrence may require a change in the dose or the drug. The health care provider should be notified if any adverse reactions occur. In some instances, a patient may have to tolerate mild adverse reactions, such as dry mouth or mild anorexia.

ALERT

Discontinuing Use of an Antihypertensive

Should it be necessary to discontinue antihypertensive therapy, withdrawal should never happen abruptly. The dosage is gradually reduced over 2 to 4 days to avoid rebound hypertension (a rapid rise in blood pressure).

Managing Fluid Volume Deficit

A patient receiving a diuretic is observed for dehydration and electrolyte imbalances. A fluid volume deficit is most likely to occur if the patient fails to drink a sufficient amount of fluid. This is especially true in elderly or confused patients. To prevent a fluid volume deficit, patients should be encouraged to drink adequate amounts of fluids (up to 3000 mL/d, unless contraindicated).

Electrolyte imbalances that may occur during therapy with a diuretic include **hyponatremia** (low blood sodium) and **hypokalemia** (low blood potassium), although other imbalances may also occur. See Chapter 32 for the signs and symptoms of electrolyte imbalances. The health care provider should be notified if any signs or symptoms of an electrolyte imbalance occur.

(text continued on page 240)

SUMMARY DRUG TABLE   Antihypertensive Drugs

Generic Name	Trade Name*	Uses	Adverse Reactions	Dosage Ranges
Peripheral Vasodilators				
hydralazine HCl *hy-dral'-a-zeen*	Apresoline, *generic*	Hypertension	Dizziness, drowsiness, headache, hypotension, diarrhea, nausea, rash, sodium retention, drug-induced lupus syndrome	10–50 mg QID PO up to 300 mg/d
minoxidil *mi-nox'-i-dill*	Loniten, *generic*	Severe hypertension	Headache, hypotension, ECG changes, tachycardia, rash, sodium and water retention, hair growth	5–100 mg/d PO; dosage greater than 5 mg given in divided doses
β-*Adrenergic Blocking Drugs*				
acebutolol HCl *a-se-byoo'-toe- lole*	Sectral, *generic*	Hypertension, ventricular arrhythmias	Fatigue, hypotension, weakness, impotence, blurred vision, hypotension, congestive heart failure (CHF), bradycardia, pulmonary edema	400–1200 mg/d in single or divided doses PO
atenolol *a-ten'-oh-lole*	Tenormin, *generic*	Angina pectoris, hypertension, myocardial infarction (MI)	Fatigue, hypotension, weakness, blurred vision, stuffy nose, impotence, decreased libido, rash, CHF, bradycardia, pulmonary edema	50–100 mg/d PO in single dose; 5 mg IV; may repeat every 10 min up to 2 times
betaxolol HCl *be-tax'-oh-lol*	Kerlone	Hypertension, glaucoma (ophthalmic)	Fatigue, weakness, drowsiness, impotence, hypotension, CHF, bradycardia, pulmonary edema	10–20 mg once daily PO
bisoprolol fumarate *bis-oh'-pro-lole*	Zebeta	Hypertension	Fatigue, hypotension, weakness, blurred vision, stuffy nose, rash, CHF, bradycardia, pulmonary edema	2.5–20 mg once daily PO
carteolol HCl *kar'-tee-oh-lole*	Cartrol	Hypertension, glaucoma (ophthalmic)	Fatigue, orthostatic hypotension, weakness, blurred vision, stuffy nose, impotence, rash, CHF, bradycardia, pulmonary edema	2.5–10 mg/d once daily PO
carvedilol *kar-ve'-di-lole*	Coreg	Essential hypertension, CHF	Fatigue, dizziness, orthostatic hypotension, diarrhea, hyperglycemia, weakness, impotence, CHF, bradycardia, pulmonary edema	Hypertension: 6.25–25 mg BID PO; CHF: 3.125–25 mg BID PO
labetalol HCl *la-bet'-oh-lole*	Normodyne, Trandate, *generic*	Hypertension	Fatigue, weakness, orthostatic hypotension, impotence, drowsiness, bradycardia, pulmonary edema, CHF	200–400 mg BID up to 2400 mg/d; 20–80 mg IV; may give q 10 min up to 300 mg

Generic Name	Trade Name*	Uses	Adverse Reactions	Dosage Ranges
metoprolol *me-toe'-proe-lole*	Lopressor, Toprol XL, *generic*	Hypertension, angina pectoris, MI, heart failure (HF)	Fatigue, weakness, orthostatic hypotension, impotence, drowsiness, bradycardia, pulmonary edema, CHF	Hypertension angina, 100–400 mg/d PO; extended-release products are given once daily; MI: 25–100 mg BID PO; 5 mg q 2 min IV for 3 doses
nadolol *nay'-doe-lole*	Corgard, *generic*	Angina pectoris, hypertension	Fatigue, weakness, orthostatic hypotension, impotence, drowsiness, bradycardia, pulmonary edema, CHF	Angina: 40–80 mg/d PO; up to 240 mg/d; hypertension: 40–80 mg/d once daily PO; may increase to 320 mg/d
penbutolol sulfate *pen-byoo'-toe-lole*	Levatol	Hypertension	Fatigue, weakness, orthostatic hypotension, impotence, drowsiness, bradycardia, pulmonary edema, CHF	20 mg once daily PO
pindolol *pin'-doe-lole*	Visken, *generic*	Hypertension	Fatigue, weakness, orthostatic hypotension, impotence, drowsiness, bradycardia, pulmonary edema, CHF	5–60 mg/d, given twice daily PO
propranolol HCl *proe-pran'-oh-lole*	Inderal, Inderal LA, *generic*	MI, cardiac arrhythmias, angina pectoris, hypertension, migraine	Fatigue, weakness, orthostatic hypotension, impotence, drowsiness, bradycardia, pulmonary edema, CHF	MI: 180–240 mg/d PO; arrhythmias: 0–30 mg/d 1PO TID, QID; 1–3 mg IV, may repeat in 2 min and again in 4 h if needed; angina: 80–320 mg/din 2–4 divided doses or once daily as extended release; hypertension: 80–240 mg/d PO in divided doses; doses up to 640 mg have been given; migraine: 20 mg QID PO or 80 mg as extended release
timolol maleate *tim'-oh-lole*	Blocadren, *generic*	Hypertension, MI, migraine prophylaxis, glaucoma (ophthalmic)	Fatigue, weakness, orthostatic hypotension, impotence, drowsiness, bradycardia, pulmonary edema, CHF	Hypertension: 20 mg/d PO up to 60 mg/d; MI: 10 mg PO BID; migraine: 10–30 mg/d PO in one or divided dose
Antiadrenergics—Centrally Acting clonidine HCl (oral) *kloe'-ni-deen*	Catapres, *generic*	Hypertension	Drowsiness, sedation dizziness, headache, fatigue that tends to diminish within 4–6 weeks, dry mouth, constipation, impotence, decreased sexual activity	Individualize dosage, 0.1–0.8 mg/d PO in divided doses; maximum dosage, 2.4 mg/d

Generic Name	Trade Name*	Uses	Adverse Reactions	Dosage Ranges
clonidine HCl (transdermal) *kloe'-ni-deen*	Catapres- TTS-1, Catapres-TTS-2, Catapres-TTS-3, *generic*	Hypertension	Drowsiness, dry mouth, transient localized skin reactions, fatigue, headache, constipation, nausea	0.1 mg system–0.3 mg system q7d, may increase up to two 0.3-mg systems per 24 hours
guanabenz acetate *gwahn'-a-benz*	Wytensin, *generic*	Hypertension	Dizziness, weakness, lassitude, syncope, postural or exertional hypotension, diarrhea, bradycardia, fluid retention and edema, inhibition of ejaculation, CHF	Individualize dosage, 4–8 mg BID PO; may increase up to 64 mg/d
guanfacine HCl *gwahn'-fa-seen*	Tenex	Hypertension	Sedation, weakness, dizziness, dry mouth, constipation, impotence	1–3 mg PO HS
methyldopa and methyldopate HCl *meth-ill-doe'-pa*	Aldomet	Hypertension	Sedation, headache, asthenia, weakness, nausea, vomiting, distention, constipation, bradycardia	Methyldopa: 250 mg–3 g/d PO in divided doses; methyldopate: 250 mg–1g q6h IV
Antiadrenergics—Peripherally Acting guanadrel *gwahn'-a-drel*	Hylorel	Hypertension	Fatigue, headache, faintness, drowsiness, visual disturbances, confusion, increased bowel movements, indigestion, constipation, anorexia, shortness of breath on exertion, palpitations, chest pain, coughing, nocturia, urinary urgency or frequency, peripheral edema, ejaculation disturbances, weight loss or gain	10–75 mg/d PO
guanethidine monosulfate *gwahn-eth'-i-deen*	Ismelin	Hypertension	Dizziness, weakness, lassitude, syncope, postural exertional hypotension, or diarrhea, bradycardia, fluid retention and edema, CHF, inhibition of ejaculation	10–50 mg/d PO
reserpine *re-ser'-peen*	*Generic*	Hypertension	Drowsiness, sedation, lethargy, respiratory depression, edema, orthostatic hypotension, nasal congestion	0.5–1 mg/d PO
α-*Adrenergic Blocking Drugs* doxazosin mesylate *dox-ay'-zoe-sin*	Cardura	Hypertension, benign prostatic hypertrophy (BPH)	Headache, fatigue, dizziness, postural hypotension, dizziness, lethargy, vertigo, nausea, dyspepsia, diarrhea, tachycardia, palpitations, edema, sexual dysfunction	Hypertension: 1–16 mg/d PO once a day; BPH: 1–8 mg/d PO

Generic Name	Trade Name*	Uses	Adverse Reactions	Dosage Ranges
mecamylamine HCl *mek-a-mill'-a-meen*	Inversine	Severe hypertension	Weakness, fatigue, sedation, anorexia, dry mouth, glossitis, nausea, orthostatic hypotension	5–25 mg/d PO in 2 or 3 doses
prazosin *pra'-zoe-sin*	Minipress, *generic*	Hypertension	Dizziness, headache, drowsiness, lethargy, weakness, nausea, palpitations	1–20 mg/d PO in divided doses
terazosin *ter-ay'-zoe-sin*	Hytrin	Hypertension, BPH	Dizziness, headache, drowsiness, lack of energy, weakness, somnolence, nausea, palpitations, edema, dyspnea, nasal congestion, sinusitis	1–20 mg/d PO at HS
Angiotensin-Converting Enzyme Inhibitors benazepril HCl *ben-a'-za-pril*	Lotensin	Hypertension	Nausea, cough, vomiting, constipation, hypotension, palpitations, rash	10–40 mg/d PO in single or two divided doses
captopril *kap'-toe-pril*	Capoten, *generic*	Hypertension, HF, left ventricular dysfunction (LVD) after MI, diabetic nephropathy	Tachycardia, gastric irritation, peptic ulcer, proteinuria, rash, pruritus, cough	Hypertension: 50–450 mg/d PO in divided doses; CHF: 25–450 mg/d in divided doses; LVD: 6.25–150 mg/d PO TID; diabetic nephropathy: 25 mg PO TID
enalapril *e-nal'-a-pril*	Vasotec, Vasotec IV	Hypertension, HF, asymptomatic LVD	Headache, dizziness, fatigue, nausea, diarrhea, decreased hematocrit and hemoglobin, cough	Hypertension: 5–40 mg/d PO as a single dose or in two divided doses; 0.625–1.25 mg q6h IV; HF: 2.5–40 mg/d in two divided doses PO; LVD: 5–10 mg PO BID
fosinopril sodium *foh-sin'-oh-pril*	Monopril	Hypertension, HF	Nausea, cough, abdominal pain, vomiting, orthostatic hypotension, palpitation, rash	10–40 mg/d PO in a single dose or two divided doses
lisinopril *lyse-in'-oh-pril*	Prinivil, Zestril, *generic*	Hypertension, HF, acute MI	Headache, dizziness, insomnia, fatigue, gastric irritation, nausea, diarrhea, orthostatic hypotension, proteinuria, angioedema, cough	Hypertension: 10–40 mg/d PO as a single dose; CHF: 5–20 mg/d PO; acute MI: 5–10 mg PO
moexipril HCl *mo-ex'-ah-pril*	Univasc	Hypertension	Tachycardia, gastric irritation, peptic ulcers, diarrhea, diarrhea, proteinuria, rash, pruritus, flushing, flu-like syndrome, dizziness, cough	7.5–30 mg PO in one or two divided doses

Generic Name	Trade Name*	Uses	Adverse Reactions	Dosage Ranges
perindopril erbumine *pur-in'-doh-pril*	Aceon	Essential hypertension	Orthostatic hypotension, headache, dizziness, insomnia, fatigue, proteinuria, gastric irritation, nausea, cough	4–16 mg/d PO
quinapril HCl *kwin'-ah-pril*	Accupril	Hypertension, HF	Nausea, cough, abdominal pain, vomiting, orthostatic hypotension, palpitation, rash	Hypertension: 10–80 mg/d PO as a single dose or two divided doses; CHF: 5–20 mg PO BID
ramipril *ra-mi'-prill*	Altace	Hypertension, HF, decrease risk of cardiovascular disease, coronary artery disease (CAD)	Nausea, cough, abdominal pain, vomiting, orthostatic hypotension, palpitation, rash	Hypertension: 2.5–20 mg/d PO as a single dose or in two divided doses; CHF: 2.5–5 mg PO BID; CAD risk: 10 mg/d PO
Angiotensin II Receptor Antagonists				
candesartan cilexetil *can-dah-sar'-tan*	Atacand	Hypertension	Diarrhea, abdominal pain, nausea, headache, dizziness, upper respiratory infection (URI) symptoms, hypotension, rash	16–32 mg/d PO in divided doses
eprosartan mesylate *ep-row-sar'-tan*	Teveten	Hypertension	Abdominal pain, fatigue, depression, URl symptoms, hypotension	400–800 mg/d PO in divided doses BID
irbesartan *er-bah-sar'-tan*	Avapro	Hypertension	Headache, dizziness, diarrhea, abdominal pain, nausea, hypotension, URl symptoms, cough, fatigue	75–300 mg/d PO as one dose
losartan potassium *low-sar'-tan*	Cozaar	Hypertension	Diarrhea, abdominal pain, nausea, headache, dizziness, hypotension, URl symptoms, cough	25–100 mg/d PO in one or two doses
telmisartan *tell-mah-sar'-tan*	Micardis	Hypertension	Diarrhea, abdominal pain, nausea, headache, dizziness, light-headedness, URl symptoms, hypotension	40–80 mg/d PO
valsartan *val-sar'-tan*	Diovan	Hypertension	Headache, dizziness, diarrhea, abdominal pain, nausea, URl symptoms, cough	80–320 mg/d PO
Drugs Used for Hypertensive Crisis diazoxide, parenteral *di-az-ok'-side*	Hyperstat IV, *generic*	Hypertensive crisis	Dizziness, weakness, nausea, vomiting, sodium and water retention, hypotension, myocardial ischemia	1–3 mg/kg IV bolus; maximum dosage: 150 mg

Generic Name	Trade Name*	Uses	Adverse Reactions	Dosage Ranges
nitroprusside sodium *nye-troe-pruss'-ide*	Nitropress, *generic*	Hypertensive crisis	Apprehension, headache, restlessness, nausea, vomiting, palpitations, diaphoresis	3 mcg/kg per minute, not to exceed infusion rate of 10 mcg/min (if blood pressure is not reduced within 10 min, discontinue administration)

*The term *generic* indicates the drug is available in generic form.

Minimizing the Risk for Injury

Dizziness or weakness along with postural hypotension can occur with the administration of antihypertensive drugs. If postural hypotension occurs, then the patient is advised to rise slowly from a sitting or lying position. The health care provider explains that when rising from a lying position, sitting on the edge of the bed for 1 or 2 minutes often minimizes these symptoms. The patient is also informed that rising slowly from a chair and then standing for 1 to 2 minutes also minimizes the symptoms of postural hypotension. When symptoms of postural hypotension, dizziness, or weakness occur, the patient should be assisted when getting out of bed or a chair or when walking.

Contraindications, Precautions, and Interactions of Antihypertensives

Antihypertensive drugs are contraindicated in patients with a known hypersensitivity to the individual drugs. When an antihypertensive is administered by a transdermal system (e.g., clonidine), the system is contraindicated if a patient is allergic to any component of the adhesive layer of the transdermal system. Use of the angiotensin II receptor antagonists during the second and third trimester of pregnancy is contraindicated because use may cause fetal and neonatal injury or death. These drugs are pregnancy category C during the first trimester of pregnancy and are pregnancy category D during the second and third trimesters.

Antihypertensive drugs are used cautiously in patients with renal or hepatic impairment or electrolyte imbalances, during lactation and pregnancy, and in older patients. ACE inhibitors are used cautiously in patients with sodium depletion, hypovolemia, or coronary or cerebrovascular insufficiency and those receiving diuretic therapy or dialysis. The angiotensin II receptor agonists are used cautiously in patients with renal or hepatic dysfunction, hypovolemia, or volume or salt depletion, and in patients receiving high doses of diuretics.

The hypotensive effects of most antihypertensive drugs are increased when administered with diuretics and other antihypertensives. Many drugs can interact with the antihypertensive drugs and decrease their effectiveness (e.g., antidepressants, monoamine oxidase inhibitors, antihistamines, and sympathomimetic bronchodilators). When the ACE inhibitors are administered with the NSAIDs, their antihypertensive effect may be decreased. Absorption of the ACE inhibitors may be decreased when administered with antacids. Administration of potassium-sparing diuretics or potassium supplements concurrently with the ACE inhibitors may cause hyperkalemia. When the angiotensin II receptor agonists are administered with NSAIDs or phenobarbital, their antihypertensive effects may be decreased.

Herbal Remedies

Various herbs and supplements, such as hawthorn extracts, garlic, onion, ginkgo biloba, vitamin E, and aspirin, may be used by herbalists for hypertension. Although these substances may lower blood pressure in some individuals, their use is not recommended because the effect is slight and usually too gentle to affect moderate to severe hypertension. However, several studies have demonstrated that hypertensive patients may benefit from daily doses of calcium (800 mg) or magnesium (300 mg).

Diets that are rich in fruit and vegetables are good sources of potassium and magnesium and are consistently associated with lower blood pressure. It has been suggested that blood pressure can be significantly lowered by a diet high in magnesium, calcium, and potassium and low in sodium and fat. The evidence that magnesium lowers hypertension is clear enough that the Joint Committee on Prevention, Detection, Evaluation, and Treatment of High Blood Pressure recommends adequate intake of magnesium for preventing and managing high blood pressure.

Patients should consult their health care provider before taking any herbal remedy.

Patient Management Issues with Antihypertensives

Before therapy with an antihypertensive drug is started, the health care provider obtains the blood pressure and pulse rate on both arms with a patient in standing, sitting, and lying positions. The health care provider also obtains a patient's weight, especially if a diuretic is part of therapy or if the health care provider prescribes a weight-loss regimen.

Monitoring and recording the blood pressure is an important part of patient management, especially early in therapy. The health care provider may need to adjust the dose of the drug upward or downward, try a different drug, or add another drug to the therapeutic regimen if a patient does not have an adequate response to drug therapy.

Each time the blood pressure is measured, the same arm and patient position (e.g., standing, sitting, or lying down) should be used. In some instances, the health care provider may order the blood pressure taken in one or more positions, such as standing and lying down. The patient is monitored for blood pressure and pulse every 1 to 4 hours if he or she has severe hypertension, does not have the expected response to drug therapy, or is critically ill.

ALERT
Monitoring Vital Signs After Administration of an Antihypertensive

The blood pressure and pulse rate of a hospitalized patient are obtained immediately before giving an antihypertensive drug and compared with previous readings. If the blood pressure is significantly lower than baseline values, then the drug should not be given, and the health care provider should be notified. In addition, the health care provider must be notified if there is a significant increase in the blood pressure.

The patient's weight is measured daily during the initial period of drug therapy. Patients taking an antihypertensive drug occasionally retain sodium and water, resulting in edema and weight gain. The patient's extremities are also examined for edema. A weight gain of 2 pounds or more per day and any evidence of edema in the hands, fingers, feet, legs, or sacral area are reported to the health care provider. A patient is also weighed at regular intervals if a weight-reduction diet is used to lower the blood pressure or if a patient is receiving a thiazide or related diuretic as part of antihypertensive therapy.

GERONTOLOGIC ALERT
Nitroprusside Sensitivity

Older adults are particularly sensitive to the hypotensive effects of nitroprusside. To minimize the hypotensive effects, the drug is initially given in lower dosages. Older adults require more frequent monitoring during the administration of nitroprusside.

Educating the Patient and Family

Health care workers can do much to educate others about the importance of having their blood pressure checked periodically. This includes people of all ages because hypertension does not occur only in older individuals. Once hypertension is detected, patient teaching becomes an important factor in successfully returning the blood pressure to normal or near-normal levels.

To ensure lifetime compliance with the prescribed therapeutic regimen, the importance of drug therapy is emphasized, as well as other treatments recommended by the health care provider. The adverse reactions that may occur with a particular antihypertensive drug are explained to the patient, who is advised to contact the health care provider if any should occur.

The health care provider may want the patient or family to monitor blood pressure during therapy. The health care provider teaches the technique of taking a blood pressure and pulse rate to the patient or family member, allowing sufficient time for supervised practice. The patient is instructed to keep a record of the blood pressure and to bring this record to each visit to the health care provider's office.

Many patients receiving antihypertensive therapy commonly receive more than one drug, placing them at risk for orthostatic hypotension. Patients are instructed to follow these measures:

- Change your position slowly
- Sit at the edge of the bed or chair for a few minutes before standing up
- Ask for help standing or walking when necessary
- If you feel dizzy or lightheaded, then sit or lie down immediately
- Make sure to drink adequate amounts of fluid during the day

Patient Education Box 16-1 includes key points about antihypertensives that the patient or family members should know.

PATIENT EDUCATION BOX 16-1

Key Points for Patients Taking Antihypertensive Drugs

❑ Never discontinue use of this drug except on the advice of your health care provider. These drugs control but do not cure hypertension. Skipping doses of the drug or voluntarily discontinuing the drug may cause severe, rebound hypertension.

❑ Do not use any nonprescription drugs (some may contain drugs that are capable of increasing the blood pressure) unless approved by your health care provider.

❑ Do not drink alcohol unless its use has been approved by your health care provider.

❑ Take the drug as requested by your health care provider. Some drugs, such as captopril and moexipril, are usually taken 1 hour before or 2 hours after meals to enhance absorption.

❑ This drug may produce dizziness or light-headedness when rising suddenly from a sitting or lying position. To

avoid these effects, rise slowly from a sitting or lying position.

❑ If the drug makes you drowsy, avoid hazardous tasks such as driving or performing tasks that require alertness. Drowsiness may disappear with time.

❑ If you feel weak or fatigued, contact your health care provider.

❑ Contact your health care provider if you experience adverse drug effects.

❑ Follow the diet restrictions recommended by your health care provider. Do not use salt substitutes unless a particular brand of salt substitute is approved by your health care provider.

❑ Notify your health care provider if your diastolic pressure suddenly increases to 130 mm Hg or higher; you may have malignant hypertension.

KEY POINTS

◉ Hypertension is serious because it causes the heart to work harder and contributes to atherosclerosis. It increases the risk of heart disease, congestive heart failure, kidney disease, blindness, and stroke. In the United States, blacks are twice as likely as whites to experience hypertension.

◉ Although many antihypertensive drugs are available, not all drugs may work equally well in a given patient.

◉ Antihypertensive drugs with vasodilating activity include adrenergic blocking drugs, antiadrenergic block-

ing drugs, calcium channel blocking drugs, and vasodilating drugs. Another type of antihypertensive drug is the diuetic.

◉ When any antihypertensive drug is given, postural or orthostatic hypotension may occur in some patients, especially early in therapy. Monitoring and recording the blood pressure is an important part of the ongoing assessment, especially early in therapy. Antihypertensive drugs are used cautiously in patients with renal or hepatic impairment or electrolyte imbalances, during lactation and pregnancy, and in older patients.

CASE STUDY

Mrs. Ohlin was prescribed captopril for her hypertension. You are asked to help educate Mrs. Ohlin and her family about hypertension and its treatment.

1. What is the optimal time for Mrs. Ohlin to take captopril?
   a. at meal time
   b. at bed time and on rising
   c. 1 hour before or 2 hours after meals
   d. after crushing the tablet and mixing with water

2. Mrs. Ohlin asks what to expect for side effects. She can be told:
   a. profuse sweating and flushing
   b. possible nausea and vomiting, constipation, rash
   c. headache, muscular weakness
   d. none of the above

3. Mrs. Ohlin asks whether captopril may aggravate her sensitive stomach. You reply:
   a. there are no known cases of gastric upset with this drug
   b. gastric upset is sometimes a side effect; if it occurs, she should notify her health care provider
   c. constipation may be a side effect, but gastric distress is not
   d. captopril may aggravate an existing peptic ulcer but is otherwise not known for gastric distress

WEBSITE ACTIVITIES

1. Go to the website for the National Center for Health Statistics (www.cdc.gov/nchs/fastats) and conduct a search for information on hypertension. Write a brief statement that includes current statistics on the number of office visits per year in America that are attributed to hypertension, and what percentages of Americans in various subcategories (women, elderly, black) are being treated for the disease.

2. Now go to the Center for Disease Control website (www.cdc.gov) and click on the "In the News" heading. Then, under related links, click on "Rumors/Hoaxes." Write a brief statement listing three of the topics found in this section.

REVIEW QUESTIONS

1. To prevent problems associated with orthostatic hypotension, the health care provider advises the patient to:
   a. sleep in a side-lying position
   b. avoid sitting for prolong periods
   c. change position slowly
   d. get up from a sitting position quickly

2. When discontinuing use of an antihypertensive drug, which of the following should occur?
   a. the blood pressure is monitored every hour for 8 hours after the drug therapy is discontinued
   b. the drug dosage is gradually decreased during a period of 2 to 4 days to avoid rebound hypertension
   c. the blood pressure and pulse are checked every 30 minutes after discontinuing the drug therapy
   d. the dosage is tapered during a period of 2 weeks to prevent a return of hypertension

3. In most patients, the following occurs:
   a. the systolic blood pressure increases sharply with age
   b. the systolic blood pressure decreases with age, and the diastolic pressure rises quickly
   c. both systolic and diastolic blood pressure tend to increase at approximately the same rates as age increases
   d. systolic blood pressure increases slowly until age 55 and then tends to level off

4. Common adverse effects of nadolol (Corgard) include:
   a. dizziness and impotence
   b. drowsiness, fatigue, and weakness
   c. dry mouth and a dry cough
   d. all of the above

5. Common adverse effects of diuretics include:
   a. dehydration and electrolyte imbalances
   b. salt craving
   c. pupil constriction
   d. all of the above

Bile Acid Sequestrants
Actions of Bile Acid Sequestrants
Uses of Bile Acid Sequestrants
Adverse Reactions of Bile Acid Sequestrants
Contraindications, Precautions, and Interactions of Bile Acid Sequestrants

HMG-CoA Reductase Inhibitors
Actions of HMG-CoA Reductase Inhibitors
Uses of HMG-CoA Reductase Inhibitors
Adverse Reactions of HMG-CoA Reductase Inhibitors
Contraindications, Precautions, and Interactions of HMG-CoA Reductase Inhibitors

Fibric Acid Derivatives
Actions of Fibric Acid Derivatives
Uses of Fibric Acid Derivatives
Adverse Reactions of Fibric Acid Derivatives
Contraindications, Precautions, and Interactions of Fibric Acid Derivatives

Miscellaneous Antihyperlipidemic Drug: Niacin
Actions of Niacin
Uses of Niacin
Adverse Reactions of Niacin
Contraindications, Precautions, and Interactions of Niacin

Natural Remedies: Garlic

Patient Management Issues with Antihyperlipidemic Drugs

Educating the Patient and Family

Key Points

Case Study

Website Activities

Review Questions

KEY TERMS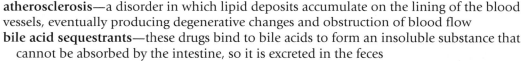

atherosclerosis—a disorder in which lipid deposits accumulate on the lining of the blood vessels, eventually producing degenerative changes and obstruction of blood flow

bile acid sequestrants—these drugs bind to bile acids to form an insoluble substance that cannot be absorbed by the intestine, so it is excreted in the feces

catalyst—a substance that accelerates a chemical reaction without itself undergoing a change

cholesterol—one of the lipids in the blood

high-density lipoproteins (HDL)—carry cholesterol from peripheral cells to the liver, where it is metabolized and excreted

HMG-CoA reductase inhibitor—an enzyme that is a catalyst in the manufacture of cholesterol

hyperlipidemia—an increase (hyper) in lipids (lipid), which are fats or fat-like substances, in the blood (-emia).

lipids—fats or fat-like substances in the blood

lipoprotein—a lipid-containing protein

low-density lipoproteins (LDL)—transport cholesterol to peripheral cells

rhabdomyolysis—a rare condition in which muscle damage results in the release of muscle cell contents into the bloodstream

triglycerides—a type of lipids in the blood

CHAPTER OBJECTIVES

On completion of this chapter, students will be able to:

1 Define the chapter's key terms.

2 Discuss the general drug actions, uses, adverse reactions, contraindications, precautions, and interactions of antihyperlipidemic drugs.

3 Discuss important points to keep in mind when educating the patient or family member about the use of an antihyperlipidemic drug.

4 Discuss cholesterol, HDL, LDL, and triglyceride levels and how they contribute to the development of heart disease.

Hyperlipidemia is an increase (hyper) in the **lipids** (lipi), which are a group of fats or fat-like substances in the blood (demia). **Cholesterol** and the **triglycerides** are the two lipids in the blood. Elevation of one or both of these lipids results in hyperlipidemia. Serum cholesterol levels above 240 mg/dL and triglyceride levels above 150 mg/dL are associated with atherosclerosis. **Atherosclerosis** is a disorder in which lipid deposits accumulate on the lining of the blood vessels, eventually producing degenerative changes and obstruction of blood flow (Fig. 17-1). Atherosclerosis is considered to be a major contributor in the development of heart disease.

FACTS ABOUT CHOLESTEROL

- 105 million Americans have a total cholesterol level of 200 mg/dL or higher, the point at which it becomes a cardiovascular risk factor
- Most people can raise their good cholesterol levels by exercising, not smoking, and maintaining a healthy weight
- The process leading to atherosclerosis can begin in children

Myths About Cholesterol

- "Using margarine instead of butter will help lower my cholesterol"–*not true!*
- "Thin people do not have to worry about high cholesterol"–*not true!*
- "Since I started taking medication for my high cholesterol, I do not have to worry about what I eat"–*not true!*
- "I am a woman so I do not have to worry. High cholesterol is a man's problem"–*not true!*

Source: American Heart Association

Triglycerides and cholesterides are insoluble in water and must be bound to a lipid-containing protein (**lipoprotein**) for transportation throughout the body. Although several lipoproteins are found in the blood, this chapter focuses on low-density lipoproteins (LDL),

high-density lipoproteins (HDL), and cholesterol. **Low-density lipoproteins** (LDL) transport cholesterol to peripheral cells. When the cells have all the cholesterol they need, the excess cholesterol is discarded into the blood. This can result in a high blood level of cholesterol, which can penetrate the walls of the arteries, leading to atherosclerotic plaque formation. Elevated levels of LDL increase the risk for heart disease. **High-density lipoproteins** (HDL) take cholesterol from peripheral cells and bring it to the liver, where it is metabolized and excreted. The higher the level of HDL, the lower the risk for development of atherosclerosis. Therefore, it is desirable to see an increase in HDL (the "good" lipoprotein), because of its protective properties against the development of atherosclerosis, and a decrease in LDL. A laboratory examination of blood lipids, called a lipoprotein profile, provides valuable information about a person's cholesterol levels, including:

- total cholesterol
- LDL (the harmful lipoprotein)
- HDL (the protective lipoprotein)
- triglycerides

Table 17-1 provides an analysis of LDL levels. HDL cholesterol protects against heart disease, so the higher the number, the better. An HDL level less than 40 mg/dL is low and considered a major risk factor for heart disease. Triglyceride levels that are borderline (150–199 mg/dL) or high (above 200 mg/dL) may require treatment in some individuals.

An increase in serum lipids is believed to contribute to or cause atherosclerosis, a disease characterized by deposits of fatty plaques on the inner walls of arteries. These deposits result in a narrowing of the lumen (inside diameter) of the artery and a decrease in blood supply to the area served by the artery. When these fatty deposits occur in the coronary arteries, the patient experiences coronary artery disease. Lowering blood cholesterol levels can arrest or reverse atherosclerosis in the vessels and can significantly decrease the person's risk for heart disease.

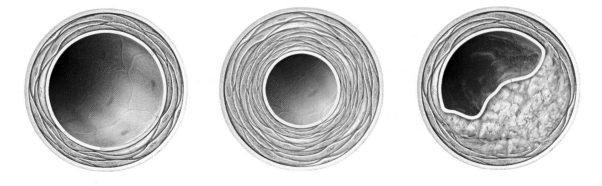

FIGURE 17-1 **Atherosclerosis** is a disorder in which lipid deposits accumulate on the lining of the blood vessels, eventually producing degenerative changes and obstruction of blood flow. (Asset provided by Anatomical Chart Co.)

TABLE 17-1 **Cholesterol Level Analysis**

Total Cholesterol Level*	Category
Less than 200 mg/dL	Desirable
200–239 mg/dL	Borderline
≥240 mg/dL	High

LDL Cholesterol Level*	LDL Cholesterol Category
<100 mg/dL	Optimal
100–129 mg/dL	Near optimal/above optimal
130–159 mg/dL	Borderline high
160–189 mg/dL	High
≥190 mg/dL	Very high

*Cholesterol levels are measured in milligrams (mg) of cholesterol per deciliter (dL) of blood.

Hyperlipidemia, particularly elevated serum cholesterol and LDL levels, is a risk factor in the development of atherosclerotic heart disease. Other risk factors, besides cholesterol levels, play a role in the development of hyperlipidemia, including:

- family history of early heart disease (father before the age of 55 years and mother before the age of 55 years)
- cigarette smoking
- hypertension (high blood pressure)
- age (men older than 45 years and women older than 55 years)
- low HDL levels
- obesity
- diabetes

In general, the higher one's LDL level and the more risk factors involved, the greater the risk for heart disease. The main goal of treatment in patients with hyperlipidemia is to lower the LDL to a level that will reduce their risk of heart disease.

The health care provider may initially seek to control the cholesterol level by encouraging therapeutic life changes. This includes a cholesterol-lowering diet, physical activity, quitting smoking (if applicable), and weight management. The diet is a plan that is low in saturated fat and low in cholesterol. It includes less than 200 mg of dietary cholesterol per day. In addition, physical activity lasting at least 30 minutes each day is recommended. Walking at a brisk pace for 30 minutes per day 5 to 7 days per week can help raise the HDL and lower LDL. Added benefits of a healthy diet and exercise program include a reduction of body weight. If these lifestyle changes do not bring blood lipids to therapeutic levels, then the health care provider may add one of the antihyperlipidemic drugs to the treatment plan. The lifestyle changes are continued along with the drug regimen.

In addition to controlling dietary intake of fat, particularly saturated fatty acids, antihyperlipidemic drug therapy is used to lower serum levels of cholesterol and triglycerides. The health care provider may use one drug or, in some instances, more than one antihyperlipidemic drug for those with poor response to therapy with a single drug. Three types of antihyperlipidemic drugs are currently in use, as well as one miscellaneous antihyperlipidemic drug (see Summary Drug Table: Antihyperlipidemic Drugs for a complete listing of the drugs):

- bile acid sequestrants
- HMG-CoA reductase inhibitors
- fibric acid derivatives
- niacin

The target LDL level for treatment is less than 130 mg/dL. If the patient's response to drug treatment is adequate, then lipid levels are monitored every 4 months. If the response is inadequate, then another drug or a combination of two drugs is used. Antihyperlipidemic drugs decrease cholesterol and triglyceride levels in several ways. Although the end result is a lower lipid blood level, each has a slightly different action.

Bile Acid Sequestrants

Actions of Bile Acid Sequestrants

Cholestyramine (Questran) and colestipol (Colestid) are examples of bile acid sequestrants. Bile, which is manufactured and secreted by the liver and stored in the gallbladder, emulsifies fat and lipids as they pass through the intestine. Once emulsified, fats and lipids are readily absorbed in the intestine. **Bile acid sequestrant** drugs bind to bile acids to form an insoluble substance that cannot be absorbed by the intestine, so it is excreted in the feces. With increased loss of bile acids, the liver uses cholesterol to manufacture more bile. This is followed by a decrease in cholesterol levels.

Uses of Bile Acid Sequestrants

Bile acid sequestrants are used as adjunctive therapy for the reduction of elevated serum cholesterol in patients with hypercholesterolemia who do not have an adequate response to a diet and exercise program. Cholestyramine may also be used to relieve pruritus associated with partial biliary obstruction.

Adverse Reactions of Bile Acid Sequestrants

A common problem associated with bile acid sequestrants is constipation. Constipation may be severe and may occasionally result in fecal impaction. Hemorrhoids may be aggravated. Additional adverse reactions include vitamin A and D deficiencies, bleeding tendencies (including gastrointestinal bleeding) caused by a

SUMMARY DRUG TABLE   Antihyperlipidemic Drugs

Generic Name	Trade Name*	Uses	Adverse Reactions	Dosage Ranges
Bile Acid Sequestrants				
cholestyramine *koe-less'-tir-a-meen*	LoCHOLEST, Prevalite, Questran, Questran Light, *generic*	Hyperlipidemia, relief of pruritus associated with partial biliary obstruction	Constipation (may lead to fecal impaction), exacerbation of hemorrhoids, abdominal pain, distention and cramping, nausea, increased bleeding related to vitamin K malabsorption, vitamin A and D deficiencies	4 g PO 1–6 times/d; individualize dosage based on response
colestipol HCl *koe-les'-ti-pole*	Colestid	Hyperlipidemia	Constipation (may lead to fecal impaction), exacerbation of hemorrhoids, abdominal pain, distention and cramping, nausea, increased bleeding related to vitamin K malabsorption, vitamin A and D deficiencies	Granules: 5–30 g/d PO in divided doses; tablets: 2–16 g/d
colesevelam HCl *ko-leh-sev'-eh-lam*	Welchol	Adjunctive therapy used alone or with an HMG-CoA inhibitor to decrease elevated LDL cholesterol	Constipation (may lead to fecal impaction), exacerbation of hemorrhoids, abdominal pain, distention and cramping, nausea, increased bleeding related to vitamin K malabsorption, vitamin A and D deficiencies	3–6 tablets/d PO
HMG-CoA Reductase				
atorvastatin *ah-tor'-va-stah-tin*	Lipitor	Hyperlipidemia, reduction of elevated total and LDL cholesterol levels; increase HDL-C in patients with hypercholesterolemia	(Usually mild) headache, flatulence, abdominal pain, cramps, constipation, nausea	10–80 mg/d PO
fluvastatin *flue-va-sta'-tin*	Lescol, Lescol XL	Hyperlipidemia and mixed dyslipidemia, reduction of elevated total and LDL cholesterol levels, to slow progression of coronary artery disease (CAD), along with diet and exercise	(Usually mild) headache, flatulence, abdominal pain, cramps, constipation, nausea	20–80 mg/d PO
lovastatin *loe-va-sta'-tin*	Mevacor	Hyperlipidemia, reduction of elevated total and LDL cholesterol levels, to slow progression of CAD along with diet and exercise	(Usually mild) headache, flatulence, abdominal pain, cramps, constipation, nausea	10–80 mg/d PO in single or divided doses

Generic Name	Trade Name*	Uses	Adverse Reactions	Dosage Ranges
pravastatin *prah-va-sta'-tin*	Pravachol	Hyperlipidemia, reduction of elevated total and LDL cholesterol levels, prevention of first MI, to slow progression of CAD, reduce risk of stroke, TIA, and MI	(Usually mild) headache, flatulence, abdominal pain, cramps, constipation, nausea	10–40 mg/d PO
simvastatin *sim-va-stah'-tin*	Zocor	Hyperlipidemia, reduction of elevated total and LDL cholesterol levels	(Usually mild) headache, flatulence, abdominal pain, cramps, constipation, nausea	5–80 mg/d PO
Fibric Acid Derivatives clofibrate *klo-fye'-brate*	Atromid-S, *generic*	Hyperlipidemia	Nausea, vomiting, GI upset, impotence, myalgia (muscle cramping and aching), increased or decreased angina, cardiac arrhythmias, fatigue, rash	2 g/d PO in divided doses
fenofibrate *fen-oh-figh'-brate*	Tricor	Hyperlipidemia, hypertriglyceridemia	Nausea, constipation, diarrhea, abnormal liver function tests, respiratory problems, rhinitis, abdominal pain, back pain, headache, asthenia, flu syndrome	54–160 mg/d PO
gemfibrozil *jem-fi'-broe-zil*	Lopid, *generic*	Hyperlipidemia, hypertriglyceridemia, reduction of coronary heart disease risk	Dyspepsia, abdominal pain, diarrhea, nausea, vomiting, rash, vertigo, headache	1200 mg/d PO in 2 divided doses 30 min before morning and evening meal
Miscellaneous Preparations niacin *nye'-a-sin* (nicotinic acid)	Niaspan	Adjunctive treatment for hyperlipidemia	Generalized flushing sensation of warmth, severe itching and tingling, nausea, vomiting, abdominal pain	1–2 g PO BID, TID; extended release: 500–2000 mg/d PO

* The term *generic* indicates the drug is available in generic form.

depletion of vitamin K, nausea, abdominal pain, and abdominal distention.

Managing Adverse Reactions of Bile Acid Sequestrants

Patients taking antihyperlipidemic drugs, particularly bile acid sequestrants, may experience constipation. The drugs can produce or severely worsen preexisting constipation. Patients are instructed to drink more fluids, eat foods high in dietary fiber, and exercise daily to help prevent constipation. If the problem persists or becomes severe, then a stool softener or laxative may be required.

Some patients require a decreased dosage or discontinuation of the drug therapy.

GERONTOLOGIC ALERT

Bile Acid Sequestrants and Constipation

Older adults are particularly prone to constipation when taking bile acid sequestrants. Older adults should be monitored for hard dry stools, difficulty passing stools, and any reports of constipation. An accurate record of bowel movements should be kept.

Contraindications, Precautions, and Interactions of Bile Acid Sequestrants

Bile acid sequestrants are contraindicated in patients with known hypersensitivity to the drugs. Bile acid sequestrants are also contraindicated in those with complete biliary obstruction. These drugs are used cautiously in patients with a history of liver or kidney disease. Bile acid sequestrants are used cautiously during pregnancy (pregnancy category C) and lactation (decreased absorption of vitamins may affect the infant).

Bile acids sequestrants, particularly cholestyramine, can decrease the absorption of numerous drugs. For this reason, bile acid sequestrants should be administered alone and other drugs given at least 1 hour before or 4 hours later. The patient has an increased risk of bleeding when bile acid sequestrants are administered with oral anticoagulants; the dosage of the anticoagulant is usually decreased. Bile acid sequestrants may bind with digoxin, thiazide diuretics, penicillin, propranolol, tetracyclines, folic acid, and thyroid hormones, resulting in decreased effects of these drugs.

HMG-CoA Reductase Inhibitors

Actions of HMG-CoA Reductase Inhibitors

Another group of antihyperlipidemic drugs is called **HMG-CoA reductase inhibitors**. HMG-CoA (3-hydroxy-3-methyglutaryl coenzyme A) reductase is an enzyme that is a **catalyst** in the manufacture of cholesterol. (A catalyst is a substance that accelerates a chemical reaction without itself undergoing a change.) These drugs appear to inhibit the manufacture of cholesterol or promote the breakdown of cholesterol. This drug activity lowers the blood levels of cholesterol and serum triglycerides and increases blood levels of HDL. Examples of these drugs are fluvastatin (Lescol), lovastatin (Mevacor), and simvastatin (Zocor).

Uses of HMG-CoA Reductase Inhibitors

These drugs, along with a diet restricted in saturated fat and cholesterol, are used to treat hyperlipidemia when diet and other nonpharmacologic treatments alone have not resulted in lowered cholesterol levels.

Adverse Reactions of HMG-CoA Reductase Inhibitors

HMG-CoA reductase inhibitors are usually well tolerated. Adverse reactions, when they do occur, are often mild and transient and do not require discontinuing therapy. Common adverse reactions include nausea, vomiting, constipation, abdominal pain or cramps, and headache. A rare but more serious adverse reaction is rhabdomyolysis.

Managing Adverse Reactions of HMG-CoA Reductase Inhibitors

Antihyperlipidemic drugs, particularly HMG-CoA reductase inhibitors, have been associated with skeletal muscle effects leading to rhabdomyolysis. **Rhabdomyolysis** is a very rare condition in which muscle damage results in the release of muscle cell contents into the bloodstream. Rhabdomyolysis may precipitate renal dysfunction or acute renal failure. It is important to be alert for unexplained muscle pain, muscle tenderness, or weakness, especially if accompanied by malaise or fever. These symptoms should be reported to the health care provider because it may be necessary to discontinue the drug.

Contraindications, Precautions, and Interactions of HMG-CoA Reductase Inhibitors

HMG-CoA reductase inhibitors are contraindicated in individuals with hypersensitivity to the drugs, patients with serious liver disorders, and during pregnancy (pregnancy category X) and lactation. HMG-CoA reductase inhibitors are used cautiously in patients with a history of alcoholism, acute infection, hypotension, trauma, endocrine disorders, visual disturbances, or myopathy.

HMG-CoA reductase inhibitors have an additive effect when used with bile acid sequestrants, which may provide an added benefit in treating hypercholesterolemia that does not respond to a single-drug regimen. The patient has an increased risk of myopathy (disorders of the striated muscle) if taking an HMG-CoA reductase inhibitor along with erythromycin, niacin, or cyclosporine. When the HMG-CoA reductase inhibitors are given with oral anticoagulants, the anticoagulant effect is increased.

Fibric Acid Derivatives

Actions of Fibric Acid Derivatives

Fibric acid derivatives, the third group of antihyperlipidemic drugs, work in a variety of ways. Clofibrate (Atromid-S) acts to stimulate the liver to increase the breakdown of very-low-density lipoproteins (VLDL) to low-density lipoproteins (LDL), decreasing the liver synthesis of VLDL and inhibiting cholesterol formation. Fenofibrate (Tricor) acts by reducing VLDL and stimulating the catabolism of triglyceride-rich lipoproteins, resulting in a decrease in plasma triglyceride and cholesterol. Gemfibrozil (Lopid) increases the excretion of cholesterol in the feces and reduces the production of triglycerides by the liver, thus lowering serum lipid levels.

Uses of Fibric Acid Derivatives

Although fibric acid derivatives have antihyperlipidemic effects, their use varies depending on the drug. For example, Clofibrate (Atromid-S) and gemfibrozil (Lopid) are used to treat individuals with very-high-serum triglyceride levels who have a risk of abdominal pain and pancreatitis and who do not experience a response to diet modifications. Clofibrate is not used to treat other types of hyperlipidemia and is not thought to be effective for prevention of coronary heart disease. Fenofibrate (Tricor) is used as adjunctive treatment for the reduction of LDL, total cholesterol, and triglycerides in patients with hyperlipidemia.

Adverse Reactions of Fibric Acid Derivatives

The adverse reactions of fibric acid derivatives include nausea, vomiting, gastrointestinal upset, and diarrhea. Clofibrate, fenofibrate, and gemfibrozil may increase cholesterol excretion into the bile, leading to cholelithiasis (stones in the gallbladder) or cholecystitis (inflammation of the gallbladder). If cholelithiasis occurs, then use of the drug is discontinued. Fenofibrate may also result in abnormal liver function tests, respiratory problems, back pain, and headache. Gemfibrozil may cause dyspepsia, skin rash, vertigo, and headache. See the Summary Drug Table: Antihyperlipidemic Drugs for additional adverse reactions.

Managing Adverse Reactions of Fibric Acid Derivatives

Although rhabdomyolysis is a very rare condition, it may be associated with fibric acid derivative use. Rhabdomyolysis may precipitate renal dysfunction or acute renal failure. Those providing patient care should be alert for unexplained muscle pain, tenderness, or weakness, especially if accompanied by malaise or fever. These symptoms should be reported to the health care provider because it may be necessary to discontinue the drug.

Contraindications, Precautions, and Interactions of Fibric Acid Derivatives

Fibric acid derivatives are contraindicated in patients with hypersensitivity to the drugs and those with significant hepatic or renal dysfunction or primary biliary cirrhosis because these drugs may increase the already elevated cholesterol. The drugs are used cautiously during pregnancy (pregnancy category C) and lactation and in patients with peptic ulcer disease or diabetes. Although rare, when a fibric acid derivative, particularly gemfibrozil, is given along with an HMG-CoA reductase inhibitor, the patient has an increased risk for rhabdomyolysis. When clofibrate, fenofibrate, or gemfibrozil is administered with anticoagulants, the patient is at an increased risk for bleeding.

Miscellaneous Antihyperlipidemic Drug: Niacin

Actions of Niacin

The mechanism by which niacin (nicotinic acid) lowers blood lipids is not fully understood.

Uses of Niacin

Niacin is used as adjunctive therapy for the treatment of very-high-serum triglyceride levels in patients who present a risk of pancreatitis (inflammation of the pancreas) and who do not adequately respond to dietary control.

Adverse Reactions of Niacin

Nicotinic acid may cause nausea, vomiting, abdominal pain, diarrhea, severe generalized flushing of the skin, a sensation of warmth, and severe itching or tingling. Although these reactions are most often seen at higher dose levels, some patients may experience them even when small doses of nicotinic acid are administered. The sudden appearance of these reactions may frighten the patient. The health care provider should be informed before the next dose is due if the patient experiences an adverse reaction. If the patient is in severe discomfort, then the health care provider should be notified immediately.

Contraindications, Precautions, and Interactions of Niacin

Niacin is contraindicated in patients with a known hypersensitivity to it and in those with active peptic ulcer, hepatic dysfunction, or arterial bleeding. The drug is used cautiously in patients with renal dysfunction, high alcohol consumption, unstable angina, gout, and pregnancy (category C).

Natural Remedies: Garlic

Garlic, an herb, is commonly used as a food product and an herbal supplement. It has been used for many years throughout the world. Although garlic has many medicinal purposes, its positive effect on cardiovascular health is the most well-known and has been extensively researched. Other benefits of garlic are that it helps to lower serum cholesterol and triglyceride levels, improves the ratio of HDL to LDL cholesterol, lowers blood pressure, and helps to prevent atherosclerosis. It is often used as an antioxidant, to protect the liver, as an effective antifungal, antiviral, and antibiotic, to reduce blood sugar levels, to strengthen the immune system, and to reduce menstrual pain. Garlic has also been used topically to treat warts, corns, calluses, ear infections, muscle pain, nerve pain, arthritis, and sciatica.

The recommended dosages of garlic are 600 to 900 mg/day of the garlic powder tablets, 10 mg of garlic oil "Perles," or one medium fresh clove of garlic per day. Generally, garlic taken orally is in the form of enteric-coated odorless garlic or fresh pressed garlic. Adverse reactions include mild stomach upset or irritation, which can usually be alleviated by taking the supplements with food. Although no serious reactions have occurred in pregnant women taking garlic, its use is not recommended. Garlic is excreted in breast milk and may cause colic in some infants.

Patient Management Issues with Antihyperlipidemic Drugs

In many individuals, hyperlipidemia has no symptoms and the disorder is not discovered until laboratory tests reveal elevated cholesterol and triglyceride levels, elevated LDL levels, and decreased HDL levels. Antihyperlipidemic drugs are often initially prescribed on an outpatient basis but may be given also to hospitalized patients. Serum cholesterol levels (i.e., a lipid profile) and liver function tests are obtained before the drugs are administered.

Patient assessment includes a dietary history, focusing on the types of foods in the patient's usual diet. Vital signs and weight are recorded. The patient's skin and eyelids are inspected for evidence of xanthomas (flat or elevated yellow deposits), which may occur in the more severe forms of hyperlipidemia.

Patients usually take these drugs as outpatients and then are seen by the health care provider for periodic monitoring. Blood cholesterol and triglyceride levels are monitored as a part of the ongoing therapy.

ALERT

Elevation of Blood Lipid Levels

Sometimes a paradoxical elevation of blood lipid levels occurs with drug therapy. Should this happen, the health care provider is notified, and a different antihyperlipidemic drug may be prescribed.

During therapy, vital signs and bowel functioning are assessed to watch for the adverse reaction constipation. Constipation may become serious if not treated.

Because hyperlipidemia is often treated on an outpatient basis, patient education is important. The health care provider explains the drug regimen and possible adverse reactions. Printed dietary guidelines may be given to a patient, and the importance of fol-

lowing these recommendations is emphasized. Drug therapy usually is discontinued or modified if the antihyperlipidemic drug is not effective after 3 months of treatment.

Bile acid sequestrants may interfere with the digestion of fats and prevent the absorption of the fat-soluble vitamins (vitamins A, D, E, and K) and folic acid. When a bile acid sequestrant is used for long-term therapy, vitamins A and D may be given in a water-soluble form or administered parenterally. If the patient has bleeding tendencies as the result of vitamin K deficiency, then parenteral vitamin K is administered for immediate treatment, and oral vitamin K is given for prevention of a deficiency in the future.

Educating the Patient and Family

It is important to stress the importance of following the recommended diet because drug therapy alone cannot significantly lower cholesterol and triglyceride levels. If necessary, the patient or family member are referred to a teaching dietitian, a dietary teaching session, or a lecture provided by a hospital or community agency.

When using diet and drugs to control high blood cholesterol levels, the health care provider does the following:

- Reviews the reasons for the drug and prescribed drug therapy, including the drug's name, form, correct dose, and frequency of administration.
- Emphasizes that drug therapy alone will not significantly lower blood cholesterol levels.
- Stresses importance of taking drug exactly as prescribed.
- Reinforces the importance of adhering to the prescribed diet.
- Provides a written copy of dietary plan and reviews its contents.
- Answers the patient's questions and offers suggestions for ways to reduce dietary fat intake.
- Instructs the patient about possible adverse reactions and signs and symptoms to report to the health care provider.
- Reviews measures to minimize gastrointestinal upset.
- Explains the possible need for vitamin A and D therapy and high-fiber foods if the patient is receiving bile acid sequestrant.
- Reassures the patient that the results of therapy will be monitored by periodic laboratory and diagnostic tests and follow-up with the health care provider.

Patient Education Box 17-1 includes key points about antihyperlipidemic drugs the patient or family should know.

PATIENT EDUCATION BOX 17-1

Key Points for Patients Taking Antihyperlipidemic Drugs

BILE ACID SEQUESTRANTS:

❑ Take the drug before meals unless your health care provider directs otherwise.

❑ Cholestyramine powder: The prescribed dose must be mixed in 4 to 6 fluid ounces of water or noncarbonated beverage and shaken vigorously. The powder can also be mixed with highly fluid soups or pulpy fruits (applesauce, crushed pineapple). The powder should not be ingested in the dry form. Other drugs are taken 1 hour before or 4 to 6 hours after cholestyramine. Cholestyramine is available combined with the artificial sweetener aspartame (Questran Light) for patients with diabetes or those concerned with weight gain.

❑ Colestipol granules: The prescribed dose must be mixed in liquids, soup, cereals, carbonated beverages, or pulpy fruits. Because the granules do not dissolve, the preparation should be slowly stirred until it is ready to drink. Take the entire drug, then rinse the glass with a small amount of water and drink it.

❑ Colesevelam: Mix the granules in liquids, soups, cereals, or pulpy fruits. Do not take it dry. Mix the prescribed amount in a glassful of liquid. Carbonated beverages should be stirred slowly in a large glass. The tablets are taken twice daily without regard to meals.

❑ Constipation, flatulence, nausea, and heartburn may occur and may disappear with continued therapy. Notify your health care provider if these effects become bothersome or if you experience unusual bleeding.

HMG-CoA INHIBITORS:

❑ Take Lovastatin once daily, preferably with the evening meal. Fluvastatin, pravastatin, and simvastatin are taken, without regard to meals, once daily in the evening or at bedtime.

❑ If fluvastatin or pravastatin is prescribed with a bile acid sequestrant, then take fluvastatin 2 hours after the bile acid sequestrant and pravastatin at least 4 hours afterward.

❑ Contact your health care provider as soon as possible if you experience nausea; vomiting; muscle pain, tenderness, or weakness; fever; upper respiratory infection; rash; itching; or extreme fatigue.

FIBRIC ACID DERIVATIVES:

❑ Clofibrate: If you experience gastrointestinal upset, then take the drug with food. Notify your health care provider if you experience chest pain, shortness of breath, palpitations, nausea, vomiting, fever, chills, or sore throat.

❑ Gemfibrozil: Dizziness or blurred vision may occur. Observe caution when driving or performing hazardous tasks. Notify your health care provider if you experience epigastric pain, diarrhea, nausea, or vomiting.

❑ Nicotinic acid: Take this drug with meals. This drug may cause mild to severe facial flushing, a feeling of warmth, severe itching, or headache. These symptoms usually subside with continued therapy, but contact your health care provider as soon as possible if your symptoms are severe. Your health care provider may prescribe aspirin (325 mg) to be taken approximately 30 minutes before nicotinic acid to decrease the flushing reaction. If you become dizzy, avoid sudden changes in posture.

KEY POINTS

● Bile acid sequestrants are used as adjunctive therapy to reduce elevated serum cholesterol in patients with hypercholesterolemia who do not adequately respond to a diet and exercise program. Constipation is a common adverse effect. Bile acid sequestrants are contraindicated in those with complete biliary obstruction and are used cautiously in patients with a history of liver or kidney disease.

● HMG-CoA reductase inhibitors, along with a diet restricted in saturated fat and cholesterol, are used to treat hyperlipidemia when diet and other nonpharmacologic treatments alone have not resulted in lowered cholesterol levels. HMG-CoA reductase inhibitors are usually well-tolerated. A rare but serious adverse reaction is rhabdomyolysis. HMG-CoA reductase inhibitors are contraindicated in individuals with hypersensitivity to the drugs or a serious liver disorder, and during pregnancy (pregnancy category X) and lactation.

● Although the fibric acid derivatives have antihyperlipidemic effects, their use varies depending on the drug. Clofibrate (Atromid-S) and gemfibrozil (Lopid) are used to treat individuals with very-high-serum triglyceride levels who have a risk of abdominal pain and pancreatitis and who do not experience a response to diet modifications. Fibric acid derivatives are contraindicated in patients with hypersensitivity to the drugs and those with significant hepatic or renal dysfunction or primary biliary cirrhosis because these drugs may increase the already elevated cholesterol.

● Niacin is used as adjunctive therapy for the treatment of very-high-serum triglyceride levels in patients at risk for pancreatitis. Nicotinic acid may cause nausea, vomiting, abdominal pain, diarrhea, severe generalized flushing of the skin, a sensation of warmth, and severe itching or tingling.

CASE STUDY

1. Mr. Braden, age 62, is taking Colestid. He has questions about his exercise plan and the adverse effects he is experiencing. Which of the following elements will most help his overall health?
   a. lowering the amount of saturated fat he consumes
   b. eating more fruits and vegetables
   c. exercising at least 5 days per week
   d. all of the above; no single element alone is sufficient

2. Mr. Braden says he hates going to the gym to exercise and asks what other options you would suggest. You tell him:
   a. he must continue with heavy cardiovascular workouts
   b. walking at a brisk pace for at least 30 minutes per day 5 to 7 days per week has proven effective
   c. walking 3 times per week for 10 minutes at a brisk pace has proven effective
   d. none of the above; exercise for someone on Colestid is ineffective

3. Mr. Braden wonders why his formerly regular bowel movements have become irregular and whether his headaches are attributable to the Colestid. You advise him that:
   a. the constipation is a common adverse effect, and you ask him for more specific information
   b. the headache is an adverse effect, but constipation is not a known effect of Colestid
   c. neither of these symptoms is associated with Colestid use
   d. both of these symptoms are associated with Colestid

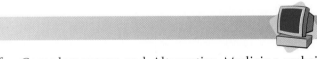

WEBSITE ACTIVITIES

1. Go to the National Center for Complementary and Alternative Medicine website (http://nccam.nih.gov) and click on "Clinical Trials." Next, click on NCCAM Clinical Trials "By Treatment or Therapy." Search for garlic. Write a brief statement describing any clinical trials that are underway involving garlic.

2. Go to the MEDLINEplus website (http://medlineplus.gov). Click on "Health Topics" and search for cholesterol. Write a brief statement about one of the current "News" articles on the MEDLINEplus site involving cholesterol.

REVIEW QUESTIONS

1. Lovastatin (Mevacor) is best taken:
   a. once daily, preferably with the evening meal
   b. three times daily with meals
   c. at least 1 hour before or 2 hours after meals
   d. twice daily without regard to meals

2. A patient taking cholestyramine (Questran) who has vitamin K deficiency should:
   a. be checked for bruising
   b. keep a record of fluid intake and output
   c. be monitored for myalgia
   d. keep a dietary record of foods eaten

3. A patient taking niacin reports flushing after each dose of the niacin. Which of the following drugs might be prescribed to help alleviate the flushing?
   a. Demerol
   b. aspirin
   c. vitamin K
   d. Benadryl

4. Which of the following points should be included when teaching a patient about drug and diet therapy for hyperlipidemia?
   a. fluids should be taken in limited amounts when eating a low-fat diet
   b. the medication should be taken at least 1 hour before meals
   c. the medication alone will not lower cholesterol levels
   d. meat is not allowed on a low-fat diet

5. Which of the following is/are a risk factor(s) in the development of atherosclerotic heart disease?
   a. cigarette smoking
   b. obesity
   c. diabetes
   d. all of the above

18 Anticoagulant, Thrombolytic, and Antianemia Drugs

KEY TERMS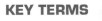

anemia—a decrease in the number of red blood cells (RBCs), a decrease in the amount of hemoglobin in RBCs, or both a decrease in the number of RBCs and hemoglobin
fibrolytic drugs—another name for thrombolytic drugs
folinic acid or leucovorin rescue—the technique of administering leucovorin after a large dose of methotrexate to rescue normal cells and allow them to survive
hemostasis—a process that stops bleeding in a blood vessel
intrinsic factor—a substance produced by cells in the stomach that is necessary for the absorption of vitamin B_{12} in the intestine

255

iron deficiency anemia—condition that results when the body does not have enough iron to supply the body's needs

megaloblastic anemia—a type of anemia that results from a deficiency of folic acid and certain other causes

pernicious anemia—a type of megaloblastic anemia that results from a deficiency of intrinsic factor

prothrombin—a substance that is essential for the clotting of blood

thrombolytic drugs—drugs designed to dissolve blood clots that have already formed within a blood vessel

thrombosis—the formation of a clot

thrombus—blood clot

CHAPTER OBJECTIVES

On completion of this chapter, students will be able to:

1 Define the chapter's key terms.

2 Describe the general drug actions, uses, adverse reactions, contraindications, precautions, and interactions of anticoagulant, thrombolytic, and antianemia drugs

3 Discuss important points to keep in mind when educating the patient or family members about the use of an anticoagulant, thrombolytic, or antianemia drug.

Anticoagulants are used to prevent the formation and extension of a **thrombus** (blood clot). Anticoagulants have no direct effect on an existing thrombus and do not reverse any damage from the thrombus. However, once a thrombus has been established, anticoagulant therapy can prevent additional clots from forming. Although they do not thin the blood, they are sometimes called blood thinners by patients. Anticoagulants are a group of drugs that include warfarin (a coumarin derivative), anisindione (an indandione derivative), and fractionated and unfractionated heparin.

Whereas the anticoagulants prevent thrombus formation, **thrombolytic drugs** dissolve blood clots that have already formed within a blood vessel. These drugs can reopen blood vessels after they become occluded. Another term for thrombolytic drugs is **fibrocytic drugs**. A basic understanding of hemostasis and thrombus formation is a foundation for understanding these drugs.

Hemostasis

Hemostasis is the body's process of stopping bleeding in a blood vessel. Normal hemostasis involves a complex process of extrinsic and intrinsic factors. Figure 18-1 shows the coagulation pathway and factors involved. The coagulation cascade is so named because as each factor is activated, it acts as a catalyst that enhances the next reaction, and the net result is a large collection of fibrin that forms a plug in the vessel. Fibrin is the insoluble protein that is essential to clot formation.

Thrombosis

Thrombosis is the formation of a clot. A thrombus may form in any vessel, artery, or vein when blood flow is impeded. For example, a venous thrombus can develop as the result of venous stasis (decreased blood flow), injury to the vessel wall, or altered blood coagulation. Venous thrombosis most often occurs in the lower extremities and is associated with venous stasis. Deep vein thrombosis occurs in the lower extremities and is the most common type of venous thrombosis. Arterial thrombosis can occur because of atherosclerosis or arrhythmias, such as atrial fibrillation. The thrombus may begin small, but fibrin, platelets, and red blood cells attach to the thrombus, increasing its size and shape. When a thrombus detaches from the wall of the vessel and is carried along through the bloodstream, it becomes an embolus. The embolus travels until it reaches a vessel that is too small to permit its passage. If the embolus goes to the lung and obstructs a pulmonary vessel, then it is called a pulmonary embolism. If the embolus occludes a vessel supplying blood to the heart, then it can cause a myocardial infarction. Anticoagulant drugs therefore are used prophylactically in patients who are at high risk for clot formation.

Coumarin and Indandione Derivatives

Warfarin (Coumadin), a coumarin derivative, is the oral anticoagulant most commonly prescribed. Warfarin can also be administered parenterally. Because it can be given orally, it is the drug of choice for patients requiring long-term therapy with an anticoagulant. Peak activity is reached 1.5 to 3 days after therapy is initiated. Anisindione (Miradon), an indandione derivative, is less frequently used but is an effective anticoagulant. For more information on anisindione, see the Summary Drug Table: Anticoagulants.

Generic Name	Trade Name*	Uses	Adverse Reactions	Dosage Ranges
Coumadin and Indandione Derivatives				
anisindione *ah-nis-in-dye'-on*	Miradon	Prophylaxis and treatment of venous thrombosis and its extension; prevention and treatment of atrial fibrillation with embolization, prophylaxis and treatment of pulmonary embolism	Hemorrhage, nausea, alopecia, dermatitis, vomiting, anorexia, abdominal cramping, nausea	25–300 mg/d PO, dose individualized based on PT or INR
warfarin sodium *war'-far-in*	Coumadin, *generic*	Venous thrombosis, atrial fibrillation with embolism, pulmonary embolism (PE), prophylaxis of systemic embolism after acute MI	Nausea, alopecia, hemorrhage, urticaria, dermatitis, vomiting, anorexia, abdominal cramping, priapism	2–10 mg/d PO, IV; individualized dose based on PT or INR
Unfractionated Heparin				
heparin *hep'-ah-rin*	Generic	Thrombosis/embolism, diagnosis and treatment of disseminated intravascular coagulation (DIC), prophylaxis of deep vein thrombosis (DVT), clotting prevention	Hemorrhage, chills, fever, urticaria, local irritation, erythema, mild pain, hematoma or ulceration at the injection site (IM or SC), bruising	10,000–20,000 units SC in divided doses q8–12h; 5000–10,000 units q4–6h intermittent IV; 5000–40,000 units/d IV infusion; 5000 units SC q2h before surgery and 5000 units SC after surgery q8–12h
heparin sodium lock flush solution *hep'-ah-rin*	Generic	Clearing intermittent infusion lines (heparin lock) to prevent clot formation at site	None significant	10–100 units/mL heparin solution
Fractionated Heparins: Low-Molecular-Weight Heparins (LMWHs)				
dalteparin sodium *dal-tep'-a-rin*	Fragmin	Unstable angina/non–Q-wave MI, DVT prophylaxis	Hemorrhage, bruising, thrombocytopenia, chills, fever, pain, erythema and irritation at site of injection	Angina/MI: 120 IU/kg, SC q12h with concurrent oral aspirin; DVT: 2500 IU SC daily
danaparoid sodium *da-nap'-a-royd*	Orgaran	Prophylaxis of DVT, after hip replacement surgery	Hemorrhage, bruising, thrombocytopenia, hyperkalemia, hypersensitivity, fever, pain and erythema at injection site	750 anti-Xa units BID SC
enoxaparin sodium *en-ocks'-a-par-in*	Lovenox	DVT and prophylaxis, DVT and pulmonary embolism (PE) treatment, unstable angina/non–Q-wave MI	Hemorrhage, bruising, thrombocytopenia, hyperkalemia, hypersensitivity, fever, pain and erythema at injection site	DVT prophylaxis: 30 mg q12h SC or 40 mg once daily SC; in abdominal surgery for patients at risk for thromboembolic complications: 40 mg/d SC; DVT/PE treatment: 1 mg/kg SC q12h; unstable angina, non–Q-wave MI: 1 mg/kg SC q12h

Generic Name	Trade Name*	Uses	Adverse Reactions	Dosage Ranges
tinzaparin sodium *ten-zah'-pear-in*	Innohep	Treatment of acute, symptomatic DVT with or without pulmonary emboli when given with warfarin sodium	Hemorrhage, bruising, thrombocytopenia, hyperkalemia, hypersensitivity, fever, pain and erythema at injection site	175 anti-Xa IU/kg/d SC once daily; 175 IU/kg/d SC once daily until the patient has been successfully anticoagulated with warfarin
Anticoagulant Antagonists phytonadione (vitamin K) *fye-toe-na-dye'-on*	Aqua-mephyton, Mephyton, *generic*	Prevention and treatment of hypoprothrombinemia associated with excessive doses of oral anticoagulants	Gastric upset, unusual taste, flushing, rash, urticaria, erythema, pain and/or swelling at injection site	PO, IM, 2.5–10 mg, may repeat PO in 12–48 h or in 6–8 h after parenteral dose
protamine sulfate *proe'-ta-meen*	*Generic*	Acute management of heparin overdosage (neutralizes heparin)	Dyspnea, bradycardia, hypotension, hypertension, bleeding, hypersensitivity reactions	Dose is determined by amount of heparin in body and the time that has elapsed since the heparin was given; the longer the interval, the smaller the dose required. Adult and pediatric: 1mg IV neutralizes 90 USP units of heparin derived from lung tissue or 115 USP units of heparin derived from intestinal mucosa

*The term *generic* indicates the drug is available in generic form.

All anticoagulants interfere with the clotting mechanism of the blood. Warfarin and anisindione interfere with the manufacturing of vitamin K-dependent clotting factors by the liver. This results in the depletion of clotting factors II (prothrombin), VII, IX, and X.

Actions of Warfarin

It is the depletion of **prothrombin** (see Fig. 18-1), a substance that is essential for the clotting of blood, that accounts for most of the action of warfarin.

Uses of Warfarin

Warfarin is used for:

- Prevention (prophylaxis) and treatment of deep vein thrombosis
- Prevention and treatment of atrial fibrillation with embolization
- Prevention and treatment of pulmonary embolism
- As part of the treatment of myocardial infarction
- Prevention of thrombus formation after valve replacement

In most situations, warfarin is the drug of choice, with anisindione reserved for those who are unable to take warfarin.

Adverse Reactions of Warfarin

The principal adverse reaction of warfarin is bleeding, which may range from very mild to severe. Bleeding may be seen in many areas of the body, such as the bladder, bowel, stomach, uterus, and mucous membranes. Other adverse reactions are rare but may include nausea, vomiting, alopecia (loss of hair), urticaria (severe skin rash), abdominal cramping, diarrhea, rash, hepatitis (inflammation of the liver), jaundice (yellow discoloration of the skin and mucous membranes), and blood dyscrasias (disorders).

Managing Adverse Reactions of Warfarin

Bleeding can occur any time during therapy with warfarin, even when the patient's prothrombin time (PT) appears to be within a safe limit. (Prothrombin time is a test of the blood's clotting time. International Normalized Ratio [INR] is another measure of clotting time.) All

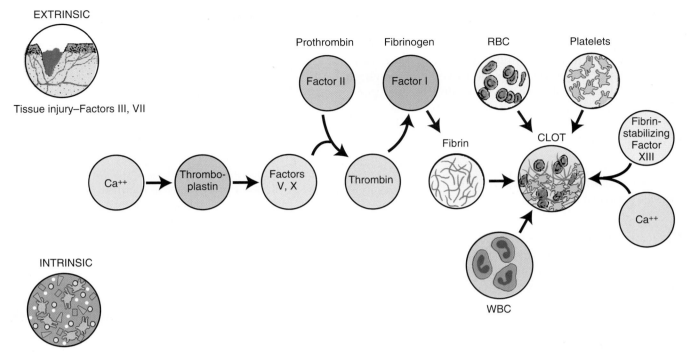

FIGURE 18-1 The blood-clotting pathway. Blood coagulation results in the formation of a stable fibrin clot. Formation of this clot involves a cascade of interactions of clotting factors, platelets, and other substances. Clotting factors exist in the blood in inactive form and must be converted to an active form before the next step in the clotting pathway can occur. Each factor is stimulated in turn until the process is complete and a fibrin clot is formed. In the intrinsic pathway, all of the components necessary for clot formation are in the circulating blood. Clot formation in the intrinsic pathway is initiated by factor XII. In the extrinsic pathway, coagulation is initiated by release of tissue thromboplastin, a factor not found in circulating blood. (From Roach SS. *Introductory Clinical Pharmacology*, 7th ed. Baltimore: Lippincott Williams & Wilkins; 2004.)

health care team members should be made aware of any patient receiving warfarin and help observe for bleeding. The following are signs of bleeding in hospitalized patients:

- Urinal, bedpan, catheter drainage unit: Inspect the patient's urine for a pink to red color and inspect the stool for signs of gastrointestinal bleeding (bright red to black stools). Visually check for catheter drainage every 2 to 4 hours and when the unit is emptied. Oral anticoagulants may impart a red–orange color to alkaline urine, making hematuria difficult to detect visually. A urinalysis may be necessary to determine if blood is in the urine.
- Emesis basin, nasogastric suction units: Visually check the nasogastric suction unit every 2 to 4 hours and when the unit is emptied. Check the emesis basin each time it is emptied.
- Skin, mucous membranes: Inspect a patient's skin daily for evidence of easy bruising or bleeding. Be alert for bleeding from minor cuts and scratches, nosebleeds, or excessive bleeding after intramuscular (IM), subcutaneous (SC), or intravenous (IV) injections, or after a venipuncture. After oral care, check the patient's toothbrush and gums for signs of bleeding.

ALERT

Adverse Reactions to Warfarin

The drug should be withheld and the health care provider contacted immediately if any of the following occurs:

- the PT exceeds 1.5–times the control value
- there is evidence of bleeding
- the INR is greater than 3

Warfarin Overdosage

Symptoms of overdosage of warfarin include:

- blood in the stool (melena)
- petechiae (pinpoint-size red hemorrhagic spots on the skin)
- oozing from superficial injuries, such as cuts from shaving or bleeding from the gums after brushing the teeth
- excessive menstrual bleeding

Any adverse reactions or evidence of bleeding must be immediately reported to the health care provider. Because warfarin interferes with the synthesis of vitamin

K_1-dependent clotting factors, the administration of vitamin K_1 reverses the effects of warfarin by providing the necessary ingredient to enhance clot formation and stop bleeding. However, withholding one or two doses of warfarin may quickly bring the PT to an acceptable level. The PT generally returns to a safe level within 6 hours of administration of vitamin K_1. Administration of whole blood or plasma may be necessary if severe bleeding occurs because the vitamin K_1 is delayed.

Contraindications, Precautions, and Interactions of Warfarin

Warfarin is contraindicated in patients with a known hypersensitivity, hemorrhagic disease, tuberculosis, leukemia, uncontrolled hypertension, gastrointestinal ulcers, recent surgery of the eye or central nervous system, aneurysms, or severe renal or hepatic disease, and during pregnancy and lactation. Use during pregnancy (pregnancy category X) can cause fetal death.

Warfarin is used cautiously in patients with fever, heart failure, diarrhea, malignancy, hypertension, renal or hepatic disease, psychoses, or depression. Women of childbearing age must use a reliable contraceptive to prevent pregnancy.

The effects of warfarin may increase when administered with acetaminophen, NSAIDs, beta blockers, disulfiram, isoniazid, chloral hydrate, loop diuretics, aminoglycosides, cimetidine, tetracyclines, and cephalosporins. Oral contraceptives, ascorbic acid, barbiturates, diuretics, and vitamin K decrease the effects of warfarin. Because the effects of warfarin are influenced by many drugs, the patient should notify the health care provider when taking a new drug or discontinuing use of any drug, both prescription and over-the-counter preparations.

Patient Management Issues with Warfarin

Before the first dose of warfarin is administered, the patient is questioned about all drugs taken during the previous 2 to 3 weeks.

Because deep vein thrombosis usually occurs in the leg, the health care provider examines the patient's legs for color and skin temperature. The rate and strength of the pedal pulse are checked, noting any difference between the affected leg and the unaffected leg. Areas of redness or tenderness are noted. The affected leg may appear edematous and exhibit a positive Homans sign (pain in the calf when the foot is dorsiflexed). A positive Homans sign is suggestive of deep vein thrombosis.

During the course of therapy, a patient is continually assessed for any signs of bleeding and hemorrhage. Areas of assessment include the gums, nose, stools, urine, or nasogastric drainage.

The skin temperature and color in a patient with a deep vein thrombosis are monitored for signs of improvement. Vital signs are taken and recorded every 4 hours or more frequently if needed.

Patients receiving warfarin for the first time often require daily adjustment of the dose.

ALERT

Vitamin K

Studies indicate that diet can influence patients' PT. In patients receiving warfarin, a diet high in vitamin K may increase the risk of clot formation. A diet low in vitamin K may increase the risk of hemorrhage. Significant changes in vitamin K intake may necessitate warfarin dosage adjustment. The key to vitamin K management for patients receiving warfarin is maintaining a consistent daily intake of vitamin K. To avoid large fluctuations in vitamin K intake, patients receiving warfarin should be aware of the vitamin K content of food. For example, green leafy vegetables and some vegetable oils (soybean and canola oil) are high in vitamin K. Root vegetables, fruits, cereals, dairy products, and meats are generally low in vitamin K.

Although the drug is most often administered orally, warfarin injection may be used as an alternative route for patients who are unable to receive oral drugs. The intravenous dosage is the same as that for the oral drug.

Educating the Patient and Family About Warfarin

The health care provider gives a full explanation of the drug regimen to patients taking warfarin, including an explanation of the problems that can occur during therapy. A thorough review of the dose regimen, possible adverse drug reactions, and early signs of bleeding tendencies help a patient cooperate with the prescribed therapy. Patient Education Box 18-1 includes key points about warfarin that the patient and family members should know.

Herbal Remedies: Warfarin Interaction

Warfarin has a narrow therapeutic index (the difference between the minimum therapeutic and minimum toxic drug concentrations is small), making any interactions very important. Warfarin interacts with many herbal remedies. For example, warfarin should not be combined with any of the following herbs because they may have additive or synergistic activity and increase the risk for bleeding: celery, chamomile, clove, dong quai, feverfew, garlic, ginger, ginkgo biloba, ginseng, green tea, onion, passion flower, red clover, St. John's wort, and tumeric. Any herbal remedy should be used with caution in patients taking warfarin.

Much of the available information about drug–herb interactions is speculative. Herb–drug interactions are

Key Points for Patients Taking Warfarin

❑ Follow the dosage schedule prescribed by your health care provider.

❑ You will have periodic blood tests to monitor your condition. Keep all health care provider and laboratory appointments because dosage changes may be necessary during therapy.

❑ Do not take or stop taking other drugs except on the advice of your health care provider. This includes nonprescription drugs as well as those prescribed by your health care provider or dentist.

❑ Inform your dentist and other health care providers of your therapy with this drug before any treatment or procedure is started or drugs are prescribed.

❑ Take the drug at the same time each day.

❑ Do not change brands of anticoagulants without consulting a physician or pharmacist.

❑ Do not drink alcohol unless it is approved by your health care provider. You should limit intake of foods high in vitamin K, such as leafy green vegetables, beans, broccoli, cabbage, cauliflower, cheese, fish, and yogurt.

❑ If you see evidence of bleeding, such as unusual bleeding or bruising, bleeding gums, blood in the urine or stool, black stool, or diarrhea, then omit the next dose of the drug and contact your health care provider immediately. (Anisindione may cause a red–orange discoloration of alkaline urine.)

❑ Use a soft toothbrush and consult a dentist regarding routine oral hygiene, including the use of dental floss. Use an electric razor when possible to avoid small skin cuts.

❑ If you are a woman of childbearing age, use a reliable contraceptive to prevent pregnancy.

❑ Wear or carry identification, such as a medical alert tag, to inform medical personnel and others of your therapy with this drug.

sporadically reported and difficult to determine. Because herbal supplements are not regulated by the Food and Drug Administration (FDA), many products lack standardization, purity, and potency. In addition, multiple ingredients in products and batch-to-batch variation make it difficult to determine if reactions occur as the result of the herb. To assist with the identification of herb–drug interactions, health care providers should report any potential interactions to the FDA through its MedWatch program (Appendix D). Because the absorption, metabolism, distribution, and elimination characteristics of most herbal products are poorly understood, many herb–drug interactions are speculative. It is especially important to take special care when patients are taking any drugs with a narrow therapeutic index and herbal supplements.

Fractionated and Unfractionated Heparin

Heparin preparations to prevent clot formation are available as heparin sodium and the low-molecular-weight heparins (fractionated heparins). Heparin is not a single drug, but rather a mixture of high- and low-molecular-weight drugs. Drugs with low molecular weights are available as low-molecular-weight heparin (LMWH). Examples of LMWHs are dalteparin (Fragmin), enoxaparin (Lovenox), and tinzaparin (Innohep). LMWHs produce very stable responses when administered at the recommended doses. Because of this stability, frequent laboratory monitoring is not necessary. In addition, bleeding is less likely to occur with LMWHs than with heparin sodium.

Actions of Heparin

Heparin inhibits the formation of fibrin clots, inhibits the conversion of fibrinogen to fibrin, and inactivates several of the factors necessary for the clotting of blood. Heparin cannot be taken orally because it is inactivated by gastric acid in the stomach; therefore, it must be given by injection. Heparin has no effect on clots that have already formed and aids only in preventing the formation of new blood clots (thrombi). The LMWHs act to inhibit clotting reactions by binding to antithrombin III, which inhibits the synthesis of factor Xa and the formation of thrombin.

Uses of Heparin

Heparin is used for:

- prevention and treatment of venous thrombosis, pulmonary embolism, and peripheral arterial embolism
- atrial fibrillation with embolus formation
- prevention of postoperative venous thrombosis and pulmonary embolism in certain patients undergoing surgical procedures, such as major abdominal surgery
- prevention of clotting in arterial and heart surgery, in blood transfusions and dialysis procedures, and in blood samples for laboratory purposes
- prevention of a repeat cerebral thrombosis in some patients who have experienced a stroke
- treatment of coronary occlusion, acute myocardial infarction, and peripheral arterial embolism
- prevention of clotting in equipment used for extracorporeal (outside the body) blood circulation
- treatment of disseminated intravascular coagulation, a severe hemorrhagic disorder
- maintenance of patency of IV catheters (very low doses of 10 to 100 units [U])

The LMWHs are used to prevent deep vein thrombosis after certain surgical procedures, such as hip or knee replacement surgery or abdominal surgery. These drugs are also used for ischemic complications of unstable angina and myocardial infarction (for specific uses of each drug, see the Summary Drug Table: Anticoagulants).

Adverse Reactions of Heparin

Hemorrhage is the chief complication of heparin administration. Hemorrhage can range from minor local bruising to major hemorrhaging from any organ. Thrombocytopenia (low levels of platelets in the blood) may occur, causing bleeding from the small capillaries and resulting in easy bruising, petechiae, and hemorrhage into the tissues.

Other adverse reactions include local irritation when heparin is given by SC injection. Hypersensitivity reactions may also occur with any route of administration and include fever, chills, and urticaria. More serious hypersensitivity reactions include an asthma-like reaction and an anaphylactoid reaction.

The LMWHs cause fewer adverse reactions than heparin. Bleeding related to the LMWHs is possible but has generally been low. See the Summary Drug Table: Anticoagulants for additional adverse reactions associated with the LMWHs.

Managing Adverse Reactions of Heparin

Bleeding at virtually any site can occur during therapy with any heparin preparation, even the LMWHs. A patient's vital signs are monitored every 2 to 4 hours or as ordered by the health care provider.

ALERT

Heparin and Patient Bleeding

In any patient receiving heparin, evidence of bleeding should be immediately reported: bleeding gums, epistaxis (nosebleed), easy bruising, black tarry stools, hematuria (blood in the urine), oozing from wounds or IV sites, or a decrease in blood pressure.

GERONTOLOGIC ALERT

Heparin and Patient Bleeding

Bleeding is more common in individuals older than 60 years (particularly older women) when heparin is administered. Older patients should be carefully monitored for evidence of bleeding.

Heparin Overdosage

If a patient has a significant decrease in blood pressure or increase in pulse rate, then the health care provider should be notified because this may indicate internal bleeding. Because hemorrhage may begin as a slight bleeding or bruising tendency, the patient is frequently observed for these. At times, hemorrhage can occur without warning. If bleeding should occur, then the health care provider may decrease the dose, discontinue the heparin therapy for a time, or order the administration of protamine sulfate.

In most instances, discontinuation of the drug is sufficient and corrects the overdosage because the duration of action of heparin is short. However, if hemorrhaging is severe, then the health care provider may order protamine sulfate, the specific heparin antagonist, or antidote. Protamine sulfate is also used to treat overdosage of the LMWHs. Protamine sulfate has an immediate onset of action and a duration of 2 hours. It counteracts the effects of heparin. The drug is given slowly via the IV route during a period of 10 minutes.

ALERT

Protamine Sulfate

Protamine sulfate can result in severe hypotension and anaphylactic reaction. Resuscitation equipment must be readily available.

If administration of protamine sulfate is necessary, then the patient's blood pressure and pulse rate are monitored every 15 to 30 minutes for 2 hours or more. The health care provider should be immediately notified of any sudden decrease in blood pressure or increase in pulse rate. The patient is observed for new evidence of bleeding until blood coagulation tests are within normal limits. To replace blood loss, the health care provider may order blood transfusions or fresh-frozen plasma.

Contraindications, Precautions, and Interactions of Heparin

Heparin preparations are contraindicated in patients with a known hypersensitivity, active bleeding (except when caused by disseminated intravascular coagulation), hemorrhagic disorders, severe thrombocytopenia, or recent surgery (except for the LMWHs used after certain surgical procedures to prevent thromboembolic complications), and during pregnancy (pregnancy category C).

The LMWHs are contraindicated in patients with a hypersensitivity to the drug, to heparin, or to pork products, and in inpatients with active bleeding or thrombocytopenia.

Treatment with heparin preparations is approached cautiously in the elderly; in patients with severe renal or kidney disease, diabetes, diabetic retinopathy, ulcer disease, or uncontrolled hypertension; and in all patients with a potential site for bleeding or hemorrhage. The LMWHs are used with caution in patients who are at increased risk for hemorrhage, such as those with severe uncontrolled hypertension, diabetic retinopathy, bacterial endocarditis, congenital or acquired bleeding disorders, gastrointestinal disease, or hemorrhagic stroke, and in patients soon after brain, spinal, or ophthalmologic surgery.

When heparin is administered with an NSAID, aspirin, penicillin, or cephalosporin, there may be an increase in clotting times, thereby increasing the risk for bleeding. During heparin administration, serum transaminase (aspartate, alanine) levels may be falsely elevated; careful interpretation is required because these laboratory tests may be used to help diagnose certain disorders, such as liver disease or myocardial infarction. Protamine sulfate, a heparin antagonist, is incompatible with certain antibiotics such as penicillin and the cephalosporins. Use of the LMWHs with any of these drugs may increase the risk of bleeding: aspirin, salicylates, NSAIDs, and thrombolytics.

Patient Management Issues with Heparin

The most commonly used test to monitor heparin's effects is activated partial thromboplastin time (APTT). Blood is drawn for laboratory studies before giving the first dose of heparin to obtain baseline data. The dosage of heparin is adjusted according to daily APTT monitoring. Periodic platelet counts, hematocrit, and tests for occult blood in the stool should also be performed throughout the course of heparin therapy.

Patients receiving heparin require close observation and careful monitoring. Vital signs are taken every 2 to 4 hours or more frequently. It is also important that a patient be monitored for any indication of hypersensitivity reaction. Reactions, such as chills, fever, or hives, are reported to the health care provider. When heparin is given to prevent the formation of a thrombus, a patient is observed for signs of thrombus formation every 2 to 4 hours. Because the signs and symptoms of thrombus formation vary and depend on the area or organ involved, the health care provider should evaluate and report any symptom the patient may have or any change in a patient's condition.

Heparin preparations, unlike warfarin, must be given by the parenteral route, preferably SC or IV. The onset of anticoagulation is almost immediate after a single dose. Maximum effects occur within 10 minutes of administration. Clotting time returns to normal within 4 hours unless subsequent doses are given. Heparin may be given by intermittent IV administration, continuous IV infusion, and the SC route. Intramuscular administration is avoided because of the possibility of the development of local irritation, pain, or hematoma (a collection of blood in the tissue).

Educating the Patient and Family About Heparin

Although heparin is given in the hospital, the LMWHs can be administered at home by a home health care provider, the patient, or a family member. The patient or a family member is taught how to administer the drug by the SC route. Prefilled syringes are available, making administration more convenient. The health care provider instructs the patient to apply firm pressure after the injection to prevent hematoma formation. Each time the drug is given, all recent injection sites are inspected for signs of inflammation (redness, swelling, tenderness) and hematoma formation. Patient Education Box 18-2 includes key points about heparin that the patient and family members should know.

Thrombolytic Drugs

Thrombolytics are drugs that dissolve certain types of blood clots and reopen blood vessels after they have been occluded. Examples of thrombolytics include alteplase recombinant (Activase), reteplase recombinant (Retavase), streptokinase (Streptase), tenecteplase (TNKase), and urokinase (Abbokinase). Before these drugs are used,

---

PATIENT EDUCATION BOX 18-2

Key Points for Patients Taking Heparin

- ❑ Report any signs of active bleeding to your health care provider immediately.
- ❑ Regular blood tests are critical for safe monitoring of the drug's effects (except the LMWHs).
- ❑ Avoid any IM injections while receiving anticoagulant therapy.
- ❑ Use a soft toothbrush when cleaning your teeth and use an electric razor for shaving (to avoid nicks and cuts).
- ❑ Do not take any prescription or nonprescription drugs without consulting your health care provider. Drugs containing alcohol, aspirin, or ibuprofen may alter the effects of heparin.
- ❑ Advise your dentist or other health care providers that you are on anticoagulant therapy before any procedure or surgery.
- ❑ Carry appropriate identification with information concerning your drug therapy, or wear a medical alert tag at all times.

their potential benefits must be carefully weighed against the potential dangers of bleeding.

Actions of Thrombolytic Drugs

Although the exact action of different thrombolytic drugs vary slightly, all these drugs break-down fibrin clots by converting plasminogen to plasmin (fibrinolysin). Plasmin is an enzyme that breaks down the fibrin of a blood clot. This reopens blood vessels after their occlusion and thereby prevents tissue necrosis.

Uses of Thrombolytic Drugs

Thrombolytic drugs are used to treat an acute myocardial infarction by lysing (dissolving) a blood clot in a coronary artery. These drugs are also effective in lysing clots causing pulmonary embolism and deep vein thrombosis. Urokinase is also used to treat pulmonary embolism and to clear IV catheter cannulas obstructed by a blood clot. See the Summary Drug Table: Thrombolytics for a more complete listing of the use of these drugs.

Adverse Reactions of Thrombolytic Drugs

Bleeding is the most common adverse reaction seen with the use of thrombolytic drugs. Bleeding may be internal and involve areas such as the gastrointestinal tract, genitourinary tract, or the brain. Bleeding may also be external (superficial) and may occur in areas of broken skin, such as venipuncture sites and recent surgical wounds. Allergic reactions may also occur.

Managing Adverse Reactions of Thrombolytic Drugs

Bleeding is the most common adverse reaction. Throughout therapy with a thrombolytic drug, the patient is monitored for signs of bleeding and hemorrhage (see earlier discussion of warfarin). Internal bleeding may occur in the gastrointestinal tract, genitourinary tract, intracranial sites, or respiratory tract. Symptoms of internal bleeding may include abdominal pain, coffee-ground emesis, black tarry stools, hematuria, joint pain, and spitting or coughing-up of blood. Superficial bleeding may occur at venous or arterial puncture sites or recent surgical incision sites. As fibrin is lysed during therapy, bleeding from recent injection sites may occur. All potential bleeding sites (including catheter insertions sites, arterial and venous puncture sites, cutdown sites, and needle puncture sites) are carefully monitored. For minor bleeding at a puncture site, bleeding can usually be controlled by applying pressure for at least 30 minutes at the site, followed by the application of a pressure dressing. The puncture site is then checked frequently for evidence of further bleeding.

ALERT

Combining Heparin and a Thrombolytic Drug

Heparin may be given along with or after administration of a thrombolytic drug to prevent another thrombus from forming. However, administration of an anticoagulant increases the risk for bleeding. The patient must be monitored closely for internal and external bleeding.

If uncontrolled bleeding is noted or if the bleeding appears to be internal, then the drug is stopped and the health care provider immediately contacted because whole blood, packed red cells, or fresh-frozen plasma may be required. Vital signs are monitored every hour or more frequently for at least 48 hours after the drug is discontinued. The health care provider should be notified if there is a marked change in any of the patient's vital signs. Any signs of an allergic (hypersensitivity) reaction, such as difficulty breathing, wheezing, hives, skin rash, or hypotension, are reported immediately to the health care provider.

Contraindications, Precautions, and Interactions of Thrombolytic Drugs

Thrombolytic drugs are contraindicated in patients with known hypersensitivity, active bleeding, history of stroke, aneurysm, or recent intracranial surgery.

These drugs are used cautiously in patients who have recently undergone major surgery (within 10 days or less), such as coronary artery bypass graft, or experienced stroke, trauma, vaginal or cesarean section delivery, gastrointestinal bleeding, or trauma within the past 10 days; those who have hypertension, diabetic retinopathy, or any condition in which bleeding is a significant possibility; and patients currently receiving oral anticoagulants. All of the thrombolytic drugs discussed in this chapter are classified in pregnancy category C, with the exception of urokinase, which is a pregnancy category B drug.

Administration of a thrombolytic drug along with aspirin, dipyridamole, or an anticoagulant may increase the risk of bleeding.

Patient Management Issues with Thrombolytic Drugs

The patient's history is checked for any conditions that might contraindicate the use of a thrombolytic drug, including any history of bleeding tendencies, heart disease, or allergic reactions to any drugs. In addition, a history of any drugs currently being taken is obtained. Most of these patients are admitted or transferred to an inten-

SUMMARY DRUG TABLE   Thrombolytics

Generic Name	Trade Name*	Uses	Adverse Reactions	Dosage Ranges
alteplase, recombinant *al'-te-plaz*	Activase	Acute myocardial infarction (AMI), acute ischemic stroke, pulmonary embolism (PE)	Bleeding (GU, gingival, retroperitoneal), and epistaxis, ecchymosis	AMI: total dose of 100 mg IV given as 60 mg 1st h, 20 mg 2nd h and 20 mg over 3rd h; for patients < 65 kg, decrease dose to 1.25 mg/kg
reteplase, recombinant *ret'-ah-plaze*	Retavase	AMI	Bleeding (GI, GU, or at injection site), intracranial hemorrhage, anemia	10 plus 10 U double bolus IV over 2 min each with the 2nd bolus given 30 min after the 1st
streptokinase *strep-toe-kye'-nase*	Streptase	AMI, DVT, PE, embolism	Minor bleeding (superficial and surface) and major bleeding (internal and severe)	Lysis of coronary artery thrombosis, 20,000 IU directly into vein; PE, DVT, embolism: 250,000 IU IV over 30 min followed by 100,000 IU for 24–72 h
tenecteplase *teh-nek'-ti-plaze*	TNKase	AMI	Bleeding (GI, GU, or at injection site), intracranial hemorrhage, anemia	Dosage based on weight, not to exceed 50 mg IV
urokinase *yoor-oh'-kye-nase*	Abbokinase	PE, lysis of coronary artery thrombi, IV catheter clearance	Minor bleeding (superficial and surface) and major bleeding (internal and severe)	PE: 4400 IU/kg IV over 10 min, followed by 4400 IU/kg/hr for 12 h; lysis of thrombi: 6000 IU/min IV for 2 h; IV catheter clearance: see packaged instructions

*The term *generic* indicates that drug is available in generic form.

sive care unit because close monitoring is necessary for 48 hours or more after therapy begins.

During drug therapy, the patient must also be continually assessed for an anaphylactic reaction (difficulty breathing, wheezing, fever, swelling around the eyes, hives, or itching), particularly with anistreplase or streptokinase. Resuscitation equipment must be immediately available.

For optimal therapeutic effect, the thrombolytic drugs are used as soon as possible after the formation of a thrombus, preferably within 4 to 6 hours or as soon as possible after the symptoms are identified. The greatest benefit occurs when the drugs are administered within 4 hours, but studies indicate that significant benefit can still occur when the drug is used within the first 24 hours. If the patient is in pain, then the health care provider may order a narcotic analgesic. Once the clot is dissolved and blood flows freely through the obstructed blood vessel, severe pain usually decreases.

Educating the Patient and Family About Thrombolytic Drugs

Patient Education Box 18-3 includes key points about thrombolytic drugs that the patient and family members should know.

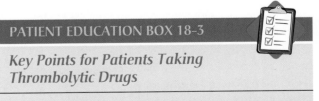

PATIENT EDUCATION BOX 18-3

Key Points for Patients Taking Thrombolytic Drugs

❏ It is normal for the health care team to continuously monitor you before and after administering the drug to watch for any potential adverse effects.
❏ Report any evidence of hypersensitivity reaction (rash, difficulty breathing) or evidence of bleeding or bruising to your health care provider.
❏ Bed rest is important during therapy.

Anemia

Anemia is a decrease in the number of red blood cells (RBCs), a decrease in the amount of hemoglobin in RBCs, or both. Anemia occurs when there is an insufficient amount of hemoglobin to deliver oxygen to the tissues. There are various types and causes of anemia. For example, anemia can result from blood loss, excessive destruction of RBCs, inadequate production of RBCs, or deficits in various nutrients, such as in iron deficiency anemia. Once the type and cause have been identified in a patient, the health care provider selects the appropriate treatment.

The anemias discussed in this chapter include iron deficiency anemia, anemia in patients with chronic renal disease, pernicious anemia, and anemia resulting from a folic acid deficiency. Table 18-1 defines these anemias. Drugs used in treatment of anemia are summarized in the Summary Drug Table: Drugs Used in the Treatment of Anemia.

Drugs for Iron Deficiency Anemia

Iron deficiency anemia is by far the most common type of anemia. Iron is a component of hemoglobin, which is present in RBCs. It is the iron in the hemoglobin of RBCs that takes oxygen from the lungs and carries it to all body tissues. Iron is stored in the body and is found mainly in the reticuloendothelial cells of the liver, spleen, and bone marrow. When the body does not have enough iron to supply the body's needs, the resulting condition is **iron deficiency anemia.**

Actions of Drugs for Iron Deficiency Anemia

Iron preparations act by elevating the serum iron concentration, which replenishes hemoglobin and depleted iron stores.

Uses of Drugs for Iron Deficiency Anemia

Iron salts, such as ferrous sulfate or ferrous gluconate, are used in the treatment of iron deficiency anemia, which occurs when there is a loss of iron that is greater than the available iron stored in the body.

Iron dextran is a parenteral iron that is also used for the treatment of iron deficiency anemia. It is primarily used when the patient cannot take oral drugs or when the patient experiences gastrointestinal intolerance to oral iron administration. Other iron preparations, both oral and parenteral, for iron deficiency anemia can be found in the Summary Drug Table: Drugs Used in the Treatment of Anemia.

Adverse Reactions of Drugs for Iron Deficiency Anemia

Iron salts occasionally cause gastrointestinal irritation, nausea, vomiting, constipation, diarrhea, headache, backache, and allergic reactions. The stools usually appear darker or black. Iron dextran is given by the parenteral route. Hypersensitivity reactions, including fatal anaphylactic reactions, have been reported with the use of this form of iron. Additional adverse reactions include soreness, inflammation, and sterile abscesses at the intramuscular (IM) injection site. Intravenous (IV) administration may result in phlebitis at the injection

TABLE 18-1   **Anemias**

Type of Anemia	Description
Iron deficiency	Anemia characterized by an inadequate amount of iron in the body to produce hemoglobin
Anemia in chronic renal failure (CRF)	Anemia resulting from a reduced production of erythropoietin, a hormone secreted by the kidney that stimulates the production of red blood cells (RBCs)
Pernicious anemia	Anemia resulting from lack of secretions by the gastric mucosa of the intrinsic factor essential to the formation of RBCs and the absorption of vitamin B_{12}
Folic acid deficiency	A slowly progressive type of anemia occurring because of the lack of folic acid, a component necessary in the formation of RBCs

SUMMARY DRUG TABLE   Drugs Used in the Treatment of Anemia

Generic Name	Trade Name*	Uses	Adverse Reactions	Dosage Ranges
darbepoetin alfa *dar-bah-poe-e'-tin*	Aranesp	Anemia associated with chronic renal failure	Hypertension, hypotension, headache, diarrhea, vomiting, nausea, myalgia, infection, cardiac arrhythmias, cardiac arrest	0.45 mcg/kg IV, SC weekly
epoetin alfa (Erythropoietin; (EPO) *e-po-e'-tin*	Epogen, Procrit	Anemia associated with chronic renal failure, anemia related to zidovudine therapy in HIV-infected patients, anemia in cancer patients receiving chemotherapy, anemia in patients who undergo elective nonvascular surgery	Hypertension, headache, tachycardia, nausea, vomiting, skin rashes, fever, skin reaction at injection site	Individualized dosage CRF 50–100 U/kg (3 times weekly IV or SC), maintenance based on HCT, generally 25 U/kg 3 times weekly; zidovudine-treated HIV-infected patients: 100 U/kg 3 times weekly; cancer: 150 U/kg 3 times weekly; surgery: 300 U/kg/d SC × 10 d before surgery, on day of surgery and 4 days after surgery
ferrous fumarate (33% elemental iron) *fair'-us*	Feostat, *generic*	Prevention and treatment of iron deficiency anemia	GI irritation, nausea, vomiting, constipation, diarrhea, allergic reactions	Daily requirements: males, 10 mg/d PO; females, 18 mg/d PO; during pregnancy and lactation, 30–60 mg/d PO; replacement in deficiency states, 90–300 mg/d (6 mg/kg/d) PO for 6–10 mo
ferrous gluconate (11.6% elemental iron)	Fergon, *generic*	Prevention and treatment of iron deficiency anemia	GI irritation, nausea, vomiting, constipation, diarrhea, allergic reactions	Daily requirements: males, 10 mg/d PO; females, 18 mg/d PO; during pregnancy and lactation, 30–60 mg/d PO; replacement in deficiency states, 90–300 mg/d (6 mg/kg/d) PO for 6–10 mo
ferrous sulfate (20% elemental iron)	Feosol, Fer-In-Sol, *generic*	Prevention and treatment of iron deficiency anemia	GI irritation, nausea, vomiting, constipation, diarrhea, allergic reactions	Daily requirements: males, 10 mg/d PO; females, 18 mg/d PO; during pregnancy and lactation, 30–60 mg/d PO; replacement in deficiency states, 90–300 mg/d (6 mg/kg/d) PO for 6–10 mo

Generic Name	Trade Name*	Uses	Adverse Reactions	Dosage Ranges
folic acid *foe'-lik*	Folvite, *generic*	Megaloblastic anemia due to deficiency of folic acid	Allergic sensitization	Up to 1 mg/d PO, IM, IV, SC
iron dextran	DexFerrum, INFeD, *generic*	Iron deficiency anemia	Anaphylactoid reactions, soreness and inflammation at injection site, chest pain, arthralgia, backache, convulsions, pruritus, abdominal pain, nausea, vomiting, dyspnea	Dosage based on body weight and grams percent (g/dL) of hemoglobin IV, IM
iron sucrose	Venofer	Iron deficiency anemia	Hypotension, cramps, leg cramps, nausea, headache, vomiting, diarrhea, dizziness	100 mg elemental iron slow IV or during dialysis session
leucovorin calcium *loo-koe-vor'-in*	Wellcovorin, *generic*	Treatment of megaloblastic anemia; leucovorin rescue after high-dose methotrexate therapy in osteosarcoma	Allergic sensitization, urticaria, anaphylaxis	Megaloblastic anemia: 1 mg/d IM; rescue after methotrexate therapy: 12–15 g/m^2 PO or parenterally then 10 mg/m^2 q6h for 72 h; check serum creatinine after 24 h; if 50% greater than the pretreatment level, increase leucovorin dose to 100 mg/m^2 until serum methotrexate level is <5 × 10^{-8} M
sodium ferric gluconate complex	Ferrlecit	Iron deficiency	Flushing, hypotension, syncope, tachycardia, dizziness, pruritus, dyspnea, conjunctivitis, hyperkalemia	125 mg of elemental iron IV over at least 10 min
vitamin B$_{12}$ (cyanocobalamin) *sye-an-oh-koe- bal'- a-min*	*generic*	B$_{12}$ deficiencies as seen in pernicious anemia, GI pathology; also used when requirements for the vitamin are increased; Schilling's test	Mild diarrhea, itching, edema, anaphylaxis	Schilling test: 100–1000 mcg/d × 2 wk, then 100–1000 mcg IM q mo

*The term *generic* indicates the drug is available in generic form.
GI, gastrointestinal; HIV, human immunodeficiency virus.

site. When iron is administered by IM injection, a brown discoloration of the skin may occur. Patients with rheumatoid arthritis may experience an acute exacerbation of joint pain, and swelling may occur when iron dextran is administered.

Managing Adverse Reactions

Patients receiving iron dextran are monitored closely for a hypersensitivity reaction. Epinephrine is kept on standby in the event of severe anaphylactic reaction.

ALERT

Parenteral Iron

Parenteral iron has resulted in fatal anaphylactic-type reactions. Any of the following adverse reactions are reported to the health care provider: dyspnea, urticaria, rashes, itching, or fever.

Constipation may be a problem with oral iron preparations. The patient is instructed to increase fluid intake to 10 to 12 glasses of water per day (if permitted), to eat a diet high in fiber, and to increase activity. An active lifestyle and regular exercise help to decrease the constipating effects of iron. If constipation persists, then the health care provider may prescribe a stool softener.

A balanced diet with an emphasis on foods that are high in iron (e.g., organ meats, lean red meats, cereals, dried beans, and leafy green vegetables), folic acid (e.g., green leafy vegetables, liver, and yeast), or vitamin B_{12} (e.g., beef, pork, organ meats, eggs, milk, and milk products) is recommended. The amount of food eaten at meals is monitored. If the patient's appetite is poor or if the patient's eating habits are inadequate to maintain normal nutrition, then consultation with the dietitian may be necessary. Small portions of food may be more appealing than large or moderate portions. A pleasant atmosphere and ample time for eating help encourage good eating habits.

Contraindications, Precautions, and Interactions of Drugs for Iron Deficiency Anemia

Drugs used to treat anemia are contraindicated in patients with known hypersensitivity to the drug or any component of the drug. Iron compounds are contraindicated in patients with any anemia except iron deficiency anemia. Iron compounds are used cautiously in patients with tartrazine or sulfite sensitivity because some iron compounds contain these substances. Oral iron preparations are pregnancy category B drugs; iron dextran is a pregnancy category C drug. Iron preparations are used cautiously during pregnancy and lactation. Iron dosages of 15 to 30 mg per day are sufficient to meet the needs of pregnancy. Iron dextran is used cautiously in patients with cardiovascular disease, a history

of asthma or allergies, or rheumatoid arthritis (may exacerbate joint pain).

The absorption of oral iron is decreased when the agent is administered with an antacid, tetracycline, penicillamine, or fluoroquinolone. When iron is administered with levothyroxine, the effectiveness of levothyroxine may be decreased. When administered orally, iron decreases the absorption of levodopa. Ascorbic acid increases the absorption of oral iron. Iron dextran administered concurrently with chloramphenicol increases serum iron levels.

Drugs for Anemia Associated with Chronic Renal Failure

Anemia may occur in patients with chronic renal failure because the kidneys do not produce enough erythropoietin. Erythropoietin is a glycoprotein hormone synthesized mainly in the kidneys and used to stimulate and regulate the production of erythrocytes or red blood cells (RBCs). Failure to produce the needed erythrocytes results in anemia. Two examples of drugs used to treat anemia associated with chronic renal failure are epoetin alfa (Epogen) and darbepoetin alfa (Aranesp).

Actions of Drugs for Anemia Associated with Chronic Renal Failure

Epoetin alfa is a drug that is produced using recombinant DNA technology. Epoetin alfa acts in a manner similar to that of natural erythropoietin. Darbepoetin alfa (Aranesp) is an erythropoiesis-stimulating protein produced in Chinese hamster ovary cells using recombinant DNA technology. Darbepoetin stimulates erythropoiesis by the same manner as natural erythropoietin. These drugs elevate or maintain RBC levels and decrease the need for transfusions.

Uses of Drugs for Anemia Associated with Chronic Renal Failure

Epoetin alfa is used to treat anemia associated with chronic renal failure, anemia in patients with cancer who are receiving chemotherapy, and in patients with anemia who are undergoing elective nonvascular surgery.

Darbepoetin is used to treat anemia associated with chronic renal failure in patients receiving dialysis, as well as other patients.

Adverse Reactions of Drugs for Anemia Associated with Chronic Renal Failure

Epoetin alfa (erythropoietin [EPO]) and darbepoetin alfa are usually well-tolerated. The most common adverse reactions include hypertension, headache, tachycardia, nausea, vomiting, diarrhea, skin rashes, fever, myalgia, and skin reaction at the injection site. See the Summary Drug Table: Drugs Used in the Treatment of Anemia for more information on these drugs.

Contraindications, Precautions, and Interactions of Drugs for Anemia Associated with Chronic Renal Failure

Epoetin alfa is contraindicated in patients with uncontrolled hypertension, those needing an emergency transfusion, or those with a hypersensitivity to human albumin. Darbepoetin alfa (Aranesp) is contraindicated in patients with uncontrolled hypertension or in those allergic to the drug.

Epoetin alfa and darbepoetin alfa are used with caution in patients with hypertension, heart disease, congestive heart failure, or a history of seizures. Both of these drugs are pregnancy category C drugs and are used cautiously during pregnancy and lactation.

Drugs for Folic Acid Deficiency Anemia

Folic acid is required for the manufacture of RBCs in the bone marrow. Folic acid is found in leafy green vegetables, fish, meat, poultry, and whole grains. A deficiency of folic acid results in **megaloblastic anemia**. Megaloblastic anemia is characterized by the presence of large, abnormal, immature erythrocytes circulating in the blood.

Actions of Drugs for Folic Acid Deficiency Anemia

Although not related to anemia, studies indicate there is a decreased risk for neural tube defects if folic acid is taken before conception and during early pregnancy. Neural tube defects occur during early pregnancy, when the embryonic folds forming the spinal cord and brain join together. Defects of this type include anencephaly (congenital absence of brain and spinal cord), spina bifida (defect of the spinal cord), and meningocele (a sac-like protrusion of the meninges in the spinal cord or skull).

Leucovorin "rescues" normal cells from the destruction caused by methotrexate and allows them to survive. This technique of administering leucovorin after a large dose of methotrexate is called **folinic acid rescue** or **leucovorin rescue**.

Uses of Drugs for Folic Acid Deficiency Anemia

Folic acid is used in the treatment of megaloblastic anemias that are caused by a deficiency of folic acid. The United States Public Health Service recommends the use of folic acid for all women of childbearing age to decrease the incidence of neural tube defects. Dosages during pregnancy and lactation are as great as 0.8 mg per day.

Leucovorin is a derivative (and active reduced form) of folic acid. The oral and parenteral forms of this drug are used in the treatment of megaloblastic anemia. Leucovorin may also be used to diminish the hematologic effects of (intentional) massive doses of methotrexate, a drug used in the treatment of certain types of cancer (see Chapter 28). Occasionally, high doses of methotrexate are administered to select patients. Leucovorin is then used either at the same time or after the methotrexate has been given to decrease the toxic effects of the methotrexate.

Adverse Reactions of Drugs for Folic Acid Deficiency Anemia

Few adverse reactions are associated with the administration of folic acid and leucovorin. Rarely, parenteral administration may result in allergic hypersensitivity.

Contraindications, Precautions, and Interactions of Drugs for Folic Acid Deficiency Anemia

Folic acid and leucovorin are contraindicated for the treatment of pernicious anemia or for other anemias for which vitamin B_{12} is deficient. Folic acid is a pregnancy category A drug and is generally considered safe for use during pregnancy. Pregnant women are more likely to experience folate acid deficiency because folic acid requirements are increased during pregnancy. Pregnant women with a folate deficiency are at increased risk for complications of pregnancy and fetal abnormalities. The recommended daily allowance (RDA) of folate during pregnancy is 0.4 mg per day, and during lactation the RDA of folate is 0.26 to 0.28 mg per day. Although the risk of fetal harm appears small, the drug should be used cautiously and only within the RDAs.

Use of aminosalicylic with folic acid may decrease serum folate levels. Folic acid utilization is decreased when folate is administered with methotrexate. Signs of folic acid deficiency may occur when sulfasalazine is administered concurrently. An increase in seizure activity may occur when folic acid is administered with a hydantoin.

Leucovorin is a pregnancy category C drug and is used cautiously during pregnancy.

Leucovorin decreases the effectiveness of anticonvulsants. The patient has an increased risk of 5-fluorouracil toxicity when that drug is administered with leucovorin.

Drugs for Pernicious Anemia

Vitamin B_{12} is essential for growth, cell reproduction, the manufacture of myelin (which surrounds some nerve fibers), and blood cell manufacture. The substance called **intrinsic factor**, which is produced by cells in the stomach, is necessary for the absorption of vitamin B_{12} in the intestine. A deficiency of intrinsic factor results in abnormal formation of erythrocytes because of the body's failure to absorb vitamin B_{12}, a necessary component for blood cell formation. The resulting anemia is a type of megaloblastic anemia called **pernicious anemia**.

Actions of Drugs for Pernicious Anemia

Vitamin B_{12} (cyanocobalamin) acts by replenishing the diminished level of vitamin B_{12} in the body.

Uses of Drugs for Pernicious Anemia

Vitamin B_{12} (cyanocobalamin) is used to treat a vitamin B_{12} deficiency. A vitamin B_{12} deficiency may be seen in:

- strict vegetarians
- people who have had a total gastrectomy or subtotal gastric resection (when the cells producing intrinsic factor are totally or partially removed)
- people who have intestinal diseases, such as ulcerative colitis or sprue
- people who have gastric carcinoma
- people who have a congenital decrease in the number of gastric cells secreting intrinsic factor

Vitamin B_{12} is also used to perform the Schilling test, which is used to diagnose pernicious anemia.

ALERT

Pernicious Anemia

Pernicious anemia must be diagnosed and treated as soon as possible because a vitamin B_{12} deficiency that is allowed to progress for more than 3 months may result in degenerative lesions of the spinal cord.

Vitamin B_{12} deficiency caused by a low dietary intake of vitamin B_{12} is rare because the vitamin is found in meats, milk, eggs, and cheese. Because the body can store this vitamin, a deficiency from any cause will not occur for 5 to 6 years.

Adverse Reactions of Drugs for Pernicious Anemia

Mild diarrhea and itching have been reported with the administration of vitamin B_{12}. Other adverse reactions include a marked increase in RBC production, acne, peripheral vascular thrombosis, congestive heart failure, and pulmonary edema.

Contraindications, Precautions, and Interactions of Drugs for Pernicious Anemia

Vitamin B_{12} is contraindicated in patients allergic to cobalt. Vitamin B_{12} is a pregnancy category A drug if administered orally and a pregnancy category C drug if

given parenterally. Vitamin B_{12} is administered cautiously during pregnancy and in patients with pulmonary disease and anemia. Alcohol, aminosalicylic acid, neomycin, and colchicine may decrease the absorption of oral vitamin B_{12}.

Patient Management Issues with Antianemia Drugs

Laboratory tests are often used to determine the type, severity, and possible cause of anemia. Sometimes it is easy to identify the cause of the anemia, but in some instances the cause of the anemia is obscure.

Vital signs are taken to provide a baseline during therapy. Patients may be evaluated for their ability to perform the activities of daily living. General symptoms of anemia include fatigue, shortness of breath, sore tongue, headache, and pallor.

If iron dextran is to be given, then an allergy history is necessary because this drug is given only with caution to those with significant allergies or asthma. The patient's weight and hemoglobin level are required for calculating the dosage.

During drug therapy, patients may be monitored, especially those who are moderately to acutely ill and those taking epoetin alfa (because of the increased risk of hypertension). The patient is monitored for adverse reactions, and any adverse reactions are reported to the health care provider before taking the next dose. Severe adverse reactions are reported immediately.

A patient on iron salt therapy should be told that the color of the stool will become darker or black. If diarrhea or constipation occurs, then the health care provider must be notified.

Patients being given iron dextran should be told that they might feel soreness at the injection site. Injection sites are checked daily for signs of inflammation, swelling, or abscess formation.

All patients are monitored for relief of the symptoms of anemia (fatigue, shortness of breath, sore tongue, headache, pallor). Some patients may note a relief of symptoms after a few days of therapy. Periodic laboratory tests are necessary to monitor the results of therapy.

Educating the Patient and Family About Antianemia Drugs

Patient Education Box 18-4 includes key points about antianemia drugs that the patient and family members should know.

PATIENT EDUCATION BOX 18–4

Key Points for Patients Taking Antianemia Drugs

IRON SALT

❑ Take this drug with water on an empty stomach. If you experience gastrointestinal upset, then take the drug with food or meals.

❑ Do not take antacids, tetracyclines, penicillamine, or fluoroquinolones at the same time or 2 hours before or after taking iron without first checking with your health care provider.

❑ This drug may cause a darkening of your stools, constipation, or diarrhea. If constipation or diarrhea becomes severe, then contact your health care provider.

❑ Mix the liquid iron preparation with water or juice and drink it through a straw to prevent staining of your teeth.

❑ Do not indiscriminately use advertised iron products. If you have a true iron deficiency, then its cause must be determined and your therapy should be guided by a health care provider.

❑ Have periodic blood tests during therapy to determine how you are responding to treatment.

❑ Patients with rheumatoid arthritis may experience an acute exacerbation of joint pain and swelling may occur with iron dextran therapy.

EPOETIN ALFA

❑ Strict compliance with antihypertensive drug regimen is important if you are being treated for known hypertension during epoetin therapy.

❑ Report to your health care provider any numbness, tingling of extremities, severe headache, dyspnea, or chest pain, dizziness, fatigue, joint pain, nausea, vomiting, or diarrhea. Joint pain may occur but can be controlled with analgesics.

❑ Keep all your appointments for blood testing, which is necessary to determine the effects of the drug on the blood count and to determine the correct dosage.

FOLIC ACID

❑ Avoid the use of multivitamin preparations unless they are approved by your health care provider.

❑ Follow the diet recommended by your health care provider, because both diet and the drug are necessary to correct a folic acid deficiency.

LEUCOVORIN

❑ Megaloblastic anemia: Adhere to the diet prescribed by your health care provider. If the purchase of foods high in protein (which can be expensive) becomes a problem, then discuss this with your health care provider.

❑ Folinic acid rescue: Take this drug at the exact prescribed intervals. If nausea and vomiting occur, then contact your health care provider immediately.

VITAMIN B$_{12}$

❑ Nutritional deficiency of vitamin B$_{12}$: Eat a balanced diet that includes seafood, eggs, meats, and dairy products.

❑ Pernicious anemia: Lifetime therapy is necessary. Eat a balanced diet that includes seafood, eggs, meats, and dairy products. Try to avoid contact with people who have infections, and report any signs of infection to your health care provider immediately because an increase in dosage may be necessary.

❑ Adhere to the treatment regimen and keep all appointments with your health care provider. The drug is given at periodic intervals (usually monthly for life). In some instances, parenteral self-administration or parenteral administration by a family member is allowed (instruction in administration is necessary).

KEY POINTS

◉ Anticoagulants include warfarin (a coumarin derivative), anisindione (an indandione derivative), and fractionated and unfractionated heparin.

◉ Warfarin (Coumadin) is the oral anticoagulant most commonly prescribed. The principal adverse reaction of warfarin is bleeding, which may range from very mild to severe. Warfarin is contraindicated in patients with known hypersensitivity to the drug, hemorrhagic disease, tuberculosis, leukemia, uncontrolled hypertension, gastrointestinal ulcers, recent surgery of the eye or central nervous system, aneurysms, or severe renal or hepatic disease, and during pregnancy and lactation. Use during pregnancy (pregnancy category X) can cause fetal death.

◉ Heparin inhibits the formation of fibrin clots, inhibits the conversion of fibrinogen to fibrin, and inactivates several of the factors necessary for the clotting of blood. Hemorrhage is the chief complication of heparin administration. Heparin preparations are contraindicated in patients with known hypersensitivity to the drug, active bleeding (except when caused by disseminated intravascular coagulation), hemorrhagic disorders, severe thrombocytopenia, or recent surgery (except for the LMWHs used after certain surgical procedures to prevent thromboembolic complications) and during pregnancy (pregnancy category C).

◉ Thrombolytics are a group of drugs used to dissolve certain types of blood clots and reopen blood vessels after they have been occluded. Bleeding is the most common adverse reaction seen with the use of these drugs. Bleeding may be internal and involve areas such as the gastrointestinal tract, genitourinary tract, and the brain. Thrombolytic drugs are contraindicated in patients with known hypersensitivity, active bleeding, history of stroke, aneurysm, or recent intracranial surgery.

⬤ Iron deficiency anemia is by far the most common type of anemia. Iron salts, such as ferrous sulfate or ferrous gluconate, are used in the treatment of iron deficiency anemia, which occurs when there is a loss of iron that is greater than the available iron stored in the body. Iron salts occasionally cause gastrointestinal irritation, nausea, vomiting, constipation, diarrhea, headache, backache, and allergic reactions. Drugs used to treat anemia are contraindicated in patients with known hypersensitivity to the drug or any component of the drug. Iron compounds are contraindicated in patients with any anemia except iron deficiency anemia.

⬤ Anemia may occur in patients with chronic renal failure as the result of the inability of the kidney to produce erythropoietin. Epoetin alfa is used to treat anemia associated with chronic renal failure, anemia in patients with cancer who are receiving chemotherapy, and in patients with anemia who are undergoing elective nonvascular surgery. Darbepoetin is used to treat anemia associated with chronic renal failure in patients receiving dialysis and other patients. The most common adverse reactions include hypertension, headache, tachycardia, nausea, vomiting, diarrhea, skin rashes, fever, myalgia, and skin reaction at the injection site.

⬤ Folic acid is required for the manufacture of RBCs in the bone marrow. Folic acid is used in the treatment of megaloblastic anemias that are caused by a deficiency of folic acid. Folic acid and leucovorin are contraindicated for the treatment of pernicious anemia or for other anemias for which vitamin B_{12} is deficient.

⬤ A deficiency of the intrinsic factor results in abnormal formation of erythrocytes because of the body's failure to absorb vitamin B_{12}, a necessary component for blood cell formation. The resulting anemia is pernicious anemia. There is a decreased risk for neural tube defects if folic acid is taken before conception and during early pregnancy. Folic acid and leucovorin are contraindicated for the treatment of pernicious anemia or for other anemias for which vitamin B_{12} is deficient.

CASE STUDY

Mr. Harris, age 72 years, is a widower who has lived alone since his wife died 5 years ago. He has been prescribed warfarin to take at home after his dismissal from the hospital. Mr. Harris has questions about caring for himself to prevent any complications with his treatment.

1. Mr. Harris wonders about potential adverse effects. You tell him:
   a. side effects are minimal but may include diarrhea
   b. bleeding is the only adverse reaction
   c. bleeding is the principal adverse reaction, and although other adverse reactions are rare, nausea, vomiting, and alopecia may occur
   d. none of the above

2. Mr. Harris wonders aloud whether the loop diuretic he is taking will impact his use of warfarin. You tell him:
   a. that the diuretic may increase the effects of warfarin
   b. that the diuretic may decrease the effects of warfarin
   c. that the diuretic will have no impact on the effectiveness of the warfarin
   d. that there would be cause for concern only if he were combining a diuretic, warfarin, and passion flower

3. Mr. Harris asks if he needs to modify his diet in any way because of warfarin use. He should be told:
   a. do not drink alcohol unless his health care provider approves it
   b. do not drink alcohol or eat lots of foods high in vitamin K
   c. do not take vitamin supplements containing vitamin B_{12}, which can impact the absorption of warfarin
   d. there are no known dietary restrictions

WEBSITE ACTIVITIES

1. Go to the University of Pennsylvania's health website (http://pennhealth.com/hi.html) and click on the link "Encyclopedia." Search the "Diseases and Conditions" subsection

for the article on pernicious anemia. Read the treatment section. In addition to vitamin B_{12}, what else is necessary for healthy blood cell development?

2. At the same website, return to the Encyclopedia section and click on "Nutrition." Search for the article on vitamin B_{12}. What are two other reasons, in addition to helping form red blood cells, why vitamin B_{12} is important in the body?

REVIEW QUESTIONS

1. The patient receiving heparin has an increased risk for bleeding when also taking:
   a. allopurinol
   b. an NSAID
   c. digoxin
   d. furosemide

2. In which of the following situations would a LMWH to be prescribed?
   a. to prevent deep vein thrombosis
   b. to treat disseminated intravascular coagulation
   c. to prevent hemorrhage
   d. to treat atrial fibrillation

3. If uncontrolled bleeding occurs while a patient is receiving a thrombolytic drug, then the patient may receive:
   a. heparin
   b. whole blood or fresh-frozen plasma
   c. a diuretic
   d. protamine sulfate

4. Which is the most common type of anemia?
   a. iron deficiency anemia
   b. folic acid anemia
   c. pernicious anemia
   d. megaloblastic anemia

5. Which of the following substances would decrease the absorption of oral iron?
   a. antacids
   b. levothryoxine
   c. ascorbic acid
   d. vitamin B_{12}

19 | Diuretics

Carbonic Anhydrase Inhibitors
Actions of Carbonic Anhydrase Inhibitors
Uses of Carbonic Anhydrase Inhibitors
Adverse Reactions of Carbonic Anhydrase Inhibitors
Contraindications, Precautions, and Interactions of Carbonic Anhydrase Inhibitors

Loop Diuretics
Actions of Loop Diuretics
Uses of Loop Diuretics
Adverse Reactions of Loop Diuretics
Contraindications, Precautions, and Interactions of Loop Diuretics

Osmotic Diuretics
Actions of Osmotic Diuretics
Uses of Osmotic Diuretics
Adverse Reactions of Osmotic Diuretics
Contraindications, Precautions, and Interactions of Osmotic Diuretics

Potassium-Sparing Diuretics
Actions of Potassium-Sparing Diuretics
Uses of Potassium-Sparing Diuretics
Adverse Reactions of Potassium-Sparing Diuretics
Contraindications, Precautions, and Interactions of Potassium-Sparing Diuretics

Thiazides and Related Diuretics
Actions of Thiazides and Related Diuretics
Uses of Thiazides and Related Diuretics
Adverse Reactions of Thiazides and Related Diuretics
Contraindications, Precautions, and Interactions of Thiazides and Related Diuretics

Patient Management Issues with Diuretics
Carbonic Anhydrase Inhibitors
Osmotic Diuretics
Potassium-Sparing Diuretics
Thiazide and Related Diuretics
Patients with Edema
Patients with Hypertension

Managing Adverse Reactions of Diuretics
Electrolyte Imbalance
Cardiac Arrhythmias and Dizziness

Herbal Remedies: Diuretics

Educating the Patient and Family About Diuretics

Key Points

Case Study

Website Activities

Review Questions

KEY TERMS

dehydration—loss of too much water from the body

diuretic—a drug that increases the secretion of urine (water, electrolytes, and waste products) by the kidneys

edema—retention of excess fluid

filtrate—fluid removed from the blood through kidney function

glaucoma—an increase in intraocular pressure (pressure within the eye)

hyperkalemia—high blood level of potassium

hypokalemia—low blood level of potassium

nephron—long tubular structure that is the functional part of the kidney

orthostatic hypotension—dizziness and light-headedness after standing in one place for a long time

postural hypotension—dizziness and light-headedness when rising suddenly from a sitting or lying position

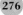

CHAPTER OBJECTIVES

On completion of this chapter, students will be able to:

1 Define the chapter's key terms.

2 Define the general drug actions, uses, adverse reactions, contraindications, precautions, and interactions of diuretics.

3 Discuss important points to keep in mind when educating the patient or family members about the use of diuretics.

A diuretic is a drug that increases the secretion of urine (i.e., water, electrolytes, and waste products) by the kidneys. Many conditions or diseases, such as heart failure, endocrine disturbances, and kidney and liver diseases, can cause retention of excess fluid (**edema**). When a patient shows signs of edema, the health care provider may order a diuretic, selecting one that best suits a patient's needs and effectively reduces the amount of excess fluid in body tissues.

The different types of diuretic drugs are:

- carbonic anhydrase inhibitors
- loop diuretics
- osmotic diuretics
- potassium-sparing diuretics
- thiazides and related diuretics

The Summary Drug Table: Diuretics lists examples of the different types of diuretic drugs. Most diuretics act on the tubules of the kidney **nephron** (Figure 19-1), the functional unit of the kidney. Each kidney contains approximately one million nephrons, which filter the bloodstream to remove waste products. During this process, water and electrolytes are also selectively removed. The **filtrate** (the fluid removed from the blood) normally contains ions (potassium, sodium, chloride), waste products (ammonia, urea), water, and, at times, other substances that are being excreted, such as drugs. The filtrate then passes through the proximal tubule, the loop of Henle, and the distal tubules. At these points, selective reabsorption of amino acids, glucose, some electrolytes, and water occurs. Ions and water that are required by the body to maintain fluid and electrolyte balance are returned to the bloodstream by means of the minute capillaries that surround the distal and proximal tubules and the loop of Henle. Ions and water that are not needed are excreted in the urine.

Diuretics are used for a variety of medical disorders. The health care provider selects the type of diuretic that will most likely be effective for treatment of a specific disorder. In some instances, hypertension may be treated with the administration of an antihypertensive drug and a diuretic. The diuretics used for this combination therapy include the loop diuretics and the thiazides and related diuretics.

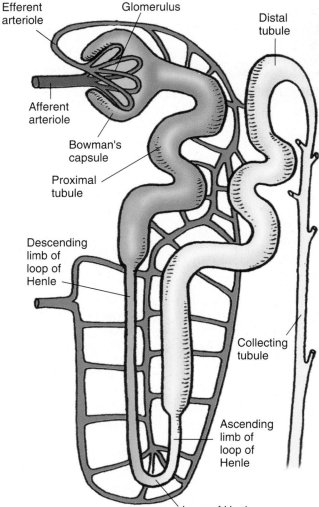

FIGURE 19-1   The nephron is the functional unit of the kidney. Note the various tubules, the site of most diuretic activity. The loop of Henle is the site of action for the loop diuretics. Thiazide diuretics act at the ascending portion of the loop of Henle and the distal tube of the nephron. (From Roach SS. *Introductory Clinical Pharmacology*, 7th ed. Baltimore: Lippincott Williams & Wilkins; 2004.)

Carbonic Anhydrase Inhibitors

Actions of Carbonic Anhydrase Inhibitors

Carbonic anhydrase is an enzyme that produces free hydrogen ions, which are then exchanged for sodium ions in the kidney tubules. Carbonic anhydrase inhibitors inhibit the action of the enzyme carbonic anhydrase. This effect results in the excretion of sodium, potassium, bicarbonate, and water. Carbonic anhydrase inhibitors also decrease the production of aqueous humor in the eye, which in turn decreases intraocular pressure (the pressure within the eye).

SUMMARY DRUG TABLE   Diuretics

Generic Name	Trade Name*	Uses	Adverse Reactions	Dosage Ranges
Carbonic Anhydrase Inhibitors				
acetazolamide *a-set-a-zole'-a-mide*	Diamox, *generic*	Open-angle glaucoma, secondary glaucoma, preoperatively to lower intraocular pressure (IOP), edema due to CHF, drug-induced edema, centrencephalic epilepsy	Fever, rash, paresthesias, photosensitivity, crystalluria, acidosis, urticaria, pruritus, hematuria, weakness, malaise, anorexia, hematologic changes, convulsions	Glaucoma: up to 1 g/d PO in divided doses; acute glaucoma: 500 mg initially then 125–250 mg PO q4h; epilepsy: 8–30 mg kg/d in divided doses; CHF and edema: 250–375 mg/d PO
methazolamide *meth-a-zoe'-la-mide*	Neptazane	Glaucoma	Same as acetazolamide	50–100 mg PO BID, TID
Loop Diuretics				
bumetanide *byoo-met'-a-nide*	Bumex, *generic*	Edema due to CHF, cirrhosis of the liver, renal disease, acute pulmonary edema (IV)	Electrolyte imbalances, anorexia, nausea, vomiting, dizziness, rash, photosensitivity reactions, postural or orthostatic hypotension, glycosuria	0.5–10 mg/d PO, IV, IM
ethacrynic acid *eth-a-krin-ik*	Edecrin, Edecrin Sodium	Same as bumetanide plus ascites due to malignancy, idiopathic edema, lymphedema	Electrolyte imbalances, anorexia, nausea, vomiting, fever, chills, anxiety, confusion, hematologic changes	50–200 mg/d PO; 0.5–1 mg/kg IV
furosemide *fur-oh'-se-mide*	Lasix, *generic*	Same as bumetanide plus hypertension (PO)	Same as bumetanide	Edema: up to 600 mg/d PO in single or divided doses, 20–40 mg IM, IV; hypertension: up to 40 mg PO BID; acute pulmonary edema: 40–80 mg IV
torsemide *tor'-se-myde*	Demadex	Same as bumetanide	Headache, dizziness, diarrhea, electrolyte imbalances, ECG abnormalities, nausea, anorexia, drowsiness	CHF: 10–20 mg/d PO, IV; renal failure: 20 mg/d PO, IV; cirrhosis, hypertension: 5–10 mg/d PO, IV
Osmotic Diuretics				
glycerin (glycerol) *gli-ser-in*	Osmoglyn	Glaucoma, before and after surgery	Fluid and electrolyte imbalance	1–2 g/kg PO
isosorbide *eye-soe-sor'-bide*	Ismotic	Same as glycerin	Same as glycerin	1–3 mg/kg BID-QID PRN PO
mannitol *man'-i-tole*	Osmitrol, *generic*	To promote diuresis in acute renal failure, reduction of IOP, treatment of cerebral edema	Edema, fluid and electrolyte imbalance, headache, blurred vision, nausea, vomiting, diarrhea, urinary retention	50–200 g/24 h IV; IOP: 1.5–2 g/kg IV

Generic Name	Trade Name*	Uses	Adverse Reactions	Dosage Ranges
urea *your-ee'-a*	Ureaphil	Reduction of IOP, reduction of intracranial pressure	Headache, nausea, vomiting, fluid and electrolyte imbalance, syncope	Up to 120 g/d IV
Potassium-Sparing Diuretics				
amiloride hydrochloride *a-mill'-oh-ride*	Midamor	CHF, hypertension, hypokalemia from other diuretics, prevention of hypokalemia in at-risk patients	Headache, nausea, anorexia, diarrhea, vomiting, weakness, hyperkalemia, dizziness, rash, hypotension	5–20 mg/d PO
spironolactone *speer-on-oh-lak'-tone*	Aldactone, *generic*	Hypertension, edema due to CHF, cirrhosis, renal disease; hypokalemia, prophylaxis of hypokalemia in those taking digitalis, hyperaldosteronism	Cramping, diarrhea, drowsiness, lethargy, rash, drug fever, hyperkalemia, gastritis, headache, inability to achieve an erection, gynecomastia	Up to 400 mg/d PO in single dose or divided doses
triamterene *trye-am'-ter-een*	Dyrenium	Prevention of hypokalemia, edema due to CHF, cirrhosis, renal disease	Diarrhea, nausea, vomiting, hyperkalemia, photosensitivity reactions, azotemia, thrombocytopenia	Up to 300 mg/d PO in divided doses
Thiazides and Related Diuretics				
bendroflume-thiazide *ben-droe-floo-me-thye'-a-zide*	Naturetin	Edema associated with CHF, hypertension	Hypotension, dizziness, vertigo, light-headedness, anorexia, gastric distress, nausea, hematologic changes, photosensitivity reactions, weakness, hyperglycemia, fluid and electrolyte imbalances, diarrhea, constipation, rash	Edema: 5–20 mg/d; hypertension: 5–20 mg/d PO
benzthiazide *benz-thye'-a-zide*	Exna	Edema associated with CHF, hypertension	Same as bendroflume-thiazide	5–200 mg/d PO
chlorothiazide *klor-oh-thye'-a-zide*	Diuril, *generic*	Hypertension, edema due to CHF, cirrhosis, corticosteroid and estrogen therapy	Same as bendroflume-thiazide	Hypertension: up to 2 g/d PO in divided doses; edema: 0.5–2 g PO, IV QID or BID
chlorthalidone *klor-thal'-I-done*	Hygroton, *generic*	Same as chlorothiazide	Same as chlorothiazide	Hypertension: 25–100 mg/d PO; edema: 50–200 mg/d PO
hydrochloroth-iazide *hye-droe-klor-oh-thye'-a-zide*	HydroDIURIL, *generic*	Same as chlorothiazide	Same as chlorothiazide	Hypertension: 25–50 mg/d PO; edema: 25–200 mg/d PO

Generic Name	Trade Name*	Uses	Adverse Reactions	Dosage Ranges
hydroflume-thiazide *hye-droe-floo-me-thye'-a-zide*	Diucardin, Saluron	Same as chlorothiazide	Same as chlorothiazide	Hypertension: 50–200 mg/d PO; edema: 25–200 mg/d PO
indapamide *in-dap'-a-mide*	Lozol, *generic*	Hypertension, edema due to CHF	Same as chlorothiazide	Hypertension: 2.5–5 mg/d PO; edema: 2.5–5 mg/d PO
metolazone *me-tole'-a-zone*	Mykrox, Zaroxolyn	Edema in CHF, cirrhosis, corticosteroids, estrogen therapy, renal dysfunction	Same as bendroflume-thiazide	Zaroxolyn: hypertension 2.5–5 mg/d PO; Mykrox: hypertension, 0.5–1 mg/d PO
methyclothiazide *meth-i-kloe-thye'-a-zide*	Aquatensen, Enduron, *generic*	Same as chlorothiazide	Same as chlorothiazide	Hypertension: 2.5–5 mg/d PO; edema: 2.5–10 mg/d PO
polythiazide *pol-i-thye'-a-zide*	Renese	Same as chlorothiazide	Same as chlorothiazide	Hypertension: 2–4 mg/d PO; edema: 1–4 mg/d PO
quinethazone *kwin-eth'-a-zone*	Hydromox	Same as bendroflume-thiazide	Same as bendroflume-thiazide	50–200 mg/d PO
trichlormethi-azide *trye-klor-meth-eye'-a-zide*	Diurese, Metahy-drin, Naqua, *generic*	Same as bendroflume-thiazide	Same as bendroflume-thiazide	Edema: 2–4 mg/d PO; hypertension: 2–4 mg/d PO

Uses of Carbonic Anhydrase Inhibitors

Glaucoma causes an increase in intraocular pressure that, if left untreated, can result in blindness. Normally the eye is filled with aqueous humor in an amount that is carefully regulated to maintain the shape of the eyeball. In glaucoma, aqueous humor is increased, which causes the intraocular pressure to rise and can, without treatment, damage the retina.

Acetazolamide (Diamox) is used in the treatment of simple (open-angle) glaucoma, secondary glaucoma, and preoperatively in acute angle-closure glaucoma when the intraocular pressure is to be lowered before surgery. These drugs are also used in the treatment of edema caused by congestive heart failure, drug-induced edema, and some forms of epilepsy. Methazolamide (Neptazane) is used in the treatment of glaucoma.

Adverse Reactions of Carbonic Anhydrase Inhibitors

Adverse reactions associated with short-term therapy with carbonic anhydrase inhibitors are rare. Long-term use of these drugs may result in fever, rash, paresthesia (numbness, tingling), photosensitivity reactions (exaggerated sunburn reaction when the skin is exposed to sunlight or ultraviolet light), anorexia, and crystalluria (crystals in the urine). On occasion, acidosis may occur, and oral sodium bicarbonate may be used to correct this imbalance.

Contraindications, Precautions, and Interactions of Carbonic Anhydrase Inhibitors

The carbonic anhydrase inhibitors are contraindicated in patients with known hypersensitivity, electrolyte imbalances, severe kidney or liver dysfunction, or anuria, and for long-term use in patients with chronic noncongestive angle-closure glaucoma (may mask worsening glaucoma).

Diuretics are used cautiously in patients with renal dysfunction. The diuretics are pregnancy category C drugs and must be used cautiously during pregnancy and lactation. The safety of these drugs for use during pregnancy and lactation has not been established, so they should be used only when the drug is clearly needed and when the potential benefits to a patient outweigh the potential hazards to the fetus.

The patient has an increased risk of cyclosporine toxicity when the drug is administered with acetazolamide. Decreased serum and urine concentrations of primidone occur when the drug is administered with acetazolamide.

Loop Diuretics

Actions of Loop Diuretics

The loop diuretics, furosemide (Lasix) and ethacrynic acid (Edecrin), increase the excretion of sodium and chloride by inhibiting reabsorption of these ions in the distal and proximal tubules and in the loop of Henle. This mechanism of action at these three sites appears to increase their effectiveness as diuretics. Torsemide (Demadex) also increases urinary excretion of sodium, chloride, and water but acts primarily in the ascending portion of the loop of Henle. Bumetanide (Bumex) primarily increases the excretion of chloride but also has some sodium-excreting ability. This drug acts primarily on the proximal tubule of the nephron.

Uses of Loop Diuretics

Loop diuretics are used in the treatment of edema associated with chronic heart failure, cirrhosis of the liver, and renal disease. These drugs are particularly useful when a greater diuretic effect is desired. Furosemide is the drug of choice when a rapid diuresis is needed or if a patient has renal insufficiency. Furosemide and torsemide are also used to treat hypertension. Ethacrynic acid is also used for the short-term management of ascites (accumulation of serous fluid in the peritoneal cavity) caused by a malignancy, idiopathic edema, or lymphedema.

Adverse Reactions of Loop Diuretics

Adverse reactions seen with the loop diuretics may include anorexia, nausea, vomiting, dizziness, rash, **postural hypotension** (dizziness and light-headedness when rising suddenly from a sitting or lying position), **orthostatic hypotension** (hypotension after standing in one place for a long time), photosensitivity reactions, and glycosuria (glucose in the urine). Patients with diabetes who take these drugs may experience an elevated blood glucose level.

Contraindications, Precautions, and Interactions of Loop Diuretics

Loop diuretics are contraindicated in patients with known hypersensitivity to the loop diuretics or to the sulfonamides, severe electrolyte imbalances, hepatic coma, or anuria, and in infants (ethacrynic acid).

Loop diuretics are used cautiously in patients with renal dysfunction. The loop diuretics are pregnancy category B (ethacrynic acid and torsemide) and C drugs (furosemide and bumetanide) and must be used cautiously during pregnancy and lactation. Furosemide should be used cautiously in children and in patients with liver disease, diabetes, lupus erythematosus (may

exacerbate or activate the disease), or diarrhea. Patients with sensitivity to the sulfonamides may have allergic reactions to furosemide, torsemide, or bumetanide. Additive hypotensive effects occur when the loop diuretics are given with alcohol, other antihypertensive drugs, or nitrates. Loop diuretics may increase the effectiveness of the anticoagulants or the thrombolytics. There is an increased risk of glycoside toxicity and digitalis-induced arrhythmias if a patient experiences **hypokalemia** (low blood potassium) while taking a loop diuretic. Ototoxicity (damage to the hearing organs from a toxic substance) is more likely to occur if a loop diuretic is given with an aminoglycoside. Plasma levels of propranolol may increase when the drug is administered with furosemide. The patient has an increased risk of lithium toxicity when it is administered with a loop diuretic. Hydantoins (phenytoin) may reduce the diuretic effects of furosemide. The effects of loop diuretics may be decreased when they are administered with an NSAID.

Osmotic Diuretics

Actions of Osmotic Diuretics

Osmotic diuretics increase the density of the filtrate in the glomerulus (Figure 19-1). This prevents selective reabsorption of water, which allows the water to be excreted. Sodium and chloride excretion is also increased.

Uses of Osmotic Diuretics

Mannitol (Osmitrol) is used for the promotion of diuresis in the prevention and treatment of the oliguric phase (low urine production) of acute renal failure, as well as for the reduction of intraocular pressure and the treatment of cerebral edema. Urea (Ureaphil) is used to reduce cerebral edema and to reduce intraocular pressure. Glycerin (Osmoglyn) and isosorbide (Ismotic) are used in the treatment of acute glaucoma and to reduce intraocular pressure before and after eye surgery.

Adverse Reactions of Osmotic Diuretics

The osmotic diuretics urea and mannitol are administered intravenously, whereas glycerin and isosorbide are administered orally. Administration by the intravenous route may result in a rapid fluid and electrolyte imbalance, especially when these drugs are administered before surgery to a patient in a fasting state.

Contraindications, Precautions, and Interactions of Osmotic Diuretics

The osmotic diuretics are contraindicated in patients with known hypersensitivity to the drugs, electrolyte imbalances, severe dehydration, or anuria, and those who experience progressive renal damage after using mannitol. Mannitol is contraindicated in patients with active intracranial bleeding (except during craniotomy).

Osmotic diuretics are used cautiously in patients with renal or kidney impairment or electrolyte imbalances. The osmotic diuretics are pregnancy category B (isosorbide) and C (glycerin, mannitol, and urea) drugs and must be used cautiously during pregnancy and lactation. Additive hypotensive effects occur when the osmotic diuretic is given with another antihypertensive drug or nitrate.

Potassium-Sparing Diuretics

Actions of Potassium-Sparing Diuretics

Potassium-sparing diuretics work in either of two ways. Triamterene (Dyrenium) and amiloride (Midamor) depress the reabsorption of sodium in the kidney tubules, therefore increasing sodium and water excretion. Both drugs additionally depress the excretion of potassium and therefore are called potassium-sparing (or potassium-saving) diuretics. Spironolactone (Aldactone), also a potassium-sparing diuretic, antagonizes the action of aldosterone. Aldosterone, a hormone produced by the adrenal cortex, enhances the reabsorption of sodium in the distal convoluted tubules of the kidney. When this activity of aldosterone is blocked, sodium (but not potassium) and water are excreted.

Uses of Potassium-Sparing Diuretics

Amiloride (Midamor) is used in the treatment of chronic heart failure and hypertension and is often used with a thiazide diuretic. Spironolactone and triamterene are also used in the treatment of hypertension and edema caused by chronic heart failure, cirrhosis, and the nephrotic syndrome. Amiloride, spironolactone, and triamterene are also available with hydrochlorothiazide, a thiazide diuretic that enhances the antihypertensive and diuretic effects of the drug combination while still conserving potassium.

Adverse Reactions of Potassium-Sparing Diuretics

Hyperkalemia (increased potassium in the blood), a serious event, may occur with the administration of potassium-sparing diuretics. Hyperkalemia is most likely to occur in patients with an inadequate fluid intake and urine output, those with diabetes or renal disease, the elderly, and severely ill patients. In patients taking spironolactone, gynecomastia (breast enlargement in the male) may occur. This reaction appears to be related to both dosage and duration of therapy. The gynecomastia usu-

ally reverses when therapy is discontinued, but in rare instances some breast enlargement may remain.

Additional adverse reactions of these drugs are listed in the Summary Drug Table: Diuretics. When a potassium-sparing diuretic and a thiazide diuretic are given together, the adverse reactions associated with both drugs may occur.

Contraindications, Precautions, and Interactions of Potassium-Sparing Diuretics

Potassium-sparing diuretics are contraindicated in patients with known hypersensitivity to the drugs, serious electrolyte imbalances, significant renal impairment, or anuria, and those receiving another potassium-sparing diuretic. Potassium-sparing diuretics are contraindicated in patients with hyperkalemia and are not recommended for children. Potassium-sparing diuretics are used cautiously in patients with renal or kidney impairment. These drugs are pregnancy category B (amiloride, triamterene) and D (spironolactone) drugs and must be used cautiously during pregnancy and lactation. Potassium-sparing diuretics are used cautiously in patients with liver disease, diabetes, or gout.

Additive hypotensive effects occur when a potassium-sparing diuretic is given with alcohol, another antihypertensive drug, or nitrate. When a potassium-sparing diuretic is administered to a patient taking an angiotensin-converting enzyme (ACE) inhibitor (see Chapter 16), the patient has an increased risk for hyperkalemia. When a potassium-sparing diuretic is administered with a potassium preparation, severe hyperkalemia may occur, possibly causing a cardiac arrhythmia or cardiac arrest. When spironolactone is administered with an anticoagulant drug or NSAID, the anticoagulant or NSAID has decreased effectiveness. When spironolactone or triamterene is administered with an ACE inhibitor, significant hyperkalemia may occur.

Thiazides and Related Diuretics

Actions of Thiazides and Related Diuretics

Thiazides and related diuretics inhibit the reabsorption of sodium and chloride ions in the ascending portion of the loop of Henle and the early distal tubule of the nephron. This action results in the excretion of sodium, chloride, and water.

Uses of Thiazides and Related Diuretics

Thiazides and related diuretics are used in the treatment of hypertension, edema caused by chronic heart failure, hepatic cirrhosis, corticosteroid and estrogen therapy, and renal dysfunction.

Adverse Reactions of Thiazides and Related Diuretics

Thiazides and related diuretics may be associated with numerous adverse reactions. However, many patients take these drugs without experiencing adverse reactions other than excessive fluid and electrolyte loss, which often can be corrected with an adequate fluid intake, a balanced diet, supplemental oral electrolytes, or ingesting foods or fluids high in the electrolytes that are being lost. Some of the adverse reactions that may occur, in addition to those listed in the Summary Drug Table: Diuretics, include gastric irritation, abdominal bloating, reduced libido, dizziness, vertigo, headache, photosensitivity, and weakness.

Contraindications, Precautions, and Interactions of Thiazides and Related Diuretics

The thiazide diuretics are contraindicated in patients with known hypersensitivity to the thiazides or related diuretics, electrolyte imbalances, renal decompensation, hepatic coma, or anuria. A cross-sensitivity reaction may occur with thiazides and sulfonamides. Some of the thiazide diuretics contain tartrazine, which may cause allergic reactions or bronchial asthma in individuals sensitive to tartrazine.

All of the thiazide diuretics are pregnancy category B drugs, with the exception of bendroflumethiazide, benzthiazide, hydroflumethiazide, methyclothiazide, which are pregnancy category C drugs. The thiazide diuretics must be used cautiously during pregnancy and lactation. These drugs should be used cautiously in children and in patients with liver or kidney disease, lupus erythematosus (may exacerbate or activate the disease), or diabetes.

Additive hypotensive effects occur when the thiazides are given with alcohol, other antihypertensive drugs, or nitrates. Concurrent use of the thiazides with allopurinol may increase the incidence of hypersensitivity to allopurinol. The effects of anesthetics may be increased by thiazide administration. The effects of anticoagulants may be diminished when administered with a thiazide diuretic. Because thiazide diuretics may raise blood uric acid levels, dosage adjustments of antigout drugs may be necessary. Thiazide diuretics may prolong antineoplastic-induced leukopenia. Hyperglycemia may occur when a thiazide is administered with an antidiabetic drug. Synergistic effects may occur when a thiazide diuretic is administered concurrently with a loop diuretic, causing profound diuresis (excretion of urine) and serious electrolyte abnormalities. There is an increased risk of glycoside toxicity if a patient experiences hypokalemia while taking a thiazide diuretic. The administration of a thiazide diuretic and a digitalis glycoside may result in cardiac arrhythmias.

Patient Management Issues with Diuretics

Before the first dose of a diuretic is given, the purpose of the drug, when diuresis may be expected to occur, and how long diuresis will last are explained to the patient (Table 19-1). These drugs are administered early in the day to prevent nighttime sleep disturbances caused by frequent urination.

TABLE 19-1   Examples of Onset and Duration of Activity of Diuretics

Drug	Onset	Duration of Activity
acetazolamide tablets	1–1.5 h	8–12 h
sustained-release capsules	2 h	18–24 h
IV	2 min	4–5 h
amiloride	2 h	24 h
bumetanide	30–60 min	4–6 h
ethacrynic acid		
PO	Within 30 min	6–8 h
IV	Within 5 min	2 h
furosemide		
PO	Within 1 h	6–8 h
IV	Within 5 min	2 h
mannitol (IV)	30–60 min	6–8 h
spironolactone	24–48 h	48–72 h
thiazides and related diuretics	1–2 h	Varies*
triamterene	2–4 h	12–16 h
urea (V)	30–45 min	5–6 h

*Duration varies with drug used. Average duration is 12–24 h with polythiazide and chlorthalidone. Indapamide has a duration of more than 24 h.

Some patients may feel anxious because they will have to urinate more frequently than usual. To reduce anxiety, the purpose and effects of the drug are thoroughly explained, including the fact that the need to urinate frequently will probably decrease. For some patients, the need to urinate frequently decreases after a few weeks of therapy. A hospitalized patient on bed rest must have a call light and, when necessary, a bedpan or urinal within easy reach. The patient should know that the drug will be given early in the day so nighttime sleep will not be interrupted. Although the duration of activity of most diuretics is approximately 8 hours or less, some diuretics have a longer activity, which may result in a need to urinate during the nighttime. This is especially true early in therapy.

Carbonic Anhydrase Inhibitors

If a carbonic anhydrase inhibitor is given for glaucoma, then the patient's response to drug therapy (relief of eye pain) is monitored every 2 hours. The health care provider should be notified immediately if eye pain increases or if it has not begun to decrease 3 to 4 hours after the first dose. If the patient has acute closed-angle glaucoma, then the pupils of the affected eye are checked every 2 hours for dilation and response to light. A patient who can walk but has reduced vision because of glaucoma may need help walking and with self-care activities.

If a carbonic anhydrase inhibitor is being given to control epileptic seizures, then the patient is checked frequently for the occurrence of seizures, especially early in therapy and in patients known to experience seizures frequently. If a seizure does occur, then it should be documented in the patient's chart, including time of onset and duration. Accurate descriptions of seizures help the health care provider plan future therapy and adjust drug dosages as needed.

Osmotic Diuretics

When an osmotic is prescribed, the disease or disorder and the symptoms being treated are closely monitored. For example, if the patient has a low urinary output and the osmotic diuretic is given to increase urinary output, then the intake and output ratio and symptoms the patient is experiencing are recorded. In addition, the patient is weighed and vital signs are taken before starting drug therapy.

Mannitol is administered only intravenously. The patient's urine output is monitored hourly.

When a patient is receiving the osmotic diuretic mannitol or urea for treatment of increased intracranial pressure caused by cerebral edema, the blood pressure, pulse, and respiratory rate are monitored every 30 to 60 minutes or as ordered by the health care provider. Any increase in blood pressure, decrease in the pulse or res-

piratory rate, or any change in the patient's neurologic status should be reported.

Potassium-Sparing Diuretics

Patients taking potassium-sparing diuretics are at risk for hyperkalemia. Serum potassium levels are monitored frequently, particularly during initial treatment.

ALERT

Potassium-Sparing Diuretics and Hyperkalemia

Patients taking potassium-sparing diuretics are at risk for hyperkalemia. Symptoms of hyperkalemia include paresthesia (numbness, tingling, or prickling sensation), muscular weakness, fatigue, flaccid paralysis of the extremities, bradycardia, shock, and electrocardiographic (ECG) abnormalities (see Box 19-1 for additional symptoms). The drug is discontinued and the health care provider notified immediately if the patient experiences these symptoms.

Thiazide and Related Diuretics

When the thiazide diuretics are administered, the patient's renal function is monitored periodically. These drugs may precipitate azotemia (accumulation of nitrogenous wastes in the blood). If the patient's level of nonprotein nitrogen or blood urea nitrogen rises, then the health care provider may consider withholding or discontinuing the drug. In addition, serum uric acid concentrations are monitored periodically during treatment with the thiazide diuretics because these drugs may precipitate an acute attack of gout. The patient also is monitored for joint pain or discomfort. Because hyperglycemia may occur, insulin or oral antidiabetic drug dosages may require alterations. Serum glucose concentrations are monitored periodically.

Patients with Edema

Patients with edema caused by heart failure or other causes are weighed daily or as ordered by the health care provider to monitor fluid loss. A weight loss of approximately 2 pounds per day is desirable to prevent dehydration and electrolyte imbalances. Fluid intake and output are measured and recorded every 8 hours. A critically ill patient or a patient with renal disease may require more frequent measurements of urinary output. Blood pressure, pulse, and respiratory rate are taken every 4 hours or as ordered by the health care provider.

Areas of edema are examined daily to evaluate the effectiveness of drug therapy.

Patients with Hypertension

The blood pressure, pulse, and respiratory rate of patients with hypertension receiving a diuretic, or a diuretic along with an antihypertensive drug, are taken before the administration of the drug. More frequent monitoring may be necessary if the patient is critically ill or the blood pressure excessively high.

Managing Adverse Reactions of Diuretics

Electrolyte Imbalance

The most common adverse reaction of diuretics is the loss of fluid and electrolytes (see Box 19-1), especially during initial therapy. In some patients the diuretic effect is moderate, whereas in others a large volume of fluid is lost. Regardless of the amount of fluid lost, there is always the possibility of excessive electrolyte loss, which is potentially serious.

The most common imbalances are a loss of potassium and water. Other electrolytes, such as magnesium, sodium, and chlorides, are also lost. When too much potassium is lost, hypokalemia (low blood level of potassium) occurs. In certain patients, such as those also receiving a digitalis glycoside or those with a cardiac arrhythmia, hypokalemia may cause a more serious arrhythmia. Hypokalemia is treated with potassium supplements or foods with high potassium content, or by changing the diuretic to a potassium-sparing diuretic. In addition to hypokalemia, patients taking loop diuretics are prone to magnesium deficiency (see Box 19-1). If too much water is lost, then **dehydration** occurs, which also can be serious, especially in elderly patients.

Whether a fluid or electrolyte imbalance occurs depends on the amount of fluid and electrolytes lost and the patient's ability to replace them. For example, if a patient receiving a diuretic eats poorly and does not drink extra fluids, an electrolyte and water imbalance is likely to occur, especially during initial therapy with the drug. However, even when a patient drinks adequate amounts of fluid and eats a balanced diet, an electrolyte imbalance may still occur and require electrolyte replacement (see Chapter 32 for further discussion of fluid and electrolyte imbalances).

ALERT

Older Patients and Electrolyte Imbalances

Older adults are particularly prone to fluid volume deficits and electrolyte imbalances (see Box 19-1) while taking a diuretic. An older adult is carefully monitored for hypokalemia (when taking a loop or thiazide diuretic) and hyperkalemia (with a potassium–sparing diuretic).

> **Box 19-1   Signs and Symptoms of Common Fluid and Electrolyte Imbalances Associated With Diuretic Therapy**
>
> **Dehydration (Excessive Water Loss)**
> - Thirst
> - Poor skin turgor
> - Dry mucous membranes
> - Weakness
> - Dizziness
> - Fever
> - Low urine output
>
> **Hyponatremia (Excessive Loss of Sodium)**
> - Cold, clammy skin
> - Decreased skin turgor
> - Confusion
> - Hypotension
> - Irritability
> - Tachycardia
>
> **Hypomagnesemia (Low Levels of Magnesium)**
> - Leg and foot cramps
> - Hypertension
> - Tachycardia
> - Neuromuscular irritability
> - Tremor
> - Hyperactive deep tendon reflexes
> - Confusion
> - Visual or auditory hallucinations
> - Paresthesias
>
> **Hypokalemia (Low Blood Potassium)**
> - Anorexia
> - Nausea
> - Vomiting
> - Depression
> - Confusion
> - Cardiac arrhythmias
> - Impaired thought processes
> - Drowsiness
>
> **Hyperkalemia (High Blood Potassium)**
> - Irritability
> - Anxiety
> - Confusion
> - Nausea
> - Diarrhea
> - Cardiac arrhythmias
> - Abdominal distress

To prevent a fluid volume deficit, oral fluids are encouraged at frequent intervals during waking hours. A balanced diet may help prevent electrolyte imbalances. Patients are encouraged to eat and drink all food and fluids served at mealtime. All patients, especially the elderly, are encouraged to eat or drink between meals and in the evening (when allowed). Their fluid intake and output are monitored and the health care provider is notified if the patient fails to drink an adequate amount of fluid, if the urinary output is low, if the urine appears concentrated, if the patient appears dehydrated, or if signs and symptoms of an electrolyte imbalance are apparent.

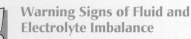

ALERT

Warning Signs of Fluid and Electrolyte Imbalance

Warning signs of a fluid and electrolyte imbalance include dry mouth, thirst, weakness, lethargy, drowsiness, restlessness, muscle pains or cramps, confusion, gastrointestinal disturbances, hypotension, oliguria (decreased urinary output), tachycardia, and seizures.

Cardiac Arrhythmias and Dizziness

Patients concurrently receiving a diuretic (particularly a loop or thiazide diuretic) and a digitalis glycoside require frequent monitoring of the pulse rate and rhythm because of the possibility of cardiac arrhythmias. Any significant changes in the pulse rate and rhythm should be immediately reported to the health care provider.

Some patients experience dizziness or light-headedness, especially during the first few days of therapy or when a rapid diuresis has occurred. Patients who are dizzy but are allowed out of bed should be helped with walking activities until these adverse drug effects disappear.

Herbal Remedies: Diuretics

Numerous herbal diuretics are available as over-the-counter (OTC) products. Most plants and herbal extracts available as OTC diuretics are nontoxic. However, most are either ineffective or no more effective than caffeine. The following are some of the herbals reported to have diuretic activity: celery, chicory, sassafras, juniper berries, St. John's wort, foxglove, horsetail, licorice, dandelion, digitalis purpurea, ephedra, hibiscus, parsley, and elderberry.

There is very little and in many instances no scientific evidence to justify the use of these plants as diuretics. For example, dandelion root is a popular preparation once thought to be a strong diuretic, but scientific research has found dandelion root, although safe, to be ineffective as a diuretic. No herbal diuretic should be taken unless approved by the health care provider.

Diuretic teas such as juniper berries and shave grass or horsetail should be avoided. Juniper berries have

been associated with renal damage, and horsetail contains severely toxic compounds. Teas with ephedrine should also be avoided, especially by individuals with hypertension.

Educating the Patient and Family About Diuretics

The patient or a family member should be given a full explanation of the prescribed drug therapy, including when to take the drug (diuretics taken once per day are best taken early in the morning), if the drug is to be taken with food, and the importance of following the dosage schedule. The onset and duration of the drug's diuretic effect are also explained. The patient and family must also be made aware of the signs and symptoms of fluid and electrolyte imbalances and adverse reactions that may occur when using a diuretic. To ensure compliance with the prescribed drug regimen, the importance of diuretic therapy in the treatment of the patient's disorder should be emphasized. Patient Education Box 19-1 includes key points about diuretics that the patient and family members should know.

PATIENT EDUCATION BOX 19-1

Key Points for Patients Taking Diuretics

- ❑ Do not stop taking the drug and do not skip doses except on the advice of your health care provider.
- ❑ If you experience gastrointestinal upset, take the drug with food or milk.
- ❑ Take the drug early in the morning (with a once-a-day dosage) unless directed otherwise to minimize the effects on nighttime sleep. Twice-a-day dosing should be administered early in the morning (e.g., 7:00 AM) and early afternoon (e.g., 2:00 PM) or as directed by your health care provider. These drugs initially cause more frequent urination, which should subside after a few weeks.
- ❑ Avoid alcohol and nonprescription drugs unless your health care provider approves. Hypertensive patients should be careful to avoid medications that increase blood pressure, such as over-the-counter drugs for appetite suppression or cold symptoms.
- ❑ Notify your health care provider if you experience any of the following: muscle cramps or weakness, dizziness, nausea, vomiting, diarrhea, restlessness, excessive thirst, general weakness, rapid pulse, increased heart rate or pulse, or gastrointestinal distress.
- ❑ If you feel dizzy or weak, be careful while driving or performing hazardous tasks, rise slowly from a sitting or lying position, and avoid standing in one place for an extended time.

PATIENT EDUCATION BOX 19-1

Key Points for Patients Taking Diuretics (continued)

❏ Weigh yourself weekly or as recommended by your health care provider. Keep a record of these weekly weights and contact your health care provider if your weight loss exceeds 3 to 5 pounds per week.

❏ If your health care provider recommends foods or fluids high in potassium, then eat the amount recommended. Do not exceed this amount or eliminate these foods from your diet for more than 1 day, except when told to do so by your health care provider. These foods include beef, chicken, pork, turkey, veal, flounder, haddock, halibut, salmon, flounder, canned sardines, scallops, tuna, apricots, bananas, dates, raisins, fresh orange juice, tomato juice, oranges, dried fruit, cantaloupe, peaches, prunes, avocado, carrots, lima beans, potatoes, radishes, spinach, sweet potatoes, tomatoes, gingersnaps, graham crackers, molasses, peanuts, peanut butter, coffee, tea, and nuts.

❏ After a time, the diuretic effect of the drug may be minimal because most of the body's excess fluid has been removed. Continue taking the drug as directed to prevent further accumulation of fluid.

❏ If you are taking a thiazide or related diuretic, loop diuretic, potassium-sparing diuretic, carbonic anhydrase inhibitor, or triamterene, then avoid exposure to sunlight or ultraviolet light (sunlamps, tanning beds) because exposure may cause exaggerated sunburn (photosensitivity reaction). Wear sunscreen and protective clothing until your tolerance is determined.

❏ If you are taking a loop or thiazide diuretic and have diabetes mellitus, your blood glucometer test results for glucose may be elevated or your urine positive for glucose. Contact your health care provider if the results of your home testing of blood glucose levels increase or if your urine tests positive for glucose.

❏ If you are taking a potassium-sparing diuretic, avoid eating foods high in potassium and avoid salt substitutes containing potassium. Read food labels carefully. Do not use a salt substitute unless your health care provider approves the particular brand. Do not take potassium supplements. Male patients taking spironolactone may experience gynecomastia (excessive development of mammary glands), which usually reverses when therapy is discontinued.

❏ If you are taking a thiazide diuretic, it may cause gout attacks. Contact your health care provider if you experience significant, sudden joint pain.

❏ If you are taking a carbonic anhydrase inhibitor for glaucoma, contact your health care provider immediately if your eye pain is not relieved or if it increases. If you are being treated for seizures, a family member should keep a record of all seizures that occur. Bring this record to your health care provider at your next visit. Contact your health care provider immediately if your seizures increase.

KEY POINTS

◉ Diuretics are used for a variety of medical disorders. Diuretics are administered early in the day to prevent any nighttime sleep disturbance caused by increased urination.

◉ Carbonic anhydrase inhibitors cause the excretion of sodium, potassium, bicarbonate, and water. These drugs are commonly used in the treatment of glaucoma. Carbonic anhydrase inhibitors are contraindicated in patients with known hypersensitivity, electrolyte imbalances, severe kidney or liver dysfunction, or anuria, and for long-term use in chronic noncongestive angle-closure glaucoma.

◉ The loop diuretics, furosemide (Lasix) and ethacrynic acid (Edecrin), increase the excretion of sodium and chloride by inhibiting reabsorption of these ions in the distal and proximal tubules and in the loop of Henle. Loop diuretics are used to treat edema associated with chronic heart failure, cirrhosis of the liver, and renal disease. These drugs are contraindicated in patients with known hypersensitivity to the loop diuretics or to the sulfonamides, severe electrolyte imbalances, hepatic coma, or anuria, and in infants (ethacrynic acid).

◉ Osmotic diuretics increase the density of the filtrate in the glomerulus (Figure 19-1), thereby preventing selective reabsorption of water. Sodium and chloride excretion are increased. Administration by the intravenous route may result in a rapid fluid and electrolyte imbalance, especially when these drugs are administered before surgery to a patient in a fasting state.

◉ Potassium-sparing diuretics work in two ways. Triamterene (Dyrenium) and amiloride (Midamor) depress the reabsorption of sodium, therefore increasing sodium and water excretion. Both drugs depress the excretion of potassium and therefore are called potassium-sparing (or potassium-saving) diuretics. Spironolactone (Aldactone), also a potassium-sparing diuretic, antagonizes the action of aldosterone, causing sodium (but not potassium) and water to be excreted. Hyperkalemia, a serious event, may occur with the administration of potassium-sparing diuretics.

◉ Thiazides and related diuretics inhibit the reabsorption of sodium and chloride. Thiazides and related diuretics are used to treat hypertension, edema caused by chronic heart failure, hepatic cirrhosis, corticosteroid and estrogen therapy, and renal dysfunction. The thiazide diuretics are contraindicated in patients with known hypersensitivity to the thiazides or related diuretics, electrolyte imbalances, renal decompensation, hepatic coma, or anuria.

CASE STUDY

> Mr. Rodriguez, age 68 years, is taking amiloride for hypertension. He and his wife have stopped by the clinic for a routine blood pressure check. Mrs. Rodriguez states that her husband has been confused and very irritable for the past 2 days. He reports nausea and has had several "loose" stools.
>
> 1. Mrs. Rodriguez asks about the adverse effects of amiloride. She should be told that:
>   a. irritability and confusion are not caused by amiloride unless it is combined with certain other drugs
>   b. nausea and loose stools may be adverse reactions to amiloride
>   c. there are no known adverse effects of amiloride use
>   d. both a and b are correct
>
> 2. You ask Mrs. Rodriguez if her husband is taking any other prescription drug. She nods and says ACE. You know the health care provider has already considered that:
>   a. amiloride and ACE inhibitors have no known interactive effects
>   b. there is an increased risk of hyperkalemia when the two drugs are combined
>   c. there is an increased risk of hypokalemia when the two drugs are combined
>   d. none of the above
>
> 3. Mr. Rodriguez asks if he should change his diet in any way because of his prescription drug use. He should be told:
>   a. do not drink alcohol unless his health care provider approves it
>   b. when taking both an ACE inhibitor and amiloride, avoid foods high in potassium
>   c. drinking adequate fluids is an important component of diuretic use
>   d. all of the above

WEBSITE ACTIVITIES

1. Go to the National Institute of Health website (http://www.nlm.nih.gov/medlineplus/edema.html) and scan the names of the listed articles. What, if any, information is available about the DASH eating plan, which is often recommended for patients with hypertension? Does this information seem sufficient for patients to start using the DASH diet?

2. Some loop diuretics are used to treat pulmonary edema. At this same website, look for general information about pulmonary edema. Why is it considered a medical emergency?

REVIEW QUESTIONS

1. When evaluating the effectiveness of acetazolamide (Diamox) given for acute glaucoma, the patient is questioned about:
   a. the amount of urine at each voiding
   b. the relief of eye pain
   c. the amount of fluid being taken
   d. occipital headaches

2. When taking spironolactone (Aldactone), a patient is closely monitored for which of the following electrolyte imbalances?
   a. hypernatremia
   b. hyponatremia
   c. hyperkalemia
   d. hypokalemia

3. When a diuretic is being given for heart failure, which of the following would be most indicative of an effective response to diuretic therapy?
   a. low urine flow
   b. daily weight loss of 2 pounds
   c. increased blood pressure
   d. increasing edema in the legs and feet

4. Which electrolyte imbalance would most likely develop in a patient receiving a loop or thiazide diuretic?
   a. hypernatremia
   b. hyponatremia
   c. hyperkalemia
   d. hypokalemia

5. Which of the following foods should patients include in their daily diet to prevent hypokalemia?
   a. green beans
   b. apples
   c. bananas
   d. corn

Urinary Anti-Infectives and Miscellaneous Urinary Drugs

KEY TERMS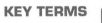

anti-infective—a drug used to treat infection
bactericidal—a drug that kills bacteria
bacteriostatic—a drug or agent that slows or retards bacteria
dysuria—painful or difficult urination
neurogenic bladder—altered bladder function caused by a nervous system abnormality
overactive bladder—involuntary contractions of the detrusor or bladder muscle
urge incontinence—accidental loss of urine caused by a sudden and unstoppable need to urinate
urinary tract infection—an infection caused by pathogenic microorganisms of one or more structures of the urinary tract
urinary frequency—frequent urination day and night
urinary urgency—sudden strong need to urinate

CHAPTER OBJECTIVES

On completion of this chapter, students will be able to:

1 Define the chapter's key terms.

2 Describe the general drug actions, uses, adverse reactions, contraindications, precautions, and interactions of urinary anti-infectives and miscellaneous urinary drugs.

3 Discuss important points to keep in mind when educating the patient or family members about the use of urinary anti-infectives and miscellaneous urinary drugs.

This chapter discusses drugs used to treat urinary tract infections and certain other drugs used to relieve the symptoms associated with an **overactive bladder** (involuntary contractions of the detrusor, or bladder, muscle). Overactive bladder is estimated to affect more than 16 million individuals in the United States. The drugs reviewed in this chapter also help control the discomfort associated with irritation of the lower urinary tract mucosa caused by infection, trauma, surgery, and endoscopic procedures.

Urinary system infections may involve the bladder (cystitis), prostate gland (prostatitis), kidney and renal pelvis (pyelonephritis), or the urethra (urethritis) (see Figure 20-1). Symptoms of an overactive bladder include **urinary urgency**, **urinary frequency**, and urge incontinence, which is an accidental loss of urine caused by a sudden and unstoppable need to urinate.

Urinary tract infection is an infection caused by pathogenic microorganisms of one or more structures of the urinary tract. The most common structure affected is the bladder (Fig. 20-1). Symptoms of a urinary tract infection of the bladder (cystitis) include urgency, frequency, burning and pain on urination, and pain caused by spasm in the region of the bladder and lower abdominal area.

Some drugs used in the treatment of urinary tract infections do not belong to the antibiotic or sulfonamide groups of drugs. The drugs discussed in this chapter are **anti-infectives** (against infection) used in the treatment of urinary tract infections. These drugs have an effect on bacteria in the urinary tract. Taken orally or by parenteral route, the drugs do not achieve significant levels in the bloodstream and are of no value in the treatment of systemic infections. They are primarily excreted by the kidneys and exert their major antibacterial effects in the urine. (See Summary Drug Table: Urinary Anti-infectives for a listing of these and other drugs used to treat problems associated with the urinary system.)

Examples of urinary anti-infectives include cinoxacin (Cinobac), fosfomycin (Monurol), methenamine mandelate (Mandelamine), nalidixic acid (NegGram), and nitrofurantoin (Furadantin). The anti-infectives work on various strains of bacteria. When a urinary tract infection is diagnosed, sensitivity tests are performed to determine bacterial sensitivity to various antibiotics and urinary anti-infectives to determine which will best control the infection.

Additional drugs can be used in the treatment of urinary tract infections. Examples of these drugs include ampicillin, cephalosporins, sulfonamides, and norfloxacin (see Chapter 25). Combination drugs are also available. The Summary Drug Table: Urinary Anti-infectives gives examples of the combination drugs used to treat urinary tract infections.

Actions, Uses, and Adverse Reactions of Urinary Anti-Infectives and Miscellaneous Urinary Drugs

Cinoxacin

Cinoxacin appears to act by disrupting the replication of DNA in susceptible Gram-negative bacteria, thereby interfering with bacterial multiplication. It accomplishes this through a high concentration in the urine. Like the sulfonamides and other anti-infectives, the systemic anti-infectives, such as cinoxacin, are used to treat urinary tract infections caused by susceptible microorganisms. Nausea, abdominal pain, vomiting, anorexia, diarrhea, perineal burning, headache, photophobia, and dizziness may be adverse reactions of cinoxacin.

Methenamine and Methenamine Salts

Methenamine and methenamine salts break down and form ammonia and formaldehyde, which are bactericidal.

Use of methenamine and methenamine salts may result in gastrointestinal disturbances, such as anorexia, nausea, vomiting, stomatitis, and cramps. Large doses may result in burning on urination and bladder irritation.

Nalidixic Acid

Nalidixic acid appears to act by interfering with bacterial multiplication through interruption of the replication of bacterial DNA. It accomplishes this through a high concentration in the urine.

Abdominal pain, nausea, vomiting, anorexia, diarrhea, rash, drowsiness, dizziness, photosensitivity reactions, blurred vision, weakness, and headache may result from nalidixic acid. Visual disturbances often occur after each dose and usually disappear after a few days of therapy.

Nitrofurantoin

Nitrofurantoin may be **bacteriostatic** (slows or retards the multiplication of bacteria) or **bactericidal** (destroys bacteria), depending on the concentration of the drug in the urine. Nitrofurantoin is used to treat urinary tract infections caused by strains of bacteria susceptible to it.

Nitrofurantoin use may result in nausea, vomiting, anorexia, rash, peripheral neuropathy, headache, brown discoloration of the urine, and hypersensitivity reactions, which may range from mild to severe. Acute and chronic pulmonary reactions may occur.

Fosfomycin

Fosfomycin is a bactericidal that interferes with bacterial cell wall synthesis. Fosfomycin is used for urinary tract

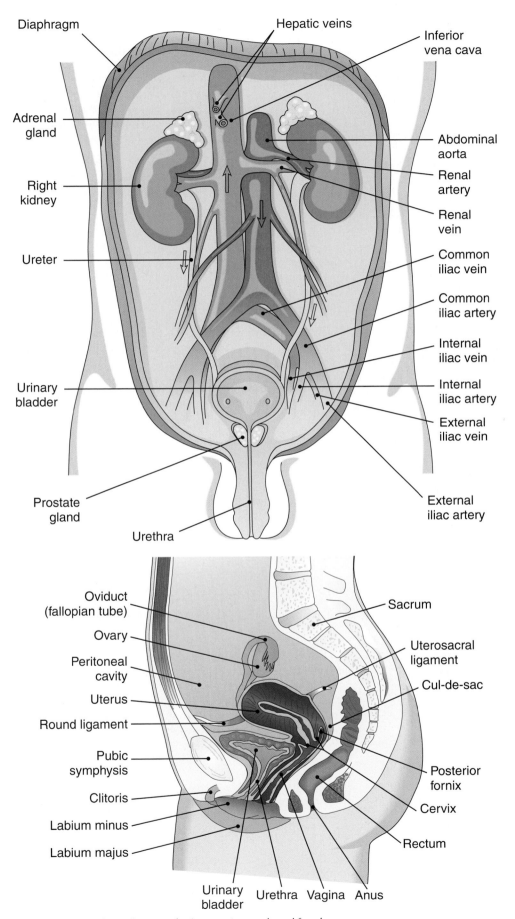

FIGURE 20-1A and B   The normal urinary system, male and female.

SUMMARY DRUG TABLE   Urinary Anti-Infectives

Generic Name	Trade Name*	Uses	Adverse Reactions	Dosage Ranges
cinoxacin *sin-ox'-a-sin*	Cinobac, *generic*	Initial or recurrent UTIs	Nausea, abdominal pain, vomiting, anorexia, diarrhea, perineal burning, headache, photophobia, dizziness, rash	1 g/d PO in 2–4 divided doses for 7–14 d
fosfomycin tromethamine *foss-fo-my'-sin tro-meth-a-meen*	Monurol	UTIs caused by susceptible microorganisms	Diarrhea, vaginitis, rhinitis, nausea, headache, back pain	3-g packet PO
methenamine hippurate *meth-en'-a-meen*	Hiprex, Urex	Suppression or elimination of bacteriuria associated with pyelonephritis, cystitis, or other chronic UTIs, infected residual urine	Anorexia, nausea, vomiting, stomatitis, cramps, rash, bladder irritation, headache	1 g PO BID
methenamine mandelate *meth-en'-a-meen*	Mandelamine, *generic*	Same as methenamine hippurate	Same as methenamine hippurate	1 g PO QID
nalidixic acid *nal-i-dix'-ic*	NegGram	UTIs caused by susceptible microorganisms	Abdominal pain, nausea, vomiting, anorexia, diarrhea, rash, drowsiness, dizziness, photosensitivity reactions, blurred vision, weakness, headache	1 g QID for 1–2 wk; may reduce to 2 g/d for prolonged therapy
nitrofurantoin *nye-troe-fyoor-an'-toyn*	Furadantin, *generic*	UTIs caused by susceptible microorganisms	Nausea, vomiting, anorexia, rash, peripheral neuropathy, headache, brown discoloration of urine, hypersensitivity reactions, superinfection	50–100 mg PO QID
nitrofurantoin macrocrystals	Macrobid, Macrodantin, *generic*	Same as nitrofurantoin	Same as nitrofurantoin	50–100 mg PO QID; SR 100 mg BID
Miscellaneous Urinary Drugs flavoxate HCl *fla-vox'-ate*	Urispas	Symptomatic relief of dysuria, urgency, nocturia, suprapubic pain, frequency and incontinence due to cystitis, prostatitis, urethritis	Nausea, vomiting, dry mouth, nervousness, vertigo, headache, drowsiness, blurred vision, mental confusion (especially in the elderly)	100–200 mg TID, QID PO
oxybutynin chloride *ox-i-byoo'-ti-nin*	Ditropan, Ditropan XL, *generic*	Bladder instability, treatment of overactive bladder	Dry mouth, constipation, headache, dizziness, diarrhea, nausea, blurred vision, drowsiness, decreased sweating, heat prostration	5 mg BID, TID PO; maximum dosage, 5 mg QID; extended release: 5–30 mg once daily

Generic Name	Trade Name*	Uses	Adverse Reactions	Dosage Ranges
phenazopyridine *fen-az-oh-peer'-i-deen*	Pyridate, Pyridium, Urogesic, *generic*	Relief of pain associated with irritation of the lower genitourinary tract	Headache, rash, pruritus, GI disturbances, red-orange discoloration of the urine, yellowish discoloration of the skin or sclera	200 mg TID PO
tolterodine tartrate *toll-tear'-oh-dyne*	Detrol, Detrol LA	Overactive bladder with symptoms of urinary frequency, urgency or urge incontinence	Nausea, vomiting, constipation, dry mouth, headache, dizziness, blurred vision, dysuria	2 mg BID PO; extended release: 2–4 mg once daily PO
trimethoprim (TMP) *trye-meth'-oh-prim*	Proloprim, Trimpex, *generic*	UTIs caused by susceptible microorganisms	Rash, pruritus, epigastric distress, nausea, vomiting	100 mg PO q12h or 200 mg PO q24h for 10 d
Urinary Anti-Infective Combinations sulfamethizole *sul-fa-meth'-i-zole*	Thiosulfil Forte	UTIs caused by susceptible microorganisms	Headache, nausea, vomiting, abdominal pain, crystalluria	0.5–1 g PO TID, QID
trimethoprim and sulfamethoxazole (TMP-SMZ) *trye-meth'-oh-prim sul-fa-meth-ox'-a-zole*	Bactrim, Bactrim DS, Septra, Septra DS, *generic*	UTIs caused by susceptible microorganisms, shigellosis and acute otitis media	Gastrointestinal disturbances, allergic skin reactions, headache, anorexia, glossitis, hypersensitivity	160 mg TMP/800 SMZ PO q12h; 8–10 mg/kg/d (based on TMP) IV in 2–4 divided doses

*The term *generic* indicates the drug is available in generic form.
UTI, urinary tract infection.

infections caused by microorganisms susceptible to its effects. Adverse reactions of fosfomycin include headache, dizziness, nausea, abdominal cramps, and vaginitis.

Trimethoprim

Trimethoprim (Trimpex) interferes with the ability of bacteria to metabolize folinic acid. Trimethoprim use may result in rash, pruritus, epigastric distress, nausea, and vomiting. When trimethoprim is combined with sulfamethoxazole (Septra), the adverse effects of sulfonamide may also occur. The adverse reactions of other anti-infectives, such as sulfonamides, ampicillin, and cephalosporins are covered in other chapters.

Flavoxate

Flavoxate (Urispas) counteracts smooth muscle spasm of the urinary tract by relaxing the detrusor and other muscles through action at the parasympathetic receptors. Flavoxate is used to relieve symptoms of **dysuria** (painful or difficult urination), urinary urgency (a strong and sudden desire to urinate), nocturia (excessive urination during the night), lower abdominal pain, fre-

quency, and **urge incontinence** (accidental loss of urine caused by a sudden and unstoppable urge to void). Flavoxate can cause blurred vision, drowsiness, nausea and vomiting, nervousness, vertigo, headache, and mental confusion, particularly in the elderly.

Oxybutynin

Oxybutynin (Ditropan) acts by relaxing the bladder muscle and reducing spasm. Oxybutynin is used to treat bladder instability (urgency, frequency, leakage, incontinence, and painful or difficult urination) caused by a **neurogenic bladder** (altered bladder function caused by a nervous system abnormality). Adverse reactions may include dry mouth, constipation or diarrhea, decreased production of tears, decreased sweating, gastrointestinal disturbances, dim vision, and urinary hesitancy.

Phenazopyridine

Phenazopyridine (Pyridium) is a dye that exerts a topical analgesic effect on the lining of the urinary tract. It has no anti-infective activity. Phenazopyridine is available as a separate a urinary analgesic drug but is also included in some urinary anti-infective combination drugs. It is used to relieve the pain, burning, urgency, frequency, and irritation caused by infection, trauma, catheters, or surgical procedures of the urinary tract. Adverse reactions may include headache, rash, and gastrointestinal upset.

Tolterodine

Tolterodine (Detrol) is an anticholinergic drug that inhibits bladder contractions and delays the urge to void. Tolerodine tartrate is used to treat symptoms of overactive bladder, such as urinary frequency, urgency, or urge incontinence. Tolterodine may cause anticholinergic adverse reactions such as dry mouth (the most common adverse reaction), drowsiness, decreased sweating, blurred vision, nausea, vomiting, dizziness, and abdominal pain. Because tolterodine acts more specifically on the bladder, adverse reactions are less pronounced than those of other anticholinergic drugs.

Miscellaneous Drugs

A number of miscellaneous drugs are used to relieve the symptoms associated with an overactive bladder (involuntary contractions of the bladder muscle) that sometimes occur because of disorders such as cystitis, prostatitis, or other affected structures, such as the kidney or the urethra. These drugs also help control the discomfort of irritated lower urinary tract mucosa caused by infection, trauma, surgery, and endoscopic procedures.

Managing Adverse Drug Reactions of Urinary Anti-infectives and Miscellaneous Urinary Drugs

Urinary Anti-Infectives

If an adverse reaction occurs, then the health care provider should be contacted before the next dose of the drug is taken. Serious drug reactions, such as a pulmonary reaction, are reported immediately.

Pulmonary reactions have been reported with the use of nitrofurantoin and may occur within hours and up to 3 weeks after therapy with this drug begins. Signs and symptoms of an acute pulmonary reaction include dyspnea (difficulty breathing), chest pain, cough, fever, and chills. If these reactions occur, then the health care provider is contacted and the next dose of the drug is not taken until the patient is seen by the health care provider. Signs and symptoms of chronic pulmonary reactions, which may occur with prolonged therapy, include dyspnea, nonproductive cough, and malaise.

Miscellaneous Urinary Drugs

Common adverse reactions of flavoxate, oxybutynin, and tolterodine include dry mouth, dizziness, blurred vision, and constipation. For patients with dry mouth, sucking on hard candy, sugarless lozenges, or small pieces of ice may help to ease discomfort. This effect sometimes lessens with continued use of the drug. Hospitalized patients experiencing drowsiness or blurred vision may need help walking. Increased fluids, a high-fiber diet, and walking or exercise (if the patient's condition allows) may help patients with constipation. If constipation persists, then the health care provider may prescribe a mild laxative or stool softener.

Phenazopyridine may cause a red–orange discoloration of the urine and may stain fabrics or contact lenses. This is normal and subsides when the drug is discontinued.

Contraindications, Precautions, and Interactions of Urinary Anti-infectives and Miscellaneous Urinary Drugs

Cinoxacin

Cinoxacin is contraindicated in patients with known hypersensitivity to the drug and in patients with anuria. Cinoxacin is a pregnancy category B drug and should be used with caution during pregnancy and lactation, and in patients with a liver condition. When cinoxacin is administered with probenecid, there is a risk for lowered urine concentration of cinoxacin.

Methenamine and Methenamine Salts

Methenamine is contraindicated in patients with hypersensitivity to the drug or a liver condition, and during pregnancy (pregnancy category C) and lactation. Patients who are allergic to tartrazine should not take methenamine hippurate (Hiprex). The drug is used cautiously in patients with liver or kidney disease or gout (may cause crystals to form in the urine). No serious interactions have been reported. An increased urinary pH decreases the effectiveness of methenamine. Therefore, to avoid raising the urine pH when taking methenamine, the patient should not use antacids containing sodium bicarbonate or sodium carbonate.

Nalidixic Acid

Nalidixic acid is contraindicated in patients who are hypersensitive to the drug or any of its components, patients with convulsive disorders, and during pregnancy (pregnancy category C) and lactation. Nalidixic acid is used cautiously in patients with liver or kidney disease, cerebral arteriosclerosis, or glucose-6-phosphate dehydrogenase deficiency. When nalidixic acid is administered with the oral anticoagulants, the patient has an increased risk of bleeding.

Nitrofurantoin

Nitrofurantoin is contraindicated in patients with kidney disease or hypersensitivity to the drug, and in lactating women. Nitrofurantoin is classified as a pregnancy category B drug and is used with caution during pregnancy. The drug is also used with caution in patients with a glucose-6-phosphate dehydrogenase deficiency, anemia, or diabetes. There is a decreased absorption of nitrofurantoin when the drug is administered with magnesium trisilicate or magaldrate. When nitrofurantoin is administered with anticholinergics, there is a delay in the rate at which nitrofurantoin leaves the stomach, increasing the amount absorbed.

Fosfomycin

Fosfomycin is contraindicated in patients with a hypersensitivity to the drug. Fosfomycin is used cautiously during pregnancy (pregnancy category B) and lactation. Lowered plasma concentration and urinary tract excretion occur when fosfomycin is administered with metoclopramide.

Trimethoprim

Trimethoprim is contraindicated in patients with a hypersensitivity to the drug or a lowered creatine clearance (rate at which creatinine is excreted from the urine over time). The drug is used cautiously in patients with liver or kidney disease and in patients with megaloblastic anemia caused by folate deficiency. Trimethoprim is classified as a pregnancy category C drug and is not recommended during pregnancy and lactation. No significant interactions have been reported.

Flavoxate

Flavoxate is contraindicated in patients with intestinal or gastric blockage, abdominal bleeding, or urinary tract blockage. It is used cautiously in patients with glaucoma, and during pregnancy (pregnancy category C) and lactation. No significant interactions with other drugs have been reported.

Oxybutynin

Oxybutynin is contraindicated in patients with a hypersensitivity to the drug, glaucoma, partial or complete blockage of the gastrointestinal tract, myasthenia gravis, or urinary tract obstruction. It is used cautiously in patients with kidney or liver disease, heart failure, irregular or rapid heart rate, hypertension, or enlarged prostate, and during pregnancy (pregnancy category C) and lactation. Phenothiazines are less effective when administered with oxybutynin. Haloperidol may have a decreased response and cause an increased risk of tardive dyskinesia (involuntary movements of face and/or extremities) when administered with oxybutynin.

Phenazopyridine

Phenazopyridine is contraindicated in patients with renal impairment or undiagnosed urinary tract pain. Phenazopyridine is used cautiously during pregnancy (pregnancy category C) and lactation.

Phenazopyridine treats the symptom of pain but does not treat the cause of the disorder. No significant interactions have been reported.

ALERT

Phenazopyridine

When used in combination with an antibacterial drug to treat a urinary tract infection, phenazopyridine should not be administered for more than 2 days, because it may mask the symptoms of a more serious disorder.

Tolterodine

Tolterodine is contraindicated in patients with urinary retention (inability to urinate), gastric retention, uncontrolled narrow-angle glaucoma, or hypersensitivity to the drug. Tolterodine is used with caution in patients with significant bladder outflow blockage or slow urinary stream, pyloric stenosis (a narrowing of the opening where the stomach contents are emptied into the small intestine), or liver or kidney disease. This drug is classified as a pregnancy category C drug and should not be used during pregnancy or lactation. No significant interactions have been reported.

Patient Management Issues with Urinary Anti-Infectives and Miscellaneous Urinary Drugs

When a urinary tract infection is diagnosed, sensitivity tests are performed to determine bacterial sensitivity to drugs (antibiotics and urinary anti-infectives) that may control the infection. The color and appearance of the patient's urine and vital signs are recorded, and a urine sample is obtained for culture and sensitivity before the first dose of the drug is given.

When the miscellaneous drugs are administered, patient symptoms such as pain, urinary frequency, and bladder distension are recorded to provide a baseline for future assessment.

Many urinary tract infections are treated on an outpatient basis, and hospitalization usually is not required. Urinary tract infections may occur in hospitalized or nursing home patients with an indwelling urethral catheter or a disorder such as a stone in the urinary tract.

The vital signs of a hospitalized patient with a urinary tract infection are taken every 4 hours or as ordered by the health care provider. Any significant rise in temperature is reported, because it may be necessary to reduce the fever or repeat the culture and sensitivity tests.

The patient's response to therapy is monitored daily. If after several days the symptoms have not improved or have become worse, then the health care provider is notified as soon as possible. Periodic urinalysis and urine culture and sensitivity tests may be ordered to monitor the effects of drug therapy.

When any of the miscellaneous drugs are administered, the patient is monitored for a reduction in symptoms such as dysuria (painful or difficult urination), urinary frequency, urgency, nocturia (excessive urination at night), and relief of pain associated with irritation of the lower urinary tract.

Educating the Patient and Family About Urinary Anti-infectives and Miscellaneous Urinary Drugs

Patient Education Box 20-1 includes key points about urinary anti-infectives and miscellaneous urinary drugs that the patient and family members should know.

Natural Remedies: Cranberry

Cranberry juice has long been recommended for preventing and treating urinary tract infections. Clinical studies have confirmed that cranberry juice is beneficial to individuals with frequent urinary tract infections. Cranberries inhibit bacteria from attaching to the walls of the urinary tract and prevent certain bacteria from forming dental plaque in the mouth. Cranberry juice is safe for use as a food and for urinary tract health. Cranberry juice and capsules have no contraindications, no known adverse reactions, and no drug interactions. The recommended dosage is 9 to 15 capsules per day (400–500 mg/d) or 4 to 8 ounces of juice per day. (See Chapter 25 for more information.)

Although cranberry may help to prevent the occurrence and relieve the symptoms of a urinary tract infection, no evidence suggests it works as a cure. If a urinary tract infection is thought to be present, then it is necessary to seek medical treatment.

PATIENT EDUCATION BOX 20-1

Key Points for Patients Taking Urinary Anti-infectives and Miscellaneous Urinary Drugs

- ❑ Take the drug with food or meals (nitrofurantoin must be taken with food or milk). If you experience stomach upset despite taking the drug with food, contact your health care provider.
- ❑ Take the drug at the prescribed intervals and complete the full course of therapy. Do not stop taking the drug when your symptoms disappear unless directed to do so by your health care provider.
- ❑ Continue therapy until all of drug is finished or until your health care provider discontinues the therapy.
- ❑ Try to drink fluids every hour. Drinking extra fluids aids in the physical removal of bacteria from your urinary tract and is an important part of treatment. When your fluid intake is increased, your urine should appear clear or barely yellow.
- ❑ Continue your increased fluid intake even when your symptoms subside.
- ❑ Notify your health care provider if your urine output is low, your urine appears dark or concentrated during the daytime, or your symptoms do not improve after 3 to 4 days.
- ❑ If you are elderly, you may have a decreased thirst sensation, but it is important nonetheless to increase fluid intake.
- ❑ If you experience drowsiness or dizziness, avoid driving and performing tasks that require alertness.
- ❑ During therapy with this drug, do not drink alcoholic beverages and do not take any nonprescription drug unless your health care provider approves it.
- ❑ Nitrofurantoin: Take this drug with food or milk to improve absorption. Continue therapy for at least 1 week or for 3 days after the urine shows no signs of infection. Notify your health care provider immediately if you experience any of the following: fever, chills, cough, shortness of breath, chest pain, or difficulty breathing. Do not take the next dose of the drug until you talk with your health care provider. The urine may appear brown during therapy with this drug; this is not abnormal.
- ❑ Nalidixic acid: Take this drug with food to prevent stomach upset. Avoid prolonged exposure to sunlight or ultraviolet light (tanning beds or lamps) because exaggerated sunburn may occur.
- ❑ Methenamine, methenamine salts: Avoid excessive intake of citrus products, milk, and milk products.
- ❑ Fosfomycin comes in dry form as a one-dose packet to be dissolved in 90 to 120 mL water (not hot water). Drink it immediately after mixing with food to prevent gastric upset.

MISCELLANEOUS DRUGS

- ❑ For dry mouth, suck on hard candy, sugarless lozenges, or small pieces of ice, and brush your teeth regularly.

PATIENT EDUCATION BOX 20-1

❏ These drugs may cause drowsiness or blurred vision. Do not drive or operate dangerous machinery or participate in any activity that requires full mental alertness until you know how the medication affects you.

❏ If you experience constipation, drink plenty of fluids, eat a high-fiber diet, and exercise (if your condition allows). If constipation persists, your health care provider may prescribe a mild laxative or stool softener.

❏ Flavoxate: Take this drug three to four times daily as prescribed. This drug is used only to treat symptoms; other drugs are given to treat the cause.

❏ Oxybutynin: Take this drug with or without food. Oxybutynin (Ditropan XL) contains an outer coating that may not disintegrate and which may be seen in the stool. This is not a cause for concern. This drug can cause heat prostration (fever and heat stroke caused by decreased sweating) in high temperatures. If you live in a hot climate or will be exposed to high temperatures, take appropriate precautions.

❏ Phenazopyridine: This drug may cause a red–orange discoloration of the urine and may stain fabrics or contact lenses. This is normal. Take the drug after meals. Do not take this drug for more than 2 days if you are also taking an antibiotic for the treatment of a urinary tract infection.

❏ Tolterodine: If you experience difficulty voiding, take the drug immediately after voiding. If urinating is difficult or your pain persists, notify your health care provider.

KEY POINTS

◉ A urinary tract infection is an infection caused by pathogenic microorganisms of one or more structures of the urinary tract. The most common structure affected is the bladder, with the urethra, prostate, and kidney also affected.

◉ Anti-infectives are used in the treatment of urinary tract infections and have an effect on bacteria in the urinary tract. Taken orally or by parenteral route, they do not achieve significant levels in the bloodstream and are of no value in the treatment of systemic infections.

◉ Examples of urinary anti-infectives include cinoxacin (Cinobac), fosfomycin (Monurol), methenamine mandelate (Mandelamine), nalidixic acid (NegGram), and nitrofurantoin (Furadantin). Each drug works best on certain strains of bacteria. When a urinary tract infection is diagnosed, sensitivity tests are performed to determine bacterial sensitivity to drugs (antibiotics and urinary anti-infectives) that may control the infection.

◉ When any of these drugs is administered, the patient is monitored for a reduction in symptoms such as dysuria, urinary frequency, urgency, nocturia, and relief of any pain associated with irritation of the lower urinary tract.

CASE STUDY

Mr. Elliott, 42 years old, had a urinary tract infection 8 weeks ago. He failed to see his health care provider for a follow-up urine sample 2 weeks after completing his course of drug therapy. Mr. Elliot is now seeing his health care provider because his symptoms of a urinary tract infection have recurred. The health care provider suspects that Mr. Elliott may not have followed treatment instructions.

1. What course of action is taken to determine whether Mr. Elliott's urinary tract infection has recurred?
   a. a review of symptoms
   b. laboratory testing of a urine sample
   c. ask Mr. Elliott whether he completed the full course of drug therapy
   d. all of the above

2. Mr. Elliott is confirmed to have a urinary tract infection. What information should be reviewed with Mr. Elliott to ensure successful treatment?
   a. drink plenty of fluids until the pain subsides
   b. drink plenty of fluids throughout the course of treatment
   c. emphasize the importance of follow-up visits and laboratory tests
   d. b and c

3. Mr. Elliott asks about the effectiveness of cranberry juice for treating urinary tract infections. He is told:
   a. clinical studies confirm its effectiveness in treating and preventing urinary tract infections
   b. cranberry juice is a reliable substitute for drug therapy
   c. cranberry juice is effective in the treatment of dental plaque in the mouth but has little therapeutic value for urinary tract infections
   d. none of the above

WEBSITE ACTIVITIES

1. Go to the NIH website (www.niddk.nih.gov) and in the search box at the top of the screen, enter "Urinary Tract Infections in Children" to find the article with that title. Scan this article for information on the potential long-term effects of urinary tract infections in children. What serious problem can result from untreated UTIs?

2. Continuing with this article, what two sources are suggested for more information on urinary tract infections in children?

REVIEW QUESTIONS

1. Nitrofurantoin (Macrodantin) is best taken:
   a. with food
   b. no longer than 7 days
   c. without regard to food
   d. no longer than 2 days

2. When taking methenamine (Mandelamine), the patient is advised to:
   a. use an antacid before taking the drug
   b. take an antacid immediately after taking the drug
   c. avoid antacids containing sodium bicarbonate or sodium carbonate
   d. avoid the use of antacids 1 hour before or 2 hours after taking the drug

3. What instruction would be most important to give a patient prescribed fosfomycin (Monurol)?
   a. drink one to two glasses of cranberry juice daily to promote healing of the urinary tract
   b. you may take the drug without regard to meals
   c. this drug comes in a one-dose packet that must be dissolved in 90 mL or more of fluids
   d. this drug may cause mental confusion

4. Which of the following would be included in information provided a patient taking phenazopyridine (Pyridium)?
   a. there is a danger of heat prostration or heat stroke when taking phenazopyridine in a hot climate
   b. this drug may turn the urine dark brown, which is an indication of a serious condition and should be reported immediately
   c. this drug may cause photosensitivity; take precautions when out in the sun by wearing sunscreen, a hat, and long-sleeved shirts for protection
   d. this drug may turn the urine red–orange; this is a normal occurrence that will disappear when the drug is discontinued

5. Which of the following are potential side effects of Ditropan?
   a. arrhythmia
   b. yellow discoloration of the skin
   c. blurred vision
   d. photosensitivity

21 Drugs That Affect the Gastrointestinal System

KEY TERMS

antacids—drugs that neutralize or reduce the acidity of stomach and duodenal contents
antiflatulents—drugs that remove flatus or gas in the intestinal tract
emetic—a drug that induces vomiting
gallstone-solubilizing—gallstone-dissolving
gastric stasis—failure to move food normally out of the stomach
gastroesophageal reflux disease—a reflux or backup of gastric contents into the esophagus
Helicobacter pylori—bacteria that causes a type of chronic gastritis and peptic and duodenal ulcers
hydrochloric acid—a substance the stomach secretes that aids in the digestive process
hypersecretory—excessive gastric secretion of hydrochloric acid
paralytic ileus—lack of peristalsis or movement of the intestines
photophobia—aversion to bright lights
proton pump inhibitors—drugs with antisecretory properties

CHAPTER OBJECTIVES

On completion of this chapter, students will be able to:

1 Define the chapter's key terms.

2 Describe the general drug actions, uses, adverse reactions, contraindications, precautions, and interactions of drugs that affect the gastrointestinal system.

3 Discuss important points to keep in mind when educating the patient or family members about the use of drugs that affect the gastrointestinal system.

The gastrointestinal tract is subject to more diseases and disorders than any other body system. Some drugs used for gastrointestinal tract disorders are available as nonprescription drugs, potentially leading to problems of misuse and overuse and the disguising of more serious medical problems.

The drugs presented in this chapter include antacids, anticholinergics, gastrointestinal tract stimulants, proton pump inhibitors, histamine H₂ antagonists, antidiarrheals, antiflatulents, digestive enzymes, emetics, gallstone-solubilizing drugs, laxatives, and miscellaneous drugs. Some of the more common preparations are listed in the Summary Drug Table: Drugs Used in the Management of Gastrointestinal Disorders.

Antacids

Actions of Antacids

Some of the cells of the stomach secrete **hydrochloric acid**, a substance that aids in the initial digestive process. **Antacids** (against acids) neutralize or reduce the acidity of stomach and duodenal contents by combining with hydrochloric acid and producing salt and water. Examples of antacids include aluminum hydroxide gel (Amphojel), magaldrate (Riopan), and magnesia or magnesium hydroxide (Milk of Magnesia).

Uses of Antacids

Antacids are used in the treatment of hyperacidity problems such as heartburn, gastroesophageal reflux, sour stomach, acid indigestion, and in the medical treatment of peptic ulcer (Fig. 21-1). Many antacid preparations contain more than one ingredient. Additional uses for aluminum carbonate are the treatment of hyperphosphatemia (abnormally high concentration of phosphates in the circulating blood) and use with a low-phosphate diet to prevent formation of phosphate urinary stones. Calcium carbonate is also used in treating calcium deficiency states such as menopausal osteoporosis. Magnesium oxide may be used in the treatment of magnesium deficiencies or magnesium depletion from malnutrition, restricted diet, or alcoholism.

Adverse Reactions of Antacids

The magnesium- and sodium-containing antacids may have a laxative effect and produce diarrhea. Aluminum- and calcium-containing products tend to produce constipation. Some of the less common but more serious adverse reactions include:

- **Aluminum-containing antacids:** constipation, intestinal impaction, anorexia, weakness, tremors, and bone pain
- **Magnesium-containing antacids:** severe diarrhea, dehydration, and hypermagnesemia (nausea, vomiting, hypotension, decreased respirations)
- **Calcium-containing antacids:** rebound hyperacidity, metabolic alkalosis, hypercalcemia, vomiting, confusion, headache, renal calculi, and neurologic impairment
- **Sodium bicarbonate:** systemic alkalosis and rebound hypersecretion

Although antacids have the potential for serious adverse reactions, they have a wide margin of safety, especially when used as prescribed.

(text continued on page 306)

SUMMARY DRUG TABLE   Drugs Used in the Management of Gastrointestinal Disorders

Generic Name	Trade Name*	Uses	Dosage Ranges
Proton Pump Inhibitors esomeprazole magnesium *ess-oh-me'-pra-zol*	Nexium	Erosive esophagitis, gastroesophageal reflux disease (GERD), long-term treatment of pathologic hypersecretory conditions	20–40 mg/d PO
lansoprazole *lan-soe'-pra-zole*	Prevacid	Duodenal ulcer, *H. pylori* eradication in patients with duodenal ulcer, gastric ulcer, erosive esophagitis, GERD, hypersecretory conditions	15–30 mg/d PO
omeprazole *oh-me'-pra-zol*	Prilosec	Duodenal ulcer, *H. pylori* eradication, hypersecretory conditions, gastric ulcer, erosive esophagitis, GERD, hypersecretory conditions	20–40 mg/d PO; 60 mg/d up to 120 mg TID
pantoprazole sodium *pan-toe'-pray-zol*	Protonix, Protonix IV	GERD	40 mg PO daily to BID up to 120 mg/d; IV, 80 mg; maximum dosage 240 mg/d
rabeprazole sodium *rah-beh'-pray-zol*	Aciphex	Duodenal ulcer, GERD, hypersecretory conditions	2–60 mg/d
Miscellaneous Gastrointestinal Drugs bismuth subsalicylate	Bis Matrol Pepto-Bismol, Pink Bismuth	Nausea, diarrhea, abdominal cramps, *H. pylori* with duodenal ulcer	2 tablets or 30 mL PO q 30 min–1 h up to 8 doses in 24 h
balsalazide disodium *bal-sal'-a-zyde*	Colazal	Ulcerative colitis	3 750-mg capsules PO TID for 8 wk
infliximab *in-flicks'-ih-mab*	Remicade	Crohn disease, rheumatoid arthritis	RA: 3 mg/kg IV; Crohn disease: 5 mg/kg IV
mesalamine *me-sal'-a-meen*	Asacol, Rowasa, *generic*	Treatment of active to moderate ulcerative colitis, proctosigmoiditis, or proctitis	Suspension enema: 4 g once daily in 60 mL; rectal suppository: 500 mg (1 suppository) BID; oral: 800 mg TID PO
misoprostol *mye-soe-prost'-ole*	Cytotec	Prevention of gastric ulcers caused by aspirin or NSAID use (unlabeled use)	100–200 μg QID PO

Generic Name	Trade Name*	Uses	Dosage Ranges
olsalazine *ole-sal'-a-zeen*	Dipentum	Maintenance of remission of ulcerative colitis in patients intolerant of sulfasalazine	1 g/d in two divided doses PO
sucralfate *soo-kral'-fate*	Carafate, *generic*	Active duodenal ulcer	1 g/d PO in divided doses
sulfasalazine *sul-fa-sal'-a-zeen*	Azulfidine, *generic*	Ulcerative colitis, rheumatoid arthritis	1 g QID PO
Antacids aluminum carbonate gel, basic *a-loo'-mi-num*	Basaljel		2 tablets or capsules or 10 mL of regular suspension (in water or fruit juice) or 5 mL of extra strength suspension as often as every 2 h, up to 12 times daily
aluminum hydroxide gel	Alu-Tab, Amphojel, Dialume, *generic*		Tablets or capsules: 500–1500 mg 3–6 times daily PO between meals and HS; suspension: 5–15 mL as needed between meals and HS PO
calcium carbonate *kal'-see-um*	Chooz, Tums, *generic*		0.5–12 g PO as needed
magaldrate (hydroxymagnesium aluminate) *mag'-al-drate*	Riopan, *generic*		980–1080 mg PO 1 and 3 hours after meals and HS
magnesia (magnesium hydroxide) *mag-nee'-zee-ah*	Milk of Magnesia, Phillips' Chewable		Liquid: 5–15 mL PO QID with water; tablets: 650 mg–1.3 g QID PO; laxative: 15–60 mL PO taken with liquid
magnesium oxide *mag-nee'-zee-um*	Mag-Ox 400, Maox 420, Uro-mag, *generic*		Capsules: 280 mg–1.5 g QID PO; tablets: 400–820 mg/d PO
sodium bicarbonate *sow-dee'-um*	Bell/ans, *generic*		0.3–2 g 1–4 times daily PO
Anticholinergics belladonna	*Generic*		Tincture: 0.6–1 mL TID–QID
clindinium bromide *klin-din'-ee-um*	Quarzan		2.5–5 mg PO TID–QID AC and HS geriatric or debilitated patients: 2.5 mg TID AC
dicyclomine HCl *dye-sye-klo'-meen*	Bentyl, Di-Spasz, *generic*		Oral: 80–160 mg/d in 4 doses PO; parenteral: 80 mg/d IM

Generic Name	Trade Name*	Uses	Dosage Ranges
glycopyrrolate *gly-ko-pie'-roll-ate*	Robinul, Robinul Forte, *generic*		Oral: 1 mg TID or 2 mg BID–TID PO; parenteral: 0.1–0.2 mg IM or IV TID–QID
1-hyoscyamine sulfate *el-hi'-o-si-ah-meen*	Anaspaz, Donnamar, Levbid, Levsin		Oral: 0.125–0.25 mg PO TID–QID PO or sublingually; sustained release: 0.375–0.75 mg q12h PO; parenteral: 0.25–0.5 mg SC, IM, IV BID–QID
mepenzolate bromide *me-pin-zo'-late*	Cantil		25–50 mg QID with meals and HS
methantheline bromide *meth-an'-tha-leen*	Banthine, *generic*		Adult: 50–100 mg PO q6h
methscopolamine bromide *meth-sco-pol'-a-meen*	Pamine		2.5 mg 30 min AC and 2.5–5 mg HS PO
propantheline bromide *proe-pan'-the-leen*	Pro-Banthine, *generic*		15 mg PO 30 min AC and HS
tridihexethyl chloride *tri-di-hex'-eth-l*	Pathilon		25–50 mg TID–QID AC and 50 mg HS PO
Gastrointestinal Stimulants dexpanthenol *dex-pan'-the-nole*	Ilopan, *generic*		250–500 mg IM, IV
metoclopramide *met-oh-kloe-pra'-mide*	Reglan, *generic*		10–15 mg PO 30 min AC and HS; 10–20 mg IM, IV
Histamine H₂ Antagonists cimetidine *sye-met'-i-deen*	Tagamet, Tagamet HB, *generic*		300–2400 mg/d PO; 300 mg q6h IM, IV; 50 mg/h continuous IV infusion
famotidine *fa-moe'-ti-deen*	Pepcid, Pepcid IV, *generic*		20–40 mg PO, IV as one dose or BID
nizatidine *ni-za'-ti-deen*	Axid Pulvules		Gastric or duodenal ulcer: 300 mg/d PO HS or 150 mg BID PO; maintenance of healed ulcer: 150 mg/d PO HS; heartburn: 75 mg PO 30 min–1 h before food or beverages that cause the problem, taken with water
ranitidine *ra-nye'-te-deen*	Zantac		150 mg PO BID or 300 mg PO HS; 50 mg q6–8h IM, IV (do not exceed 400 mg/d)

Generic Name	Trade Name*	Uses	Dosage Ranges
Antidiarrheals difenoxin HCl with atropine *dye-fen-ox'-in a'-troe-peen*	Motofen		Initial dose 2 tablets PO, then 1 tablet after each loose stool (no more than 8 mg/d for no more than 2 days)
diphenoxylate HCl with atropine *di-fen-ox'-i'-late*	Lomotil, Lonox, *generic*		Initial dose 5 mg PO TID–QID as needed

loperamide HCl
loe-per'-a-mide
	Imodium A-D, Kaopectate
	  II, Maalox Anti-Diarrheal
	  caplets, *generic*
			Initial dose 4 mg PO then 2
			mg after each loose stool
			(no more than 16 mg/d)

Antiflatulents charcoal *char'-kole*	Liqui-Char, *generic*		520 mg PO after meals or at the first sign of discomfort (up to 4.16 g/d)
simethicone *sigh-meth'-ih-kohn*	Gas-X, Mylicon, *generic*		Capsules: 125 mg PO QID PC and HS; tablets: 40–125 mg PO QID PC and HS; drops: 40–80 mg PO QID PC and HS (up to 500 mg/d)
Digestive Enzymes pancreatin *pan-kre-at'-in*	Creon, Digepepsin, Donnazyme		1–2 tablets PO with meals or snacks

pancrelipase
pan-kre-li'-pase
	Cotazym Capsules,
	  Viokase Powder,
	  Ilozyme tablets
			4000–48,000 lipase PO with
			meals and snacks; usually
			1–3 capsules or tablets be-
			fore or with meals and
			snacks

Emetics apomorphine HCl *a-po-mor'-feen*	*Generic*		2–10 mg SC; do not repeat
ipecac syrup *ip'-e-kak*	*Generic*		15–30 mL PO, followed by 3–4 glasses of water; chil- dren's dosage based on age: 5–15 mL PO followed by 0.5–3 glasses of water
Gallstone-Solubilizing Agent ursodiol *ur-soe-dye'-ole*	Actigall, *generic*		8–10 mg/kg/d PO in 2–3 divided doses
Laxatives *Saline Laxatives* magnesium preparations *mag-nez'-e-um*	Epsom Salt, Milk of Magnesia		Follow directions given on the container

Generic Name	Trade Name*	Uses	Dosage Ranges
Irritant or Stimulant Laxatives			
cascara sagrada *kas-kar'-a-sa-grad'-a*	Aromatic Cascara, *generic*		Follow directions given on the container
sennosides *sen-oh-sides*	Agoral, Ex-Lax, Senexon, Senna-Gel, Senokot		Follow directions given on the container
bisacodyl *bis-a-koe'-dill*	Bisca-Evac, Dulcolax, Modane		Tablets: 10–15 mg daily PO Suppositories: 10 mg once daily
Bulk-Producing Laxatives			
psyllium *sill'-I-um*	Fiberall Tropical Fruit Flavor, Genfiber, Hydrocil Instant, Konsyl, Metamucil, Serutan		Follow directions on the container
polycarbophil *pol-i-kar'-boe-fil*	Equalactin, FiberCon, Mitrolan		1250 mg 1 to 4 times daily or as needed (do not exceed 5 g in 24 h)
Emollients			
mineral oil	Kondremul Plain, Milkinol, *generic*		15–45 mL PO at HS
Fecal Softeners/Surfactants			
docusate sodium (dioctyl sodium sulfosuccinate: DDS) *dok'-yoo-sate*	Colace, D-S-S, Ex-Lax Stool Softener, Modane Soft, *generic*		Follow directions on the container
docusate calcium (dioctyl calcium sulfosuccinate) *dok'-yoo-sate*	Surfak Liquigels, *generic*		240 mg/d until bowel move- ments are normal
Hyperosmotic Agents			
glycerin *gli'-ser-in*	Colace Suppositories, Sani-Supp, *generic*		Suppositories: insert 1 high in the rectum and retain 15 min; rectal liquid: insert all the liquid into rectum to- ward the navel
lactulose *lak-tyoo-los*	Chronulac, Constilac, Duphalac, *generic*		10–60 mL/d PO
Bowel Evacuants			
polyethylene glycol-electrolyte solution (PEG-ES) *pol-e-eth-i-leen*	CoLyte, GoLYTELY, NuLytely, OCL, *generic*		4 L oral solution before GI examination (do not give solid foods within 2 h be- fore administration)
polyethylene glycol (PEG) solution	MiraLax		17 g of powder/d in 8 oz of water (48–72 h may be re- quired to produce a bowel movement)

*The term *generic* indicates the drug is available in generic form.

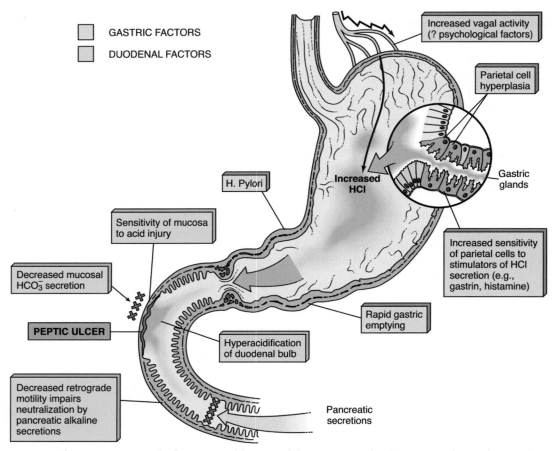

GASTRIC FACTORS

DUODENAL FACTORS

Increased vagal activity
(? psychological factors)

Parietal cell
hyperplasia

Increased
HCl

Gastric
glands

H. Pylori

Sensitivity of mucosa
to acid injury

Increased sensitivity
of parietal cells to
stimulators of HCl
secretion (e.g.,
gastrin, histamine)

Decreased mucosal
HCO₃⁻ secretion

Rapid gastric
emptying

PEPTIC ULCER

Hyperacidification
of duodenal bulb

Decreased retrograde
motility impairs
neutralization by
pancreatic alkaline
secretions

Pancreatic
secretions

FIGURE 21-1 A peptic ulcer is an erosion and inflammation of the stomach lining. (Reprinted with permission from Rubin E, Farber JL. Pathology, 3rd ed. Philadelphia: Lippincott Williams & Wilkins, 1999.)

Managing Adverse Reactions of Antacids

When antacids are given, the patient's bowel movements should be monitored because these drugs may cause constipation or diarrhea. If a hospitalized patient experiences diarrhea, then an accurate record of fluid intake and output is kept along with a description of the diarrhea stool. Changing to a different antacid usually alleviates the problem. Diarrhea may be controlled by combining a magnesium antacid with an antacid containing aluminum or calcium.

Contraindications, Precautions, and Interactions of Antacids

Antacids are contraindicated in patients with severe abdominal pain of unknown cause and during lactation. Sodium-containing antacids are contraindicated in patients with cardiovascular problems, such as hypertension or congestive heart failure, and in patients on sodium-restricted diets. Calcium-containing antacids are contraindicated in patients with renal calculi or hypercalcemia.

Aluminum-containing antacids are used cautiously in patients with gastric outlet obstruction. Magnesium- and aluminum-containing antacids are used cautiously in patients with decreased kidney function. Calcium-containing antacids are used cautiously in patients with respiratory insufficiency, renal impairment, or cardiac disease. Antacids are classified as pregnancy category C drugs and should be used with caution during pregnancy.

Antacids may interfere with other drugs in three ways:

1. By increasing the gastric pH, which causes a decrease in absorption of weakly acidic drugs and results in a decreased drug effect (e.g., digoxin, phenytoin, chlorpromazine, and isoniazid)
2. By absorbing or binding drugs to their surface, resulting in a decrease in the amount of drug being absorbed into the bloodstream (e.g., tetracycline)
3. By affecting the rate of drug elimination by increasing urinary pH (e.g., the excretion of salicylates is increased, whereas excretion of quinidine and amphetamines is decreased)

The following drugs have a decreased pharmacologic effect when administered with an antacid: corticosteroids, digoxin, chlorpromazine, oral iron products, isoniazid, phenothiazines, ranitidine, phenytoin, valproic acid, and tetracyclines.

Anticholinergics

Actions of Anticholinergics

Anticholinergics (cholinergic blocking drugs) reduce gastric motility and decrease the amount of acid secreted by the stomach (see Chapter 4). Examples of anticholinergics used for gastrointestinal tract disorders include propantheline (Pro-Banthine) and glycopyrrolate (Robinul).

Uses of Anticholinergics

Specific anticholinergic drugs are occasionally used in the medical treatment of peptic ulcer. These drugs have been largely replaced by histamine H_2 antagonists, which appear to be more effective and have fewer adverse drug reactions.

Adverse Reactions of Anticholinergics

Dry mouth, blurred vision, urinary hesitancy, urinary retention, nausea, vomiting, palpitations, and headache are some of the adverse reactions that may occur with anticholinergic drugs (see Chapter 4).

Managing Adverse Reactions of Anticholinergics

Urinary retention or hesitancy may occur during therapy with these drugs. The patient can prevent this problem by voiding before taking the drug. If urinary retention is suspected, then fluid intake and output are monitored. These drugs also may cause drowsiness, dizziness, and blurred vision, which may interfere with activities such as reading or watching television. If dizziness occurs, the patient will need help with walking and self-care activities. If **photophobia** (aversion to bright light) occurs, then the room may be kept semidark.

Contraindications, Precautions, and Interactions of Anticholinergic Drugs

Contraindications, precautions, and interactions of anticholinergic drugs are discussed in Chapter 4.

Gastrointestinal Stimulants

Actions of Gastrointestinal Stimulants

Metoclopramide (Reglan) and dexpanthenol (Ilopan) increase the strength of the spontaneous movement of the upper gastrointestinal tract. The exact mode of action of these drugs is unclear.

Uses of Gastrointestinal Stimulants

Oral preparations of metoclopramide are used in the treatment of symptomatic **gastroesophageal reflux disease** (a reflux or backup of gastric contents into the esophagus) and **gastric stasis** (failure to move food normally out of the stomach) in patients with diabetes. This drug is given intravenously to prevent nausea and vomiting associated with cancer chemotherapy and to prevent nausea and vomiting during the immediate postoperative period. Dexpanthenol may be given intravenously immediately after major abdominal surgery to reduce the risk of **paralytic ileus** (lack of peristalsis or movement of the intestines).

Adverse Reactions of Gastrointestinal Stimulants

The adverse reactions of metoclopramide are usually mild. Higher doses or prolonged administration may produce central nervous system symptoms, such as drowsiness, dizziness, Parkinson-like symptoms (tremor, mask-like facial expression, muscle rigidity), depression, facial grimacing, motor restlessness, and involuntary movements of the eyes, face, or limbs. Dexpanthenol administration may cause itching, difficulty breathing, and urticaria.

Managing Adverse Reactions of Gastrointestinal Stimulants

If drowsiness or dizziness occurs when taking metoclopramide, then the patient will need help walking and with self-care activities. Patients receiving high or prolonged doses of this drug should be monitored for adverse reactions related to the central nervous system (extrapyramidal reactions or tardive dyskinesia, see Chapter 5). Any sign of extrapyramidal reaction or tardive dyskinesia should be reported to the health care provider before the next dose of metoclopramide is taken, because the drug therapy may be discontinued. These reactions are irreversible if therapy is continued.

Dexpanthenol is administered to prevent a lack of intestinal movement immediately postoperative. If a lack of intestinal movement occurs, then bowel sounds will be diminished or absent, and dexpanthenol may be taken. Adverse reactions, such as nausea, vomiting, diarrhea, and a slight drop in blood pressure, may occur. A common adverse reaction is intestinal colic that may occur within 30 minutes after administration of the drug.

Contraindications, Precautions, and Interactions of Gastrointestinal Stimulants

Gastrointestinal tract stimulants are contraindicated in patients with a known hypersensitivity, gastrointestinal tract obstruction, gastric perforation or hemorrhage, or epilepsy. These drugs are secreted in breast milk and should not be used during lactation, and are used cautiously in patients with diabetes and cardiovascular disease. Metoclopramide is a pregnancy category B drug; dexpanthenol is a pregnancy category C drug.

The effects of metoclopramide are compromised by concurrent administration of anticholinergics or narcotic analgesics. Metoclopramide may decrease the absorption of digoxin and cimetidine and increase absorption of acetaminophen, tetracyclines, and levodopa. Metoclopramide may alter the body's insulin requirements.

Histamine H₂ Antagonists

Actions of Histamine H₂ Antagonists

These drugs inhibit the action of histamine at histamine H₂ receptor cells of the stomach, which then reduces the secretion of gastric acid and reduces total pepsin output. The decrease in acid allows ulcerated areas to heal. Examples of histamine H₂ antagonists include cimetidine (Tagamet), famotidine (Pepcid), nizatidine (Axid Pulvules), and ranitidine (Zantac).

Uses of Histamine H₂ Antagonists

Histamine H₂ antagonists are used for the medical treatment of gastric and duodenal ulcers, gastric **hypersecretory** (excessive gastric secretion of hydrochloric acid) conditions, and gastroesophageal reflux disease. These drugs may also be used to prevent stress-related ulcers and acute upper gastrointestinal tract bleeding in critically ill patients.

Adverse Reactions of Histamine H₂ Antagonists

Adverse reactions of the histamine H₂ antagonists include dizziness, somnolence (a tendency to sleep), headache, confusion, hallucinations, diarrhea, and impotence (reversible when the drug is discontinued). Adverse reactions are usually mild and transient.

Managing Adverse Reactions of Histamine H₂ Antagonists

During early therapy with these drugs, the patient may experience dizziness or drowsiness and may require help walking and with self-care activities. These reactions usually must be tolerated, but they will disappear after several days of therapy.

Adverse reactions, such as skin rash, sore throat, fever, unusual bleeding, or hallucinations, should be reported immediately, because the health care provider may want to discontinue the drug therapy.

ALERT

Older Adults and H₂ Antagonists

Older adults are particularly sensitive to the effects of the histamine H₂ antagonists. Older adults must be carefully monitored for confusion and dizziness. Dizziness increases the risk for falls.

These patients often need help walking and with self-care activities. Throw rugs or small pieces of furniture should be removed. Any change in the patient's orientation should be reported to the health care provider.

Contraindications, Precautions, and Interactions of Histamine H₂ Antagonists

Histamine H₂ antagonists are contraindicated in patients with a known hypersensitivity. These drugs are used cautiously in patients with renal or hepatic impairment and in severely ill or debilitated patients. Cimetidine is used cautiously in patients with diabetes. Histamine H₂ antagonists are used cautiously in older adults because they may cause confusion, and a dosage reduction may be required. Histamine antagonists are pregnancy category B (cimetidine, famotidine, and ranitidine) drugs or pregnancy category C (nizatidine) drugs and should be used with caution during pregnancy and lactation.

Many drugs may interact with the H₂ antagonists, but only some of the more common interactions can be described here. Antacids and metoclopramide may decrease absorption of H₂ antagonists if administered concurrently. Concurrent use of cimetidine and digoxin may decrease serum digoxin levels. The patient may have a decreased white blood cell count when an H₂ an antagonist is administered along with an alkylating drugs or antimetabolite. The patient has an increased risk for toxicity of oral anticoagulants, phenytoin, quinidine, lidocaine, or theophylline when administered with H₂ antagonists. Concurrent use of cimetidine and morphine increases the risk of respiratory depression.

Antidiarrheals

Actions of Antidiarrheals

Antidiarrheals decrease intestinal peristalsis, which is usually increased in a patient with diarrhea. Examples of these drugs include difenoxin with atropine (Motofen), diphenoxylate with atropine (Lomotil), and loperamide (Imodium).

Uses of Antidiarrheals

Antidiarrheals are used in the treatment of diarrhea.

Adverse Reactions of Antidiarrheals

Diphenoxylate use may result in anorexia, nausea, vomiting, constipation, rash, dizziness, drowsiness, sedation, euphoria, and headache. This is a narcotic-related drug that has no analgesic activity but has sedative and euphoric effects and a potential for drug dependence. To discourage abuse, it is combined with atropine (an anticholinergic or cholinergic blocking drug), which causes dry mouth and other mild adverse reactions. Loperamide is not a narcotic-related drug, and minimal adverse reactions are associated with its use. Occasionally, abdominal discomfort, pain, and distention occur, but these symptoms also occur with severe diarrhea and are difficult to distinguish from an adverse drug reaction.

Managing Adverse Reactions of Antidiarrheals

If the patient has an elevated temperature, severe abdominal pain, or abdominal rigidity or distention, then the health care provider should be notified immediately because this may indicate a complication of the disorder, such as infection or intestinal perforation. If diarrhea is severe, then additional treatment measures, such as intravenous fluids and electrolyte replacement, may be necessary.

Drowsiness or dizziness may occur, and the patient may need help walking and with self-care activities. For chronic diarrhea, the patient is encouraged to drink extra fluids. Fluids such as weak tea, water, bouillon, or a commercial electrolyte preparation may be used. Fluid intake and output should be closely monitored. In some instances, the health care provider may prescribe an oral electrolyte supplement to replace electrolytes lost by frequent loose stools. For perianal irritation caused by loose stools, the area may be cleaned with mild soap and water after each bowel movement, dried with a soft cloth, and an emollient applied, such as petrolatum.

Contraindications, Precautions, and Interactions of Antidiarrheals

These drugs are contraindicated in patients whose diarrhea is associated with organisms that can harm the intestinal mucosa (*Escherichia coli*, *Salmonella*, *Shigella*) and in patients with pseudomembranous colitis, abdominal pain of unknown origin, or obstructive jaundice. Antidiarrheals are contraindicated in children younger than 2 years.

Antidiarrheals are used cautiously in patients with severe liver disease or inflammatory bowel disease. Antidiarrheals are classified as pregnancy category B drugs and should be used cautiously during pregnancy and lactation.

Antidiarrheals cause an additive central nervous system depression when administered with alcohol, antihistamines, narcotics, and sedatives or hypnotics. The patient has additive cholinergic effects when they are administered with other drugs having anticholinergic activity, such as antidepressants or antihistamines. Concurrent use of an antidiarrheal with a monoamine oxidase inhibitor increases the risk of a hypertensive crisis.

Antiflatulents

Actions of Antiflatulents

Simethicone (Mylicon) and charcoal are used as **antiflatulents** (reducing flatus or gas in the intestinal tract). Simethicone has a defoaming action that disperses and prevents the formation of mucus-surrounded gas pockets in the intestine. Charcoal is an absorbent that reduces the amount of intestinal gas.

Uses of Antiflatulents

Antiflatulents are used for the relief of painful symptoms of excess gas in the digestive tract. These drugs are useful as adjunctive treatment for any condition in which gas retention is a problem (e.g., postoperative gaseous distention, air swallowing, dyspepsia, peptic ulcer, irritable colon, or diverticulosis). Charcoal may also be used to prevent nonspecific pruritus (itching) associated with kidney dialysis treatment and as an antidote in poisoning. Simethicone is included in some antacid products, such as Mylanta Liquid and Di-Gel Liquid.

Adverse Reactions of Antiflatulents

No adverse reactions have been reported with the use of antiflatulents.

Contraindications, Precautions, and Interactions of Antiflatulents

Antiflatulents are contraindicated in patients with known hypersensitivity to any components of the drug. The pregnancy category of simethicone is unknown; charcoal is a pregnancy category C drug. A decreased effectiveness of other drugs may occur because of adsorption by charcoal, which can also adsorb other drugs in the gastrointestinal tract. There are no known interactions with simethicone.

Digestive Enzymes

Actions of Digestive Enzymes

The enzymes pancreatin and pancrelipase, which are manufactured and secreted by the pancreas, are responsible for the breakdown and digestion of fats, starches, and proteins in food. Both enzymes are available as oral supplements.

Uses of Digestive Enzymes

These drugs are prescribed as replacement therapy for those with pancreatic enzyme insufficiency. Conditions or diseases that may cause a decrease in or absence of pancreatic digestive enzymes include cystic fibrosis, chronic pancreatitis, cancer of the pancreas, malabsorption syndrome, surgical removal of all or part of the stomach, and surgical removal of all or part of the pancreas.

Adverse Reactions of Digestive Enzymes

No adverse reactions have been reported with the use of digestive enzymes; however, high doses may cause nausea and diarrhea.

Managing Adverse Reactions of Digestive Enzymes

The patient should be monitored for nausea and diarrhea. If these occur, then the health care provider should be notified before the next dose is due, because the dosage may need to be reduced. Digestive enzymes come in regular capsule-form or as delayed-released capsules. The capsules are taken before or with meals. If necessary, the capsules may be opened and sprinkled over soft foods that can be swallowed without chewing, such as gelatin, applesauce, or ice cream. It is particularly important that enteric-coated beads from the time-released capsules be swallowed and not chewed. The patient should be weighed weekly (or as ordered) and the health care provider alerted if there is any significant or steady weight loss.

Periodic stool examinations help the health care provider determine the effectiveness of therapy.

Contraindications, Precautions, and Interactions of Digestive Enzymes

Digestive enzymes are contraindicated in patients with a hypersensitivity to hog or cow proteins and in patients with acute pancreatitis. The digestive enzymes are used cautiously in patients with asthma (an acute asthmatic attack can occur), hyperuricemia (increased concentrations of uric acid in the blood), and during pregnancy and lactation. These drugs are pregnancy category C drugs; safe use in pregnancy has not been established.

Calcium carbonate or magnesium hydroxide antacids may decrease the effectiveness of the digestive enzymes. When administered concurrently with an iron preparation, the digestive enzymes decrease the absorption of oral iron preparations.

Emetics

Actions of Emetics

The **emetic** (a drug that induces vomiting) ipecac causes vomiting because of its local irritating effect on the stomach and by stimulating the vomiting center in the medulla.

Uses of Emetics

Emetics are used to cause vomiting to empty the stomach rapidly when an individual has accidentally or intentionally ingested a poison or drug overdose. Not all poison ingestions or drug overdoses are treated with emetics.

Adverse Reactions of Emetics

There are no apparent adverse reactions to ipecac. Although not an adverse reaction, a danger associated with any emetic is the aspiration (inhalation) of stomach contents.

Contraindications, Precautions, and Interactions of Emetics

Emetics are contraindicated in patients who are unconscious, semiconscious, or convulsing, and in poisonings caused by corrosive substances, such as strong acids or petroleum products. Ipecac is a pregnancy category C drug; safe use in pregnancy has not been established. Activated charcoal may absorb ipecac, negating its effects.

Gallstone-Solubilizing Drugs

Actions of Gallstone-Solubilizing Drugs

Gallstone-solubilizing (gallstone-dissolving) drugs, such as ursodiol (Actigall), suppress the manufacture of cholesterol and cholic acid by the liver. This may ultimately result in a decrease in the size of radiolucent gallstones.

Uses of Gallstone-Solubilizing Drugs

These drugs are used in the nonsurgical treatment of radiolucent gallstones. They are not effective for all types of gallstones and require many months of use to produce results. Because of the potential toxic effects associated with long-term use, these drugs are recommended only for carefully selected and closely monitored patients.

Adverse Reactions of Gallstone-Solubilizing Drugs

Diarrhea, cramps, nausea, and vomiting are the most common adverse drug reactions. A reduction in the dose may reduce or eliminate these problems. Prolonged use of these drugs may result in hepatotoxicity (toxic to the liver).

Contraindications, Precautions, and Interactions of Gallstone-Solubilizing Drugs

Ursodiol is used cautiously in patients with a known hypersensitivity to it or to bile salts, and in patients with liver impairment, calcified stones, radiopaque stones or radiolucent bile pigment stones, severe acute cholecystitis, biliary obstruction, or gallstone pancreatitis. Ursodiol is used cautiously during pregnancy (pregnancy category B) and lactation. Absorption of ursodiol is decreased if the agent is taken with bile acid-sequestering drugs or aluminum-containing antacids. Clofibrate, estrogens, and oral contraceptives increase hepatic cholesterol secretion and encourage cholesterol gallstone formation, and may counteract the effectiveness of ursodiol.

Laxatives

Actions of Laxatives

There are various types of laxatives (see the Summary Drug Table: Drugs Used in the Management of Gastrointestinal Disorders). The action of each laxative is somewhat different, but they produce the same result: the relief of constipation (Box 21-1).

Uses of Laxatives

A laxative is most often prescribed for short-term relief or prevention of constipation. Certain stimulant, emollient, and saline laxatives are used to empty the colon for

---

Box 21-2 **Drugs That May Cause Constipation**

- Anticholinergics
- Antihistamines
- Phenothiazines
- Tricyclic antidepressants
- Opiates
- Non–potassium-sparing diuretics
- Iron preparations
- Barium sulfate
- Clonidine
- Antacids containing either calcium carbonate or aluminum hydroxide

---

rectal and bowel examinations. Fecal softeners or mineral oil are used to prevent constipation in patients who should not strain during defecation, such as after anorectal surgery or a myocardial infarction. Psyllium may be used in patients with irritable bowel syndrome and diverticular disease. Polycarbophil may be prescribed for constipation or diarrhea associated with irritable bowel syndrome and diverticulosis. Mineral oil is useful for the relief of fecal impaction. Docusate is used to prevent dry, hard stools.

Constipation may occur as an adverse drug reaction. When the patient has constipation as an adverse reaction to another drug, the health care provider may prescribe a stool softener or another laxative to prevent constipation during the drug therapy. Box 21-2 lists the names of some drugs and drug classifications that may cause constipation.

Adverse Reactions of Laxatives

Laxative use, especially high doses or prolonged use, can cause diarrhea and a loss of water and electrolytes. For some patients, this may be a serious adverse reaction. Laxatives may also cause abdominal pain or discomfort, nausea, vomiting, perianal irritation, fainting, bloating, flatulence, cramps, and weakness. Prolonged use of a laxative can result in serious electrolyte imbalances, as well as the "laxative habit," that is, a dependency on a laxative to have a bowel movement. Some of these products contain tartrazine, which may cause allergic-type reactions (including bronchial asthma) in susceptible individuals.

Obstruction of the esophagus, stomach, small intestine, and colon may occur when bulk-forming laxatives are administered without adequate fluid intake or in patients with intestinal stenosis (narrowing).

Managing Adverse Reactions of Laxatives

If excessive bowel movements or severe prolonged diarrhea occur, or if the laxative is ineffective, then the health care provider should be notified. If a laxative is ordered for constipation, then a liberal fluid intake and

---

Box 21-1 **Actions of Different Types of Laxatives**

- **Bulk-producing laxatives** are not digested by the body and therefore add bulk and water to the contents of the intestines. The added bulk in the intestines stimulates peristalsis, moves the products of digestion through the intestine, and encourages evacuation of the stool. Examples of bulk-forming laxatives are psyllium (Metamucil) and polycarbophil (FiberCon).
- **Emollient laxatives** lubricate the intestinal walls and soften the stool, thereby enhancing passage of fecal material. Mineral oil is an emollient laxative.
- **Fecal softeners** promote water retention in the fecal mass and soften the stool. One difference between emollient laxatives and fecal softeners is that the emollient laxatives do not promote the retention of water in the stool. Examples of fecal softeners include docusate sodium (Colace) and docusate calcium (Surfak).
- **Hyperosmolar drugs** dehydrate local tissues, which causes irritation and increased peristalsis, with consequent evacuation of the fecal mass. Glycerin is a hyperosmolar drug.
- **Irritant or stimulant laxatives** increase peristalsis by direct action on the intestine. Examples of irritant laxatives are cascara sagrada and senna (Senokot).
- **Saline laxatives** attract or pull water into the intestine, thereby increasing pressure in the intestine, followed by an increase in peristalsis. Magnesium hydroxide (Milk of Magnesia) is a saline laxative.

an increase in foods high in fiber is encouraged to prevent a repeat of the problem.

Contraindications, Precautions, and Interactions of Laxatives

Laxatives are contraindicated in patients with a known hypersensitivity and those with persistent abdominal pain, nausea, or vomiting of unknown cause or signs of acute appendicitis, fecal impaction, intestinal obstruction, or acute hepatitis. These drugs must be used only as directed because excessive or prolonged use may cause dependence. Magnesium hydroxide is used cautiously in patients with any degree of renal impairment. Laxatives are used cautiously in patients with rectal bleeding, in pregnant women, and during lactation. The following are pregnancy category C drugs: cascara, sagrada, docusate, glycerin, phenolphthalein, magnesium hydroxide, and senna. These drugs are used during pregnancy only when the benefits clearly outweigh the risks to the fetus.

Mineral oil may impair the gastrointestinal tract absorption of fat-soluble vitamins (A, D, E, and K). Laxatives may reduce absorption of other drugs present in the gastrointestinal tract by combining with them chemically or hastening their passage through the intestinal tract. When surfactants are administered with mineral oil, surfactants may increase mineral oil absorption. Milk, antacids, H_2 antagonists, and proton pump inhibitors should not be administered 1 to 2 hours before bisacodyl tablets, because the enteric coating may dissolve early (before reaching the intestinal tract), resulting in gastric lining irritation or dyspepsia and decreasing the laxative effect of the drug.

Proton Pump Inhibitors

Actions of Proton Pump Inhibitors

Proton pump inhibitors, such as lansoprazole, omeprazole, pantoprazole, and rabeprazole, belong to a group of drugs with antisecretory properties. These drugs suppress gastric acid secretion by blocking the last step of acid production.

The proton pump inhibitors suppress gastric acid secretion by blocking the final step in the production of gastric acid by the gastric mucosa.

Uses of Proton Pump Inhibitors

Proton pump inhibitors are used for treatment or symptomatic relief of various gastric disorders, including gastric and duodenal ulcers, gastroesophageal reflux disease, or pathological hypersecretory conditions. Painful, persistent heartburn 2 or more days per week may indicate acid reflux disease, which can erode the delicate lining of the esophagus, causing erosive esophagitis.

Esomeprazole (Nexium) or Omeprazole (Prilosec) may provide 24-hour relief from the heartburn associated with gastroesophageal reflux disease or erosive esophagitis while healing occurs.

Proton pump inhibitors are particularly important in the treatment of *Helicobacter pylori* in patients with active duodenal ulcers. **H. pylori** have been implicated as bacteria that cause a type of chronic gastritis and in a large number of cases of peptic and duodenal ulcers. Infection with *H. pylori* is often treated with a triple-drug treatment regimen, such as one of the proton pump inhibitors (e.g., omeprazole or lansoprazole) and two anti-infectives (e.g., amoxicillin and clarithromycin). Another treatment regimen includes bismuth subsalicylate plus two anti-infective drugs. Helidac, a treatment regimen of three drugs (bismuth subsalicylate, metronidazole, and tetracycline), may be given along with a histamine H_2 antagonist to treat disorders of the gastrointestinal tract infected with *H. pylori*. Table 21-1 lists various combinations used in the treatment of *H. pylori*. Additional information concerning the anti-infectives listed is in Chapter 25. The Summary Drug Table: Drugs Used in the Management of Gastrointestinal Disorders provides information on the drugs used in the treatment of *H. pylori*.

Adverse Reactions of Proton Pump Inhibitors

The most common adverse reactions of the proton pump inhibitors include headache, diarrhea, and abdominal pain. Other less common adverse reactions include nausea, flatulence, constipation, and dry mouth.

Managing Adverse Reactions of Proton Pump Inhibitors

Adverse reactions of proton pump inhibitors are usually mild. The most common adverse reactions are headache, diarrhea, and abdominal pain. Headache may be treated with analgesics. The number, color, and consistency of the stools are recorded, and any excessive diarrhea or severe headache should be reported to the health care provider.

Contraindications, Precautions, and Interactions of Proton Pump Inhibitors

Proton pump inhibitors are contraindicated in patients who have a known hypersensitivity. Omeprazole (pregnancy category C) and lansoprazole, rabeprazole, and pantoprazole (pregnancy category B) are contraindicated during pregnancy and lactation. Proton pump inhibitors are used cautiously in older adults and in patients with liver disease.

There is a decreased absorption of lansoprazole when it is administered with sucralfate. Lansoprazole may decrease the effects of ketoconazole, iron salts, and digoxin. When lansoprazole is administered with theo-

TABLE 21-1   Agents Used to Treat *H. Pylori* in Patients With Duodenal Ulcers

Drug	Use for Eradication of *H. Pylori* in Patients with Duodenal Ulcer	Dosage Range
amoxicillin *a-mocks'-ih-sill-in*	In combination with lansoprazole and clarithromycin or lansoprazole alone	1 g BID for 14 d (triple therapy) or 1 g TID (double therapy)
bismuth *bis'-muth*	In combination with other products	525 mg QID in combination with other products
bismuth subsalicylate (Bis Matrol) *bis'-muth sub-sa-li'-si-late*	*H. pylori* eradication in patients with duodenal ulcer	525-mg chewable tablets QID in combination with at least two anti-infectives
bismuth subsalicylate, metronidazole *me-troe-ni'-da-zole* tetracycline *tet-ra-sye'-cleen* (Helidac)	*H. pylori* eradication in patients with duodenal ulcer	525-mg chewable tablets, 250 mg metronidazole, 500 mg tetracycline QID P0
clarithromycin (Biaxin) *clair-ith'-row-my-sin*	In combination with amoxicillin	500 mg TID
lansoprazole (Prevacid) *lan-sew-prah'-zoll*	In combination with clarithromycin and/or amoxicillin	30 mg BID for 14 d (triple therapy) or 30 mg TID for 14 d (double therapy)
metronidazole (Flagyl) *meh-trow-nye'-dah-zoll*	In combination with other products	250 mg QID
omeprazole (Prilosec) *oh-mep'-rah-zole*	In combination with clarithromycin	40 mg BID for 4 wk and 20 mg/d for 15–28 d
ranitidine bismuth citrate (Tritec) *rah-nih'-tih-deen*	In combination with clarithromycin	400 mg BID for 4 wk in combination with clarithromycin
tetracycline *tet-rah-si'-cleen*	In combination with other products	500 mg QID

phylline, there is an increase in theophylline clearance requiring dosage changes of the theophylline. When omeprazole is administered with clarithromycin, there is a risk for an increase in plasma levels of both drugs. Omeprazole may prolong the elimination of warfarin when the two drugs are administered together. Increased serum levels and the risk for toxicity of benzodiazepines, phenytoin, and warfarin may occur if any of these drugs is used with omeprazole.

Miscellaneous Drugs

Actions of Miscellaneous Drugs

The miscellaneous gastrointestinal tract drugs include bismuth subsalicylate, mesalamine, misoprostol, olsalazine, sucralfate, and sulfasalazine.

Bismuth disrupts the integrity of the bacterial cell wall. Misoprostol (Cytotec) inhibits gastric acid secretion and increases the protective property of the mucosal lining of the gastrointestinal tract by increasing the production of mucus by the lining of the tract. Sucralfate (Carafate) exerts a local action on the lining of the stomach. The drug forms a complex with the fluid from the inflamed tissue of the stomach lining. This complex

forms a protective layer over a duodenal ulcer, thus aiding in healing of the ulcer. Mesalamine (Asacol), olsalazine (Dipentum), and sulfasalazine (Azulfidine) exert a topical anti-inflammatory effect in the bowel. The exact mechanism of action of these drugs is unknown.

Uses of Miscellaneous Drugs

Bismuth subsalicylate is used in combination with other drugs to treat gastric and duodenal ulcers caused by *H. pylori* bacteria. Mesalamine is used in the treatment of chronic inflammatory bowel disease. Misoprostol is used to prevent gastric ulcers in those taking aspirin or nonsteroidal anti-inflammatory drugs in high doses for a prolonged time. Olsalazine is used in the treatment of ulcerative colitis in those allergic to sulfasalazine. Sulfasalazine is used in the treatment of Crohn disease and ulcerative colitis. Sucralfate is used in the treatment of duodenal ulcers.

Adverse Reactions of Miscellaneous Drugs

Adverse reactions of bismuth subsalicylate include a temporary and harmless darkening of the tongue and stool and constipation. Salicylate toxicity (e.g., tinnitus and rapid respirations; see Chapter 10) may also occur, particularly when the drug is used for an extended period of time.

Oral administration of mesalamine may cause abdominal pain, nausea, headache, dizziness, fever, and weakness. The adverse reactions associated with rectal administration are less than those with oral administration, but headache, abdominal discomfort, flu-like syndrome, and weakness may still occur. Olsalazine administration may result in diarrhea, abdominal discomfort, and nausea. Sulfasalazine is a sulfonamide with adverse reactions that are the same as for the sulfonamide drugs (see Chapter 25).

The adverse reactions of sucralfate are usually mild, but constipation may occur in some patients. Misoprostol administration may result in diarrhea, abdominal pain, nausea, gastrointestinal tract distress, and vomiting.

Contraindications, Precautions, and Interactions of Miscellaneous Drugs

The miscellaneous gastrointestinal tract drugs are given with caution to patients with a known hypersensitivity. In addition, mesalamine, olsalazine, and sulfasalazine are contraindicated in patients who have hypersensitivity to the sulfonamides and salicylates or intestinal obstruction, and in children younger than 2 years. There is a possible cross-sensitivity of mesalamine, olsalazine, and sulfasalazine with furosemide, sulfonylurea antidiabetic drugs, and carbonic anhydrase inhibitors. Misoprostol is contraindicated in those with an allergy to the prostaglandins and during pregnancy (pregnancy category X) and lactation.

Misoprostol is used cautiously in women of childbearing age. Mesalamine, olsalazine, sucralfate, and sulfasalazine are pregnancy category B drugs; all are used with caution during pregnancy (safety has not been established) and lactation.

A patient has an increased risk of diarrhea when taking misoprostol along with a magnesium-containing antacid. Sulfasalazine may increase the risk of toxicity of oral hypoglycemic drugs, zidovudine, methotrexate, and phenytoin. There is also an increased risk of crystalluria (the excretion of crystalline materials in the urine) when sulfasalazine is administered with methenamine. A decrease in the absorption of iron and folic acid may occur when these agents are administered with sulfasalazine. When bismuth subsalicylate is administered with an aspirin-containing drug, the patient is at risk for salicylate toxicity. The patient has an increased risk of toxicity of valproic acid and methotrexate and decreased effectiveness of corticosteroids when these agents are administered with bismuth subsalicylate.

Patient Management Issues with Drugs that Affect the Gastrointestinal System

When a patient receives a drug that affects the gastrointestinal system, monitoring for relief of symptoms (such as diarrhea, pain, or constipation) is important. The health care provider should be notified if the drug fails to relieve the patient's symptoms. Vital signs are monitored daily or more frequently if the patient has a bleeding peptic ulcer, severe diarrhea, or other condition that may warrant it. The patient is observed for adverse drug reactions associated with the prescribed drug, and any adverse reactions are reported to the health care provider before the next dose is given. The effectiveness of drug therapy is evaluated by a daily comparison of symptoms with those experienced before therapy began. In some instances, frequent evaluation of the patient's response to therapy may be necessary.

Antacids

Antacids should not be given within 2 hours before or after administration of other oral drugs. Liquid antacid preparations must be shaken thoroughly immediately before administration. If tablets are given, then the patient is told to chew the tablets thoroughly before swallowing and to then drink a full glass of water or milk. Liquid antacids are followed by a small amount of water. The health care provider should be notified if the patient dislikes the taste of the antacid or has difficulty chewing the tablet form. A flavored antacid may be ordered if the taste is a problem, and a liquid form may be ordered if the patient has difficulty chewing a tablet. The antacid may be administered hourly for the first 2 weeks when used to treat acute peptic ulcer. After the first 2 weeks, the drug is administered 1 to 2 hours after meals and at bedtime.

ALERT

Antacid Interaction with Other Drugs
Because of the possibility of an antacid interfering with the activity of other oral drugs, no oral drug should be administered within 1 to 2 hours of an antacid.

Gastrointestinal Stimulants

The administration of oral metoclopramide should be carefully timed to occur 30 minutes before each meal. Dexpanthenol is administered intramuscularly or intravenously, and the patient is told that an intestinal colic may occur within 30 minutes. This is not abnormal and will pass within a short time.

Histamine H$_2$ Antagonists

Ranitidine and oral cimetidine are administered before or with meals and at bedtime. Nizatidine and famotidine are given in single doses at bedtime or, with twice-per-day doses, in the morning and at bedtime. These drugs are usually given concurrently with an antacid to relieve pain.

Antidiarrheals

The health care provider may request these drugs to be given after each loose bowel movement. Each bowel movement is inspected before a decision is made to administer the drug.

Digestive Enzymes

When digestive enzymes are given in capsule or enteric-coated tablet form, the patient is instructed not to bite or chew the capsule or tablet. If the patient has difficulty swallowing, then the capsule can be opened and sprinkled on a small amount of soft food served at room temperature, such as applesauce or flavored gelatin.

Emetics

Before an emetic is given, it is extremely important to know the chemicals or substances the patient ingested, the time they were ingested, and what symptoms occurred before seeking medical treatment. This information is often obtained from a family member or friend. The health care provider may also contact the local poison control center for more information.

The patient's blood pressure, pulse, and respiratory rate are measured, and a brief physical examination is performed to determine what other damages or injuries, if any, may have occurred.

After the administration of an emetic, the patient is closely observed for signs of shock, respiratory depression, or other signs and symptoms associated with the specific poison or drug.

Laxatives

Bulk-producing or fecal-softening laxatives are taken with a full glass of water or juice. A bulk-producing laxative is followed by an additional full glass of water. Mineral oil is preferably given to the patient with an empty stomach in the evening. Laxatives in powder, flake, or granule-form are mixed or stirred immediately before administration. The laxative may have an un-

pleasant or salty taste that may be disguised by chilling, adding to juice, or pouring over cracked ice.

Antiflatulents

Activated charcoal can adsorb drugs while they are in the gastrointestinal tract. Charcoal is administered 2 hours before or 1 hour after other medications. If diarrhea persists or lasts longer than 2 days or is accompanied by fever, then the health care provider should be notified. Simethicone is administered after each meal and at bedtime.

Proton Pump Inhibitors

Omeprazole is taken before meals. The drug should be swallowed whole and not chewed or crushed. Esomeprazole magnesium must be swallowed whole and taken at least 1 hour before meals. For patients who have difficulty swallowing, the capsule may be broken open and the granules mixed lightly with applesauce and eaten immediately without chewing. Likewise, lansoprazole may be sprinkled on approximately 1 tablespoon of applesauce, cottage cheese, pudding, yogurt, or strained pears. The drug may also be administered through a nasogastric tube. The granules are mixed with a small amount of apple juice and injected through a tube. The tube is flushed with fluid afterward.

Educating the Patient and Family About Drugs that Affect the Gastrointestinal System

When a gastrointestinal tract drug must be taken for a long time, there is a possibility that the patient may begin to skip doses or stop taking the drug. Patients are encouraged to take the prescribed drug as directed by the health care provider, emphasizing the importance of not omitting doses or stopping the therapy unless advised to do so by the health care provider.

Patient Education Box 21-1 includes key points about drugs that affect the gastrointestinal system that the patient and family members should know.

Natural Remedies

Ginger

Ginger has been used safely as a food by millions of individuals for hundreds of years. It is a medicinal herb derived from the root of the ginger plant. When dried for consumption, it resembles an ash-colored powder, smells like pepper, and has a spicy taste. Ginger is

Key Points for Patients Taking Drugs that Affect the Gastrointestinal System

ANTACIDS

❏ Do not use the drug indiscriminately. Check with your health care provider before using an antacid if you have other medical problems, such as a cardiac condition, because some laxatives contain sodium.

❏ Chew tablets thoroughly before swallowing, and then drink a full glass of water.

❏ Allow effervescent tablets to completely dissolve in water. Allow most of the bubbling to stop before drinking.

❏ Follow the dosage schedule recommended by your health care provider. Do not increase the frequency of use or the dose if your symptoms become worse; instead, see your health care provider as soon as possible.

❏ Antacids impair the absorption of some drugs. Do not take other drugs within 2 hours before or after taking the antacid unless your health care provider recommends use of an antacid with the drug.

❏ If your pain or discomfort remains the same or becomes worse, if your stools turn black, or if you vomit a substance that resembles coffee grounds, then contact your health care provider as soon as possible.

❏ Antacids may change the color of your stool (white, white streaks); this is normal.

❏ Magnesium-containing products may produce a laxative effect and may cause diarrhea; aluminum- or calcium-containing antacids may cause constipation.

❏ If you take too much antacid, then it may cause your stomach to secrete excess stomach acid. Consult your health care provider or pharmacist about an appropriate dose. Do not use the maximum dose for more than 2 weeks, except under the supervision of your health care provider.

ANTICHOLINERGICS

❏ If your eyes become sensitive to light, wear sunglasses when outside, keep rooms dimly lit, and schedule outdoor activities (when necessary) before taking the first dose, such as early in the morning.

❏ If you experience dry mouth, then take frequent sips of cool water during the day, several sips of water before taking oral drugs, and frequent sips of water during meals.

❏ Constipation may be avoided by drinking plenty of fluids during the day.

❏ Drowsiness may occur with these drugs. Schedule tasks requiring alertness during times when drowsiness does not occur, such as early in the morning before taking the first dose of the drug.

GASTROINTESTINAL STIMULANTS

❏ Take metoclopramide 30 minutes before meals. If you experience drowsiness or dizziness, then be cautious while driving or performing hazardous tasks. Immediately report any of the following signs: difficulty speaking or swallowing; a mask-like facial expression; shuffling gait; muscle rigidity or tremors; uncontrolled movements of the mouth, face, or extremities; and uncontrolled chewing or unusual movements of the tongue.

HISTAMINE H₂ ANTAGONISTS

❏ Keep your health care provider informed of relief of pain or discomfort.

❏ Take as directed on the prescription container, for example, with meals or at bedtime.

❏ Follow your health care provider's recommendations regarding additional treatment, such as eliminating certain foods or avoiding the use of alcohol and additional drugs such as antacids.

❏ If you become drowsy, then avoid driving or performing other hazardous tasks.

❏ Notify your health care provider of the following adverse reactions: sore throat, rash, fever, unusual bleeding, black or tarry stools, easy bruising, or confusion.

❏ Regular follow-up appointments are required while taking these drugs. These drugs may need to be taken for 4 to 6 weeks or longer.

❏ With cimetidine, inform your health care provider if you smoke. Cigarette smoking may decrease the effectiveness of the drug.

ANTIDIARRHEALS

❏ Do not exceed the recommended dosage.

❏ The drug may cause drowsiness. Be cautious when you are driving or performing other hazardous tasks.

❏ Do not drink alcohol or use other central nervous system depressants (tranquilizers, sleeping pills) and other nonprescription drugs unless use has been approved by your health care provider.

❏ Notify your health care provider if diarrhea persists or becomes more severe.

ANTIFLATULENTS

❏ Take simethicone after each meal and at bedtime. Thoroughly chew tablets to enhance the antiflatulent action.

❏ Take charcoal 2 hours before or 1 hour after meals.

❏ Notify your health care provider if your symptoms are not relieved within several days.

DIGESTIVE ENZYMES

❏ Take the drugs as directed by your health care provider. Do not exceed the recommended dose.

❏ Do not chew tablets or capsules. Swallow the whole form of the drug quickly while sitting upright to improve swallowing and to prevent mouth and throat irritation. Eat immediately after taking the drug.

❏ If the capsules are difficult to swallow, then you may open them and sprinkle the contents over small quantities of food, but not with hot foods. You should eat all the food sprinkled with the powder.

❏ Do not change brands without consulting with your health care provider or pharmacist.

❏ Do not inhale the powder dosage form or powder from capsules because it may irritate the skin or mucous membranes.

EMETICS (IPECAC SYRUP)

❏ Ipecac is available without a prescription for use at home. The instructions for use and the recommended dose are printed on the label.

❏ Read the directions on the label and be familiar with these instructions before an emergency occurs.

❏ In case of accidental or intentional poisoning, contact the nearest poison control center before using or giving this drug. Not all poisonings can be treated with this drug.

❏ Do not give this drug to anyone who is semiconscious, unconscious, or convulsing.

❏ Vomiting should occur in 20 to 30 minutes after taking this drug. Seek medical attention immediately after contacting the poison control center and giving this drug.

GALLSTONE-SOLUBILIZING DRUGS

❏ Periodic laboratory tests (liver function studies) and ultrasound or radiologic examinations of the gallbladder may be scheduled by your health care provider.

❏ If you experience diarrhea, then contact your health care provider. If symptoms of gallbladder disease (pain, nausea, or vomiting) occur, then immediately contact your health care provider.

❏ Never take these drugs with aluminum-containing antacids. If you need an antacid, then take it 2 to 3 hours after ursodiol.

LAXATIVES

❏ Avoid long-term use of these products unless use of the product has been recommended by your health care provider. Long-term use may result in the "laxative habit," which is a dependence on a laxative to have a bowel movement. Constipation may also occur with overuse of these drugs. Read and follow the directions on the label.

❏ Avoid long-term use of mineral oil. Daily use of this product may interfere with the absorption of some vitamins (vitamins A, D, E, K). Take it when your stomach is empty, preferably at bedtime.

❏ Do not use these products if you are having abdominal pain, nausea, or vomiting.

❏ Notify your health care provider if your constipation is not relieved or if rectal bleeding or other symptoms occur.

❏ To avoid constipation, drink plenty of fluids, get exercise, and eat foods high in bulk or roughage.

❏ Bulk-producing or fecal-softening laxatives: Drink a full glass of water or juice, followed by more glasses of fluid in the next few hours.

❏ Bisacodyl (Dulcolax): Do not chew the tablets or take them within 1 hour of taking an antacid or milk.

❏ Cascara sagrada or senna: Your urine may turn pink–red, red–violet, red–brown, yellow–brown, or black when taking this drug.

PROTON PUMP INHIBITORS

❏ Esomeprazole: Swallow whole at least 1 hour before eating. If you have difficulty swallowing, then the capsule may be opened and the granules sprinkled on a small amount of applesauce.

❏ Omeprazole: Swallow tablets whole; do not chew them. You will take this drug for up to 8 weeks or a prolonged period. Regular medical check-ups are required.

❏ Lansoprazole: Take before meals. Swallow the capsules whole. You should not chew, open, or crush them. If you have difficulty swallowing the capsule, then open and sprinkle granules on gelatin or applesauce. You will need regular medical check-ups while taking this drug.

H. PYLORI COMBINATION DRUGS

❏ Helidac: Each dose includes four tablets: two round, chewable, pink tablets (bismuth), one white tablet (metronidazole), and one pale orange and white capsule (tetracycline). Take each dose four times per day with meals and at bedtime for 14 days. Chew and swallow the bismuth subsalicylate tablets; swallow the metronidazole tablet and tetracycline capsule with a full glass of water. Take prescribed H_2 antagonist therapy as directed. Drink an adequate amount of fluid to reduce the risk of esophageal irritation and ulceration. Missed doses may be made up by continuing the formal dosing schedule until the medication is gone. Do not take double doses. If you miss more than four doses, contact your health care provider.

❏ Bismuth subsalicylate: Immediately report any symptoms of salicylate toxicity (ringing in the ears, rapid respirations) to your health care provider. Chew tablets thoroughly or dissolve them in the mouth. Do not swallow tablets whole. Stools may become dark; this is normal and will disappear when the drug therapy is discontinued. Do not take this drug with aspirin or aspirin products.

MISCELLANEOUS DRUGS

❏ Olsalazine: If you experience diarrhea, then contact your health care provider as soon as possible.

❏ Mesalamine: Swallow the tablets whole; do not chew them. Partially intact tablets may be found in the stool; if this occurs, you should notify your health care provider. To use the suppository, remove the foil wrapper and immediately insert the pointed end of the suppository into the rectum without using force. For the suspension form, instructions are included with the product. Shake well, remove the protective sheath from the applicator tip, and gently insert the tip into the rectum.

❏ Misoprostol: Take this drug four times per day with meals and at bedtime. Continue to take the NSAID while taking misoprostol. Take it with meals to decrease the severity of diarrhea. Taking antacids before or after misoprostol may decrease the pain. Avoid magnesium-containing antacids because of the risk of increasing the diarrhea.

❏ Misoprostol may cause spontaneous abortion. Women of childbearing age must use a reliable contraceptive while taking this drug. If pregnancy is suspected, then discontinue use and notify your health care provider. Report severe menstrual pain, bleeding, or spotting.

❏ Sucralfate: Take on an empty stomach 1 hour before meals. Antacids may be taken for pain but not within 30 minutes before or after sucralfate. Your sucralfate dosage will continue for 4 to 8 weeks. Keep all follow-up appointments with your health care provider.

usually taken to reduce nausea, vomiting, and indigestion. In addition, it is recommended for the pain and inflammation of arthritis and may help lower cholesterol. Clinical studies suggest that ginger is effective in preventing the nausea associated with motion sickness, seasickness, and anesthesia. Results are unclear regarding whether ginger helps people already experiencing the symptoms of seasickness. In the United States, the Food and Drug Administration (FDA) classifies it as a dietary supplement rather than a drug. It is commercially available over the counter as dried ginger (chopped, powdered, powdered extract), candied ginger, and tea.

Ginger is not recommended for morning sickness associated with pregnancy or for patients with gallstones or hypertension. Small amounts present in food preparation are generally regarded as safe. Further, it is suggested that medicinal use of ginger should cease 2 to 3 weeks before surgery to reduce the risk of bleeding. The only known side effects of ginger are heartburn and heightened taste sensitivity.

Chamomile

Chamomile is an herb extracted from two varieties of chamomile plant. When taken orally, it reduces flatulence and diarrhea caused by a nervous stomach, reduces stomach upset, helps to control travel sickness, reduces restlessness and irritability, treats the common cold and fever, reduces cough, liver, and gallbladder symptoms, increases appetite, and acts as a mild sedative. It has also been used for menstrual cramps and, when applied topically, soothes skin irritation and inflammation.

Chamomile is on the United States Food and Drug Administration (FDA) list of herbs generally regarded as safe. It is available in pill, liquid, and tea formulations. When used as a tea, chamomile appears to produce an antispasmodic effect of the smooth muscle of the gastrointestinal tract and to protect against the development of stomach ulcers. It is one of the most popular teas in Europe. Although the herb is generally safe and nontoxic, the tea is prepared from the pollen-filled flower heads and has resulted in mild symptoms of contact dermatitis to severe anaphylactic reactions in individuals hypersensitive to ragweed, asters, and chrysanthemums.

Although uncommon, allergic reaction to any form of chamomile is possible. Symptoms include difficulty breathing, closing of the throat, swelling lips, tongue, or face, and hives or vomiting. A physician should be consulted before consuming chamomile if a patient is being treated with warfarin (Coumadin), ardeparin (Normflo), dalteparin (Fragmin), danaparoid (Orgarin), enoxaparin (Lovenox), heparin, or any other blood thinner, or if a patient is hypersensitive to ragweed, asters, and chrysanthemums.

KEY POINTS

⊙ Antacids neutralize or reduce the acidity of stomach and duodenal contents by combining with hydrochloric acid and producing salt and water. They are used in the treatment of hyperacidity, such as heartburn, gastroesophageal reflux, sour stomach, acid indigestion, and in the medical treatment of peptic ulcer. Antacids are contraindicated in patients with severe abdominal pain of unknown cause and during lactation. Sodium-containing antacids are contraindicated for patients who have cardiovascular problems, such as hypertension or congestive heart failure, or are on sodium-restricted diets. Calcium-containing antacids are contraindicated in patients with renal calculi or hypercalcemia. Adverse reactions to various antacids include constipation, intestinal impaction, anorexia, weakness, tremors, and bone pain, severe diarrhea, dehydration, and hypermagnesemia.

⊙ Anticholinergics reduce gastric motility and decrease the amount of acid secreted by the stomach. Specific anticholinergic drugs are occasionally used in the medical treatment of peptic ulcer. Dry mouth, blurred vision, urinary hesitancy, urinary retention, nausea, vomiting, palpitations, and headache are some of the adverse reactions that may occur.

⊙ Gastrointestinal stimulants increase the strength of the spontaneous movement of the upper gastrointestinal tract. Metoclopramide is used in the treatment of symptomatic gastroesophageal reflux disease and gastric stasis in patients with diabetes. Dexpanthenol may be given immediately after major abdominal surgery to reduce the risk of paralytic ileus. Gastrointestinal tract stimulants are contraindicated in patients with a known hypersensitivity, gastrointestinal tract obstruction, gastric perforation or hemorrhage, or epilepsy. These drugs are secreted in breast milk and should not be used during lactation, and are used cautiously in patients with diabetes and cardiovascular disease. The adverse reactions of metoclopramide are usually mild. Dexpanthenol administration may cause itching, difficulty breathing, and urticaria.

⊙ Histamine H_2 antagonists inhibit the action of histamine at histamine H_2 receptor cells of the stomach, which then reduces the secretion of gastric acid and reduces total pepsin output. The decrease in acid allows the ulcerated areas to heal. These drugs are used mainly to treat gastric and duodenal ulcers, gastric hypersecretory conditions, and gastroesophageal reflux disease. Adverse reactions are usually mild and transient and include dizziness, sleeplessness, and diarrhea. These drugs are used cautiously in patients with liver or kidney disease, in severely ill or debilitated patients, and in older adults because they may cause confusion and a dosage reduction may be required. These drugs interact with a wide array of drugs, and drug combinations must be closely monitored.

◎ Antidiarrheals are used to treat diarrhea by decreasing intestinal peristalsis. Diphenoxylate is a narcotic-related drug with adverse reactions that include anorexia, nausea, vomiting, constipation, rash, dizziness, drowsiness, sedation, euphoria, and headache. Loperamide is not a narcotic-related drug, and minimal adverse reactions are associated with its use. These drugs are contraindicated in patients whose diarrhea is associated with organisms that can harm the intestinal mucosa (*E. coli*, *Salmonella*, *Shigella*) and in patients with pseudomembranous colitis, abdominal pain of unknown origin, or obstructive jaundice. Antidiarrheal drugs are contraindicated in children younger than 2 years.

◎ Antiflatulents are used for the relief of painful symptoms of excess gas in the digestive tract. These drugs are useful as adjunctive treatment of any condition in which gas retention may be a problem. Simethicone (Mylicon) and charcoal are both antiflatulents. Simethicone has a defoaming action that disperses and prevents the formation of mucus-surrounded gas pockets in the intestine. Charcoal is an absorbent that reduces the amount of intestinal gas. No adverse reactions have been reported with the use of antiflatulents; they are contraindicated in patients with a known hypersensitivity to any components of the drug.

◎ The digestive enzymes pancreatin and pancrelipase, which are manufactured and secreted by the pancreas, are responsible for the breakdown of fats and starches in food. Both enzymes are available as oral supplements and are prescribed as replacement therapy for those with pancreatic enzyme insufficiency. No adverse reactions have been reported, but high doses may cause nausea and diarrhea, and use of these drugs is contraindicated in patients with a hypersensitivity to hog or cow proteins and in patients with acute pancreatitis.

◎ Emetics are used to cause vomiting to empty the stomach rapidly when an individual has accidentally or intentionally ingested a poison or drug overdose. Not all poison ingestions or drug overdoses are treated with emetics. There are no apparent adverse reactions to ipecac. Although not an adverse reaction, a danger of any emetic is the aspiration of vomit. Emetics are contraindicated in patients who are unconscious, semiconscious, or convulsing and in poisonings caused by corrosive substances, such as strong acids or petroleum products.

◎ Gallstone-solubilizing drugs are used in the nonsurgical treatment of radiolucent gallstones. They are not effective for all types of gallstones and require many months of use to produce results. Because of the potential toxic effects with long-term use, these drugs are recommended for only carefully selected and closely monitored patients. Diarrhea, cramps, nausea, and vomiting are the more common adverse drug reactions. The drug ursodiol is used cautiously in patients with known hypersensitivity to it or bile salts, and in patients with liver impairment, calcified stones, radiopaque stones or radiolucent bile pigment stones, severe acute cholecystitis, biliary obstruction, or gallstone pancreatitis.

◎ A laxative is used primarily for the short-term relief or prevention of constipation. Certain stimulant, emollient, and saline laxatives are used to evacuate the colon for rectal and bowel examinations. The action of each laxative is somewhat different, but they produce the same result: the relief of constipation. Laxative use, especially high doses or use over a long time, can cause diarrhea and a loss of water and electrolytes. For some patients, this may be a serious adverse reaction. Laxatives may also cause abdominal pain or discomfort, nausea, vomiting, perianal irritation, fainting, bloating, flatulence, cramps, and weakness. Laxatives are contraindicated in patients with a known hypersensitivity and those with persistent abdominal pain, nausea, or vomiting of unknown cause or signs of acute appendicitis, fecal impaction, intestinal obstruction, or acute hepatitis.

◎ Proton pump inhibitors suppress gastric acid secretion by blocking the last step of acid production and are used for treatment or symptomatic relief of various gastric disorders, including gastric and duodenal ulcers, gastroesophageal reflux disease, or pathological hypersecretory conditions. Proton pump inhibitors are particularly important in the treatment of *H. pylori*, which has been implicated as a cause of a type of chronic gastritis and most cases of peptic and duodenal ulcers. These drugs are often used in combination therapy for the treatment of *H. pylori* in patients with duodenal ulcers. The most common adverse reactions of proton pump inhibitors include headache, diarrhea, and abdominal pain. Other less common adverse reactions include nausea, flatulence, constipation, and dry mouth. Proton pump inhibitors are contraindicated in patients who have a known hypersensitivity.

◎ Miscellaneous gastrointestinal tract drugs include bismuth subsalicylate, mesalamine, misoprostol, olsalazine, sucralfate, and sulfasalazine. Bismuth disrupts the integrity of the bacterial cell wall. Misoprostol (Cytotec) inhibits gastric acid secretion and increases the protective property of the mucosal lining of the gastrointestinal tract by increasing the production of mucus by the lining of the tract. Sucralfate (Carafate) exerts a local action on the lining of the stomach, forming a protective layer over a duodenal ulcer, thus aiding in healing of the ulcer. Mesalamine (Asacol), olsalazine (Dipentum), and sulfasalazine (Azulfidine) exert a topical anti-inflammatory effect in the bowel. The exact mechanism of action of these drugs is unknown.

◎ Several miscellaneous drugs are used to treat gastrointestinal disorders. Bismuth subsalicylate is used in combination with other drugs to treat gastric and duodenal ulcers caused by *H. pylori* bacteria. Mesalamine is used in the treatment of chronic inflammatory bowel disease. Misoprostol is used to prevent gastric ulcers in those taking aspirin or nonsteroidal anti-inflammatory drugs in high doses for a prolonged time. Olsalazine is used in the treatment of ulcerative colitis in those allergic to sulfasalazine. Sulfasalazine is used in the treatment of Crohn disease and ulcerative colitis. Sucralfate is used in the treatment of duodenal ulcer. Adverse reactions to the various drugs in this group range from a temporary and harmless darkening of the tongue and stool and constipation to tinnitus and rapid respirations. The miscellaneous gastrointestinal tract drugs are given with caution to patients with a known hypersensitivity. In addition, mesalamine, olsalazine, and sulfasalazine are contraindicated in patients with hypersensitivity to the sulfonamides and salicylates or intestinal obstruction, and in children younger than 2 years.

CASE STUDY

Mr. Eldridge, your neighbor, has been given a prescription for diphenoxylate with atropine (Lomotil) to be taken if he should experience diarrhea while he is traveling in a foreign country.

1. Mr. Eldridge asks what potential adverse reactions Lomotil may cause. He should be told:
   a. nausea
   b. vomiting
   c. headache
   d. all of the above

2. Mr. Eldridge wonders if drinking an occasional alcoholic beverage might interfere with Lomotil use. He should be aware that:
   a. there are no known adverse reactions from combining alcohol and Lomotil
   b. the combination of Lomotil and alcohol may suppress the central nervous system
   c. the combination of Lomotil and alcohol may cause anorexia
   d. none of the above

3. Mr. Eldridge tells you that he is also being treated for inflammatory bowel disease. He wonders if Lomotil is safe for use with his condition. He should be told:
   a. to consult his health care provider
   b. Lomotil has no known adverse reaction on inflammatory bowel disease
   c. that if he is on drug therapy, it will prevent the chance of a drug reaction to Lomotil
   d. none of the above

WEBSITE ACTIVITIES

1. Go to the Centers for Disease Control and Prevention website (www.cdc.gov) and follow the links through "Health Topics A–Z" to look for information about ulcers. Look for the information about Ulcer Awareness Week. What kinds of information could a patient gain from this web page on ulcer awareness?

2. What percentage of ulcers are thought to result from *H. pylori*?

REVIEW QUESTIONS

1. An antacid should be taken:
   a. with other drugs
   b. 3 minutes before or after administration of other drugs
   c. 2 hours before or after administration of other drugs
   d. during early morning and at bedtime

2. Fecal softeners relieve constipation by:
   a. stimulating the walls of the intestine
   b. promoting the retention of sodium in the fecal mass
   c. promoting water retention in the fecal mass
   d. lubricating the intestinal walls

3. When an anticholinergic drug is prescribed for the treatment of a peptic ulcer, which of the following adverse reactions may occur?
   a. dry mouth, urinary retention
   b. edema, tachycardia
   c. weight gain, increased respiratory rate
   d. diarrhea, anorexia

4. Antidiarrheal drugs are administered:
   a. hourly until diarrhea ceases
   b. after each loose bowel movement
   c. with food
   d. twice per day, in the morning and at bedtime

5. When an emetic is administered, the patient may:
   a. become violent
   b. experience severe diarrhea
   c. retain fluid
   d. aspirate (inhale) vomit

Unit VI • Drugs That Affect the Endocrine and Reproductive Systems

22 Antidiabetic Drugs

KEY TERMS

diabetes mellitus—a chronic disorder characterized either by insufficient insulin production in the beta cells of the pancreas or by cellular resistance to insulin

diabetic ketoacidosis—a potentially life-threatening deficiency of insulin (hypoinsulinism), resulting in severe hyperglycemia and requiring prompt diagnosis and treatment

glucagon—a hormone produced by the alpha cells of the pancreas that increases blood sugar by stimulating the conversion of glycogen to glucose in the liver

glucometer—a device used to monitor blood glucose levels

hyperglycemia—elevated blood glucose level

hypoglycemia—low blood glucose level

insulin—a hormone produced by the pancreas that helps maintain blood glucose levels within normal limits

lipodystrophy—atrophy of subcutaneous fat

secondary failure—a gradual increase in blood sugar levels that can be caused by an increase in the severity of diabetes or a decreased response to a drug

CHAPTER OBJECTIVES

On completion of this chapter, students will be able to:

1 Define the chapter's key terms.

2 Describe the general drug actions, uses, adverse reactions, contraindications, precautions, and interactions of antidiabetic drugs.

3 Discuss important points to keep in mind when educating the patient or family members about the use of antidiabetic drugs.

Insulin, a hormone produced by the pancreas, acts to maintain blood glucose levels within normal limits. This is accomplished by the release of small amounts of insulin into the bloodstream throughout the day in response to changes in blood glucose levels. Insulin is essential for using glucose in cellular metabolism and for the metabolism of protein and fat.

Diabetes mellitus is a complicated, chronic disorder characterized either by insufficient insulin production in the beta cells of the pancreas or by cellular resistance to insulin. Insulin insufficiency results in elevated blood glucose levels, or hyperglycemia. Individuals with diabetes are at greater risk for a number of disorders, including myocardial infarction, cerebrovascular accident (stroke), blindness, kidney disease, and lower limb amputations.

Insulin and the oral antidiabetic drugs, along with diet and exercise, are the cornerstones of treatment for diabetes mellitus. They are used to prevent episodes of hyperglycemia and to normalize carbohydrate metabolism.

There are two major types of diabetes mellitus:

* Type 1: Insulin-dependent diabetes mellitus. (Former names include juvenile diabetes, juvenile-onset diabetes, and brittle diabetes.)
* Type 2: Noninsulin-dependent diabetes mellitus. (Former names include maturity-onset diabetes, adult-onset diabetes, and stable diabetes.)

Those with type 1 diabetes mellitus produce insulin in insufficient amounts and therefore must have insulin supplementation to survive. Type 1 diabetes usually has a rapid onset, occurs before the age of 20 years, produces more severe symptoms than type 2 diabetes, and is more difficult to control. Major symptoms of type 1 diabetes include hyperglycemia, polydipsia (increased thirst), polyphagia (increased appetite), polyuria (increased urination), and weight loss. Treatment of type 1 diabetes is particularly difficult because of the lack of insulin production by the pancreas. Treatment requires a strict regimen that typically includes a carefully calculated diet, planned physical activity, home glucose testing several times per day, and multiple daily insulin injections.

Approximately 90% to 95% of individuals with diabetes have type 2. Those with type 2 either have a decreased production of insulin by the beta cells of the pancreas or have a decreased sensitivity of the cells to insulin, making the cells insulin-resistant. Although type 2 diabetes mellitus may occur at any age, the disorder occurs most often after the age of 40 years. The onset of type 2 diabetes is usually insidious, and the symptoms are less severe than in type 1 diabetes mellitus. Because it tends to be more stable, it is easier to control than type 1 diabetes. Risk factors for type 2 diabetes include:

* obesity
* older age
* family history of diabetes
* history of gestational diabetes (diabetes that develops during pregnancy but disappears when pregnancy is over)
* impaired glucose tolerance
* minimal or no physical activity
* race/ethnicity (more common in blacks, Hispanic/Latino Americans, American Indians, and some Asian Americans)

Obesity is thought to contribute to type 2 diabetes by placing additional stress on the pancreas, which makes it less able to respond and produce adequate insulin to meet the body's metabolic needs.

Many individuals with type 2 diabetes are able to control the disorder with diet, exercise, and oral antidiabetic drugs. However, approximately 40% of those with type 2 diabetes do not have a good response to the oral antidiabetic drugs and require the addition of insulin to control the diabetes.

Insulin

Insulin is a hormone manufactured by the beta cells of the pancreas. It is the principal hormone required for the proper use of glucose (carbohydrate) by the body. Insulin also controls the storage and use of amino acids and fatty acids. Insulin lowers blood glucose levels by inhibiting liver glucose production.

Insulin developed from purified extracts from beef and pork pancreas is biologically similar to human insulin. However, these animal source insulins are used less frequently today than in years past. Synthetic insulins, including human insulin or insulin analogs, are replacing them.

Human insulin is derived from a biosynthetic process using strains of *Escherichia coli* (a nonpathogenic colon bacteria). Human insulin appears to cause fewer allergic reactions than insulin obtained from animal sources. Insulin analogs, insulin lispro, and insulin aspart are newer forms of human insulin made by using recombinant DNA technology and are structurally similar to human insulin.

Actions of Insulin

Insulin appears to activate a process that helps glucose molecules enter the cells of striated muscle and adipose tissue. Figure 22-1 depicts normal glucose metabolism. Insulin also stimulates the synthesis of glycogen by the liver. In addition, insulin promotes protein synthesis and helps the body store fat by preventing its breakdown for energy.

Various insulin preparations have been developed with a more gradual onset and prolonged duration of effect. Insulin preparations are classified as rapid-acting, intermediate-acting, or long-acting. The Summary Drug Table: Insulin Preparations gives information concerning the onset, peak, and duration of various insulins.

Uses of Insulin

Insulin is necessary for controlling type 1 diabetes mellitus that is caused by a marked decrease in the amount of insulin produced by the pancreas. Insulin is also used to control the more severe and complicated forms of type 2 diabetes mellitus. However, many patients can control type 2 diabetes with diet and exercise alone or with diet, exercise, and an oral antidiabetic drug (see later section). Insulin may also be used in the treatment of severe diabetic ketoacidosis (a type of metabolic acidosis caused by an accumulation of ketone bodies in the blood) or diabetic coma. Insulin is also used in combination with glucose to treat hypokalemia by shifting potassium from the blood into the cells.

Adverse Reactions of Insulin

The two major adverse reactions seen with insulin administration are **hypoglycemia** (low blood glucose or sugar) and **hyperglycemia** (elevated blood glucose or sugar). The symptoms of hypoglycemia and hyperglycemia are listed in Table 22-1.

Hypoglycemia may occur when there is too much insulin in the bloodstream in relation to the available glucose (hyperinsulinism). Hypoglycemia may occur:

- when the patient eats too little food
- when the insulin dose is incorrectly measured and is greater than that prescribed
- when the patient drastically increases physical activity

Hyperglycemia may occur if there is too little insulin in the bloodstream in relation to the available glucose (hypoinsulinism). Hyperglycemia may occur:

- when the patient eats too much food
- when too little or no insulin is used
- when the patient experiences emotional stress, infection, surgery, pregnancy, or an acute illness

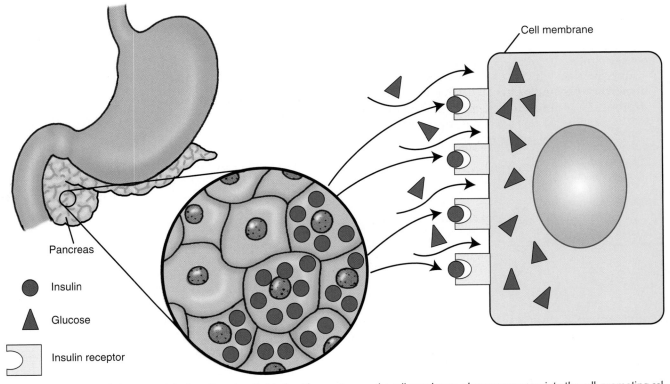

Pancreas

● Insulin

▲ Glucose

⊐ Insulin receptor

Cell membrane

FIGURE 22-1   Normal glucose metabolism. Once insulin binds with receptors on the cell membrane, glucose can move into the cell, promoting cellular metabolism and energy production. (From Roach SS. *Introductory Clinical Pharmacology*, 7th ed. Baltimore: Lippincott Williams & Wilkins; 2004.)

SUMMARY DRUG TABLE Insulin Preparations

Types of Insulin	Trade Name	Activity		
		Onset	Peak	Duration
Rapid-Acting Insulins				
insulin injection (regular)	Humulin R, Iletin II Regular, Novolin R, Novolin R PenFill, Novolin R Prefilled, Velosulin BR	30–60 min	2–4 h	6–8 h
insulin lispro (insulin analog)	Humalog, Humalog Mix 50/50, Humalog Mix 75/25	45 min 30–60 min, then 1–2 h	0.1 h 2–4 h, then 6–12 h	3.5–4.5 h 6–8 h, then 8–24 h
insulin aspart solution (insulin analog)	NovoLog	5–10 min	30–60 min	2–3 h
Intermediate-Acting Insulin				
isophane insulin suspension (NPH)	Humulin N, Novolin N, Novolin N PenFill, Novolin N Prefilled, NPH Iletin II	1–2 h	6–12 h	18–24 h
insulin zinc suspension (Lente)	Humulin L, Lente Iletin II, Novolin L	1–2.5 h	6–12 h	18–24 h
Long-Acting Insulins				
insulin glargine solution	Lantus	30–60 min	none	8 h
extended insulin zinc suspension (Ultralente)	Humulin U	4–8 h	8–20 h	24–48 h
Mixed Insulins				
isophane insulin suspension and insulin injections (NPH)	Humulin 70/30, Novolin 70/30, Novolin 70/30 PenFill, Novolin 70/30 Prefilled	30–60 min, then 1–2 h	2–4 h, then 6–12 h	6–8 h, then 18–24 h
isophane insulin suspension and insulin injection	Humulin 50/50	30–60 min, then 1–2 h	2–4 h, then 6–12 h	6–8 h, then 18–24 h
High-Potency Insulin				
insulin injection concentrated	Humulin R Regular U-500			24 h

Another potential adverse reaction may occur if the patient has an allergy to the animal (pig or cow) from which the insulin is obtained or to the protein or zinc added to insulin to increase its duration of action. To minimize the possibility of an allergic reaction, some health care providers prescribe human insulin or purified insulin. However, on rare occasions, some patients also become allergic to the human and purified insulins.

A patient can also become insulin-resistant because of the development of antibodies against insulin.

TABLE 22-1   Hypoglycemia Versus Hyperglycemia

Symptoms	Hypoglycemia (Insulin Reaction)	Hyperglycemia (Diabetic Coma, Ketoacidosis)
Onset	Sudden	Gradual (hours or days)
Blood glucose	<60 mg/dL	>200 mg/dL
Central nervous system	Fatigue, weakness, nervousness, agitation, confusion, headache, diplopia, convulsions, dizziness, unconsciousness	Drowsiness, dim vision
Respirations	Normal to rapid, shallow	Deep, rapid (air hunger)
Gastrointestinal	Hunger, nausea	Thirst, nausea, vomiting, abdominal pain, loss of appetite, excessive urination
Skin	Pale, moist, cool, diaphoretic	Dry, flushed, warm
Pulse	Normal or uncharacteristic	Rapid, weak
Miscellaneous	Numbness, tingling of the lips or tongue	Acetone breath

Managing Adverse Reactions of Insulin

Hypoglycemic Reactions. Close observation of a patient with diabetes is important, especially when diabetes is newly diagnosed, the insulin dosage is changed, or the patient is pregnant, has a medical illness or has had surgery, or fails to adhere to the prescribed diet. Episodes of hypoglycemia are corrected as soon as the symptoms are recognized.

ALERT

Hypoglycemia

Hypoglycemia, which can develop suddenly, may indicate a need for an adjustment in the insulin dosage or other changes in treatment, such as a change in diet. Hypoglycemic reactions can occur at any time but are most likely to occur when insulin is at its peak activity.

Methods of ending a hypoglycemic reaction include taking one or more of the following:

- orange juice or other fruit juice
- hard candy or honey
- commercial glucose products
- glucagon by the subcutaneous, intramuscular, or intravenous route
- glucose 10% or 50% via intravenous route

Use of any one or more of these methods for terminating a hypoglycemic reaction depends on the written order of the health care provider or hospital policy. Oral fluids or substances (such as candy) used to terminate a hypoglycemic reaction should never be given to a patient without intact swallowing and gag reflexes. Ab-

sence of these reflexes may result in aspiration of the oral fluid or substance into the lungs, which can result in extremely serious consequences and even death. If a patient's swallowing and gag reflexes are absent, or if the patient is unconscious, then glucose or glucagon is given by the parenteral route.

The health care provider should be notified of any hypoglycemic reaction, the substance and amount used to terminate the reaction, blood samples drawn (if any), the length of time required for the symptoms of hypoglycemia to disappear, and the current status of the patient. After a hypoglycemic reaction, the patient is closely observed for additional hypoglycemic reactions.

ALERT

Hypoglycemia and Animal-Based Products

Hypoglycemic symptoms are more pronounced in patients taking animal-based products than in patients taking human insulin.

Contraindications, Precautions, and Interactions of Insulin

Insulin is contraindicated in patients with hypersensitivity to any ingredient of the product (e.g., beef or pork) and when a patient is hypoglycemic.

Insulin is used cautiously in patients with liver or kidney disease and during pregnancy (pregnancy category B and category C, insulin glargine, and insulin aspart). Insulin appears to inhibit milk production in lactating women and could interfere with breastfeeding. Lactating women may require adjustment of their insulin dose and diet.

ALERT

Pregnancy and Insulin

Pregnancy makes diabetes more difficult to manage. Insulin requirements usually decrease in the first trimester, increase during the second and third trimester, and decrease rapidly after delivery. A patient with diabetes or a history of gestational diabetes must be encouraged to maintain good metabolic control before conception and throughout pregnancy. Frequent monitoring is necessary.

When certain drugs are administered with insulin, a decrease or increase in hypoglycemic effect can occur. Following are some drugs that decrease the hypoglycemic effect of insulin:

- AIDS antivirals
- albuterol
- contraceptives, oral
- corticosteroids
- diltiazem
- diuretics
- dobutamine
- epinephrine
- estrogens
- lithium
- morphine sulfate
- niacin
- phenothiazines
- thyroid hormones

Following are some drugs that, when administered with insulin, may increase the hypoglycemic effect of insulin:

- alcohol
- angiotensin-converting enzyme (ACE) inhibitors
- antidiabetic drugs, oral
- beta blocking drugs
- calcium
- clonidine
- disopyramide
- lithium
- monoamine oxidase inhibitors (MAOIs)
- salicylates
- sulfonamides
- tetracycline

Patient Management Issues with Insulin

If a patient has recently had diabetes mellitus diagnosed and has not received insulin, then the initial physical assessment before giving the first dose of insulin includes vital signs and weight. The skin, mucous membranes, and extremities are checked, with special attention given to any sores or cuts that appear to be infected or healing poorly, or any ulcerations or other skin or mucous membrane changes are noted. The patient is asked about dietary habits, any family history of diabetes, and the type and duration of symptoms experienced.

The number of daily insulin injections, the dosage, times of administration, and diet and exercise requirements require continual monitoring. Dosage adjustments may be necessary when changing types of insulin, particularly when changing from the single-peak to the more pure Humulin insulins.

The patient is assessed for signs and symptoms of hypoglycemia and hyperglycemia throughout insulin therapy. A patient on insulin is particularly prone to hypoglycemic reactions at the time of peak insulin action or when the patient has not eaten for some time or has skipped a meal. Patients in acute care settings have frequent blood glucose monitoring. Testing usually occurs before meals and at bedtime.

There is no standard dose of insulin as there is for most other drugs. Insulin dosage is highly individualized. Some patients achieve the best control with one injection of insulin per day; others may require two or more injections per day. In addition, two different types of insulin may be combined, such as a rapid-acting and a long-acting preparation. The number of insulin injections, dosage, times of administration, and type of insulin are determined by the health care provider after careful evaluation of a patient's metabolic needs and response to therapy.

ALERT

Changing Insulin Requirements

Insulin requirements may change when a patient experiences any form of stress and with any illness, particularly illnesses resulting in nausea and vomiting.

Insulin must be given parenterally, usually subcutaneously. Insulin cannot be administered orally because it is a protein and is readily destroyed in the gastrointestinal tract. Regular insulin is the only insulin preparation given intravenously. Regular insulin is given 30 to 60 minutes before a meal to achieve optimal results. Other forms of insulin are given on different schedules.

Insulin is injected into the arms, thighs, abdomen, or buttocks. Sites of insulin injection are rotated to prevent **lipodystrophy** (atrophy of subcutaneous fat), a problem that can interfere with the absorption of insulin from the injection site. Lipodystrophy appears as a slight dimpling or pitting of the subcutaneous fat. Because absorption rates vary at the different sites, with the abdomen having the most rapid rate of absorption, followed by the upper arm, thigh, and buttocks, some health care providers recommend rotating the injection sites within one specific area, rather than rotating areas.

Localized allergic reactions, signs of inflammation, or other skin changes must be reported to the health care provider as soon as possible because a different type of insulin may be necessary. Patients who give their own injections need to be taught how to rotate sites (Patient Education Box 22-1).

In addition to injection by syringe and needle, the insulin pump used by some patients, such as a pregnant woman with diabetes with early long-term complications and those with, or candidates for, renal transplantation. This system uses only regular insulin, is battery-powered, and requires insertion of a needle into subcutaneous tissue. The amount of insulin injected can be adjusted according to blood glucose monitoring, which is usually performed 4 to 8 times per day.

Blood glucose levels are monitored often in patients with diabetes. The health care provider may order blood glucose levels to be tested before meals, after meals, and at bedtime. Less frequent monitoring may be performed if the patient's glucose levels are well controlled. The **glucometer** is a device used to monitor blood glucose levels. Patients must be taught to monitor their blood glucose levels at home.

Diabetic ketoacidosis is a potentially life-threatening deficiency of insulin (hypoinsulinism), resulting in severe hyperglycemia. Dangerously high levels of glucose build up in the blood (hyperglycemia). The body, unable to use the glucose but needing energy, begins to break-down fat for energy. As fats are broken down, the liver produces ketones. As more and more fat is used for energy, higher levels of ketones accumulate in the blood. This increase in ketones disrupts the acid–base balance within the body, leading to diabetic ketoacidosis. This condition is treated with fluids, correction of acidosis and hypotension, and low doses of regular insulin.

ALERT

Symptoms of Hyperglycemia

Any of the following symptoms of hyperglycemia must be immediately reported to the health care provider: elevated blood glucose levels, headache, increased thirst, epigastric pain, nausea, vomiting, restlessness, diaphoresis (sweating), or hot, dry, flushed skin.

A patient with newly diagnosed diabetes often has many concerns regarding the diagnosis. For some, initially coping with diabetes and the methods required for controlling the disorder creates many problems. They may have concerns or fears about giving themselves an injection, having to follow a diet, weight control, the

---

PATIENT EDUCATION BOX 22-1

Key Points for Rotating Insulin Injection Sites

- ❑ Site rotation is crucial to prevent injury to the skin and fatty tissue. The following sites are acceptable for injection:
  - ❑ upper arms, outer portion
  - ❑ stomach, except for a 2-inch margin around the umbilicus (belly button)
  - ❑ back, right, and left sides just below the waist
  - ❑ upper thighs, both front and side
- ❑ To rotate sites, you should do the following:
  - ❑ note the site of your last injection
  - ❑ place the side of your thumb at the old site and measure across its width—approximately 1 inch
  - ❑ select a site on the other side of your thumb for the next injection
  - ❑ repeat the procedure for each subsequent 10 to 15 injections and then move to another area

---

complications associated with diabetes, and changes in eating times and habits. An effective education program helps relieve some of this anxiety.

Educating the Patient and Family About Insulin

Noncompliance is a problem with some patients with diabetes, making patient and family teaching vital to the proper management of diabetes. Patients may occasionally lapse in their adherence to the prescribed diet, such as around holidays or other special occasions. This slip may not cause a problem if it is brief and not excessive, as long as the patient immediately returns to the prescribed regimen. However, some patients frequently stray from the prescribed regimen, take extra insulin to cover dietary indiscretions, fast for several days before follow-up blood glucose determinations, and engage in other dangerous behaviors. Although some patients can be convinced that failure to adhere to the prescribed therapeutic regimen is detrimental to their health, others continue to deviate from the prescribed regimen until serious complications develop. Every effort is made to stress the importance of adherence to the prescribed treatment during all office or clinic visits.

The patient's self-monitoring of blood glucose levels using a glucometer is important. The patient must learn to obtain a small sample of blood from the finger and use the device. Printed instructions and illustrations are supplied with the device and must be reviewed with the patient. Patient Education Box 22-2 includes key points about insulin the patient and family members should know.

Oral Antidiabetic Drugs

Oral antidiabetic drugs are used to treat patients with type 2 diabetes that is not controlled by diet and exercise alone. These drugs are not effective for treating type 1 diabetes. Five types of oral antidiabetic drugs are currently in use:

- sulfonylureas (glimepiride, glyburide)
- biguanides (metformin)
- α-glucosidase inhibitors (acarbose, miglitol)
- meglitinides (nateglinide, repaglinide)
- thiazolidinediones (pioglitazone, rosiglitazone)

Additional drugs are listed in the Summary Drug Table: Antidiabetic Drugs.

Actions of Oral Antidiabetic Drugs

Actions of Sulfonylureas

Sulfonylureas appear to lower blood glucose by stimulating the beta cells of the pancreas to release insulin. The sulfonylureas are not effective if the beta cells of the pancreas are unable to release a sufficient amount of insulin to meet a patient's needs. The first-generation sulfonylureas (e.g., chlorpropamide, tolazamide, and tolbutamide) are not commonly used today because they have a long duration of action and a higher incidence of adverse reactions, and are more likely to react with other drugs. More commonly used sulfonylureas are the second- and third-generation drugs, such as glimepiride (Amaryl), glipizide (Glucotrol), and glyburide (DiaBeta, Micronase).

PATIENT EDUCATION BOX 22-2

Key Points for Patients Taking Insulin

❑ Use the home test method recommended by your health care provider for blood glucose or urine testing. Review the instructions included with the glucometer or the materials used for urine testing, including the technique for collecting the specimen, interpreting your test results, the number of times per day or week to test your blood or urine, and a record of test results.

❑ Your health care provider will review your dosage of insulin and how to calculate it. It is very important to use only the recommended type, source, and brand name of insulin. Do not change brands unless your health care provider approves, and keep a spare vial on hand.

❑ Keep your insulin at room temperature, away from heat and direct sunlight, if used within 1 month (and up to 3 months if refrigerated). Store vials not in use in the refrigerator. Prefilled insulin in glass or plastic syringes is stable for 1 week under refrigeration. Keep filled syringes in a vertical position with the needle pointing upward to avoid plugging the needle. Before injection, pull back the plunger and tip the syringe back and forth slightly to agitate and remix insulin.

❑ Be certain to purchase the same brand and needle size each time.

❑ Your health care provider will teach you how to hold the syringe, how to withdraw insulin from the vial, how to measure the insulin in the syringe using the syringe scale, how to mix insulin in the same syringe (when appropriate), how to eliminate air in the syringe and needle, and what to do if the syringe or needle is contaminated.

❑ Your insulin needs may change if you become ill, especially with vomiting or fever and during periods of stress or emotional disturbances. Contact your health care provider if these situations occur.

❑ It is important that you follow the prescribed diet, especially the calories allowed and the permissible food exchanges. Planning daily menus and establishing meal schedules are an important part of your care, as are selecting food from a restaurant menu, reading food labels, and the proper use of artificial sweeteners.

❑ It is important to carry an extra supply of insulin and a prescription for needles and syringes. Your health care provider will explain how to store insulin when traveling, to protect needles and syringes from theft, and the importance of discussing travel plans (especially foreign travel) before departing.

❑ Your health care provider will explain the signs and symptoms of hypoglycemia and hyperglycemia, what foods or fluids you should use to terminate a hypoglycemic reaction, and the importance of notifying your health care provider immediately if either reaction occurs.

❑ Good skin and foot care, personal cleanliness, frequent dental checkups, and routine eye examinations are an important part of treating your diabetes.

❑ Follow your health care provider's recommendations regarding physical activity.

❑ Notify your health care provider if you have an increase in blood glucose levels or your urine tests positive for ketones, if you become pregnant, if you have an occurrence of antidiabetic or hyperglycemic episodes, or if you have an illness, infection, or diarrhea (your insulin dosage may require adjustment). Tell your health care provider about any new problems (e.g., leg ulcers, numbness of the extremities, significant weight gain or loss).

❑ Wear identification, such as a medical alert tag, to inform medical personnel and others that you use insulin to control the disease

Generic Name	Trade Name*	Uses	Adverse Reactions	Dosage Ranges
Sulfonylureas acetohexamide *α-set-oh-hex'-a-mide*	Dymelor, *generic*	Adjunct to diet to lower blood glucose in type 2 diabetes; adjunct to insulin therapy in certain patients with type 1 diabetes	Anorexia, nausea, vomiting, epigastric discomfort, heartburn, hypoglycemia	250 mg–1.5 g/d PO
chlorpropamide *klor-proe'-pa-mide*	Diabinese, *generic*	Adjunct to diet in type 2 diabetes	Anorexia, nausea, vomiting, epigastric discomfort, heartburn, hypoglycemia	100–500 mg/d PO
glimepiride *glye-meh'-per-ide*	Amaryl	Adjunct to diet to lower blood glucose in type 2 diabetes; adjunct to insulin therapy in certain patients with type 1 diabetes	Anorexia, nausea, vomiting, epigastric discomfort, heartburn, diarrhea, hypoglycemia, allergic skin reactions	1–4 mg/d PO (do not exceed 8 mg/d)
glipizide *glip'-i-zide*	Glucotrol, Glucotrol XL, *generic*	Type 2 diabetes; adjunct to insulin therapy in the stabilization of certain cases of insulin-dependent diabetes (type 1)	Anorexia, nausea, vomiting, epigastric discomfort, heartburn, diarrhea, hypoglycemia, allergic skin reactions	5–40 mg/d PO
glyburide (glibenclamide) *glye-byoor-ide*	DiaBeta, Micronase, *generic*	Type 2 diabetes; adjunct to metformin when adequate results are not achieved with either drug alone; adjunct to insulin in stabilization of certain individuals with type 1 diabetes	Anorexia, nausea, vomiting, epigastric discomfort, heartburn, hypoglycemia	1.25–20 mg/d PO
tolazamide *tole-az'-a-mide*	Tolinase, *generic*	Type 2 diabetes; adjunct to insulin therapy in the stabilization of certain cases of insulin-dependent diabetes (type 1)	Anorexia, nausea, vomiting, epigastric discomfort, heartburn, hypoglycemia	100–1000 mg/d PO
tolbutamide *tole-byoo'-ta-mide*	Orinase, *generic*	Type 2 diabetes; adjunct to insulin therapy in the stabilization of certain cases of insulin-dependent diabetes (type 1)	Anorexia, nausea, vomiting, epigastric discomfort, heartburn, hypoglycemia	0.25–3 g/d PO
α-Glucosidase Inhibitors acarbose *aye-kar'-bose*	Precose	Type 2 diabetes; combination therapy with a sulfonylurea to enhance glycemic control	Flatulence, diarrhea, abdominal pain	25–100 mg TID PO
miglitol *mi'-gli-tole*	Glyset	Type 2 diabetes; combination therapy with a sulfonylurea to enhance glycemic control	Skin rash, flatulence, diarrhea, abdominal pain	25–100 mg TID PO

Generic Name	Trade Name*	Uses	Adverse Reactions	Dosage Ranges
Biguanide metformin *met-for'-min*	Glucophage, Glucophage XR generic	Type 2 diabetes; with a sulfonylurea or insulin to improve glycemic control	Anorexia, nausea, vomiting, epigastric pain, heartburn, diarrhea, hypoglycemia, allergic skin reactions	500–3000 mg/d PO; XR (extended release): 500–2000 mg/d
Meglitinides nateglinide *nah-teg'-lah-nyde*	Starlix	Type 2 diabetes; in combination with metformin to improve glycemic control	Headache, upper respiratory tract infection, back pain, flu symptoms, bronchitis	60–120 mg TID before meals
repaglinide *re-pag'-lah-nyd*	Prandin	Type 2 diabetes; in combination with metformin to improve glycemic control	Hyperglycemia, hypoglycemia, nausea, diarrhea, upper respiratory tract infection, sinusitis, headache, arthralgia, back pain	0.5–4 mg before meals PO (maximum dose is 16 mg/d)
Thiazolidinediones pioglitazone HCl *pie-oh-glit'-ah-zohn*	Actos	Type 2 diabetes; with sulfonylurea, metformin, or insulin to improve glycemic control	Headache, pain, myalgia, aggravated diabetes, infections, fatigue	15–45 mg/d PO
rosiglitazone maleate *roh-zee-glit'-ah-zohn*	Avandia	Type 2 diabetes; in combination with metformin to improve glycemic control	Headache, pain, diarrhea, hypoglycemia, hyperglycemia, fatigue, infections	4–8 mg/d PO
Antidiabetic Combination Drugs glyburide/ metformin HCl	Glucovance	Type 2 diabetes	See individual drugs	Starting dose: 1.25 mg/250 mg PO once or twice daily with meals; second-line therapy: 2.5 mg/500 mg– 5 mg/500 mg PO BID with meals; maximum daily dosage: 20 mg/2500 mg
Glucose-Elevating Agents diazoxide, oral *die-aze-ox'-ide*	Proglycem	Hypoglycemia caused by hyperinsulinism	Sodium and fluid retention, hyperglycemia, glycosuria, tachycardia, congestive heart failure	3–8 mg/kg/d PO in 2 or 3 equal doses every 8 or 12 h
glucagon *glue-kuh-gahn*	Glucagon Emergency Kit	Hypoglycemia	Nausea, vomiting, generalized allergic reactions	See instructions on the product

*The term *generic* indicates the drug is available in generic form.

Actions of Biguanides

Metformin (Glucophage), currently the only biguanide, acts by reducing hepatic glucose production and increasing insulin sensitivity in muscle and fat cells. The liver normally releases glucose by detecting the level of circulating insulin. When insulin levels are high, glucose is available in the blood and the liver produces little or no glucose. When insulin levels are low, there is little circulating glucose, so the liver produces more glucose. In type 2 diabetes, the liver may not detect levels of glucose in the blood and, instead of regulating glucose production, releases glucose despite blood sugar levels. Metformin sensitizes the liver to circulating insulin levels and reduces hepatic glucose production.

Actions of α-Glucosidase Inhibitors

The α-glucosidase inhibitors, acarbose (Precose) and miglitol (Glyset), lower blood sugar by delaying the digestion of carbohydrates and absorption of carbohydrates in the intestine.

Actions of Meglitinides

Like the sulfonylureas, the meglitinides act to lower blood glucose levels by stimulating the release of insulin from the pancreas. This action depends on the ability of the beta cell in the pancreas to produce some insulin. Examples of the meglitinides include nateglinide (Starlix) and repaglinide (Prandin).

Actions of Thiazolidinediones

The thiazolidinediones, also called glitazones, decrease insulin resistance and increase insulin sensitivity by modifying several processes, with the end result being decreasing hepatic glucogenesis (formation of glucose from glycogen) and increasing insulin-dependent muscle glucose uptake. Examples of the thiazolidinediones are rosiglitazone (Avandia) and pioglitazone (Actos).

Uses of Oral Antidiabetic Drugs

The oral antidiabetic drugs are of value only in the treatment of patients with type 2 diabetes mellitus whose condition cannot be controlled by diet alone. These drugs may also be used with insulin in the management of some patients with diabetes mellitus. Use of an oral antidiabetic drug with insulin may decrease the required insulin dosage in some individuals. Two oral antidiabetic drugs (e.g., a sulfonylurea and metformin) may also be used together when one antidiabetic drug and diet do not control blood glucose levels in type 2 diabetes mellitus.

Adverse Reactions of Oral Antidiabetic Drugs

Adverse Reactions of Sulfonylureas

Adverse reactions seen with the sulfonylureas include hypoglycemia, anorexia, nausea, vomiting, epigastric discomfort, weight gain, heartburn, and various vague neurologic symptoms, such as weakness and numbness of the extremities. Often, these can be eliminated by reducing the dosage or by giving the drug in divided doses. If these reactions become severe, then the health care provider may try another oral antidiabetic drug or discontinue the use of these drugs. If the drug therapy is discontinued, then it may be necessary to control the diabetes with insulin.

Adverse Reactions of Biguanides

Adverse reactions associated with the biguanide (metformin) include gastrointestinal upset (such as abdominal bloating, nausea, cramping, diarrhea) and a metallic taste. These adverse reactions are self-limiting and can be reduced if a patient is started on a low dose and the dosage increases slowly, and if the drug is taken with meals. Hypoglycemia rarely occurs when metformin is used alone.

Lactic acidosis (buildup of lactic acid in the blood) may also occur with metformin use. Although lactic acidosis is a rare adverse reaction, it is serious and can be fatal. Lactic acidosis occurs mainly in patients with kidney dysfunction. Symptoms of lactic acidosis include malaise (vague feeling of bodily discomfort), abdominal pain, rapid respirations, shortness of breath, and muscular pain. In some patients, vitamin B_{12} levels are decreased. This can be reversed with vitamin B_{12} supplements or with discontinuation of the drug therapy. Because weight loss can occur, metformin is sometimes recommended for obese patients or patients with insulin-resistant diabetes.

Adverse Reactions of α-Glucosidase Inhibitors

Because the α-glucosidase inhibitors, acarbose or miglitol, increase the transit time of food in the digestive tract, gastrointestinal disturbances may occur. The most common adverse reactions are bloating and flatulence. Other adverse reactions such as abdominal pain and diarrhea can occur. Although most oral antidiabetic drugs produce hypoglycemia, acarbose and miglitol, when used alone, do not cause hypoglycemia.

Adverse Reactions of Meglitinides

Adverse reactions of the meglitinides include upper respiratory infection, headache, rhinitis, bronchitis, headache, back pain, and hypoglycemia.

Adverse Reactions of Thiazolidinediones

Adverse reactions of the thiazolidinediones include aggravated diabetes mellitus, upper respiratory infections, sinusitis, headache, pharyngitis, myalgia, diarrhea, and back pain. When used alone, rosiglitazone and pioglitazone rarely cause hypoglycemia. However, patients receiving these drugs in combination with insulin or other oral hypoglycemics (e.g., the sulfonylureas) are at greater risk for hypoglycemia. A reduction in the dosage of insulin or the sulfonylurea may be required to prevent episodes of hypoglycemia.

Contraindications, Precautions, and Interactions of Oral Antidiabetic Drugs

Contraindications, Precautions, and Interactions of Sulfonylureas

Oral antidiabetic drugs are contraindicated in patients with a known hypersensitivity, diabetic ketoacidosis, severe infection, or severe endocrine disease. The first-generation sulfonylureas (chlorpropamide, tolazamide, and tolbutamide) are contraindicated in patients with coronary artery disease or liver or renal dysfunction. Other sulfonylureas are used cautiously in patients with impaired liver function because liver dysfunction can prolong the drug's effect. In addition, the sulfonylureas are used cautiously in patients with renal impairment and severe cardiovascular disease. There is a risk for cross-sensitivity with the sulfonylureas and the sulfonamides.

Many drugs may affect the action of the sulfonylureas; blood glucose must be monitored carefully when beginning therapy, discontinuing therapy, and any time any change is made in a drug regimen involving these drugs. The sulfonylureas may have an increased hypoglycemic effect when administered with the anticoagulants, chloramphenicol, clofibrate, fluconazole, histamine H_2 antagonists, methyldopa, monoamine oxidase inhibitors, salicylates, sulfonamides, and tricyclic antidepressants. The hypoglycemic effect of the sulfonylureas may be decreased when the agents are administered with beta-blockers, calcium channel blockers, cholestyramine, corticosteroids, estrogens, hydantoins, isoniazid, oral contraceptives, phenothiazines, thiazide diuretics, and thyroid agents.

Contraindications, Precautions, and Interactions of Biguanides

Metformin is contraindicated in patients with heart failure, renal disease, hypersensitivity to metformin, and acute or chronic metabolic acidosis, including ketoacidosis. The drug is also contraindicated in patients older than age 80 and during pregnancy (pregnancy category B) and lactation.

The drug is used cautiously during surgery. Metformin use is temporarily discontinued for surgical procedures. The drug therapy is restarted when a patient's oral intake has been resumed and renal function is normal.

There is a risk of acute renal failure when iodinated contrast material used for radiological studies is administered with metformin. Metformin therapy is stopped for 48 hours before and after radiological studies using iodinated material. Alcohol, amiloride, digoxin, morphine, procainamide, quinidine, quinine, ranitidine, tri-

amterene, trimethoprim, vancomycin, cimetidine, and furosemide all increase the risk of hypoglycemia. There is an increased risk of lactic acidosis when metformin is administered with the glucocorticoids.

Contraindications, Precautions, and Interactions of α–Glucosidase Inhibitors

The α-glucosidase inhibitors are contraindicated in patients with a hypersensitivity to the drug and in those with diabetic ketoacidosis, cirrhosis, inflammatory bowel disease, colonic ulceration, partial intestinal obstruction or predisposition to intestinal obstruction, or chronic intestinal diseases. Acarbose and miglitol are used cautiously in patients with renal impairment or pre-existing gastrointestinal problems such as irritable bowel syndrome and Crohn disease. These drugs are pregnancy category B drugs; safety for use during pregnancy has not been established. Digestive enzymes may reduce the effect of miglitol. The effects of acarbose may increase when administered with the loop or thiazide diuretics, glucocorticoids, oral contraceptives, calcium channel blockers, phenytoin, thyroid drugs, or the phenothiazines. Miglitol may decrease absorption of ranitidine and propranolol.

Contraindications, Precautions, and Interactions of Meglitinides

These drugs are contraindicated in patients with hypersensitivity to the drug, type 1 diabetes, and diabetic ketoacidosis. Both repaglinide and nateglinide are pregnancy category C drugs and are not recommended for use during pregnancy and lactation. These drugs are used cautiously in patients with liver or kidney disease. Certain drugs, such as NSAIDs, salicylates, MAOIs, and beta-adrenergic blocking drugs, may potentiate the hypoglycemic action of the meglitinides. Drugs such as the thiazides, corticosteroids, thyroid drugs, and sympathomimetics may decrease the hypoglycemic action of these drugs. A patient receiving one or more of these drugs along with an oral antidiabetic drug must be closely monitored.

Contraindications, Precautions, and Interactions of Thiazolidinediones

The thiazolidinediones are contraindicated in patients with a known hypersensitivity to any component of the drug and in patients with severe heart failure. These drugs are pregnancy category C drugs and should not be used during pregnancy unless the potential benefit of therapy outweighs the potential risk to the fetus. The thiazolidinediones are used cautiously in patients with edema, cardiovascular disease, and liver or kidney disease. These drugs may alter the effects of oral contraceptives.

Patient Management Issues with Oral Antidiabetic Drugs

Patients are observed every 2 to 4 hours for symptoms of hypoglycemia, particularly during the initial therapy or after a change in dosage. If both an oral antidiabetic drug and insulin are given, then the patient is observed more frequently for hypoglycemic episodes during the initial period of combination therapy. If the patient is receiving only an oral antidiabetic drug and a hypoglycemic reaction occurs, it is often (but not always) less intense than if it occurred with insulin administration.

The health care provider may order the patient weighed daily or weekly and vital signs taken daily. The patient is observed for adverse drug reactions and the health care provider notified if an adverse reaction occurs or if there is a significant weight gain or loss.

When some patients learn that diet and an oral drug can help them manage their diabetes, they have a tendency to discount the seriousness of the disorder. The importance of following the prescribed treatment regimen should be emphasized.

There is no fixed dosage for the treatment of diabetes. The drug regimen is individualized on the basis of the effectiveness and tolerance of the drug(s) used and the maximum recommended dose of the drug(s).

ALERT

Stabilizing Blood Glucose Levels
Exposure to stress, such as infection, fever, surgery, or trauma, may cause a loss of control of blood glucose levels in patients who have been stabilized with oral antidiabetic drugs. Should this occur, the health care provider might discontinue use of the oral drug and administer insulin.

Patient Management Issues with Sulfonylureas

Acetohexamide (Dymelor), chlorpropamide (Diabinese), tolazamide (Tolinase), and tolbutamide (Orinase) are given with food to prevent gastrointestinal upset. However, because food delays absorption, glipizide (Glucotrol) is given 30 minutes before a meal. Glyburide (Micronase) is administered with breakfast or with the first main meal of the day. Glimepiride is give once daily with breakfast or with the first main meal of the day.

ALERT

Older Patients and Sulfonylureas
Older adults have a greater sensitivity to the sulfonylureas and may require a dosage reduction.

After a patient has been taking sulfonylureas for a period of time, a condition called secondary failure may occur. **Secondary failure** occurs when the sulfonylurea loses its effectiveness. When a patient who has a history of good diabetes management has a gradual increase in blood sugar levels, secondary failure may be the cause. This increase in blood glucose levels can be caused by an increase in the severity of the diabetes or a decreased response to the drug. When secondary failure occurs, the health care provider may prescribe another sulfonylurea or add an oral antidiabetic drug such as metformin to the drug regimen.

Patient Management Issues with α-Glucosidase Inhibitors

Acarbose and miglitol are given three times per day with the first bite of the meal because food increases absorption. Some patients begin therapy with a lower dose once daily to minimize gastrointestinal effects such as abdominal discomfort, flatulence, and diarrhea. The dose is then gradually increased to three times daily. Periodic testing monitors the response to these drugs.

Patient Management Issues with Biguanides

Metformin is given 2 to 3 times per day with meals. If a patient has not experienced a response in 4 weeks using the maximum dose of metformin, then the health care provider may add an oral sulfonylurea while continuing metformin at the maximum dose. Glucophage XR (metformin extended release) is administered once daily with the evening meal.

Patient Management Issues with Meglitinides

Repaglinide is usually taken 15 minutes before meals but can be taken immediately, or up to 30 minutes before the meal. Nateglinide is taken up to 30 minutes before meals.

Patient Management Issues with Thiazolidinediones

The thiazolidinediones, pioglitazone and rosiglitazone, are given with or without meals. If the dose is missed at the usual meal, then the drug is taken at the next meal. If the dose is missed on one day, then the dose should not be doubled the next day. Once the drug is taken, the meal should not be delayed. Delay of a meal for as little as 30 minutes can cause hypoglycemia.

Managing Adverse Reactions of Oral Antidiabetic Drugs

Hypoglycemia

A hypoglycemic reaction must be immediately terminated. The health care provider is notified as soon as possible if hypoglycemia occurs, because the dosage of the oral antidiabetic drug (or insulin, when both insulin and an oral antidiabetic drug are given) may need to be changed.

ALERT

α-Glucosidase Inhibitors and Hypoglycemia

When hypoglycemia occurs in a patient taking an α-glucosidase inhibitor (e.g., acarbose or miglitol), the patient is given an oral form of glucose, such as glucose tablets or dextrose, rather than sugar (sucrose). Absorption of sugar is blocked by acarbose or miglitol.

When oral antidiabetic drugs are combined with other antidiabetic drugs (e.g., sulfonylureas) or insulin, the hypoglycemic effect may be enhanced. Elderly, debilitated, or malnourished patients are more likely to experience hypoglycemia.

ALERT

Hypoglycemia in Older Adults

Although elderly patients taking an oral antidiabetic drug are particularly susceptible to hypoglycemic reactions, these reactions may be difficult to detect in the elderly. The health care provider should be notified if blood sugar levels are elevated or if ketones are present in the urine.

Hyperglycemia and Ketoacidosis

Capillary blood specimens are obtained and tested in the same manner as for insulin. The health care provider should be notified if blood sugar levels are elevated or if ketones are present in the urine.

Lactic Acidosis

When taking metformin, a patient is at risk for lactic acidosis. The symptoms include unexplained hyperventilation, myalgia, malaise, gastrointestinal symptoms, or unusual somnolence. If a patient experiences these symptoms, then the health care provider should be notified at once. Elevated blood lactate levels are associated with lactic acidosis and should be reported immediately. Once a patient's diabetes is stabilized on metformin therapy, the adverse gastrointestinal tract reactions that often occur at the beginning of such therapy are unlikely to be related to the drug therapy. A later occurrence of gastrointestinal tract symptoms is more likely to be related to lactic acidosis or other serious disease.

Educating the Patient and Family About Oral Antidiabetic Drugs

Patients taking an oral antidiabetic drug may fail to comply with the prescribed treatment regimen because of the erroneous belief that not having to take insulin means that their disease is not serious. A patient may also mistakenly conclude that strict adherence to the recommended dietary plan is not required. The patient needs to understand that control of their diabetes is just as important as for patients requiring insulin and that control is achieved only when they adhere to the prescribed treatment regimen.

Although taking an oral antidiabetic drug is less complicated than self-administration of insulin, a patient with diabetes who is taking one of these drugs needs a thorough explanation of the management of the disease. Patient Education Box 22-3 includes key points about antidiabetic drugs the patient and family members should know.

PATIENT EDUCATION BOX 22-3

Key Points for Patients Taking Oral Antidiabetic Drugs

- ❑ Take the drug exactly as directed on the container; for example, with food or 30 minutes before a meal.
- ❑ To control your diabetes, follow exactly the diet and drug regimen prescribed by your health care provider.
- ❑ The drug prescribed for you is not oral insulin and cannot be substituted for insulin.
- ❑ Never stop taking this drug or increase or decrease the dose unless told to do so by your health care provider.
- ❑ Take the drug at the same time or times each day.
- ❑ Eat meals at approximately the same time each day. Erratic meal hours or skipped meals may cause you to have difficulty in controlling diabetes with this drug.
- ❑ Avoid alcohol, dieting, commercial weight-loss products, and strenuous exercise programs unless your health care provider has approved.
- ❑ Test your blood for glucose and urine for ketones as directed by your health care provider. Keep a record of your test results and bring this record to each visit to your health care provider.
- ❑ Maintain good foot and skin care and have routine eye and dental examinations for the early detection of any complications that may occur.
- ❑ Perform moderate exercise; avoid strenuous exercise and erratic periods of exercise.

Key Points for Patients Taking Oral Antidiabetic Drugs (continued)

❏ Wear identification, such as a medical alert tag, to inform medical personnel and others of your diabetes and the drug or drugs you currently use to treat the disease.

❏ Notify your health care provider if you experience any of the following: episodes of hypoglycemia, apparent symptoms of hyperglycemia, elevated blood glucose levels, positive results of urine tests for glucose or ketone bodies, or pregnancy. Also notify your health care provider of any serious illness not requiring hospitalization.

❏ Know the symptoms of hypoglycemia and hyperglycemia and your health care provider's recommended method for terminating a hypoglycemic reaction.

❏ Metformin: there is a risk of lactic acidosis when you use this drug. Discontinue the drug therapy and notify your health care provider immediately if you experience any of the following: respiratory distress, muscular aches, unusual difficulty sleeping, unexplained malaise, or nonspecific abdominal distress.

❏ α-Glucosidase Inhibitors: these drugs do not generally cause hypoglycemia. However, if sulfonylureas or insulin are used in combination with acarbose or miglitol, your blood sugar levels can be lowered enough to cause symptoms or even life-threatening hypoglycemia. Have a ready source of glucose to treat symptoms of low blood sugar when taking insulin or a sulfonylurea with these drugs.

❏ Meglitinides: if you skip a meal, do not take the drug. Similarly, if you add a meal, add a dose of the drug for that meal.

KEY POINTS

● Diabetes mellitus is a chronic disorder characterized either by insufficient insulin production in the beta cells of the pancreas or by cellular resistance to insulin. Insulin insufficiency results in elevated blood glucose levels, or hyperglycemia, and may cause other serious health conditions. Insulin and the oral antidiabetic drugs, along with diet and exercise, are the cornerstones of treatment for diabetes mellitus. They are used to prevent episodes of hypoglycemia and to normalize carbohydrate metabolism.

● Patients with type 1 diabetes mellitus produce insulin in insufficient amounts and therefore must have insulin supplementation to survive. Type 1 usually occurs before the age of 20 years, produces more severe symptoms than type 2 diabetes, and is more difficult to control. Treatment of type 1 diabetes is difficult and requires a strict regimen that typically includes a carefully calculated diet, planned physical activity, home glucose testing several times per day, and multiple daily insulin injections. The two major adverse reactions seen with insulin administration are hypoglycemia (low blood glucose or sugar) and hyperglycemia (elevated blood glucose or sugar). Insulin is contraindicated in patients with hypersensitivity to any ingredient of the product or when a patient is hypoglycemic, and is used cautiously in patients with liver or kidney disease and during pregnancy and lactation.

● Type 2 diabetes mellitus involves either a decreased production of insulin by the beta cells of the pancreas or a decreased sensitivity of the cells to insulin, making the cells insulin-resistant. The symptoms are less severe than in type 1 diabetes mellitus, and it is easier to control than type 1 diabetes. The oral antidiabetic drugs are of value only in the treatment of patients with type 2 diabetes mellitus whose condition cannot be controlled by diet alone. Both insulin and an oral antidiabetic may be prescribed, but use of an oral antidiabetic drug with insulin may decrease the insulin dosage in some patients. Two oral antidiabetic drugs may also be used together when one antidiabetic drug and diet do not control blood glucose levels in type 2 diabetes mellitus. The oral antidiabetic drugs are contraindicated in patients with a known hypersensitivity, diabetic ketoacidosis, severe infection, or severe endocrine disease.

CASE STUDY

Mr. Goddard, age 78 years, recently had type 2 diabetes mellitus diagnosed, and his health care provider has prescribed an oral antidiabetic drug. Mr. Goddard says his friend with diabetes takes insulin and he wonders why insulin was not prescribed for him.

1. What explanation should be given to Mr. Goddard's initial question?
   a. oral antidiabetics are used to treat patients with type 2 diabetes because insulin is used only for type 1 diabetes
   b. insulin is sometimes used for type 2 diabetes, but Mr. Goddard's case may not require it
   c. older patients are more responsive to oral antidiabetics than to insulin
   d. both a and c

2. As a patient with newly diagnosed disease, what topics should be reviewed with Mr. Goddard?
   a. diet
   b. diet and exercise
   c. diet, exercise, and stress reduction
   d. diet, exercise, stress reduction, and alcohol intake

3. Mr. Goddard mentions that his health care provider prescribed Tolinase. He wonders whether the nausea and occasional vomiting he has experienced could be an adverse reaction to Tolinase. He should be told:
   a. nausea and vomiting are adverse reactions to Tolinase, but he should ignore them and continue on with drug therapy
   b. nausea and vomiting are not adverse reactions to Tolinase
   c. he should contact his health care provider; older adults sometimes have sensitivity to the sulfonylurea drugs
   d. none of the above

WEBSITE ACTIVITIES

1. Go to the American Diabetes Association website (http://www.diabetes.org) and follow the link for the "Diabetes Risk Test." Read the opening material. What fraction of Americans with diabetes does not know they have it?

2. Now take the risk test and calculate your score. Although this is a simple assessment, this score can help you understand your own risk.

REVIEW QUESTIONS

1. Which of the following would most likely terminate a hypoglycemic reaction?
   a. regular insulin
   b. pH insulin
   c. orange juice
   d. crackers and milk

2. What are the adverse effects of meglitinides?
   a. photophobia
   b. aches in legs, shortness of breath
   c. skin rashes, urinary frequency
   d. headache, back pain

3. Which of the following symptoms indicate a possible hyperglycemic reaction?
   a. fatigue, weakness, confusion
   b. pale skin, elevated temperature
   c. thirst, abdominal pain, nausea
   d. rapid, shallow respirations, headache, nervousness

4. Which of the following drugs decrease the hypoglycemic effect of insulin?
   a. oral contraceptives
   b. spironolactone
   c. amoxicillin
   d. none of the above

5. In patients receiving oral hypoglycemic drugs, hypoglycemic reactions:
   a. will most likely occur 1 to 2 hours after a meal
   b. may be more intense than reactions seen with insulin administration
   c. may be less intense than reactions seen with insulin administration
   d. may occur more frequently in patients receiving oral hypoglycemic drugs

23 Hormones and Related Drugs

KEY TERMS

adrenal insufficiency—a critical deficiency of the mineralocorticoids and the glucocorticoids that requires immediate treatment

androgens—hormones that stimulate activity of the accessory male sex organs

corticosteroids—the collective name for the glucocorticoids and mineralocorticoids, hormones secreted by the adrenal cortex and essential to life

cryptorchism—failure of the testes to descend into the scrotum

Cushing syndrome—a disease caused by the overproduction of endogenous glucocorticoids

diabetes insipidus—a disease resulting from the failure of the posterior pituitary to secrete vasopressin or from surgical removal of the pituitary

estradiol—the most potent of the three endogenous estrogens

estriol—one of three endogenous estrogens

estrogens—female hormones influenced by the anterior pituitary gland

estrone—one of three endogenous estrogens

euthyroid—a normal thyroid

glucocorticoids—a hormone essential to life produced by the adrenal cortex

goiter—enlargement of the thyroid gland

gonadotropins—hormones that promote growth and function of the gonads

hyperstimulation syndrome—sudden ovarian enlargement with accumulation of serous fluid in the peritoneal cavity

hyperthyroidism— an increase in the amount of thyroid hormones secreted

hypothyroidism—a decrease in the amount of thyroid hormones secreted

iodism—excessive amounts of iodine in the body

mineralocorticoids—a hormone essential to life produced by the adrenal cortex

myxedema—a severe hypothyroidism manifested by a variety of symptoms

progesterone—female hormones influenced by the anterior pituitary gland

progestins—natural or synthetic substances that cause changes similar to those of progesterone

somatotropic hormone—a growth hormone secreted by the anterior pituitary

testosterone—the most potent naturally occurring androgen

thyroid storm—a severe form of hyperthyroidism also known as thyrotoxicosis

thyrotoxicosis—a severe form of hyperthyroidism, also known as thyroid storm

thyroxine—a hormone manufactured and secreted by the thyroid gland

triiodothyronine—a hormone manufactured and secreted by the thyroid gland

virilization—acquisition of male sexual characteristics by a woman

CHAPTER OBJECTIVES

On completion of this chapter, students will be able to:

1 Define the chapter's key terms.

2 Describe the general drug actions, uses, adverse reactions, contraindications, precautions, and interactions of hormones and related drugs.

3 Discuss important points to keep in mind when educating the patient or family members about the use of hormones and related drugs.

This chapter gives a basic overview of some of the drugs that affect the endocrine system, including drugs that affect the pituitary and adrenocortical hormones, the thyroid and antithyroid drugs, and male and female hormones.

Pituitary and Adrenocortical Hormones

The pituitary gland lies deep within the cranial vault, connected to the brain by the infundibular stalk (a downward extension of the floor of the third ventricle), and protected by an indentation of the sphenoid bone called the sella turcica (see Fig. 23-1). The pituitary gland, a small, gray, rounded structure, has two parts:

- anterior pituitary (adenohypophysis)
- posterior pituitary (neurohypophysis)

The gland secretes a number of pituitary hormones that regulate growth, metabolism, the reproductive cycle, electrolyte balance, and water retention or loss. Because the pituitary gland secretes so many hormones that regulate numerous vital processes, the gland is often referred to as the "master gland." The hormones secreted by the anterior and posterior pituitary and the organs influenced by these hormones are shown in Fig. 23-2.

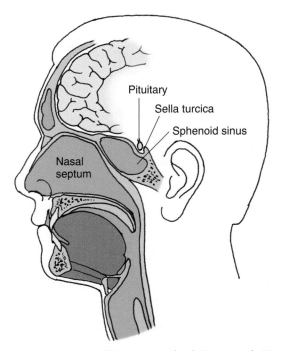

FIGURE 23-1   Location of the pituitary gland. (From Roach SS. *Introductory Clinical Pharmacology*, 7th ed. Baltimore: Lippincott Williams & Wilkins; 2004.)

Pituitary Gland

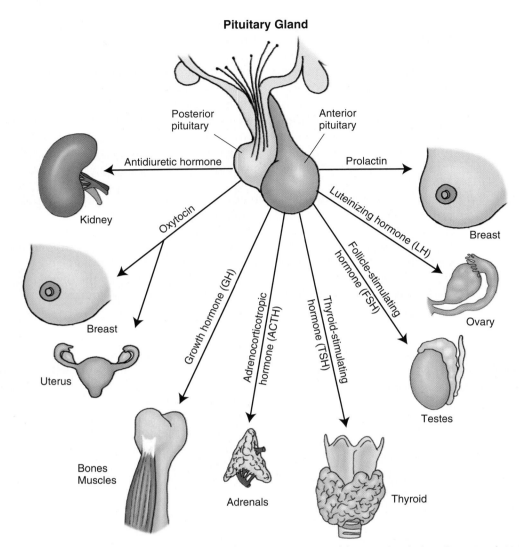

FIGURE 23-2   The pituitary gland and the hormones secreted by the anterior pituitary and the posterior pituitary. (From Roach SS. *Introductory Clinical Pharmacology*, 7th ed. Baltimore: Lippincott Williams & Wilkins; 2004.)

Anterior Pituitary Hormones

The hormones of the anterior pituitary include:

- follicle-stimulating hormone
- luteinizing hormone
- growth hormone
- adrenocorticotropic hormone
- thyroid-stimulating hormone and prolactin

This section discusses follicle-stimulating hormone, luteinizing hormone, growth hormone, and adrenocorticotropic hormone. Follicle-stimulating hormone and luteinizing hormone are called **gonadotropins** because they influence the gonads (the organs of reproduction). Growth hormone, also called somatotropin, contributes to the growth of the body during childhood, especially the growth of muscles and bones. Adrenocorticotropic hormone is produced by the anterior pituitary and stimulates the adrenal cortex to secrete the corticosteroids. The anterior pituitary hormone, thyroid-stimulating

hormone, is discussed later in the chapter. Prolactin, which is also secreted by the anterior pituitary, stimulates the production of breast milk in the postpartum patient. Additional functions of prolactin are not well understood. Prolactin is the only anterior pituitary hormone that is not used medically.

Gonadotropins: Follicle–Stimulating Hormone and Luteinizing Hormone

The gonadotropins (follicle-stimulating hormone and luteinizing hormone) influence the secretion of sex hormones, the development of secondary sex characteristics, and the reproductive cycle in both men and women. The gonadotropins discussed in this chapter include menotropins, urofollitropin, clomiphene, and chorionic gonadotropin.

Actions of Menotropins and Urofollitropin. Menotropins (Pergonal) and urofollitropin (Metrodin) are purified preparations of the gonadotropins extracted from the urine of postmenopausal women and induce ovulation and pregnancy. In men, menotropins induce the production of sperm.

Uses of Menotropins and Urofollitropin. Menotropins are used to induce ovulation and pregnancy in anovulatory (failure to produce an ovum or failure to ovulate) women. Menotropins are also used with human chorionic gonadotropin in women to stimulate multiple follicles for in vitro fertilization. In men, menotropins are used to induce the production of sperm (spermatogenesis). Urofollitropin is used to induce ovulation in women with polycystic ovarian disease and to stimulate multiple follicular development in ovulatory women for in vitro fertilization. See the Summary Drug Table: Anterior and Posterior Pituitary Hormones for additional information on the gonadotropins.

Adverse Reactions of Menotropins and Urofollitropin. The adverse reactions of the menotropins include ovarian enlargement, hemoperitoneum (blood in the peritoneal cavity), abdominal discomfort, and febrile reactions. Urofollitropin may result in mild to moderate ovarian enlargement, abdominal discomfort, nausea, vomiting, breast tenderness, and irritation at the injection site. Multiple births and birth defects have been reported with the use of both menotropins and urofollitropin.

Contraindications, Precautions, and Interactions of Menotropins and Urofollitropin. These drugs are contraindicated in patients who have a known hypersensitivity to any component of the drug. Menotropins are contraindicated in patients with high gonadotropin levels, thyroid dysfunction, adrenal dysfunction, abnormal bleeding, ovarian cysts, or those with an organic intracranial lesion. Urofollitropin is contraindicated during pregnancy (pregnancy category X). Menotropins are pregnancy category C drugs and also are contraindicated for use during pregnancy.

Actions of Clomiphene and Chorionic Gonadotropin. Clomiphene (Clomid) is a synthetic nonsteroidal compound that binds to estrogen receptors, decreasing the number of available estrogen receptors and causing the anterior pituitary to increase secretion of follicle-stimulating hormone and luteinizing hormone.

Chorionic gonadotropin is extracted from human placentas. The actions of chorionic gonadotropin are identical to those of the pituitary luteinizing hormone.

Uses of Clomiphene and Chorionic Gonadotropin. Clomiphene (Clomid) and Chorionic gonadotropin are both used to induce ovulation in anovulatory (nonovulating) women. Chorionic gonadotropin is also used for the treatment of prepubertal **cryptorchism** (failure of the testes to descend into the scrotum) and in men to treat selected cases of hypogonadotropic hypogonadism (inadequate secretion of gonadal hormones).

Adverse Reactions of Clomiphene and Chorionic Gonadotropin. Administration of clomiphene may result in vasomotor flushes (like the hot flashes of menopause), abdominal discomfort, ovarian enlargement, blurred vision, nausea, vomiting, and nervousness. Chorionic gonadotropin may result in headache, irritability, restlessness, fatigue, edema, and precocious puberty (when given for cryptorchism).

Contraindications, Precautions, and Interactions of Clomiphene and Chorionic Gonadotropin. These drugs are contraindicated in patients with a known hypersensitivity. Clomiphene is contraindicated in patients with liver disease, abnormal bleeding of undetermined origin, or ovarian cysts, and during pregnancy (pregnancy category C). Chorionic gonadotropin is contraindicated in patients with precocious puberty, prostatic cancer, or androgen-dependent neoplasm, and during pregnancy (pregnancy category X). These drugs are used cautiously in patients with epilepsy, migraine headaches, asthma, cardiac or renal dysfunction, and during lactation. There are no clinically significant known interactions with the gonadotropins.

Patient Management Issues with Gonadotropins. These drugs are almost always administered on an outpatient basis. Before prescribing any one of these drugs, the health care provider will take a thorough medical history and perform a physical examination. Additional laboratory and diagnostic tests for ovarian function and tubal patency may also be performed. A pelvic examination may be performed to rule out ovarian enlargement, pregnancy, or uterine problems.

Once drug therapy is begun, the patient is checked for signs of excessive ovarian enlargement such as abdominal distention, pain, or ascites (accumulation of serous fluid in the peritoneal cavity). The drug is discontinued at the first sign of ovarian stimulation or enlargement. The patient is usually admitted to the hospital for supportive measures.

ALERT

Clomiphene

If a patient reports visual disturbances, then the drug is discontinued and the health care provider should be notified. An examination by an ophthalmologist is usually required.

The patient is observed for symptoms of ovarian stimulation (abdominal pain, distension, sudden ovarian enlargement, ascites). The drug is discontinued and the health care provider should be notified if symptoms occur.

Menotropins, urofollitropin, and chorionic gonadotropin injections are given in the health care

SUMMARY DRUG TABLE   Anterior and Posterior Pituitary Hormones

Generic Name	Trade Name*	Uses	Adverse Reactions	Dosage Ranges
Anterior Pituitary Hormones				
chorionic gonadotropin (HCG) *sgo-nad'-oh-tro-pin*	A.P.L., Chorex, Gonic, Profasi, *generic*	Ovulatory failure, prepubertal cryptorchidism	Headache, edema, irritability, fatigue, nervousness, restlessness, precocious puberty, gynecomastia	Dosage frequency, length of treatment are individualized; ranges 5000–10,000 units dose IM
clomiphene citrate *klo'-mi-feen*	Clomid, Milophene, Serophene, *generic*	Ovulatory failure	Vasomotor flushes, breast tenderness, abdominal discomfort, blurred vision, ovarian enlargement, nausea, vomiting, nervousness	First course: 50 mg/d PO for 5 d; second and third course (if necessary) 100 mg/d for 5 d PO
corticotropin (ACTH) *kor-ti-ko-trop'-in*	Acthar, *generic*	Diagnostic testing of adrenocortical function, nonsuppurative thyroiditis, hypercalcemia associated with cancer, acute exacerbations of multiple sclerosis (MS)	Same as glucocorticoids (Box 23-2)	20 units QID IM, SC; diagnostic: 10–25 units *in 500 mL of 5% dextrose injection infused* IV over 8 h; acute exacerbations of MS: 80–120 units/d IM for 2–3 wk
menotropins *men-oh-troe'-pins*	Humegon, Pergonal	Ovulatory failure, stimulation of spermatogenesis	Ovarian enlargement, hemoperitoneum, febrile reactions, multiple pregnancies, hypersensitivity	75–150 IU IM
somatropin *soe-ma-tro'-pin*	Genotropin, Humatrope	Growth failure caused by deficiency of pituitary growth hormone in children	Failure to respond to therapy because of development of antibodies, hypothyroidism, insulin resistance, swelling of the joints, joint and/or muscle pain	Genotropin: 0.16–0.24 mg/kg/wk SC divided into 6–7 injections; Humatrope: 0.006–0.0125 mg/kg/d SC
somatrem *soe'-ma-trem*	Protropin	Growth failure	Same as somatropin	Individualize dosage based on response. Up to 0.1 mg/kg IM or SC 3 times per week.
urofollitropin *your-oh-fahl-ih-troe'-pin*	Fertinex, Metrodin	Induction of ovulation, stimulation of multiple follicle development	Ovarian enlargement, nausea, vomiting, breast tenderness, ectopic pregnancy, abdominal discomfort	75 IU IM for 7–12 d then 5000–10,000 U 1 day after last dose, may repeat sequence using 150 mg for 7–12 d followed by 5000–10,000 U HCG 1 day after last dose

Generic Name	Trade Name*	Uses	Adverse Reactions	Dosage Ranges
Posterior Hormones desmopressin acetate *des-moe-press'-in*	DDAVP, Stimate	Diabetes insipidus, hemophilia A, von Willebrand disease, nocturnal enuresis	Headache, nausea, nasal congestion, abdominal cramps	0.1–0.4 mL/d as a nasal solution as a single dose or in 2–3 divided doses; 0.5–1 mL/d SC, IV; 1 spray per nostril for a total of 300 mg; 0.05 mg PO BID (adjust according to water turnover)
lypressin *lye-press'-in*	Diapid	Diabetes insipidus	Rhinorrhea, nasal congestion, irritation of nasal passages, headache	1–2 sprays in one or both nostrils QID
vasopressin *vay-soe-press'-in*	Pitressin Synthetic	Diabetes insipidus, prevention and treatment of postoperative abdominal distension, to dispel gas interfering with abdominal x-ray examination	Tremor, sweating, vertigo, nausea, vomiting, abdominal cramps, hypersensitivity, headache	Diabetes insipidus: 5–10 U SC, IM; abdominal distension: 5–10 U IM; before abdominal x-ray: 10 U IM, SC 2 h and 30 min before procedure

*The term *generic* indicates the drug is available in generic form.

provider's office or clinic. These drugs are administered intramuscularly because they are destroyed in the gastrointestinal tract. Urofollitropin may cause pain and irritation at the injection site, and sites should be rotated and previous sites examined for redness and irritation. Female patients taking these drugs are usually examined by the health care provider every other day during treatment and at 2-week intervals to detect excessive ovarian stimulation, called **hyperstimulation syndrome** (sudden ovarian enlargement with accumulation of serous fluid in the peritoneal cavity). The patient may also experience pain. This syndrome usually develops quickly over a period of 3 to 4 days and requires hospitalization and discontinuation of the drug therapy. Abdominal pain and distention are indicators that hyperstimulation syndrome may be developing.

Managing Anxiety Patients wishing to become pregnant often experience anxiety. In addition, when taking these drugs there is the possibility of multiple births. The success rate of these drugs varies and depends on many factors. The health care provider usually discusses the value of drug therapy, as well as other approaches, with the patient and her sexual partner.

Educating the Patient and Family About Gonadotropins. Patients taking gonadotropins should keep all health care provider appointments, and adverse reactions should be reported. Patient Education Box 23-1 includes key points about gonadotropins that the patient and family members should know.

Growth Hormone

Growth hormone, also called **somatotropic hormone**, is secreted by the anterior pituitary. This hormone regulates the growth of the individual until early adulthood or the time when the person no longer gains height.

Actions of Growth Hormone. Growth hormone is available as the synthetic products somatrem (Protropin) and somatropin (Humatrope). Both are recombinant DNA products, are identical to human growth hormone, and produce skeletal growth in children.

Uses of Growth Hormone. These drugs are administered to children who have not grown because of a deficiency of pituitary growth hormone. They must be used before closure of bone epiphyses. Bone epiphyses are the ends of bones, separated from the main bone but joined to its cartilage, that allow for growth or lengthening of the bone. Growth hormone is ineffective in patients with closed epiphyses because when the epiphyses close, growth (in height) can no longer occur.

Adverse Reactions of Growth Hormone. These hormones cause few adverse reactions when administered as directed. Antibodies to somatropin may develop in a small number of patients, resulting in a failure of the drug to produce growth in the child. Some patients may experience hypothyroidism or insulin resistance. Swelling, joint pain, and muscle pain may also occur.

Contraindications, Precautions, and Interactions of Growth Hormone. Somatrem and somatropin are contraindicated in patients with known hypersensitivity to somatropin or sensitivity to benzyl alcohol, and those with epiphyseal closure or underlying cranial lesions. The drug is used cautiously in patients with thyroid disease or diabetes, and during pregnancy (pregnancy category C) and lactation. Excessive amounts of glucocorticoids may decrease response to somatropin.

Patient Management Issues with Growth Hormone. A thorough physical examination and laboratory and diagnostic tests are performed before a child is accepted into a growth program. Before therapy is started, a patient's vital signs, height, and weight are recorded.

Children may increase their growth rate from 3.5 to 4 centimeters per year before treatment to 8 to 10 centimeters per year during the first year of treatment. Each time the child visits the health care provider's office or clinic (usually every 3–6 months), the child's height and weight are measured and recorded to evaluate the response to therapy. Bone age is monitored periodically.

The bone age monitors bone growth and detects epiphyseal closure, at which time therapy must be stopped.

Periodic testing of growth hormone levels, glucose tolerance, and thyroid functioning may be performed at intervals during treatment.

Educating the Patient and Family About Growth Hormone. When the patient is receiving growth hormone, the health care provider discusses in detail the therapeutic regimen for increasing growth (height) with the child's parents or guardians. If the drug is to be given at bedtime (which most closely adheres to the body's natural release of the hormone), the parents are instructed on the proper technique to administer the injections. The parents are encouraged to keep all clinic or office visits. The child may experience sudden growth and an increase in appetite, and it is important for the parents to understand these possibilities. The parents are asked to report lack of growth, symptoms of diabetes (e.g., increased hunger, increased thirst, or frequent voiding), or symptoms of hypothyroidism (e.g., fatigue, dry skin, or intolerance to cold).

Adrenocorticotropic Hormone: Corticotropin

Actions of Corticotropin. Corticotropin is an anterior pituitary hormone that stimulates the adrenal cortex to produce and secrete adrenocortical hormones, primarily the glucocorticoids.

Uses of Corticotropin. Corticotropin is used for diagnostic testing of adrenocortical function. This drug may also be used for the management of acute exacerbations of multiple sclerosis, nonsuppurative thyroiditis, and hypercalcemia associated with cancer. It is also used as an anti-inflammatory and immunosuppressant drug when conventional glucocorticoid therapy has not been effective (see Box 23-1).

Adverse Reactions of Corticotropin. Because ACTH stimulates the release of glucocorticoids from the adrenal gland, adverse reactions of this hormone are similar to those seen with the glucocorticoids (see Box 23-2) and affect many body systems. The most common adverse reactions include:

• Central nervous system: mental depression, mood swings, insomnia, psychosis, euphoria, nervousness, and headaches
• Cardiovascular system: hypertension, edema, congestive heart failure, and thromboembolism
• Gastrointestinal system: nausea, vomiting, increased appetite, weight gain, and peptic ulcer
• Genitourinary system: amenorrhea and irregular menses
• Integumentary system: petechiae, ecchymosis, decreased wound healing, hirsutism (excessive growth of body hair), and acne
• Musculoskeletal system: weakness and osteoporosis

Box 23-1 **Uses of Glucocorticoids**

Endocrine Disorders
Primary or secondary adrenal cortical insufficiency, congenital adrenal hyperplasia, nonsuppressive thyroiditis, hypercalcemia associated with cancer

Rheumatic Disorders
Short-term management of acute ankylosing spondylitis, acute and subacute bursitis, acute nonspecific tenosynovitis, acute gouty arthritis, psoriatic arthritis, rheumatoid arthritis, post-traumatic osteoarthritis, synovitis of osteoarthritis, epicondylitis

Collagen Diseases
Lupus erythematosus, acute rheumatic carditis, systemic dermatomyositis

Dermatologic Diseases
Pemphigus, bullous dermatitis herpetiformis, severe erythema multiforme (Stevens–Johnson syndrome), exfoliative dermatitis, mycosis fungoides, severe psoriasis, severe seborrheic dermatitis, angioedema, urticaria, various skin disorders, such as lichen planus or keloids

Allergic States
Control of severe or incapacitating allergic conditions not controlled by other methods, bronchial asthma (including status asthmaticus), contact dermatitis, atopic dermatitis, serum sickness, drug hypersensitivity reactions

Ophthalmic Diseases
Severe acute and chronic allergic and inflammatory processes, keratitis, allergic corneal marginal ulcers, herpes zoster of the eye, iritis, iridocyclitis, chorioretinitis, diffuse posterior uveitis, optic neuritis, sympathetic ophthalmia, anterior segment inflammation

Respiratory Diseases
Sarcoidosis, berylliosis, fulminating or disseminating pulmonary tuberculosis, aspiration pneumonia

Hematologic Disorders
Idiopathic or secondary thrombocytopenic purpura, hemolytic anemia, red blood cell anemia, congenital hypoplastic anemia

Neoplastic Diseases
Leukemia, lymphomas

Edematous States
To induce diuresis or remission of proteinuria in the nephrotic state

Gastrointestinal Diseases
During critical period of ulcerative colitis, regional enteritis, intractable sprue

Nervous System
Acute exacerbations of multiple sclerosis

Box 23-2 **Adverse Reactions of Glucocorticoids**

Fluid and Electrolyte Disturbances
Sodium and fluid retention, congestive heart failure in susceptible patients, potassium loss, hypokalemic alkalosis, hypertension, hypocalcemia, hypotension or shocklike reactions

Musculoskeletal
Muscle weakness, loss of muscle mass, tendon rupture, osteoporosis, aseptic necrosis of femoral and humoral heads, spontaneous fractures

Cardiovascular
Thromboembolism or fat embolism, thrombophlebitis, necrotizing angiitis, syncopal episodes, cardiac arrhythmias, aggravation of hypertension

Gastrointestinal
Pancreatitis, abdominal distention, ulcerative esophagitis, nausea, increased appetite and weight gain, possible peptic ulcer with perforation, hemorrhage

Dermatologic
Impaired wound healing, thin fragile skin, petechiae, ecchymoses, erythema, increased sweating, suppression of skin test reactions, subcutaneous fat atrophy purpura, striae, hyperpigmentation, hirsutism, acneiform eruptions, urticaria, angioneurotic edema

Neurologic
Convulsions, steroid-induced catatonia, increased intracranial pressure with papilledema (usually after treatment is discontinued), vertigo, headache, neuritis or paresthesia, steroid psychosis, insomnia

Endocrine
Amenorrhea, other menstrual irregularities, development of cushingoid state, suppression of growth in children, secondary adrenocortical and pituitary unresponsive (particularly in times of stress), decreased carbohydrate tolerance, manifestation of latent diabetes mellitus, increased requirements for insulin or oral hypoglycemic agents (in diabetics)

Ophthalmic
Posterior subcapsular cataracts, increased intraocular pressure, glaucoma, exophthalmos

Metabolic
Negative nitrogen balance (caused by protein catabolism)

Other
Anaphylactoid or hypersensitivity reactions, aggravation of existing infections, malaise, increase or decrease in sperm motility and number

- Endocrine system: menstrual irregularities, hyperglycemia, and decreased growth in children
- Miscellaneous: hypersensitivity reactions, hypokalemia, hypernatremia, increased susceptibility to infection, cushingoid appearance (e.g., moon face, "buffalo hump," hirsutism), cataracts, and increased intraocular pressure

Managing Adverse Reactions of Corticotropin Corticotropin may mask signs of infection, including fungal or viral eye infections. Any symptoms of sore throat, cough, fever, malaise, sores that do not heal, or redness or irritation of the eyes should be reported. The patient may have a decreased resistance and inability to localize infection. The patient's skin should be observed daily for localized signs of infection, especially at injection sites or intravenous access sites. Visitors are monitored to protect the patient against those with infectious illness.

Corticotropin can also cause alterations in the psyche. Any evidence of behavior change, such as mental depression, insomnia, euphoria, mood swings, or nervousness must be reported. Anxiety is decreased with understanding of the therapeutic regimen.

Contraindications, Precautions, and Interactions of Corticotropin. Corticotropin is contraindicated in patients with adrenocortical insufficiency or hyperfunction, an allergy to pork or pork products (corticotropin is obtained from porcine pituitaries), systemic fungal infections, ocular herpes simplex, scleroderma, osteoporosis, or hypertension. Patients taking corticotropin also should avoid any vaccinations with live virus.

Corticotropin is used cautiously in patients with diabetes, diverticulosis, renal insufficiencies, myasthenia gravis, tuberculosis (may reactivate the disease), hypothyroidism, cirrhosis, nonspecific ulcerative colitis, heart failure, seizures, or febrile infections. The drug is classified as a pregnancy category C drug and is used cautiously during pregnancy and lactation. Corticotropin is used cautiously in children because it can inhibit skeletal growth.

When amphotericin B or diuretics are administered with corticotropin, the potential for hypokalemia is increased. There may be an increased need for insulin or oral antidiabetic drugs in a patient with diabetes who is taking corticotropin. There is a decreased effect of corticotropin when the agent is administered with a barbiturate. Profound muscular depression is possible when corticotropin is administered with an anticholinesterase drug. Live virus vaccines taken while taking corticotropin may potentiate virus replication, increase the vaccine's adverse reaction, and decrease the patient's antibody response to the vaccine.

Before administering corticotropin, the patient's weight and vital signs are taken, and skin integrity, lungs, and mental status are assessed. Additional assessments depend on the patient's condition and diagnosis.

The health care provider may order baseline diagnostic tests, such as chest x-rays, an upper gastrointestinal x-ray, serum electrolytes, complete blood count, or urinalysis. Patients receiving prolonged therapy should have periodic hematologic, serum electrolytes, and serum glucose studies performed.

Educating the Patient and Family About Corticotropin. Patient Education Box 23-2 includes key points about corticotropin that the patient and family members should know.

Posterior Pituitary Hormones

The posterior pituitary gland produces two hormones: vasopressin (antidiuretic hormone) and oxytocin (see Chapter 24). Posterior pituitary hormones are summarized in the Summary Drug Table: Anterior and Posterior Pituitary Hormones.

Actions of Vasopressin

Vasopressin (Pitressin Synthetic) and its derivatives, namely lypressin (Diapid) and desmopressin (DDAVP), regulate the reabsorption of water by the kidneys. The pituitary secretes vasopressin when body fluids must be conserved. An example of this mechanism may be seen when a patient has severe vomiting and diarrhea with little or no fluid intake. When this and similar conditions are present, the posterior pituitary releases the hormone vasopressin, water in the kidneys is reabsorbed into the blood (i.e., conserved), and the urine becomes concentrated. Vasopressin exhibits its greatest activity on the renal tubular epithelium, where it promotes water resorption and smooth muscle contraction throughout the vascular bed. Vasopressin has some vasopressor activity.

PATIENT EDUCATION BOX 23-2

Key Points for Patients Taking Corticotropin Therapy

- ☐ Report any adverse reactions to your health care provider.
- ☐ Avoid contact with those who have an infection because your resistance to infection may be decreased.
- ☐ Report any symptoms of infection immediately (e.g., sore throat, fever, cough, or sores that do not heal).
- ☐ Patients with diabetes: Monitor your blood glucose (if you are performing self-monitoring) or urine closely, and notify your health care provider if glucose appears in the urine or the blood glucose level increases significantly. An increase in the dosage of the oral antidiabetic drug or insulin may be needed.
- ☐ Notify your health care provider of a marked weight gain, swelling in the extremities, muscle weakness, persistent headache, visual disturbances, or behavior change.

Uses of Vasopressin

Vasopressin and its derivatives are used in the treatment of **diabetes insipidus**, a disease resulting from the failure of the pituitary to secrete vasopressin or from surgical removal of the pituitary. Diabetes insipidus is characterized by marked increase in urination (as much as 10 L in 24 hours) and excessive thirst. Treatment with vasopressin therapy replaces the hormone in the body and restores normal urination and thirst. Vasopressin may also be used for the prevention and treatment of postoperative abdominal distention and to dispel gas interfering with abdominal x-rays.

Adverse Reactions of Vasopressin

Local or systemic hypersensitivity reactions may occur in some patients receiving vasopressin. Tremor, sweating, vertigo, nausea, vomiting, abdominal cramps, and water intoxication (overdosage, toxicity) may also occur.

Managing Adverse Reactions of Vasopressin. The adverse reactions of vasopressin, such as skin blanching, abdominal cramps, and nausea, may be decreased by administering the agent with one or two glasses of water. If these adverse reactions occur, the patient should be told that these reactions are not serious and should disappear within a few minutes.

ALERT

Vasopressin and Water Intoxication

An excessive dosage is manifested as water intoxication (fluid overload). Symptoms of water intoxication include drowsiness, listlessness, confusion, and headache (which may precede convulsions and coma). If signs of excessive dosage occur, then the health care provider should be notified before the next dose of the drug is due, because a change in the dosage, a restriction of oral or intravenous fluids, and the administration of a diuretic may be necessary.

Contraindications, Precautions, and Interactions of Vasopressin

Vasopressin is contraindicated in patients with chronic renal failure, increased blood urea nitrogen, or an allergy to beef or pork proteins.

Vasopressin is used cautiously in patients with a history of seizures, migraine headaches, asthma, congestive heart failure, or vascular disease (may precipitate angina or myocardial infarction) and in those with perioperative polyuria. The drug is classified as a pregnancy category C drug and must be used cautiously during pregnancy and lactation.

The antidiuretic effects of vasopressin may be decreased when the agent is taken with the following drugs: lithium, heparin, norepinephrine, or alcohol. The antidiuretic effect may be increased when the drug is used with carbamazepine, clofibrate, or fludrocortisone.

Patient Management Issues with Vasopressin

Before administering the first dose of vasopressin for the management of diabetes insipidus, the patient's blood pressure, pulse, and respiratory rate and weight are measured. Serum electrolyte levels and other laboratory tests may be ordered.

Before administering vasopressin to relieve abdominal distention, the patient's blood pressure, pulse, and respiratory rate are taken, and the patient's abdominal girth is measured and recorded.

ALERT

Older Adults and Vasopressin Use

Older adults are particularly sensitive to the effects of vasopressin and should be monitored closely during administration of the drug.

Vasopressin may be given intramuscularly or subcutaneously to treat diabetes insipidus. The injection solution may also be administered intranasally on cotton pledgets or by nasal spray or dropper. The health care provider instructs the patient about intranasal administration. To prevent or relieve abdominal distention, it may be given intramuscularly.

Lypressin is administered intranasally by spraying one to two sprays in one or both nostrils usually four times per day or when the frequency of urination increases or significant thirst develops. Dosages greater than 10 sprays in each nostril every 3 to 4 hours are not recommended. Patients learn to regulate their dosage based on the frequency of urination and increase of thirst.

Desmopressin may be given orally, intranasally, subcutaneously, or intravenously. The oral dose must be individualized for each patient and adjusted according to the patient's response to therapy. When the drug is administered nasally, a nasal tube is used for administration.

Managing Fluid Volume. The symptoms of diabetes insipidus include the voiding of a large volume of urine at frequent intervals during the day and throughout the night. Accompanied by frequent urination is the need to drink large volumes of fluid because these patients are continually thirsty. Patients must be supplied with large amounts of drinking water. When the patient has limited ability to move about, water should be readily available. Until controlled by a drug, the symptoms of frequent urination and excessive thirst may cause a great deal of anxiety. The patient should be reassured that with the proper drug therapy, these symptoms will most likely be reduced or eliminated.

When a patient has diabetes insipidus, fluid intake and output are measured and the patient is monitored for signs of dehydration (dry mucous membranes, concentrated urine, poor skin turgor, flushed dry skin, confusion). This is especially important early in treatment until the optimum dosage is determined and symptoms have diminished. If the patient's output greatly exceeds intake, then the health care provider should be notified. In some instances, the health care provider may order specific gravity and volume measurements of each voiding or at hourly intervals.

Managing Abdominal Distention. If the patient is receiving vasopressin for abdominal distention, then the method of treating this problem and the necessity of monitoring drug effectiveness (i.e., auscultation of the abdomen for bowel sounds, insertion of a rectal tube, measurement of the abdomen) are fully explained.

Educating the Patient and Family About Vasopressin

Patients should be reminded of the importance of adhering to their prescribed treatment program. Patient Education Box 23-3 includes key points about vasopressin that the patient and family members should know.

Adrenocortical Hormones

The adrenal gland lies on the superior surface of each kidney. It is a double organ composed of an outer cortex and an inner medulla. In response to adrenocorticotropic hormone secreted by the anterior pituitary, the adrenal cortex secretes several hormones (the glucocor-

ticoids, the mineralocorticoids, and small amounts of sex hormones).

This section of the chapter discusses the hormones produced by the adrenal cortex or the adrenocortical hormones, which are the **glucocorticoids** and **mineralocorticoids**. These hormones are essential to life and influence many organs and structures of the body. The glucocorticoids and mineralocorticoids are collectively called **corticosteroids**.

Actions of Glucocorticoids

The glucocorticoids influence or regulate functions such as the immune response, the regulation of glucose, fat and protein metabolism, and control of the anti-inflammatory response. Table 23-1 describes the activity of the glucocorticoids within the body.

The glucocorticoids enter target cells and bind to receptors, initiating many complex reactions in the body. Some of these actions are considered undesirable, depending on the indication for which these drugs are being used. Examples of the glucocorticoids include cortisone, hydrocortisone, prednisone, prednisolone, and triamcinolone. The Summary Drug Table: Adrenocortical Hormones: Glucocorticoids and Mineralocorticoids provides information concerning these hormones.

Uses of Glucocorticoids

The glucocorticoids are used as replacement therapy for adrenocortical insufficiency and to treat allergic reactions, collagen diseases (e.g., systemic lupus erythematosus), dermatologic conditions, rheumatic disorders, shock, and other conditions (see Box 23-1). The anti-inflammatory activity of these hormones makes them valuable as anti-inflammatories and as immunosuppressants to suppress inflammation and modify the immune response.

Adverse Reactions of Glucocortitoids

The adverse reactions of glucocorticoids are given in Box 23-2. Long- or short-term high-dose therapy may also produce many of the signs and symptoms seen with **Cushing syndrome**, a disease caused by the overproduction of endogenous glucocorticoids. Some of the signs and symptoms of this Cushing-like (or cushingoid) state include a "buffalo" hump (a hump on the back of the neck), moon face, oily skin and acne, osteoporosis, purple striae on the abdomen and hips, skin pigmentation, and weight gain. When a serious disease or disorder is being treated, it is often necessary to allow these effects to occur because therapy with these drugs is absolutely necessary.

Managing Adverse Reactions of Glucocorticoids.
Adrenal Insufficiency Administration of the glucocorticoids poses the threat of adrenal gland insufficiency

PATIENT EDUCATION BOX 23-3

Key Points for Taking Vasopressin

- ❑ Drink one or two glasses of water immediately before taking the drug.
- ❑ Measure the amount of fluids you drink each day.
- ❑ Measure the amount of urine passed at each voiding, and then total the amount for each 24-hour period.
- ❑ Do not drink alcohol while taking these drugs.
- ❑ Rotate injection sites for parenteral administration.
- ❑ Contact your primary health care provider immediately if you experience any of the following: a significant increase or decrease in urinary output, abdominal cramps, blanching of the skin, nausea, signs of inflammation or infection at the injection sites, confusion, headache, or drowsiness.
- ❑ Wear a medical alert tag identifying the diabetes insipidus and your drug regimen.

TABLE 23-1   **Activity of Glucocorticoids in the Body**

Function Within the Body	Description of Bodily Activity
Anti-inflammatory	Stabilizes lysosomal membrane and prevents the release of proteolytic enzymes released during the inflammatory process
Regulation of blood pressure	Potentiates vasoconstrictor action of norepinephrine. Without glucocorticoids, the vasoconstricting action is decreased and blood pressure falls.
Metabolism of carbohydrates and protein	Facilitates the breakdown of protein in the muscle, leading to increased plasma amino acid levels. Increases activity of enzymes necessary for glucogenesis producing hyperglycemia, which can aggravate diabetes, precipitate latent diabetes, and cause insulin resistance
Metabolism of fat	A complex phenomena that promotes the use of fat for energy (a positive effect) and permits fat stores to accumulate in the body, causing buffalo hump and moon-shaped or round face (a negative effect).
Interference with the immune response	Decreases the production of lymphocytes and eosinophils in the blood by causing atrophy of the thymus gland; blocks the release of cytokines, resulting in a decreased performance of T and B monocytes in the immune response. (This action, coupled with the anti-inflammatory action, makes the corticosteroids useful in delaying organ rejection in patients with transplants.)
Stress	As a protective mechanism, the corticosteroids are released during periods of stress (e.g., injury or surgery). The release of epinephrine or norepinephrine by the adrenal medulla during stress has a synergistic effect along with the corticosteroids.
Central nervous system disturbances	Affects mood and possibly causes neuronal or brain excitability, causing euphoria, anxiety, depression, psychosis, and an increase in motor activity in some individuals

(particularly if the alternate-day therapy is not prescribed). Administration of glucocorticoids several times per day and during a short time (as little as 5–10 days) results in shutting off the pituitary release of andrenocorticotropic hormone because there are always high levels of the glucocorticoids in the plasma (caused by the body's own glucocorticoid production plus the administration of a glucocorticoid drug). Ultimately, the pituitary atrophies and ceases to release andrenocorticotropic hormone. Without andrenocorticotropic hormone, the adrenals fail to manufacture and release (endogenous) glucocorticoids. When this happens, the patient has acute adrenal insufficiency, which is a life-threatening situation until corrected with the administration of an exogenous glucocorticoid.

Adrenal insufficiency is a critical deficiency of the mineralocorticoids and the glucocorticoids that requires immediate treatment. Symptoms of adrenal insufficiency include fever, myalgia, arthralgia, malaise, anorexia, nausea, orthostatic hypotension, dizziness, fainting, dyspnea, and hypoglycemia. Death caused by circulatory collapse will result unless the condition is treated promptly. Situations producing stress (e.g., trauma, surgery, severe illness) may precipitate the need for an increase in dosage of the corticosteroids until the crisis situation is resolved.

ALERT

Ending Glucocorticoid Therapy

At no time should glucocorticoid therapy be discontinued suddenly. When administration of a glucocorticoid extends beyond 5 days and the drug therapy is to be discontinued, the dosage must be tapered off over several days. In some instances, it may be necessary to taper the dose over 7 to 10 or more days. Abrupt discontinuation of glucocorticoid therapy usually results in acute adrenal insufficiency, which, if not recognized in time, can result in death. Tapering the dosage allows normal adrenal function to return gradually, preventing adrenal insufficiency.

Managing Infection Any slight rise in temperature, sore throat, or other signs of infection should be reported to the health care provider as soon as possible because of a possible decreased resistance to infection during glucocorticoid therapy. The patient should avoid contact with anyone with any type of infection or recent exposure to an infectious disease.

Managing Mental and Emotional Changes Mental and emotional changes may occur when the glucocorticoids are administered. Mental changes should be reported to

SUMMARY DRUG TABLE   Adrenocortical Hormones: Corticosteroids and Mineralocorticoids

Generic Name	Trade Name*	Uses	Adverse Reactions	Dosage Ranges
Glucocorticoids betamethasone *bay-ta-meth'-a-zone*	Celestone	See Box 23-1	See Box 23-2	Individualize dosage: 0.6–7.2 mg/d PO
betamethasone sodium phosphate *bay-ta-meth'-a-zone*	Celestone Phosphate	See Box 23-1	See Box 23-2	Up to 9 mg/d IM, IV
budesonide *bue-des'-oh-nide*	Entocort EC	Crohn disease	See Box 23-2	9 mg once daily in AM for 8 wk
cortisone *kor'-ti-sone*	*Generic*	See Box 23-1	See Box 23-2	25–300 mg/day PO
dexamethasone *dex-a-meth'-a-sone*	Decadron, Dexameth, Dexone, Hexadrol, *generic*	Acute self-limited allergic disorder or acute exacerbations of chronic allergic disorders	See Box 23-2	Individualize dosage based on severity of condition and response; give daily dose before 9 AM to minimize adrenal suppression; after long-term therapy, reduce slowly to avoid adrenal insufficiency
dexamethasone acetate *dex-a-meth'-a-sone*	Cordostat-LA, Dalalone-LA, Decadron-LA, Dexasone-LA, Dalalone DP, *generic*	See Box 23-1	See Box 23-2	0.5–9 mg/d 10 mg IV, then 4 mg IM q6h; intra-articular: large joints 4–16 mg; soft tissue: 0.8–1.6 mg
hydrocortisone (cortisol) *hye-droe-kor'-ti-zone*	Cortef *generic*,	See Box 23-1	See Box 23-2	20–240 mg PO in single or divided doses
hydrocortisone sodium phosphate *hye-droe-kor'-ti-zone*	*Generic*	See Box 23-1	See Box 23-2	20–240 mg/d q12h
hydrocortisone sodium succinate *hye-droe-kor'-ti-zone*	A-hydro Cort, Solu-Cortef	See Box 23-1	See Box 23-2	Reduce dose based on condition and response but give no less than 25 mg/d
methylprednisolone *meth-ill-pred-niss'-oh-lone*	Medrol, *generic*	See Box 23-1	See Box 23-2	Initial dose: 4–48 mg/d PO; Dosepak 21-day therapy: follow manufacturer's directions; alternate day therapy: twice the usual dose is administered every other morning
methylprednisolone acetate *meth-ill-pred-niss'-oh-lone*	Depoject, Depo-Medrol, Depopred, *generic*	See Box 23-1	See Box 23-2	40–120 mg IM; 4–80 mg intra-articular and soft tissue injections
methylprednisolone sodium succinate *meth-ill-pred-niss'-oh-lone*	A-Methapred, Solu-Medrol, *generic*	See Box 23-1	See Box 23-2	10–40 mg IV, IM

Generic Name	Trade Name*	Uses	Adverse Reactions	Dosage Ranges
prednisolone *pred-niss'-oh-lone*	Prelone, *generic*	See Box 23-1	See Box 23-2	5–60 mg/d PO; acute exacerbations in MS: 200 mg/d for 1 wk, followed by 80 mg every other day for 1 mo PO
prednisolone acetate *pred-niss'-oh-lone*	Key-Pred 50, Predcor-50, *generic*	See Box 23-1	See Box 23-2	4–60 mg/d IM (not for IV use); MS: 200 mg/d for 1 wk, followed by 80 mg/d every other day for 1 month IM
prednisone *pred'-ni-sone*	Deltasone, Meticorten, Orasone, *generic*	See Box 23-1	See Box 23-2	Individualize dosage: initial dose usually between 5 and 60 mg/d PO
triamcinolone *trye-am-sin'-oh-lone*	Aristocort, Atolone, Kenacort *generic*	See Box 23-1	See Box 23-2	4–48 mg/d PO
triamcinolone acetonide *trye-am-sin'-oh-lone*	Kenalog-10, Tac-3, Triam-A, *generic*	See Box 23-1	See Box 23-2	Systemic: 2.5–60 mg/d IM; Intra-articular: 2.5–15 mg
Corticosteroid Retention Enemas corticosteroid intrarectal foam, hydrocortisone acetate intrarectal foam	Cortifoam	Adjunctive therapy in treatment of ulcerative proctitis of the distal portion of the rectum	Local pain or burning, rectal bleeding, apparent exacerbations or sensitivity reactions	1 applicator once or twice daily for 2 wk and every second day thereafter
Mineralocorticoid fludrocortisone acetate *floo-droe-kor'-te-sone*	Florinef Acetate	Partial replacement therapy for Addison disease, salt-losing adrenogenital syndrome	See Box 23-2	0.1 mg 3 times per week to 0.2 mg/d PO

*The term *generic* indicates the drug is available in generic form.

the health care provider. Patients who appear extremely depressed must be closely observed. Mental status, memory, and impaired thinking (e.g., changes in orientation, impaired judgment, thoughts of hopelessness, guilt) should be closely monitored.

Managing Fluid and Electrolyte Imbalances Fluid and electrolyte imbalances, particularly excess fluid volume, are common with corticosteroid therapy. The patient should be checked for visible edema, a fluid intake and output record should be kept along with a daily weight, and a sodium-restricted diet must be adhered to if prescribed by the health care provider. If signs of electrolyte imbalance or glucocorticoid drug effects occur, then the health care provider should be notified. Dietary adjustments are made for the increased loss of potassium and the retention of sodium if necessary. Consultation with a dietitian may be indicated.

Managing Fractures Patients receiving long-term glucocorticoid therapy, especially those allowed limited activity, should be observed for signs of compression fractures of the vertebrae and pathologic fractures of the long bones. If the patient reports back or bone pain, then the health care provider should be notified. Extra care is also necessary to prevent falls and other injuries when a hospitalized patient is confused or is allowed out of bed. If the patient is weak, then help is needed for walking and self-care activities. Edematous extremities must be handled with care to prevent trauma.

Managing Ulcers Peptic ulcer has been associated with glucocorticoid therapy. Any patient symptoms of epigastric burning or pain, bloody or coffee-ground emesis, or the passing of tarry stools should be reported to the health care provider. Giving oral corticosteroids with food or a full glass of water may minimize gastric irritation.

Contraindications, Precautions, and Interactions of Glucocorticoids

The glucocorticoids are contraindicated in patients with serious infections, such as tuberculosis and fungal and antibiotic-resistant infections.

The glucocorticoids are administered with caution to patients with renal or hepatic disease, hypothyroidism, ulcerative colitis, diverticulitis, peptic ulcer disease, inflammatory bowel disease, hypertension, osteoporosis, convulsive disorders, or diabetes. The glucocorticoids are classified as pregnancy category C drugs and should be used with caution during pregnancy and lactation.

Many drug interactions may occur with the glucocorticoids. Table 23-2 identifies select clinically significant interactions.

Mineralocorticoids

Actions of Mineralocorticoids

The mineralocorticoids consist of aldosterone and desoxycorticosterone, which play an important role in conserving sodium and increasing the excretion of potassium. Because of these activities, the mineralocorticoids are important in controlling salt and water balance. Aldosterone is the more potent of these two hormones. Deficiencies of the mineralocorticoids result in a loss of sodium and water and a retention of potassium. Fludrocortisone (Florinef) has both glucocorticoid and mineralocorticoid activity and is the only currently available mineralocorticoid drug.

Uses of Mineralocorticoids

Fludrocortisone is used for replacement therapy for primary and secondary adrenocortical deficiency. Even though this drug has both mineralocorticoid and glucocorticoid activity, it is used only for its mineralocorticoid effects.

Adverse Reactions of Mineralocorticoids

Adverse reactions may occur if the dosage is too high or prolonged, or if withdrawal is too rapid. Administration of fludrocortisone may cause edema, hypertension, congestive heart failure, enlargement of the heart, increased

TABLE 23-2   Select Drug Interactions of Glucocorticoids

Precipitant Drug	Object Drug	Description
Barbiturates	Corticosteroids	Decreased pharmacologic effects of the corticosteroid may be observed
Cholestyramine	Hydrocortisone	The effects of hydrocortisone may be decreased
Contraceptives, oral	Corticosteroids	Corticosteroid concentration may be increased and clearance decreased
Estrogens	Corticosteroids	Corticosteroid clearance may be decreased
Hydantoin	Corticosteroids	Corticosteroid clearance may be increased, resulting in reduced therapeutic effects
Ketoconazole	Corticosteroids	Corticosteroid clearance may be decreased
Rifampin	Corticosteroids	Corticosteroid clearance may be increased, resulting in decreased therapeutic effects
Corticosteroids	Anticholinesterases	Anticholinesterase effects may be antagonized in myasthenia gravis
Corticosteroids	Anticoagulants, oral	Anticoagulant dose requirements may be reduced; corticosteroids may decrease the anticoagulant action.
Corticosteroids	Digitalis glycosides	Co-administration may enhance the possibility of digitalis toxicity associated with hypokalemia
Corticosteroids	Isoniazid	Isoniazid serum concentrations may be decreased
Corticosteroids	Potassium-depleting diuretics	Hypokalemia may occur
Corticosteroids	Salicylates	Corticosteroids will reduce serum salicylate levels and may decrease their effectiveness
Corticosteroids	Somatrem	Growth-promoting effect of somatrem may be inhibited
Corticosteroids	Theophyllines	Alterations in the pharmacologic activity of either agent may occur

sweating, or allergic skin rash. Additional adverse reactions include hypokalemia, muscular weakness, headache, and hypersensitivity reactions. Because this drug has glucocorticoid and mineralocorticoid activity and is often given with a glucocorticoid, adverse reactions of the glucocorticoid must be closely monitored as well (see Box 23-2).

Managing Adverse Reactions of Mineralocorticoids.
Fluid and electrolyte imbalances, particularly excess fluid volume, are common with corticosteroid therapy. The patient should be checked for visible edema, a fluid intake and output record must be kept along with a daily weight, and a sodium-restricted diet adhered to if indicated by the health care provider. If signs of electrolyte imbalance or glucocorticoid drug effects occur, then the health care provider should be notified. Dietary adjustments are made for the increased loss of potassium and the retention of sodium if necessary. Consultation with a dietitian may be indicated.

Contraindications, Precautions, and Interactions of Mineralocorticoids

Fludrocortisone is contraindicated in patients with hypersensitivity to fludrocortisone and those with systemic fungal infections. Fludrocortisone is used cautiously in patients with Addison disease or infection, and during pregnancy (pregnancy category C) and lactation. Fludrocortisone decreases the effects of the barbiturates, hydantoins, and rifampin. There is a decrease in serum levels of the salicylates when those agents are administered with fludrocortisone.

Patient Management Issues with Corticosteroids

Because these drugs are used to treat a great many diseases and conditions, an evaluation of drug response is based on the patient's diagnosis and the signs and symptoms of disease.

Adverse effects of the mineralocorticoid or glucocorticoid, particularly signs of electrolyte imbalance, such as hypocalcemia, hypokalemia, and hypernatremia (see Chapter 32), are closely monitored. The patient's mental status is monitored for any change, especially if there is a history of depression or other psychiatric problems, or if high doses of the drug are being given. The patient is also monitored for signs of an infection, which may be masked by glucocorticoid therapy. The blood of patients without diabetes is checked weekly for glucose levels because glucocorticoids may aggravate latent diabetes. Those with diabetes must be checked more frequently.

When administering fludrocortisone, the patient's blood pressure is monitored at frequent intervals. Hypotension may indicate insufficient dosage. Edema, particularly swelling of the feet and hands, is closely

monitored. The lungs are auscultated for adventitious sounds (e.g., rales or crackles).

> **ALERT**
>
> **Missing a Glucocorticoid Dosage**
> A glucocorticoid dosage must never be omitted. If the patient cannot take the drug orally because of nausea or vomiting, then the health care provider must be notified immediately because the drug needs to be given parenterally. Patients who are receiving nothing by mouth for any reason must have parenteral glucocorticoid.

> **ALERT**
>
> **Older Patients and Corticosteroid Use**
> Corticosteroids are administered with caution in older adults because they are more likely to have pre-existing conditions, such as congestive heart failure, hypertension, osteoporosis, or arthritis, that may be worsened by the use of such agents. Older adults are monitored for exacerbation of existing conditions during corticosteroid therapy. In addition, lower dosages may be needed because of the effects of aging, such as decreased muscle mass, renal function, and plasma volume.

Alternate-Day Therapy

An alternate-day therapy with glucocorticoid is used in the treatment of diseases and disorders requiring long-term therapy, especially arthritic disorders. This regimen involves giving twice the daily dose of the glucocorticoid every other day. The purpose of alternate-day administration is to provide the patient requiring long-term glucocorticoid therapy with the beneficial effects of the drug while minimizing certain undesirable reactions (see Box 23-2).

Plasma levels of the endogenous adrenocortical hormones vary throughout the day and nighttime hours. They are normally higher between 2 AM and approximately 8 AM, and lower between 4 PM and midnight. When plasma levels are lower, the anterior pituitary releases andrenocorticotropic hormone, which in turn stimulates the adrenal cortex to manufacture and release glucocorticoids. When plasma levels are high, the pituitary gland does not release adrenocorticotropic hormone. The response of the pituitary to high or low plasma levels of glucocorticoids and the resulting release or nonrelease of adrenocorticotropic hormone is an example of the feedback mechanism, which may also be seen in other glands of the body, such as the thyroid gland. The feedback mechanism is how the body maintains most hormones at relatively constant levels within the bloodstream. When the hormone concentration falls, the rate of production of that hormone increases. Likewise, when the hormone level becomes too high, the body decreases production of that hormone.

Administration of a short-acting glucocorticoid on alternate days and before 9 AM, when glucocorticoid plasma levels are still relatively high, does not affect the release of adrenocorticotropic hormone later in the day, yet it gives the patient the benefit of exogenous glucocorticoid therapy.

Patients with Diabetes

Patients with diabetes who are receiving a glucocorticoid may require frequent adjustment of their insulin or oral hypoglycemic drug dosage. Blood glucose levels are monitored several times daily or as prescribed by the health care provider. If the patient's blood glucose levels increase or if the urine is positive for glucose or ketones, then the health care provider should be notified. Some patients may have latent (hidden) diabetes. In these cases, the

---

PATIENT EDUCATION BOX 23-4

Key Points for Patients Taking Corticosteroid, Glucocorticoid and Mineralocorticoid

THERAPY

❑ These drugs may cause gastrointestinal upset. To decrease gastrointestinal effects, take the oral drug with meals or snacks.

❑ Take antacids between meals to help prevent peptic ulcer.

SHORT-TERM GLUCOCORTICOID THERAPY

❑ Take the drug exactly as directed on the prescription container. Do not increase, decrease, or omit a dose unless advised to do so by your health care provider.

❑ Take single daily doses before 9:00 AM.

❑ Follow the instructions for tapering the dose because they are extremely important.

❑ If the problem does not improve, then contact your health care provider.

ALTERNATE-DAY ORAL GLUCOCORTICOID THERAPY

❑ Take this drug before 9 AM once every other day. Use a calendar or some other method to identify the days of each week to take the drug.

❑ Do not stop taking the drug unless advised to do so by your health care provider.

❑ If the problem becomes worse, especially on the days the drug is not taken, then contact your health care provider. *Most of the information below may also apply to alternate-day therapy, especially when higher doses are used and therapy extends over many months.*

LONG-TERM OR HIGH-DOSE GLUCOCORTICOID THERAPY

❑ Do not miss a dose of this drug or increase or decrease the dosage except on the advice of your health care provider.

❑ Inform your other health care providers, dentists, and all medical personnel that you are taking this drug. Wear a medical alert tag or other form of identification to alert medical personnel of your long-term therapy with a glucocorticoid.

❑ Do not take any nonprescription drug unless your health care provider has approved its use.

❑ Do not take live virus vaccinations (e.g., smallpox) because of the risk of a lack of antibody response. This does not include patients receiving the corticosteroids as replacement therapy.

❑ Whenever possible, avoid exposure to infections. Contact your health care provider if minor cuts or abrasions fail to heal or if you experience persistent joint swelling or tenderness, fever, sore throat, upper respiratory infection, or other signs of infection.

❑ If you cannot take this drug orally for any reason or if you have diarrhea, then contact your health care provider immediately. If you are unable to contact your health care provider before the next dose is due, then go to the nearest hospital emergency department (preferably where the original treatment was started or where your health care provider is on the hospital staff), because the drug has to be given by injection.

❑ Weigh yourself weekly. If you experience significant weight gain or swelling of the extremities, then contact your health care provider.

❑ Remember that dietary recommendations made by the health care provider are an important part of therapy and must be followed.

❑ Follow the health care provider's recommendations regarding periodic eye examinations and laboratory tests.

INTRA-ARTICULAR OR INTRALESIONAL ADMINISTRATIONS

❑ Do not overuse the injected joint, even if the pain is gone.

❑ Follow your health care provider's instructions concerning rest and exercise.

MINERALOCORTICOID (FLUDROCORTISONE) THERAPY

❑ Take the drug as directed. Do not increase or decrease the dosage except as instructed to do so by your health care provider.

❑ Do not stop using the drug abruptly.

❑ Inform your health care provider if you experience the following adverse reactions: edema, muscle weakness, weight gain, anorexia, swelling of the extremities, dizziness, severe headache, or shortness of breath.

❑ Carry patient identification, such as a medical alert tag, so that medical personnel will know your drug therapy during an emergency situation.

❑ Keep follow-up appointments to determine if a dosage adjustment is necessary.

corticosteroid may precipitate hyperglycemia. Therefore, all patients, those with diabetes and those without, should have frequent checks of blood glucose levels.

Educating the Patient and Family About Corticosteroid, Glucocorticoid, and Mineralocorticoid Therapy

Patient Education Box 23-4 includes key points about corticosteroid, glucocorticoid, and mineralocorticoid therapy that the patient and family members should know.

Thyroid and Antithyroid Drugs

The thyroid gland is located in the neck in front of the trachea. This highly vascular gland manufactures and secretes two hormones: **thyroxine** and **triiodothyronine**. Iodine is essential for the manufacture of both of these hormones. The activity of the thyroid gland is regulated by thyroid-stimulating hormone, produced by the anterior pituitary gland (see Figure 23-1). When the level of circulating thyroid hormones decreases, the anterior pituitary secretes thyroid-stimulating hormone, which then activates the cells of the thyroid to release stored thyroid hormones. This is an example of the feedback mechanism.

Two diseases are related to the hormone-producing activity of the thyroid gland:

- **hypothyroidism:** a decrease in the amount of thyroid hormones manufactured and secreted
- **hyperthyroidism:** an increase in the amount of thyroid hormones manufactured and secreted

The symptoms of hypothyroidism and hyperthyroidism are given in Table 23-3. A severe form of hyperthyroidism, called **thyrotoxicosis** or **thyroid storm**, is characterized by high fever, extreme tachycardia, and altered mental status. Thyroid hormones are used to treat hypothyroidism, and antithyroid drugs and radioactive iodine are used to treat hyperthyroidism.

Thyroid Hormones

Thyroid hormones used in medicine include both the natural and synthetic hormones. Synthetic hormones are generally preferred because they are more uniform in potency than the natural hormones obtained from animals. Thyroid hormones are listed in the Summary Drug Table: Thyroid and Antithyroid Drugs.

Actions of Thyroid Hormones

The thyroid hormones influence every organ and tissue of the body. These hormones are principally concerned with increasing the metabolic rate of tissues, which results in increases in the heart and respiratory rate, body temperature, cardiac output, oxygen consumption, and the metabolism of fats, proteins, and carbohydrates. The exact mechanisms by which the thyroid hormones exert their influence on body organs and tissues are not well understood.

Uses of Thyroid Hormones

Thyroid hormones are used as replacement therapy when the patient is hypothyroid. By supplementing the decreased endogenous thyroid production and secretion with exogenous thyroid hormones, an attempt is made to create a **euthyroid** (normal thyroid) state. Levothyroxine (Synthroid) is the drug of choice for hypothyroidism because it is relatively inexpensive, requires once-per-day dosages, and has a more uniform potency than other thyroid hormone replacement drugs.

Myxedema is a severe hypothyroidism manifested by lethargy, apathy, memory impairment, emotional changes, slow speech, deep coarse voice, thick dry skin, cold intolerance, slow pulse, constipation, weight gain, and absence of menses.

Thyroid hormones are also used in the treatment or prevention of various types of euthyroid **goiters** (enlargement of the thyroid gland), including thyroid nodules, subacute or chronic lymphocytic thyroiditis (Hashimoto), and multinodular goiter, and in the management of thyroid cancer. The hormone may be used with the antithyroid drugs to treat thyrotoxicosis.

TABLE 23-3   Signs and Symptoms of Thyroid Dysfunction

Body System or Function	Hypothyroidism	Hyperthyroidism
Metabolism	Decreased with anorexia, intolerance to cold, low body temperature, weight gain despite anorexia	Increased with increased appetite, intolerance to heat, elevated body temperature, weight loss despite increased appetite
Cardiovascular	Bradycardia, moderate hypotension	Tachycardia, moderate hypertension
Central nervous system	Lethargy, sleepiness	Nervousness, anxiety, insomnia, tremors
Skin, skin structures	Pale, cool, dry skin; face appears puffy; coarse hair; thick and hard nails	Flushed, warm, moist skin
Ovarian function	Heavy menses, may be unable to conceive, loss of fetus possible	Irregular or scant menses
Testicular function	Low sperm count	

SUMMARY DRUG TABLE Thyroid and Antithyroid Drugs

Generic Name	Trade Name*	Uses	Adverse Reactions	Dosage Ranges
Thyroid Hormones levothyroxine sodium (T$_4$) *lee-voe-thyerox'-een*	Eltroxin, Levo-T Levothroid, Levoxyl, Synthroid, *generic*	Hypothyroidism, thyrotoxicosis	Palpitations, tachycardia, headache, nervousness, insomnia, diarrhea, vomiting, weight loss, sweating, heat intolerance	0.025–0.3 mg/d PO; 0.05–0.1 mg IV; 0.05 mg initially, increase by 0.025 mg PO q2–3 wk; maintenance dose, 0.2 mg/d, may substitute IV IM
liothyronine sodium (T$_3$) *lye'-oh-thye'-roe-neen*	Cytomel, *generic* Trio stat	Hypothyroidism, thyrotoxicosis	Same as levothyroxine	5–75 mcg/d PO, 25–50 µg IV q4–12h
liotrix (T$_2$, T$_4$) *lye'-oh-trix*	Thyrolar	Hypothyroidism, thyrotoxicosis	Same as levothyroxine	15–120 mg/d PO
thyroid desiccated *thye'-roid*	Armour Thyroid, *generic*	Hypothyroidism, thyrotoxicosis	Same as levothyroxine	65–195 mg/d PO
Antithyroid Preparations methimazole *meth-im-a-zole*	Tapazole, *generic*	Hyperthyroidism	Agranulocytosis, headache, exfoliative dermatitis, granulocytopenia, thrombocytopenia, hepatitis, hypopro-thrombinemia, jaundice, loss of hair, nausea, vomiting	15–60 mg/d
propylthiouracil (PTU) *proe-pill-thye-oh-yoor'-a-sill*	PTU *generic*	Same as methimazole	Same as methimazole	300–900 mg/d PO, usually in divided doses at approx-imately 8-h intervals
Iodine Products strong iodine solution *eye'-oh-dine*	Lugol's Solution, Thyro-Block, *generic*	To prepare hyperthyroid patients for thyroid surgery, thyrotoxic crisis, thyroid blocking in radiation therapy	Rash, swelling of salivary glands, "iodism" (metallic taste, burning mouth and throat, sore teeth and gums, symptoms of a head cold, diarrhea, nausea), allergic reactions (fever, joint pains, swelling of parts of face and body)	2–6 drops PO TID for 10 d before surgery; 130 mg/d PO
sodium iodine (^{131}I) *so'-de-um, eye'-oh-dide*	Iodotope, *generic*	Thyrotoxicosis, selected cases of thyroid cancer	Bone marrow depression, anemia, blood dyscrasias, nausea, vomiting, tachycardia, itching, rash, hives, tenderness and swelling of the neck, sore throat, and cough	Measured by a radioactivity calibration system before administering PO 4–10 mCi; thyroid cancer: 50–150 mCi

*The term *generic* indicates the drug is available in generic form.

Thyroid hormones also may be used as a diagnostic measure to differentiate suspected hyperthyroidism from euthyroidism.

Adverse Reactions of Thyroid Hormones

During initial therapy, the most common adverse reactions seen are signs of overdose and hyperthyroidism (see Table 23-3). Adverse reactions other than symptoms of hyperthyroidism are rare.

Managing Adverse Reactions of Thyroid Hormones. The patient must be monitored for any adverse reactions, especially during the initial stages of dosage adjustment. The health care provider should be notified if the patient experiences these or any adverse drug reactions. If the dosage is inadequate, then the patient will continue to experience signs of hypothyroidism (see Table 23-3). If the dosage is excessive, then the patient will exhibit signs of hyperthyroidism.

ALERT

Signs of Hyperthyroidism

If signs of hyperthyroidism (e.g., nervousness, anxiety, increased appetite, elevated body temperature, tachycardia, moderate hypertension, or flushed, warm, moist skin) occur, then they must be reported to the health care provider before the next dose because it may be necessary to decrease the daily dosage.

Thyroid hormone replacement therapy in patients with diabetes may increase the intensity of the symptoms or the diabetes. A patient with diabetes is monitored during thyroid hormone replacement therapy for signs of hyperglycemia (see Chapter 22), and the health care provider should be notified if this problem occurs.

Patients with cardiovascular disease are closely monitored while taking thyroid hormones. The development of chest pain or worsening of cardiovascular disease should be reported to the health care provider immediately because the patient may require a reduction in dosage.

Contraindications, Precautions, and Interactions of Thyroid Hormones

These drugs are contraindicated in patients with a known hypersensitivity to any or all constituents of the drug, after a recent myocardial infarction (heart attack), or in patients with thyrotoxicosis (severe hypothyroidism). When hypothyroidism is a cause or contributing factor to myocardial infarction or heart disease, the health care provider may prescribe small doses of thyroid hormone.

These drugs are used cautiously in patients with Addison disease and during lactation. The thyroid hormones are classified as pregnancy category A and are considered safe to use during pregnancy.

When administered with cholestyramine or colestipol, there is a decreased absorption of the oral thyroid preparations. These drugs should not be administered within 4 to 6 hours of the thyroid hormones. When administered with an oral anticoagulants, there is an increased risk of bleeding; it may be advantageous to decrease the dosage of the anticoagulant. There is a decreased effectiveness of the digitalis preparation if taken with a thyroid preparation.

ALERT

Older Adults and Sensitivity to Thyroid Replacement Therapy

Older adults are more sensitive to thyroid hormone replacement therapy and are more likely to experience adverse reactions when taking the thyroid hormones. In addition, the elderly are at increased risk for adverse cardiovascular reactions when taking thyroid drugs. The initial dosage is smaller for an older adult, and increases, if necessary, are made in smaller increments over a period of approximately 8 weeks. Periodic thyroid function tests are necessary to monitor drug therapy. The dosage may need to be reduced with age. If the pulse rate is 100 beats per minute or more, then the health care provider must be notified before the drug is administered.

Patient Management Issues with Thyroid Hormones

Before therapy starts, the patient's vital signs, weight, and history are obtained. A general physical assessment is performed to determine the signs of hypothyroidism.

ALERT

Older Patients and Hypothyroidism

The symptoms of hypothyroidism may be confused with symptoms associated with aging, such as depression, cold intolerance, weight gain, confusion, or unsteady gait. The presence of these symptoms should be thoroughly evaluated and documented in the preadministration assessment and periodically throughout therapy.

The full effects of thyroid hormone replacement therapy may not be apparent for several weeks or more, but early effects may be apparent in as little as 48 hours. The patient's vital signs are monitored daily or as ordered for signs of hyperthyroidism, which is a sign of excessive drug dosage. Signs of a therapeutic response include weight loss, mild diuresis, a sense of well-being, increased appetite, an increased pulse rate, an increase in mental activity, and decreased puffiness of the face, hands, and feet.

Thyroid hormones are administered once per day, early in the morning and preferably before breakfast. An empty stomach increases the absorption of the oral preparation. Levothyroxine (Synthroid) also can be given intravenously and is prepared for administration immediately before use.

The dosage is individualized for the patient. The dose of thyroid hormones must be carefully adjusted according to the patient's hormone requirements. Several upward or downward dosage adjustments are often made until the optimal therapeutic dosage is reached and the patient becomes euthyroid.

Some patients may have anxiety related to the symptoms of their disorder, as well as concern about relief of their symptoms. A patient should be reassured that although relief may not be immediate, symptoms should begin to decrease or disappear in a few weeks.

Educating the Patient and Family About Thyroid Hormones

Patient Education Box 23-5 includes key points about thyroid hormone therapy the patient and family members should know.

PATIENT EDUCATION BOX 23-5

Key Points for Patients Taking Thyroid Hormone Drugs

❑ Replacement therapy is for life, with the exception of transient hypothyroidism seen in those with thyroiditis. Therefore, it is important to maintain the dosage as prescribed by your health care provider: do not increase, decrease, or skip a dose unless advised to do so.

❑ Take this drug in the morning, preferably before breakfast, unless advised by your health care provider to take it at a different time of day.

❑ Notify your health care provider if you experience any of the following: headache, nervousness, palpitations, diarrhea, excessive sweating, heat intolerance, chest pain, increased pulse rate, or any unusual physical change or event.

❑ The dosage of this drug may require periodic adjustments; this is normal. Dosage changes are based on your response to therapy and thyroid function tests.

❑ Therapy needs to be evaluated at periodic intervals, which may vary from every 2 weeks at the beginning of therapy to every 6 to 12 months once your symptoms are controlled. Periodic thyroid function tests are needed.

❑ Weigh yourself weekly and report any significant weight gain or loss to your health care provider.

❑ Do not change from one brand of this drug to another without consulting your health care provider.

Antithyroid Drugs

Antithyroid drugs or thyroid antagonists are used to treat hyperthyroidism. In addition to the antithyroid drugs, hyperthyroidism may be treated by the administration of strong iodine solutions, use of radioactive iodine (^{131}I), or by surgical removal of some or almost all of the thyroid gland (subtotal thyroidectomy).

Actions of Antithyroid Drugs

Antithyroid drugs inhibit the manufacture of thyroid hormones. They do not affect existing thyroid hormones that are circulating in the blood or stored in the thyroid gland. For this reason, the therapeutic effects of the antithyroid drugs may not be observed for 3 to 4 weeks. Antithyroid drugs are listed in the Summary Drug Table: Thyroid and Antithyroid Drugs.

Strong iodide solutions act by decreasing the vascularity of the thyroid gland by rapidly inhibiting the release of the thyroid hormones. Radioactive iodine is distributed within the cellular fluid and excreted. The radioactive isotope accumulates in the cells of the thyroid gland, where destruction of thyroid cells occurs without damaging other cells throughout the body.

Uses of Antithyroid Drugs

Methimazole (Tapazole) and propylthiouracil (PTU) are used for the medical management of hyperthyroidism. Not all patients respond adequately to antithyroid drugs; therefore, a thyroidectomy (removal of the thyroid gland) may be necessary. Antithyroid drugs may be administered before surgery to temporarily return a patient to a euthyroid state. When used for this reason, the vascularity of the thyroid gland is reduced and the tendency to bleed excessively during and immediately after surgery is decreased.

Strong iodine solution, also known as Lugol solution, may be given orally with methimazole or propylthiouracil to prepare the patient for thyroid surgery. Iodine solutions are also used for rapid treatment of hyperthyroidism because they can decrease symptoms in 2 to 7 days. Radioactive iodine (^{131}I) may be used for treatment of hyperthyroidism and selected cases of cancer of the thyroid.

Adverse Reactions of Antithyroid Drugs

Adverse Reactions of Methimazole and Propylthiouracil. The most serious adverse reaction associated with these drugs is agranulocytosis (decrease in the number of white blood cells, e.g., neutrophils, basophils, and eosinophils). Reactions observed with agranulocytosis include hay fever, sore throat, skin rash, fever, or headache. Other major reactions include exfoliative dermatitis, granulocytopenia, aplastic anemia, hypoprothrombinemia, and hepatitis. Minor reactions, such as nausea, vomiting, and paresthesias, also may occur.

Adverse Reactions of Strong Iodine Solutions. Reactions that may occur with strong iodine solution include symptoms of **iodism** (excessive amounts of iodine in the body), which are a metallic taste in the mouth, swelling and soreness of the parotid glands, burning of the mouth and throat, sore teeth and gums, symptoms of a head cold, and occasionally gastrointestinal upset. Allergy to iodine may occur and can be serious. Symptoms of iodine allergy include swelling of parts of the face and body, fever, joint pains, and sometimes difficulty in breathing. Difficulty breathing requires immediate medical attention.

Adverse Reactions of Radioactive Iodine (^{131}I). Reactions after administration of ^{131}I include sore throat, swelling in the neck, nausea, vomiting, cough, and pain on swallowing. Other reactions include bone marrow depression, anemia, leukopenia, thrombocytopenia, and tachycardia.

Managing Adverse Reactions of Antithyroid Drugs The patient is monitored throughout therapy for adverse drug reactions and for signs of agranulocytosis (a decrease or lack of granulocytes, a type of white blood cell). The patient must be protected from individuals with infectious disease because if agranulocytosis is present, the patient is at increased risk for contracting any infection, particularly an upper respiratory infection. The patient should be monitored for signs of infection.

A L E R T

Agranulocytosis

Agranulocytosis is potentially the most serious adverse reaction to methimazole and propylthiouracil. The health care provider should be notified if fever, sore throat, rash, headache, hay fever, yellow discoloration of the skin, or vomiting occurs.

If the patient experiences a rash while taking methimazole or propylthiouracil, then this should be reported to the health care provider. Soothing creams or lubricants may be applied, and soap is used sparingly, if at all, until the rash subsides.

When an iodine solution is administered, the patient is closely observed for symptoms of iodism and iodine allergy (see section on Adverse Reactions). If these occur, then the drug is withheld and the health care provider notified immediately. This is especially important with swelling around or in the mouth or difficulty breathing.

Contraindications, Precautions, and Interactions of Antithyroid Drugs. The antithyroid drugs are contraindicated in patients with a known hypersensitivity to them or any constituent of the drug. Methimazole and propylthiouracil are contraindicated during pregnancy and lactation. Radioactive iodine is contraindicated during pregnancy (pregnancy category X) and lactation.

Methimazole and propylthiouracil are used with extreme caution during pregnancy (pregnancy category D) because they can cause hypothyroidism in the fetus. However, if an antithyroid drug is necessary during pregnancy or lactation, propylthiouracil is often prescribed. In many pregnant women, thyroid dysfunction diminishes as the pregnancy proceeds, making a dosage reduction possible. Methimazole and propylthiouracil are used cautiously in patients older than age 40, because there is an increased risk of agranulocytosis, and in patients with a decrease in bone marrow reserve (e.g., after radiation therapy for cancer). Strong iodine preparations (except ^{131}I) are classified as pregnancy category D and are used cautiously during pregnancy.

An additive bone marrow depression occurs when methimazole or propylthiouracil is administered with other bone marrow depressants, such as the antineoplastic drugs, or with radiation therapy. When methimazole is administered with digitalis, there is an increased effectiveness of the digitalis and increased risk of toxicity. There is an additive effect of propylthiouracil when the drug is administered with lithium, potassium iodide, or sodium iodide. When iodine products are administered with lithium products, synergistic hypothyroid activity is likely to occur.

Patient Management Issues with Antithyroid Drugs. Before therapy with an antithyroid drug begins, the patient is assessed, including a history of the symptoms of hyperthyroidism, vital signs, and weight (see Table 23-3). If the patient is prescribed an iodine solution, then a careful allergy history, particularly to iodine or seafood (which contains iodine), is included.

During therapy, the patient is monitored for adverse drug effects. With short-term therapy before surgery, adverse drug reactions are usually minimal. Long-term therapy is usually on an outpatient basis. Relief of symptoms, as well as signs or symptoms indicating an adverse reaction related to the blood cells, such as fever, sore throat, easy bruising or bleeding, fever, cough, or any other signs of infection, is monitored. As the patient becomes euthyroid, signs and symptoms of hyperthyroidism become less obvious. The patient is monitored for signs of thyroid storm (high fever, extreme tachycardia, and altered mental status), which can occur in patients whose hyperthyroidism is inadequately treated.

A patient with an enlarged thyroid gland may have difficulty swallowing the tablet. In this case, strong iodine solution may be prescribed. It is measured in drops, which are added to water or fruit juice. This drug has a strong, salty taste. The patient is allowed to experiment with various types of fruit juices to determine which one best disguises the taste of the drug. Iodine solutions should be drunk through a straw because they may cause tooth discoloration.

The health care provider gives radioactive iodine orally as a single dose. The effects of iodides are evident within 24 hours, with maximum effects attained after 10 to 15 days of continuous therapy. If the patient is hospitalized, then radiation safety precautions identified by the hospital's department of nuclear medicine are followed.

Once a euthyroid state is achieved, the health care provider may add a thyroid hormone to the therapeutic regimen to prevent or treat hypothyroidism, which may develop slowly during long-term antithyroid drug therapy or after administration of ^{131}I.

A patient with hyperthyroidism is likely to have cardiac symptoms such as tachycardia or palpitations. Propranolol, an adrenergic blocking drug (see Chapter 4), may be prescribed by the health care provider as adjunctive treatment for several weeks until the therapeutic effects of the antithyroid drug occur.

Educating the Patient and Family About Antithyroid Drugs

Patient Education Box 23-6 includes key points about antithyroid drugs the patient and family members should know.

Male and Female Hormones

Male and female hormones play a vital role because they aid in the development and maintenance of secondary sex characteristics and are necessary for human reproduction. Although the body naturally produces hormones, a male or female hormone is used in the treatment of certain disorders, such as inoperable breast cancer, male hypogonadism, or male or female hormone deficiency. Hormones also are used as contraceptives and for treating the symptoms of menopause.

Male Hormones

Male hormones—**testosterone** (the most potent naturally occurring androgen) and its derivatives—are collectively called **androgens**. Androgen secretion is under the influence of the anterior pituitary gland. Small amounts of male and female hormones are also produced by the adrenal cortex, as discussed earlier in this chapter. The anabolic steroids are closely related to the androgen testosterone and have both androgenic and anabolic (stimulate cellular growth and repair) activity. Androgen hormone inhibitors inhibit the conversion of testosterone into a potent androgen.

Actions of Androgens

The male hormone testosterone and its derivatives activate reproductive potential in adolescent boys. From puberty onward, androgens continue to aid in the development and maintenance of secondary sex characteristics: facial hair, deep voice, body hair, body fat distribu-

PATIENT EDUCATION BOX 23-6

Key Points for Patients Taking Antithyroid Drugs

METHIMAZOLE AND PROPYLTHIOURACIL

❑ Take these drugs at regular intervals around the clock (e.g., every 8 hours) unless directed otherwise by your health care provider.

❑ Do not take these drugs in larger doses or more frequently than as directed on the prescription container.

❑ Notify your health care provider promptly if you experience any of the following: sore throat, fever, cough, easy bleeding or bruising, headache, or a general feeling of malaise.

❑ Record your weight twice per week and notify your health care provider if you have any sudden weight gain or loss. (Note: your health care provider may also want you to monitor your pulse rate. If so, then your health care provider will show you the proper technique and how to record the pulse rate. Bring the record to your health care provider's office or clinic.)

❑ Avoid the use of nonprescription drugs unless your health care provider has approved the use of a specific drug.

STRONG IODINE SOLUTION

❑ Dilute the solution with water or fruit juice. Fruit juice often disguises the taste more than water. Experiment with the types of fruit juice that best reduces the unpleasant taste of this drug.

❑ Discontinue the use of this drug and notify your health care provider if you experience any of the following: skin rash, metallic taste in the mouth, swelling and soreness in front of the ears, sore teeth and gums, severe gastrointestinal distress, or symptoms of a head cold.

RADIOACTIVE IODINE

❑ Follow the directions of the department of nuclear medicine regarding precautions to be taken. (Note: In some instances, the dosage is small and no special precautions may be necessary.)

❑ Thyroid hormone replacement therapy may be necessary if hypothyroidism develops.

❑ Follow-up evaluations of the thyroid gland and the effectiveness of treatment with this drug are necessary.

tion, and muscle development. Testosterone also stimulates the growth of the accessory sex organs (penis, testes, vas deferens, prostate) at the time of puberty. The androgens also promote tissue-building processes (anabolism) and reverse tissue-depleting processes (catabolism). Examples of androgens are fluoxymesterone (Halotestin), methyltestosterone (Oreton Methyl), and testosterone. Additional examples of androgens are given in the Summary Drug Table: Male Hormones.

SUMMARY DRUG TABLE Male Hormones

Generic Name	Trade Name*	Uses	Adverse Reactions	Dosage Ranges
Androgens fluoxymesterone *floo-oxi-mes'-te-rone*	Halotestin, *generic*	Males: hypogonadism; Females: inoperable breast cancer	Males: gynecomastia, testicular atrophy, inhibition of testicular function, impotence, enlargement of the penis, nausea, jaundice, headache, anxiety, male pattern baldness, acne, depression Females: amenorrhea, virilization	Males: hypogonadism 5–20 mg/d PO; Females: breast cancer, 10–40 mg/d PO in divided doses
methyltestosterone *meth-ill-tess-toss'-ter-one*	Android, Methitest, Testred, Virilon, *generic*	Males: hypogonadism, male climacteric, impotence, androgen deficiency, postpubertal cryptorchidism; Females: breast cancer	Same as fluoxymesterone	Males: 10–50 mg/d PO, 5–25 mg/d buccal tablets; Females: 50–200 mg/d PO, 25–100 mg/d buccal tablets
testosterone gel *tess-toss'-ter-one*	Androgel	Males: delayed puberty, androgen replacement theory, hypogonadism; Females: palliation of inoperable breast cancer	Same as fluoxymesterone	5–10 mg/d applied to any skin
testosterone cypionate (in oil)	Depo- Testosterone, *generic*	Males: hypogonadism, delayed puberty; Females: palliation of inoperable breast cancer	Same as fluoxymesterone	Males: 50–400 mg/dose IM; Females: 200–400 mg/dose IM
testosterone enanthate	Delastryl	Same as testosterone cypionate	Same as fluoxymesterone	50–400 mg IM q2–4 wk
testosterone transdermal system	Androderm, Testoderm, Testoderm TTS	Males: androgen replacement therapy	Same as fluoxymesterone	One system applied daily
Anabolic Steroids nandrolone decanoate *nan'-droe-lone*	Deca-Durabolin, *generic*	Management of anemia of renal insufficiency	Acne, nausea, vomiting, fluid and electrolyte imbalances, jaundice, anorexia, muscle cramps, malignant and benign liver tumors, increased risk of atherosclerosis, mental changes, testicular atrophy, virilization (females)	50–200 mg/wk IM

Generic Name	Trade Name*	Uses	Adverse Reactions	Dosage Ranges
oxymetholone	Anadrol-50	Anemia	Same as nandrolone decanoate	1–5 mg/kg/d PO
oxandrolone *oks-an-droe-lone*	Oxandrin	Promote weight gain in those with weight loss after extensive surgery, severe trauma, severe infections	Same as nandrolone decanoate	2.5 mg PO BID to QID
stanozolol	Winstrol	Hereditary angioedema	Same as nandrolone decanoate	2 mg PO TID, then reduce to 2 mg/d or to 2 mg/d every other d PO
Androgen Hormone Inhibitor finasteride *fin-as'-teh-ride*	Proscar	Benign prostatic hypertrophy, prevention of male pattern baldness	Impotence, decreased libido, decreased volume of ejaculate	5 mg/d PO

*The term *generic* indicates the drug is available in generic form.

Uses of Androgens

In male patients, androgen therapy may be given as replacement therapy for testosterone deficiency. Deficiency states in male patients, such as hypogonadism (failure of the testes to develop), selected cases of delayed puberty, and the development of testosterone deficiency after puberty may be treated with androgens. A transdermal testosterone system may be used for replacement therapy when endogenous testosterone is deficient or absent.

In female patients, androgen therapy may be used as part of the treatment for inoperable metastatic breast carcinoma in women who are 1 to 5 years past menopause. In addition, some breast carcinomas in women are "hormone-dependent" tumors; in other words, the female hormone, estrogen, influences their growth and spread. Administration of an androgen to patients with this type of malignant breast tumor counteracts the effect of estrogen on these tumors. Androgens may also be administered to premenopausal women with metastatic breast carcinoma that is believed to be hormone-dependent and whose tumor growth and spread have been slowed after an oophorectomy (removal of the ovaries). The uses of the androgens are listed in the Summary Drug Table: Male Hormones.

Adverse Reactions of Androgens

In men, administration of an androgen may result in breast enlargement (gynecomastia), testicular atrophy, inhibition of testicular function, impotence, enlargement of the penis, nausea, jaundice, headache, anxiety,

male pattern baldness, acne, and depression. Fluid and electrolyte imbalances, which include sodium, water, chloride, potassium, calcium, and phosphate retention, may also occur.

In women receiving an androgen preparation for breast carcinoma, the most common adverse reactions are amenorrhea, other menstrual irregularities, and **virilization** (acquisition of male sexual characteristics by a woman). Virilization produces facial hair, a deepening of the voice, and enlargement of the clitoris. Male pattern baldness and acne may also occur.

Contraindications, Precautions, and Interactions of Androgens

The androgens are contraindicated in patients with a known hypersensitivity, liver disorders, or serious cardiac disease, and in men with prostate gland disorders (e.g., prostate carcinoma and prostate enlargement). The androgens are classified as pregnancy category X drugs and should not be administered during pregnancy and lactation. When the androgens are administered with anticoagulants, the anticoagulant effect may be increased.

Patient Management Issues with Androgens

In most instances, androgens are administered to men on an outpatient basis. Before and during therapy, the health care provider may order electrolyte studies because these drugs can cause fluid and electrolyte imbalances.

If the androgen is to be administered as a buccal tablet, then the patient is warned not to swallow the tablet but to allow it to dissolve in the mouth. The patient should not smoke or drink water until the tablet is dissolved. Oral and parenteral androgens are often taken or given by injection on an outpatient basis. When given by injection, the injection is administered deep intramuscularly into the gluteal muscle. Oral testosterone is given with or before meals to decrease gastric upset.

When the testosterone transdermal system Testoderm is prescribed, the system is placed on clean, dry scrotal skin. Optimal skin contact of the transdermal system is achieved by dry shaving scrotal hair before placing the system.

When these drugs are given to female patients with inoperable breast carcinoma, the patient's current status (physical, emotional, and nutritional) is carefully monitored and recorded in the patient's chart. Baseline laboratory tests may include a complete blood count, hepatic function tests, serum electrolytes, and serum and urinary calcium levels.

Actions of Anabolic Steroids

The anabolic steroids are synthetic drugs chemically related to the androgens. Like androgens, they promote tissue-building processes. Given in normal doses, they have a minimal effect on the accessory sex organs and secondary sex characteristics. Examples of anabolic steroids are given in the Summary Drug Table: Male Hormones.

Uses of Anabolic Steroids

The uses of the various anabolic steroids include management of anemia of renal insufficiency, control of metastatic breast cancer in women, and promotion of weight gain in those with weight loss after surgery, trauma, or infections. Stanozolol is used prophylactically to decrease the frequency and severity of hereditary angioedema, a condition characterized by urticaria (eruption of itching wheals) and edematous areas of the skin, mucous membranes, or viscera.

A L E R T

Anabolic Steroid Abuse
The use of anabolic steroids to promote an increase in muscle mass and strength is a serious problem. Anabolic steroids are not intended for this use. Unfortunately, deaths in young, healthy individuals have been directly attributed to this use of these drugs. The illegal use of anabolic steroids to increase muscle mass should be discouraged.

Adverse Reactions of Anabolic Steroids

Virilization in women is the most common reaction associated with anabolic steroids, especially when higher doses are used. Acne occurs frequently in all age groups and both sexes. Nausea, vomiting, diarrhea, fluid and electrolyte imbalances (the same as for the androgens,

discussed previously), testicular atrophy, jaundice, anorexia, and muscle cramps may also occur. Blood-filled cysts of the liver and sometimes the spleen, malignant and benign liver tumors, an increased risk of atherosclerosis, and mental changes are the most serious adverse reactions with prolonged use.

Many serious adverse drug reactions occur in healthy individuals using anabolic steroids. There is some indication that prolonged high-dose use has resulted in psychological and possibly physical addiction, and some individuals have required treatment in drug abuse centers. Severe mental changes, such as uncontrolled rage, severe depression, suicidal tendencies, malignant and benign liver tumors, aggressive behavior, increased risk of atherosclerosis, inability to concentrate, and personality changes are common. In addition, the incidence of the severe adverse reactions cited earlier appears to be increased in those using anabolic steroids for this purpose.

Contraindications, Precautions, and Interactions of Anabolic Steroids

Anabolic steroids are contraindicated in patients with a known hypersensitivity, liver disorders, or serious cardiac disease, and in men with prostate gland disorders (e.g., prostate carcinoma or prostate enlargement). The anabolic steroids are classified as pregnancy category X drugs and should not be administered during pregnancy and lactation. Anabolic steroids are contraindicated for use to enhance physical appearance or athletic performance.

When the anabolic steroids are administered with anticoagulants, the anticoagulant effect may be increased. Administration of methyltestosterone with imipramine may cause a paranoid response in some patients. The anabolic steroids may increase the hypoglycemic action when administered with the sulfonylureas.

A L E R T

Older Men and Steroid Treatment
Older men treated with the steroids are at increased risk for prostate enlargement and prostate cancer.

Patient Management Issues with Anabolic Steroids

The patient's physical and nutritional status are recorded before therapy is started, including the patient's weight, blood pressure, pulse, and respiratory rate. Baseline laboratory studies may include a complete blood count, hepatic function tests, and serum electrolytes and serum lipid levels.

Actions of Androgen Hormone Inhibitor

The androgen hormone inhibitor finasteride (Proscar) is a synthetic compound drug that inhibits the conversion of testosterone into the potent androgen 5 alpha (α)-

dihydrotestosterone. The development of the prostate gland depends on α-dihydrotestosterone. The lowering of serum levels of α-dihydrotestosterone reduces the effect of this hormone on the prostate gland, resulting in a decrease in the size of the gland and the symptoms associated with prostatic gland enlargement.

Uses of Androgen Hormone Inhibitor

Finasteride is used in the treatment of the symptoms associated with benign prostatic hypertrophy, such as difficulty starting the urinary stream, frequent passage of small amounts of urine, and having to urinate during the night (nocturia). Several months of therapy may be required before a significant improvement occurs and the symptoms decrease. Finasteride is also used for the prevention of male pattern baldness in men with early signs of hair loss.

Adverse Reactions of Androgen Hormone Inhibitor

Adverse reactions with finasteride usually are mild and do not require discontinuing use of the drug. Adverse reactions, when they occur, are related to the sexual drive and include impotence, decreased libido, and a decreased volume of ejaculate.

Contraindications, Precautions, and Interactions of Androgen Hormone Inhibitor

Finasteride is contraindicated in patients with hypersensitivity to the drug or any component of the drug, in women who are pregnant (pregnancy category X) or women who may potentially be pregnant, and during lactation. The drug is used cautiously in patients with liver function impairment.

Patient Management Issues with Androgen Hormone Inhibitors

The patient is questioned at length about symptoms of benign prostatic hypertrophy, such as frequency of voiding during the day and night and difficulty starting the urinary stream.

Managing Adverse Reactions of Male Hormones

Patients receiving an androgen or anabolic steroid are closely observed for signs of adverse drug reactions. In women, virilization may be seen with long-term administration and in many cases must be tolerated to obtain the desired effect of the drug.

When the androgens are administered to a patient with diabetes, blood glucose measurements should be performed frequently because glucose tolerance may be altered. Adjustments may need to be made in insulin dosage, oral antidiabetic drugs, or diet. The patient is monitored for signs for hypoglycemia and hyperglycemia (see Chapter 22).

Sodium and water retention may also occur with androgen or anabolic steroids, causing the patient to become edematous. In addition, other electrolyte imbalances, such as hypercalcemia, may occur. Signs of fluid and electrolyte disturbances should be closely monitored (see Chapter 32 for signs and symptoms of electrolyte disturbance).

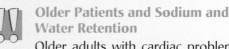

ALERT

Older Patients and Sodium and Water Retention

Older adults with cardiac problems or kidney disease are at increased risk for sodium and water retention when taking an androgen or anabolic steroid.

A daily comparison is made of the patient's preadministration weight with current weights. The presence of puffy eyelids and dependent swelling of the hands or feet (if the patient can walk) or the sacral area (if the patient is unable to walk) should be reported to the health care provider. Daily fluid intake and output are monitored to calculate fluid balance.

With long-term administration, a female patient may experience mild to moderate masculine changes (virilization), including facial hair, a deepening of the voice, and enlargement of the clitoris. Male pattern baldness, patchy hair loss, skin pigmentation, and acne may also occur. Although these adverse effects are not life threatening, they often are distressing and add to the patient's discomfort and anxiety. These problems may be easy to identify, but they are not always easy to solve. If hair loss occurs, then the wearing of a wig can be suggested. Mild skin pigmentation may be covered with makeup, but severe and widespread pigmented areas and acne are often difficult to conceal.

Educating the Patient and Family about Male Hormones

Patient Education Box 23-7 includes key points the patient and family members should know about male hormones.

Female Hormones

The two endogenous (produced by the body) female hormones are the **estrogens** and **progesterone**. Like androgens, their production is under the influence of the anterior pituitary gland. The endogenous estrogens are **estradiol**, **estrone**, and **estriol**. The most potent of these three estrogens is estradiol. Examples of estrogens used as drugs include estropipate (Ortho-Est) and estradiol (Estrace).

There are natural and synthetic progesterones, which are collectively called **progestins**. Examples of progestins used as drugs include medroxyprogesterone (Provera) and norethindrone (Aygestin). Examples of estrogens and progestins are given in the Summary Drug Table: Female Hormones.

PATIENT EDUCATION BOX 23-7

Key Points for Patients Taking Male Hormones

ANDROGENS

❑ Notify your health care provider if you experience any of the following: nausea, vomiting, swelling of the legs, or jaundice. Women should report any signs of virilization.

❑ Oral tablets: Take with food or a snack to avoid gastrointestinal upset.

❑ Buccal tablets: Place the tablet between your cheek and molars and allow it to dissolve in your mouth. Do not smoke or drink water until the tablet is dissolved.

❑ Testosterone transdermal system: Apply the patch according to the directions supplied with the product. Be sure your skin is clean and dry and the placement area is free of hair. Do not store the patch outside the pouch or use a damaged patch. Discard the patch in household trash in a safe manner to prevent ingestion by children or pets.

ANABOLIC STEROIDS

❑ These drugs may cause nausea and gastrointestinal upset. Take this drug with food or meals.

❑ Keep all health care provider visits because close monitoring of your therapy is essential.

❑ Female patients: Notify your health care provider if you experience signs of virilization.

ANDROGEN HORMONE INHIBITOR

❑ Take this drug without regard to meals.

❑ Inform your health care provider immediately if your sexual partner is or may become pregnant, because additional measures such as discontinuing the drug or use of a condom may be necessary.

Actions of Female Hormones

Actions of Estrogens. The estrogens are secreted by the ovarian follicle and in smaller amounts by the adrenal cortex. Estrogens are important in the development and maintenance of the female reproductive system and the primary and secondary sex characteristics. At puberty, they promote growth and development of the vagina, uterus, fallopian tubes, and breasts. They also affect the release of pituitary gonadotropins, as discussed earlier in this chapter.

Other actions of estrogen include fluid retention, protein anabolism, thinning of the cervical mucus, and the inhibition or facilitation of ovulation. Estrogens contribute to the conservation of calcium and phosphorus, the growth of pubic and axillary hair, and pigmentation of the breast nipples and genitals. Estrogens also stimu-late contraction of the fallopian tubes (which promotes movement of the ovum), modify the physical and chemical properties of the cervical mucus, and restore the endometrium after menstruation.

Actions of Progestins. Progesterone is secreted by the corpus luteum, by the placenta, and in small amounts by the adrenal cortex. Progesterone and its derivatives (i.e., the progestins) transform the proliferative endometrium into a secretory endometrium. Progestins are necessary for the development of the placenta and inhibit the secretion of pituitary gonadotropins, which in turn prevents maturation of the ovarian follicle and ovulation. The synthetic progestins are usually preferred for medical use because of the decreased effectiveness of progesterone when administered orally.

Uses of Female Hormones

Uses of Estrogens. Estrogen is most commonly used in combination with progesterones as contraceptives or as hormone replacement therapy in postmenopausal women. The estrogens are used to relieve moderate to severe vasomotor symptoms of menopause (flushing, sweating), female hypogonadism, atrophic vaginitis (orally and intravaginally), osteoporosis in women past menopause, palliative treatment for advanced prostatic carcinoma, and selected cases of inoperable breast carcinoma. The estradiol transdermal system is used as estrogen replacement therapy for moderate to severe vasomotor symptoms associated with menopause, for female hypogonadism, after removal of the ovaries in premenopausal women (female castration), for primary ovarian failure, and in the prevention of osteoporosis (Fig. 23-3).

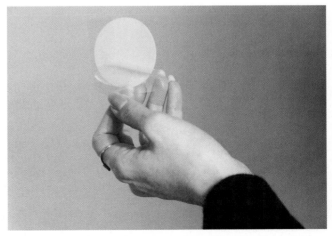

FIGURE 23-3 This low-dose estrogen transdermal patch, available as the trade name Estraderm (Estradiol Transdermal System), is transparent and approximately the size of a silver dollar. It releases small amounts of estrogen directly into the bloodstream at a constant and controlled rate to a female requiring estrogen replacement therapy for postmenopausal symptoms. (From Roach SS. *Introductory Clinical Pharmacology*, 7th ed. Baltimore: Lippincott Williams & Wilkins; 2004.)

SUMMARY DRUG TABLE   Female Hormones

Generic Name	Trade Name*	Uses	Adverse Reactions	Dosage Ranges
Estrogens conjugated estrogens	Premarin, Premarin Intravenous	Oral: vasomotor symptoms associated with menopause, atrophic vaginitis, osteoporosis, hypogonadism, castration, primary ovarian failure, breast cancer palliation, prostate cancer palliation; Parenteral: abnormal uterine bleeding due to hormonal imbalance	Headache, migraine, dizziness, mental depression, chorea, insomnia, chloasma, nausea, vomiting, abdominal cramps, pain/bloating, colitis, breakthrough bleeding, spotting, dysmenorrhea, steepening of corneal curvature, intolerance to contact lenses, edema, changes in libido, breast pain and tenderness, hypertension, gallbladder disease	0.3–1.25 mg PO QD–TID 25 mg IV or IM
esterified estrogens	Estratab, Menest	Vasomotor symptoms, atrophic vaginitis, vulva and vaginal atrophy, hypogonadism, castration, primary ovarian failure, palliation for breast cancer, palliation for prostate cancer, osteoporosis prevention	Same as conjugated estrogens	0.3–1.25 mg/d PO
estradiol, oral *ess-troe-dye'-ole*	Estrace, *generic*	Moderate to severe vasomotor symptoms associated with menopause, atrophic vaginitis, female hypogonadism, female castration, primary ovarian failure, palliative therapy for breast and prostate cancer	Same as conjugated estrogens	1–2 mg/d PO
estradiol cypionate in oil *ess-troe-dye'-ole* *sip-ee-oh-nate*	depGynogen, Depo-Estradiol, DepoGen, *generic*	Moderate to severe vasomotor symptoms associated with menopause, female hypogonadism	Same as conjugated estrogens; pain at injection site	1–5 mg IM
estradiol hemihydrate *ess-troe-dye'-ole*	Vagifem	Atrophic vaginitis	Same as conjugated estrogens	1 tablet inserted vaginally daily

Generic Name	Trade Name*	Uses	Adverse Reactions	Dosage Ranges
estradiol transdermal system *ess-troe-dye'-ole*	Alora, Climara, Estraderm, FemPatch, Vivelle	Same as conjugated estrogens	Same as conjugated estrogens	0.025–0.1 mg; therapy may be given continuously in patients with no intact uterus; in patients with uterus, treatment regimen is on a cyclic schedule (eg, 3 wk therapy, 1 wk off)
estradiol valerate in oil *ess-troc-dye'-ole val-eh-rate*	Delestrogen, Estra-L 40, Gynogen LA 20, *generic*	Same as conjugated estrogens	Same as conjugated estrogens; pain at injection site	10–20 mg IM, IV
estrone *ess-trone*	Estrone Aqueous, Kestrone 5	Moderate to severe vasomotor symptoms associated with menopause, atrophic vaginitis, female hypogonadism, female castration, primary ovarian failure, palliative therapy for breast and prostate cancer, treatment of abnormal uterine bleeding due to hormone imbalance	Same as conjugated estrogens; pain at injection site	Menopause symptoms: 0.1–0.5 mg 2–3 × wk
estropipate *ess-troe-pi'-pate*	Ogen, Ortho-Est, *generic*	Moderate to severe vasomotor symptoms associated with menopause, atrophic vaginitis, female hypogonadism, female castration, primary ovarian failure	Same as conjugated estrogens	0.625–5 mg/d PO
ethinyl estradiol *eth'-i-nil ess-troe-dye'-ole*	Estinyl	Same as conjugated estrogens	Same as conjugated estrogens	0.02–2 mg PO
synthetic conjugated estrogens, A *ess'-troe-jens*	Cenestin	Moderate to severe vasomotor symptoms associated with menopause	Same as conjugated estrogens	0.0625–1.25 mg PO
vaginal estrogens *ess'-troe-jens*	Estring, Estrace Vaginal Cream, Ogen Vaginal Cream, Premarin Vaginal Cream	Atrophic vaginitis	Rare: minor vaginal irritation or itching	1–2 applicators per day

Generic Name	Trade Name*	Uses	Adverse Reactions	Dosage Ranges
Progestins				
hydroxyprogesterone caproate in oil *hi-drox-ee-pro-jess'-te-rone cap-row'-ate*	Hylutin, *generic*	Amenorrhea, abnormal uterine bleeding, production of secretory endometrium and desquamation	Breakthrough bleeding, spotting, change in menstrual flow, amenorrhea, breast tenderness, weight gain or loss, chloasma, melasma, mental depression	125–375 mg IM
medroxyprogesterone acetate *me-drox'-ee-proe-jess'-te-rone*	Amen, Cycrin, Depo-Provera (parenteral), Provera, *generic*	Amenorrhea, abnormal uterine bleeding, reduction of endometrial hypoplasia in postmenopausal women	Same as hydroxyprogesterone caproate	5–10 mg/d PO; 400–1000 mg/wk IM
megestrol acetate *me-jess'-troll*	Megace, *generic*	Palliation of advanced carcinoma of breast or endometrium	Same as hydroxyprogesterone caproate	Breast cancer: 160 mg/d in 4 doses; endometrial cancer: 40–320 mg/d PO in divided doses
norethindrone acetate *nor-eth-in'-drone*	Aygestin, *generic*	Amenorrhea, abnormal uterine bleeding, endometriosis	Same as hydroxyprogesterone caproate	Amenorrhea, abnormal uterine bleeding: 2.5–10 mg/d PO; endometriosis: up to 15 mg/d PO
progesterone *proe-jess'-te-rone*	Crinone, Prometrium, *generic*	Amenorrhea, abnormal uterine bleeding, infertility	Same as hydroxyprogesterone caproate; Vaginal gel (Crinone): somnolence, constipation, headache, breast enlargement	5–10 mg IM, 200–400 mg PO; Crinone: 90 mg vaginally QD
Combination Products				
estrogens and progestins combined	Activella, Combi-Patch, Femhrt, Ortho-Prefest, Prempro	Treatment of moderate to severe vasomotor symptoms associated with menopause, treatment of vulval and vaginal atrophy, osteoporosis; Combination: Menopause symptoms only	Adverse reactions of both hormones; same as synthetic conjugated estrogens and progesterone	PO and Patch system: dosage varies depending on specific drug and reason for administration; follow primary health care provider's instructions
estrogen and androgen, parenteral	Depo-Testadiol	Moderate to severe vasomotor symptoms associated with menopause in patients with no response to estrogens alone	Adverse reactions of both hormones (estrogen and androgen)	Parenterally: dosage varies depending on specific drug and reason for administration; follow primary health care provider's instructions
estrogen and androgen, oral	Estratest, Estratest H.S., Syntest D. S.	Same as estrogen and androgen, parenteral	Same as estrogen and androgen, parenteral	PO dosage varies depending on reason for administration; follow primary health care provider's instructions

*The term *generic* indicates the drug is available in generic form.

Estrogen is given intramuscularly or intravenously to treat uterine bleeding caused by hormonal imbalance. When estrogen is used to treat menopausal symptoms in a woman with an intact uterus, concurrent use of progestin is recommended to decrease the risk of endometrial cancer. After a hysterectomy, estrogen alone may be used for estrogen replacement therapy.

The estrogens, in combination with a progestin, are also used as oral contraceptives (Table 23-4). The uses of individual estrogens are given in the Summary Drug Table: Female Hormones. The use of estrogens in the treatment of carcinoma is discussed in Chapter 28.

Uses of Progestins. The progestins are used in the treatment of amenorrhea, endometriosis, and functional uterine bleeding. Progestins are also used as oral contraceptives, either alone or in combination with an estrogen (see the Summary Drug Table: Female Hormones and Table 23-4).

Uses of Contraceptive Hormones. Estrogens and progestins (combination oral contraceptives) are used as oral contraceptives. There are three types of estrogen and progestin combination oral contraceptives: monophasic, biphasic, and triphasic. The monophasic oral contraceptives provide a fixed dose of estrogen and progestin throughout the cycle. The biphasic and triphasic oral contraceptives deliver hormones similar to the levels naturally produced by the body (Table 23-4). The oral contraceptives have changed a great deal since their introduction in the 1960s. Today, the levels of hormones provide lower dosages of hormones compared with the older formulations while retaining the same degree of effectiveness (>99% when used as prescribed).

Taking contraceptive hormones provides health benefits not related to contraception, such as regulating the menstrual cycle and decreased blood loss and lowering the incidence of iron deficiency anemia and dysmenorrhea. Health benefits related to the inhibition of ovulation include a decrease in ovarian cysts and ectopic pregnancies. In addition, there is a decrease in fibrocystic breast disease, acute pelvic inflammatory disease, endometrial cancer, ovarian cancer, maintenance of bone density, and symptoms related to endometriosis in women taking contraceptive hormones. Newer combination contraceptives such as norgestimate and ethinyl estradiol combinations found in Ortho Tri-Cyclen have been shown to help reduce moderate acne and maintain clear skin in women 15 years of age or older (who menstruate, want contraception, and have no response to topical anti-acne medications).

Adverse Reactions of Female Hormones

Adverse Reactions of Estrogens. Administration of estrogens by any route may result in many adverse reactions, although the incidence and intensity of these re-

actions vary. Some of the adverse reactions of estrogens include:

- Central nervous system: headache, migraine, dizziness, mental depression
- Dermatologic: chloasma (pigmentation of the skin) or melasma (discoloration of the skin), which may continue when use of the drug is discontinued
- Gastrointestinal: nausea, vomiting, abdominal cramps, dermatitis, pruritus
- Genitourinary: breakthrough bleeding, withdrawal bleeding, spotting, change in menstrual flow, dysmenorrhea, premenstrual-like syndrome, amenorrhea, vaginal candidiasis, cervical erosion, vaginitis
- Local: pain at injection site, sterile abscess, redness and irritation at the application site with transdermal system
- Ophthalmic: steepening of corneal curvature, intolerance to contact lenses
- Miscellaneous: edema, changes in libido, reduced carbohydrate tolerance, venous thromboembolism, pulmonary embolism, increase or decrease in weight, skeletal pain, and breast pain, enlargement, and tenderness

Warnings associated with the administration of estrogen include an increased risk of endometrial cancer, gallbladder disease, hypertension, hepatic adenoma (a benign tumor of the liver), cardiovascular disease, increased risk of thromboembolic disease, and hypercalcemia in those with breast cancer and bone metastases.

Adverse Reactions of Progestins. Administration of the progestins by any route may result in many adverse reactions, although the incidence and intensity of these reactions varies. Progestin may result in breakthrough bleeding, spotting, change in the menstrual flow, amenorrhea, breast tenderness, edema, weight increase or decrease, acne, chloasma or melasma, and mental depression. In addition to the adverse reactions of progestins, the use of a levonorgestrel implant system may result in bruising after insertion, scar tissue formation at the site of insertion, and hyperpigmentation at the implant site. The use of medroxyprogesterone acetate contraceptive injection may result in the same adverse reactions as those of any progestin.

Adverse Reactions of Contraceptive Hormones. When estrogen/progestin combinations are used as oral contraceptives, the adverse reactions of the estrogens and the progestins may occur. These drugs may cause adverse reactions that vary depending on their estrogen or progestin content. Table 23-5 identifies the symptoms of estrogen and progestin excess or deficiency. Adjusting the estrogen progestin balance or dosage can minimize the adverse effects.

TABLE 23-4   Oral and Implantable Contraceptives

Generic Name	Trade Name
Monophasic Oral Contraceptives	
50 mcg ethinyl estradiol acetate 1mg norethindrone	Necon 1/50, Norinyl 1+50, Ortho-Novum 1/50
50 mcg ethinyl estradiol, 1 mg ethynodiol diacetate	Demulen 1/50, Zovia 1/50E
50 mcg ethinyl estradiol, 0.5 mg norgestrel	Ogestrel, Ovral
35 mcg ethinyl estradiol, 1 mg norethindrone	Necon 1/35, Norinyl l+135, Ortho Novum 1/35
35 mcg ethinyl estradiol, 0.5 mg norethindrone	Brevicon, Modicon, Necon 0.5/35, Notrel
35 mcg ethinyl estradiol, 0.4 mg norethindrone	Ovcon-35
35 mcg ethinyl estradiol, 0.25 mg norgestimate	Ortho-Cyclen, Sprintex
35 mcg ethinyl estradiol, 1 mg ethynodiol diacetate	Demulen 1/35, Zovia 1/35 E
30 mcg ethinyl estradiol, 1.5 mg norethindrone acetate	Loestrin, 21 1.5/30, Loestrin Fe 1.5/30, Microgestin Fe 1.5/30
30 mcg ethinyl estradiol, 0.3 mg norgestrel	Lo/Ovral, Low-Ogestrel, Cryselle
30 mcg ethinyl estradiol, 0.15 mg desogestrel	Apri, Desogen, Ortho-Cept
30 mcg ethinyl estradiol, 0.15 mg levonorgestrel	Levler, Levora, Nordette, Portia
20 mcg ethinyl estradiol, 1 mg norethindrone acetate	Loestrin 21 1/20, Loestrin Fe 1/20, Microgestin Fe 1/20
20 mcg ethinyl estradiol, 0.1 mg levonorgestrel	Alesse, Aviane, Levlite
Biphasic Oral Contraceptives	
Phase one: 35 mcg ethinyl estradiol, 0.5 mg norethindrone	Necon 10/11, Ortho-Novum 10/11
Phase two: 35 mcg ethinyl estradiol, 1 mg norethindrone	
Triphasic Oral Contraceptives	
Phase one: 35 mcg ethinyl estradiol, 0.5 mg norethindrone	Tri-Norinyl
Phase two: 35 mcg ethinyl estradiol, 1 mg norethindrone	
Phase three: 35 mcg ethinyl estradiol, 0.5 mg norethindrone	
Phase one: 35 mcg ethinyl estradiol, 0.5 mg norethindrone	Ortho-Novum 7/7/7, Necon 7/7/7
Phase two: 35 mcg ethinyl estradiol, 0.75 mg norethindrone	
Phase three: 35 mcg ethinyl estradiol, 1 mg norethindrone	
Phase one: 30 mcg ethinyl estradiol, 0.05 mg levonorgestrel	Tri-Levlen, Triphasil, Trivora, Enpresse
Phase two: 40 mcg ethinyl estradiol, 0.075 mg levonorgestrel	
Phase three: 30 mcg ethinyl estradiol, 0.125 mg levonorgestrel	
Phase one: 35 mcg ethinyl estradiol, 0.18 mg norgestimate	Ortho Tri-Cyclen
Phase two: 35 mcg ethinyl estradiol, 0.215 mg norgestimate	
Phase three: 35 mcg ethinyl estradiol, 0.25 mg norgestimate	
Phase one: 25 mcg ethinyl estradiol, 0.18 mg norgestimate	Ortho Tri-Cyclen Lo
Phase two: 25 mcg ethinyl estradiol, 0.215 mg norgestimate	
Phase three: 25 mcg ethinyl estradiol, 0.25 mg norgestimate	
Phase one: 1 mg norethindrone acetate, 20 mcg ethinyl estradiol	Estrostep 21, Estrostep Fe
Phase two: 30 mcg ethinyl estradiol, 1 mg norethindrone acetate	
Phase three: 35 mcg ethinyl estradiol, 1 mg norethindrone acetate	
Phase one: 25 mcg ethinyl estradiol, 0.1 mg desogestrel	Cyclessa
Phase two: 25 mcg ethinyl estradiol, 0.125 mg norgestimate	
Phase three: 25 mcg ethinyl estradiol, 0.15 mg norgestimate	
Progestin Only Contraceptives	
0.35 mg norethindrone	Camila, Errin, Nor-QD, Nora-BE, Ortho Micronor
0.075 norgestrel	Ovrette
Implant Contraceptive Systems (Progestins)	
levonorgestrel: 6 capsules, each containing 36 mg levonorgestrel for subdermal implantation	Norplant System
progesterone: T-shaped unit containing 38 mg progesterone for insertion in the uterine cavity	Progestasert

TABLE 23-5   Estrogen and Progestin: Excess and Deficiency

Hormone*	Signs of Excess	Signs of Deficiency
estrogen	Nausea, bloating, cervical mucorrhea (increased cervical discharge), polyposis (numerous polyps), melasma (discoloration of the skin), hypertension, migraine headache, breast fullness or tenderness, edema	Early or mid-cycle breakthrough bleeding, increased spotting, hypomenorrhea
progestin	Increased appetite, weight gain, tiredness, fatigue, hypomenorrhea, acne, oily scalp, hair loss, hirsutism (excessive growth of hair), depression, monilial vaginitis, breast regression	Late breakthrough bleeding, amenorrhea, hypermenorrhea

*Hormonal balance is achieved by adjusting the estrogen/progestin dosage. Oral contraceptives have different amounts of progestin and estrogen varying the estrogenic and progestational activity in each product.

Managing Adverse Reactions of Female Hormones.
Patients prescribed female hormones usually take them for several months or years. Throughout that time, the patient must be monitored for adverse reactions. These drugs are self-administered at home. Patient education is therefore an important avenue for detecting and managing adverse reactions.

With the estrogens it is important to monitor for breakthrough bleeding. If breakthrough bleeding occurs with either estrogen or progestin, then the patient should notify the health care provider. A dosage change may be necessary.

Gastrointestinal upsets, such as nausea, vomiting, abdominal cramps, and bloating, may also occur. Nausea usually decreases or subsides within 1 to 2 months of therapy. However, until that time the discomfort may lessen if the drug is taken with food. If nausea is continual, then frequent small meals may help. If nausea and vomiting persist, then an antiemetic may be prescribed. Bloating may be lessened with light to moderate exercise or by limiting fluid intake with meals.

A patient with diabetes who is taking female hormones must be carefully monitored. The health care provider should be notified if blood glucose levels are elevated or the urine is positive for glucose or ketone bodies, because a change in the dosage of insulin or the oral hypoglycemic drug may be required. See Chapter 22 for how to manage hypoglycemic and hyperglycemic episodes.

Sodium and Water Retention Sodium and water retention may occur during female hormone therapy. Any swelling of the hands, ankles, or feet should be reported to the health care provider. A hospitalized patient is weighed daily, an accurate record of the intake and output is kept, walking is encouraged, and the patient is encouraged to eat a diet low in sodium (if prescribed by the health care provider).

Thromboembolic Effects The patient is monitored for signs of thromboembolic effects, such as pain, swelling, tenderness in the extremities, headache, chest pain, and blurred vision. These adverse effects should be reported to the health care provider. Patients with previous venous insufficiency, who are on bed rest for other medical reasons, or who smoke are at increased risk for thromboembolic effects. The patient is encouraged to elevate the lower extremities when sitting, if possible, and to exercise the lower extremities by walking.

ALERT

Postoperative Thromboembolic Complications

There is an increased risk of postoperative thromboembolic complications in women taking oral contraceptives. If possible, the drug is discontinued at least 4 weeks before a surgical procedure associated with thromboembolism or during prolonged immobilization.

Alterations in Nutrition Alterations in nutrition can occur, resulting in significant weight gain or loss. Weight gain occurs more frequently than weight loss. A low-fat diet that includes adequate amounts of protein and carbohydrates is recommended. A variety of nutritious foods (fruits, vegetables, grains, cereals, meats, and poultry) should be eaten, with portion sizes decreased to meet individual needs. A dietitian may be consulted if necessary. An exercise program is helpful for both losing weight and maintaining weight loss.

Weight loss is often as difficult to manage as weight gain. A patient taking female hormones who has a decreased appetite and loses weight should be encouraged to increase the protein, carbohydrates, and calories in the diet. Small feedings with several daily snacks are usually better-tolerated in those with a loss of appetite than are three larger meals. Patients are encouraged to eat foods that they like. Dietary supplements may be necessary if a significant weight loss occurs. A dietitian may be consulted if necessary. Patients are usually weighed weekly.

Anxiety A woman taking female hormones may have many concerns about therapy with these drugs. Although there are dangers associated with long-term use of female hormones, many of these adverse reactions are rare. When the health care provider monitors a patient closely, the dangers associated with long-term use are often minimal.

Male patients with inoperable prostatic carcinoma also may have concerns about taking a female hormone. The patient needs to be reassured that the dosage is carefully regulated and that feminizing effects, if they occur at all, are usually minimal.

Contraindications, Precautions, and Interactions of Female Hormones

Contraindications, Precautions, and Interactions of Estrogens. Estrogen therapy is contraindicated in patients with a known hypersensitivity, breast cancer (except for metastatic disease), estrogen-dependent neoplasms, undiagnosed abnormal genital bleeding, known or suspected pregnancy (pregnancy category X), or thromboembolic disorders.

Estrogens are used cautiously in patients with gallbladder disease, hypercalcemia (may lead to severe hypercalcemia in patients with breast cancer and bone metastasis), cardiovascular disease, or liver impairment.

The effects of oral anticoagulants may be decreased when administered with an estrogen. When an estrogen is combined with a tricyclic antidepressant, there is an increased risk of toxicity of the antidepressant. Barbiturates or rifampin may decrease estrogen blood levels, increasing the risk for breakthrough bleeding. When an estrogen is administered concurrently with a hydantoin, breakthrough bleeding, spotting, and pregnancy may occur. A loss of seizure control has also been reported. Cigarette smoking increases the risk for cardiovascular complications.

Contraindications, Precautions, and Interactions of Progestins. The progestins are contraindicated in patients with a known hypersensitivity, thromboembolic disorders, cerebral hemorrhage, impaired liver function, or cancer of the breast or genital organs. Both the estrogens and progestins are classified as pregnancy category X drugs and are contraindicated during pregnancy. The progestins are used cautiously in patients with a history of migraine headaches, epilepsy, asthma, or cardiac or renal impairment.

The effects of the progestins are decreased when administered with an anticonvulsant, barbiturate, or rifampin. Administration of a penicillin or tetracycline with an oral contraceptive decreases the effects of the oral contraceptive.

Contraindications, Precautions, and Interactions of Contraceptive Hormones. See the preceding sections on "Contraindications, Precautions, and Interactions" of estrogens and progestins for information regarding the combination oral contraceptives. The warnings associated with the use of oral contraceptives are the same as those for estrogens and progestins and include cigarette smoking, which increases the risk of cardiovascular side effects, such as venous and arterial thromboembolism, myocardial infarction, and thrombotic and hemorrhagic stroke. Also reported with oral contraceptive use are hepatic adenomas and tumors, visual disturbances, gallbladder disease, hypertension, and fetal abnormalities.

Patient Management Issues with Female Hormones

Before administering an estrogen or progestin, a complete patient health history is obtained including menstrual history, which includes the menarche (age of onset of first menstruation), menstrual pattern, and any changes in the menstrual pattern (including a menopause history when applicable). In patients prescribed an estrogen (including oral contraceptives), a history of thrombophlebitis or other vascular disorders, smoking history, and a history of liver diseases are included. Vital signs are taken. The health care provider usually performs a breast and pelvic examination and a Pap smear test before starting therapy. Liver function tests may be ordered.

If the male or female patient is being treated for a malignancy, then the patient's physical status and mental status are evaluated. The health care provider may also order laboratory tests, such as serum electrolytes and liver function tests.

At each office visit, the patient's vital signs and weight are recorded, along with any adverse drug effects and the result of drug therapy. If the patient is receiving an estrogen for the symptoms of menopause, then her original symptoms are compared with the symptoms she is currently experiencing, if any. A steady weight gain or loss is also noted. A periodic physical examination is performed by the health care provider and may include a pelvic examination, breast examination, Pap smear test, and laboratory tests. A patient with a prostatic or breast carcinoma usually requires more frequent evaluations of response to drug therapy.

A hospitalized patient receiving a female hormone requires careful monitoring. Vital signs are taken daily or more often, depending on the patient's physical condition and the reason for drug use. The patient is observed for any adverse drug reactions, especially those related to the liver (the development of jaundice) or the cardiovascular system (thromboembolism). The patient is weighed weekly or as ordered by the health care provider.

In patients with breast carcinoma or prostatic carcinoma, signs indicating a response to therapy are monitored, such as relief of pain, an increased appetite, or feeling of well-being. With prostatic carcinoma, the response to therapy may be rapid, but with breast carcinoma the response is usually slow.

Estrogens. Oral estrogens are administered with food or immediately after eating to reduce gastrointestinal upset. When estrogens are given vaginally for atrophic vaginitis, the patient is given instructions on proper use.

Contraceptive Hormones Monophasic oral contraceptives are administered in a 21-day regimen, with the first tablet taken on the first Sunday after the menses begins. After 21 days, the next 7 days are skipped, and then the cycle is begun again. With biphasic oral contraceptives, the first phase is 10 days of a smaller dosage of progestin, and the second phase is a larger amount of progestin. The estrogen dosage remains constant for 21 days, followed by no estrogen for 7 days. Some regimens contain seven placebo tablets for the "off days" for easier management. With triphasic oral contraceptives, the estrogen amount stays the same or may vary and the progestin amount varies throughout the 21-day cycle. Progestin-only oral contraceptives are taken daily and continuously.

Implant Contraceptive System Levonorgestrel, a progestin, is available as an implant contraceptive system (Norplant System). Six capsules, each containing levonorgestrel, are implanted under local anesthesia beneath the skin in the mid-portion of the upper arm. The capsules provide contraceptive protection for 5 years but may be removed at any time at the request of the patient.

Medroxyprogesterone Acetate Contraceptive Injection Medroxyprogesterone acetate (Depo-Provera), a synthetic progestin used in the treatment of abnormal uterine bleeding and secondary amenorrhea, is also used as a contraceptive. This drug is given intramuscularly every 3 months, with the initial dosage given within the first 5 days of menstruation or within 5 days postpartum.

A L E R T

Frequency of Medroxyprogesterone Acetate Intramuscular Injections

With an interval greater than 14 weeks between intramuscular injections, the health care provider must be certain that the patient is not pregnant before administering the next injection.

Educating the Patient and Family About Female Hormones

Each oral contraceptive product has detailed patient instruction sheets regarding starting oral contraceptive therapy, including instructions for missed doses. All instructions are discussed with the patient. The patient is given a thorough explanation of the dose regimen and adverse reactions that may occur. Patients taking oral contraceptives are reminded that skipping a dose could result in pregnancy.

The health care provider usually performs periodic examinations, including laboratory tests, a pelvic examination, or a Pap smear test. The patient is encouraged to keep all appointments for follow-up evaluation of therapy. Patient Education Box 23-8 includes key points about female hormones the patient and family members should know.

Natural Remedies

Black Cohosh

Black cohosh, an herb, grows in North America and has been used for centuries for a variety of medicinal purposes. Black cohosh is generally regarded as safe when used as directed. Today, it is used primarily for hot flashes and other menopausal symptoms, muscular and arthritic pain, headache, and eyestrain. The Food and Drug Administration (FDA) classifies it as a dietary supplement rather than a drug. It is available over the counter in the form of tablets, capsules, tinctures, and tea. Black cohosh tea is not considered as effective as other forms.

This herb is popular as an alternative to hormone alternative replacement therapy, which may increase the woman's risk of serious illness, including cancer, depression, and high blood pressure.

Black cohosh is thought to increase diminished estrogen levels in menopausal women. When taken orally it may reduce physical menopausal symptoms, including night sweats, hot flashes, headaches, heart palpitations, dizziness, vaginal atrophy, and tinnitus (ringing in the ears). It may improve the regularity of menstrual cycles by balancing hormones and reducing uterine spasms. Black cohosh may also reduce the psychological symptoms associated with menopause, including insomnia, nervousness, irritability, and depression.

In 2001 the American College of Obstetricians and Gynecologists stated that black cohosh (not to be confused with blue cohosh) may be helpful in the short-term for menopausal symptoms, although clinical trial results are mixed. Long-term data are not available.

Many natural substances can have adverse effects, particularly if they are taken in large quantities or if they interact with other medications. The primary adverse effect of black cohosh is nausea, and other possible effects include dizziness, headache, nausea, impaired vision, and vomiting. Pregnant women should not take black cohosh.

Although no specific drug interactions have been reported, women taking hormone alternative replacement therapy should consult with their health care provider before taking black cohosh.

Key Points for Taking Female Hormones

ESTROGENS AND PROGESTINS

❑ A patient package insert comes with the drug. Read the information carefully. If you have any questions about this information, discuss them with your health care provider.

❑ If you experience gastrointestinal upset, take the drug with food.

❑ Notify your health care provider if you experience any of the following: pain in the legs or groin area, sharp chest pain or sudden shortness of breath, lumps in the breast, sudden severe headache, dizziness or fainting, vision or speech disturbances, weakness or numbness in the arms or legs, severe abdominal pain, depression, or yellowing of the skin or eyes.

❑ If you think you may be pregnant or you experience abnormal vaginal bleeding, stop taking the drug and contact your health care provider immediately.

❑ If you have diabetes, check your blood glucose or urine daily, or more often. Contact your health care provider if your blood glucose is elevated or if your urine is positive for glucose or ketones. An elevated blood glucose level or urine positive for glucose or ketones may require a change in diabetic therapy (insulin, oral hypoglycemic drug) or diet; your health care provider must make these changes.

ORAL CONTRACEPTIVES

❑ A patient package comes with the drug. Read the information carefully. Begin the first dose as directed in the package insert or as directed by your health care provider. If you have any questions about this information, discuss them with your health care provider.

❑ To obtain a maximum effect, take this drug as prescribed and at intervals not exceeding once every 24 hours. An oral contraceptive is best taken with the evening meal or at bedtime. The effectiveness of this drug depends on following the prescribed dosage schedule. Failure to comply with the dosage schedule may result in a pregnancy.

❑ Use an additional method of birth control (as recommended by your health care provider) until after the first week in the initial cycle.

❑ If you miss one day's dose, take the missed dose as soon as remembered or take 2 tablets the next day. If you miss 2 days, take 2 tablets for the next 2 days and continue on with the normal dosing schedule. However, another form of birth control must be used until the cycle is completed and a new cycle is begun. If you miss 3 days in a row or more, discontinue use of the drug and use another form of birth control until a new cycle can begin. Before restarting the dosage regimen, make sure a pregnancy did not result from the break in the dosage regimen.

❑ If you have any questions regarding what to do about a missed dose, discuss the procedure with your health care provider.

❑ Do not smoke and avoid exposure to second-hand smoke while taking these drugs; cigarette smoking during estrogen therapy may increase the risk of cardiovascular effects.

❑ Report adverse reactions such as fluid retention or edema of the extremities; weight gain; pain, swelling, or tenderness in the legs; blurred vision; chest pain; yellowed skin or eyes; dark urine; or abnormal vaginal bleeding.

❑ While taking these drugs, periodic examinations by your health care provider and laboratory tests are necessary.

ESTRADIOL TRANSDERMAL SYSTEM

❑ Alora, Estraderm, Esclim, and Vivelle are applied twice per week; Climara and FemPatch are applied every 7 days.

❑ Apply the patch immediately after opening the pouch, with the adhesive side down. Apply to clean, dry skin of your trunk (not breast or waistline), buttocks, abdomen, upper inner thigh, or upper arm. (Do not apply to breasts or a site exposed to sunlight.) The area should not be oily or irritated.

❑ Press the patch firmly in place with the palm of your hand for approximately 10 seconds. Rotate the application site with at least 1-week intervals between applications to a particular site.

❑ Avoid areas that may be exposed to rubbing or where your clothing may rub the system off or loosen the edges.

❑ Remove the old patch before applying a new one unless your health care provider directs otherwise. Rotate application sites to prevent skin irritation.

❑ Follow the directions of your health care provider regarding application of the patch (e.g., continuous 3-week use followed by 1 week off, changed weekly, or applied twice weekly).

❑ If the patch falls off, then reapply it or apply a new patch. Continue the original treatment schedule.

INTRAVAGINAL APPLICATION

❑ Use the applicator correctly. Refer to the package insert for the correct procedure. The applicator is marked with the correct dosage and accompanies the drug when purchased.

❑ Wash the applicator after each use in warm water with a mild soap and rinse it well.

❑ Stay in a recumbent position for at least 30 minutes after instillation.

❑ Use a sanitary napkin or panty liner to protect your clothing if necessary.

❑ Do not double the dosage if you miss a dose. Instead, skip the dose and resume treatment the next day.

❑ When using the vaginal ring, press the ring into an oval and insert it into the upper third of the vaginal vault.

Saw Palmetto

Saw palmetto, an herb, is derived from the berries of the saw palm tree and is used to treat benign prostatic hypertrophy, commonly known as enlargement of the prostate. Half of all men older than 60 have some symptoms of benign prostatic hypertrophy and must cope with a more urgent and more frequent need to urinate, often interrupting sleep, creating urinary leaking, a feeling of not having completely emptied the bladder, and a stop-and-start flow of urine. The Food and Drug Administration (FDA) classifies saw palmetto as a dietary supplement rather than as a drug. Although commercially available over the counter in tea-form, saw palmetto should be taken as a tincture, capsule, or tablet, because the active agents in the herb are not water-soluble.

Although scientific study is far from complete, encouraging evidence reported in the *Journal of the American Medical Association* suggests that saw palmetto is effective in the treatment of benign prostatic hypertrophy, increases the flow of urine, and reduces urinary frequency and the sleep interruption associated with it. It often takes 1 to 3 months of treatment before an improvement in symptoms occurs. After 6 months of treatment with saw palmetto, a health care provider should assess the person's condition.

The only known adverse effect of this herb is upset stomach.

KEY POINTS

◉ The pituitary gland secretes a number of hormones that regulate growth, metabolism, the reproductive cycle, electrolyte balance, and water retention or loss. The hormones of the anterior pituitary include follicle-stimulating hormone, luteinizing hormone, growth hormone, adrenocorticotropic hormone, thyroid-stimulating hormone, and prolactin.

◉ The gonadotropins (follicle-stimulating hormone and luteinizing hormone) influence the secretion of sex hormones, development of secondary sex characteristics, and the reproductive cycle in both men and women. The gonadotropins include menotropins, urofollitropin, clomiphene, and chorionic gonadotropin.

◉ Menotropins (Pergonal) and urofollitropin (Metrodin) are purified preparations of the gonadotropins extracted from the urine of postmenopausal women and induce ovulation and pregnancy. Menotropins are used to induce ovulation and pregnancy in anovulatory women and are also used with human chorionic gonadotropin in women to stimulate multiple follicles for in vitro fertilization. In men, menotropins are used to induce the production of sperm (spermatogenesis). Urofollitropin is used to induce ovulation in women with polycystic ovarian disease and to stimulate multiple follicular developments in ovulatory women for in vitro fertilization. Adverse reactions associated with the menotropins include ovarian enlargement, hemoperitoneum (blood in the peritoneal cavity), abdominal discomfort, and febrile reactions. Urofollitropin use may result in mild to moderate ovarian enlargement, abdominal discomfort, nausea, vomiting, breast tenderness, and irritation at the injection site. Multiple births and birth defects have been reported with the use of both menotropins and urofollitropin.

◉ Clomiphene (Clomid) is a synthetic nonsteroidal compound that decreases the number of available estrogen receptors and causes the anterior pituitary to increase secretion of follicle-stimulating hormone and luteinizing hormone. The actions of chorionic gonadotropin are identical to those of the pituitary luteinizing hormone. Clomiphene (Clomid) and chorionic gonadotropin are both used to induce ovulation in anovulatory women. Chorionic gonadotropin is also used for the treatment of prepubertal cryptorchism and in men to treat selected cases of hypogonadotropic hypogonadism. Clomiphene may result in vasomotor flushes, abdominal discomfort, ovarian enlargement, blurred vision, nausea, vomiting, and nervousness. Chorionic gonadotropin may result in headache, irritability, restlessness, fatigue, edema, and precocious puberty (when given for cryptorchism).

◉ Growth hormone is secreted by the anterior pituitary and regulates the growth of the individual until early adulthood. Growth hormone is available as the synthetic products somatrem (Protropin) and somatropin (Humatrope). Both produce skeletal growth in children and are administered to children who have not grown because of a deficiency of pituitary growth hormone. These hormones cause few adverse reactions when administered as directed.

◉ Corticotropin is an anterior pituitary hormone that stimulates the adrenal cortex to produce and secrete adrenocortical hormones, primarily glucocorticoids. It is used for diagnostic testing of adrenocortical function. This drug may also be used for the management of acute exacerbations of multiple sclerosis, nonsuppurative thyroiditis, or hypercalcemia associated with cancer, and as an anti-inflammatory and immunosuppressant drug when conventional glucocorticoid therapy has not been effective. Adverse reactions may affect many body systems, including the central nervous, cardiovascular, gastrointestinal, genitourinary, integumentary, musculoskeletal, and endocrine systems.

◉ Vasopressin, a posterior pituitary gland hormone, and its derivatives regulate the resorption of water by the kidneys. Vasopressin and its derivatives are used in the treatment of diabetes insipidus. Treatment with vasopressin replaces the hormone in the body and restores normal urination and thirst. Vasopressin may also be used for the prevention and treatment of postoperative abdominal distention and to dispel gas interfering with abdominal x-rays. Local or systemic hypersensitivity reactions may occur in some patients receiving vasopressin. Tremor, sweating, vertigo, nausea, vomiting, abdominal cramps, and water intoxication may also occur.

◉ The adrenal cortex secretes several hormones (the glucocorticoids, the mineralocorticoids, and small amounts of sex hormones). The glucocorticoids and mineralocorticoids are collectively called corticosteroids.

◉ The glucocorticoids influence or regulate functions such as the immune response system, the regulation of glucose, fat and protein metabolism, and control of the anti-inflammatory response. Examples of the glucocorticoids include cortisone, hydrocortisone, prednisone, prednisolone, and triamcinolone. The glucocorticoids are used as replacement therapy for adrenocortical insufficiency and to treat allergic reactions, collagen diseases, dermatologic conditions, rheumatic disorders, shock, and other conditions. The anti-inflammatory activity of these hormones makes them valuable as anti-inflammatories and as immunosuppressants to suppress inflammation and modify the immune response. High-dose therapy may produce many of the signs and symptoms seen with Cushing syndrome, including a "buffalo" hump, moon face, oily skin and acne, osteoporosis, purple striae on the abdomen and hips, skin pigmentation, and weight gain.

◉ The mineralocorticoids aldosterone and desoxycorticosterone play an important role in conserving sodium and increasing the excretion of potassium, and are important in controlling salt and water balance. Deficiencies of the mineralocorticoids result in a loss of sodium and water and a retention of potassium. Fludrocortisone (Florinef) has both glucocorticoid and mineralocorticoid activity and is the only currently available mineralocorticoid drug. Adverse reactions may occur if the dosage is too high or prolonged or if withdrawal is too rapid, and may cause edema, hypertension, congestive heart failure, enlargement of the heart, increased sweating, or allergic skin rash, hypokalemia, muscular weakness, headache, and hypersensitivity reactions.

◉ The thyroid gland secretes thyroxin and triiodothyronine. Two diseases related to the hormone-producing activity of the thyroid gland are hypothyroidism and hyperthyroidism. Thyroid hormones used in medicine include both natural and synthetic hormones. The synthetic hormones are generally preferred because they are more uniform in potency than are the natural hormones obtained from animals. Thyroid hormones increase the metabolic rate of tissues, which results in increases in the heart and respiratory rate, body temperature, cardiac output, oxygen consumption, and the metabolism of fats, proteins, and carbohydrates. Thyroid hormones are used as replacement therapy when the patient is hypothyroid. The most common adverse reactions seen are signs of overdose and hyperthyroidism; other adverse reactions are rare.

◉ Antithyroid drugs or thyroid antagonists are used to treat hyperthyroidism. Hyperthyroidism may also be treated by the administration of strong iodine solutions, use of radioactive iodine (^{131}I), or by surgical removal of some or almost all of the thyroid gland (subtotal thyroidectomy). Antithyroid drugs inhibit the manufacture of thyroid hormones. Strong iodide solutions act by decreasing the vascularity of the thyroid gland by rapidly inhibiting the release of the thyroid hormones. Methimazole (Tapazole) and propylthiouracil (PTU) are used for the medical management of hyperthyroidism. Strong iodine solution, also known as Lugol solution, may be given orally with methimazole or propylthiouracil to prepare for thyroid surgery. Iodine solutions are also used for rapid treatment of hyperthyroidism. Radioactive iodine (^{131}I) may be used for treatment of hyperthyroidism and selected cases of cancer of the thyroid. The most serious adverse reaction agranulocytosis; other reactions include exfoliative dermatitis, granulocytopenia, aplastic anemia, hypoprothrombinemia, and hepatitis. Reactions to strong iodine solution include symptoms of iodism (excessive amounts of iodine in the body), such as a metallic taste in the mouth, swelling and soreness of the parotid glands, burning of the mouth and throat, sore teeth and gums, symptoms of a head cold, and occasionally gastrointestinal upset. Iodine allergy can be serious. Reactions to ^{131}I include sore throat, swelling in the neck, nausea, vomiting, cough, pain on swallowing, marrow depression, anemia, leukopenia, thrombocytopenia, and tachycardia.

◉ Male and female hormones aid in development and maintenance of secondary sex characteristics and are necessary for human reproduction. A male or female hormone may be used to treat certain disorders, such as inoperable breast cancer, male hypogonadism, or a male or female hormone deficiency, and are used as contraceptives and for treating the symptoms of menopause.

◉ Testosterone, the most potent naturally occurring androgen, and its derivatives are called androgens. The anabolic steroids are closely related to testosterone and have both androgenic and anabolic activity. Testosterone and its derivatives activate the reproductive potential in adolescent boys, and stimulate the growth of accessory sex organs at the time of puberty. The androgens also promote tissue-building processes anabolism and reverse tissue-depleting processes catabolism. Androgens include fluoxymesterone (Halotestin), methyltestosterone (Oreton Methyl), and testosterone. Androgen therapy may be given as replacement therapy for testosterone deficiency. In female patients, androgen therapy may be used as part of the treatment for inoperable metastatic breast carcinoma in women who are 1 to 5 years past menopause. Androgens may also be given to premenopausal women with metastatic breast carcinoma that is believed to be hormone-dependent and whose tumor growth and spread have been slowed after an oophorectomy (removal of the ovaries). In men, androgens may result in breast enlargement (gynecomastia), testicular atrophy, inhibition of testicular function, impotence, enlargement of the penis, nausea, jaundice, headache, anxiety, male pattern baldness, acne, and depression. Fluid and electrolyte imbalances may also occur. In women receiving an androgen preparation for breast carcinoma, the most common adverse reactions are amenorrhea, other menstrual irregularities, and virilization.

◉ Anabolic steroids, synthetic drugs chemically related to the androgens, promote tissue-building processes. Given in normal doses, they have a minimal effect on the accessory sex organs and secondary sex characteristics. Anabolic steroids are used to treat anemia of renal insufficiency, to control metastatic breast cancer in women, and to promote weight gain in those with weight loss after surgery, trauma, or infections. Stanozolol is used prophylactically to decrease the frequency and severity of hereditary angioedema. Virilization in women is the most common reaction associated with anabolic steroids, especially with higher doses. Nausea, vomiting, diarrhea, fluid and electrolyte imbalances, testicular atrophy, jaundice, anorexia, and muscle cramps may occur. Blood-filled cysts of the liver and sometimes the spleen, malignant and benign liver tumors, an increased risk of atherosclerosis, and mental changes are the most serious adverse reactions with prolonged use. Abuse of anabolic steroids for muscle tissue development is a growing problem and should be discouraged.

◉ Androgen hormone inhibitor finasteride (Proscar) is a synthetic compound drug that inhibits the conversion of testosterone into the potent androgen 5-α-dihydrotestosterone. Finasteride is used to treat the symptoms of prostatic hypertrophy, such as difficulty starting the urinary stream, frequent passage of small amounts of urine, and having to urinate during the night. Finasteride is also used for the prevention of male pattern baldness in men with early signs of hair loss. Adverse reactions with finasteride usually are mild and do not require discontinuing use of the drug. Adverse reactions, when they occur, are related to the sexual drive and include impotence, decreased libido, and a decreased volume of ejaculate.

◉ The two female hormones are the estrogens and progesterone. The endogenous estrogens are estradiol, estrone, and estriol. Examples of estrogens used as drugs include estropipate (Ortho-Est) and estradiol (Estrace). Natural and synthetic progesterones are collectively called progestins. Examples of progestins used as drugs include medroxyprogesterone (Provera) and norethindrone (Aygestin).

◉ Estrogens are important in the development and maintenance of the female reproductive system and the primary and secondary sex characteristics. Other actions include fluid retention, protein anabolism, thinning of the cervical mucus, and the inhibition or facilitation of ovulation. Estrogen is most commonly used in combination with progesterones as contraceptives or as hormone replacement therapy in postmenopausal women. The estrogens are used to relieve moderate to severe vasomotor symptoms of menopause (flushing, sweating), female hypogonadism, atrophic vaginitis (orally and intravaginally), osteoporosis in women past menopause, as palliative treatment for advanced prostatic carcinoma, and in selected cases of inoperable breast carcinoma. The estradiol transdermal system is used as estrogen replacement therapy for moderate to severe vasomotor symptoms associated with menopause, for female hypogonadism, after removal of the ovaries in premenopausal women (female castration), primary ovarian failure, and to prevent osteoporosis. Estrogens have many adverse reactions. Warnings include an increased risk of endometrial cancer, gallbladder disease, hypertension, hepatic adenoma, cardiovascular disease, increased risk of thromboembolic disease, and hypercalcemia in those with breast cancer and bone metastases.

◉ Progestins are necessary for the development of the placenta and inhibit the secretion of pituitary gonadotropins, which in turn prevents maturation of the ovarian follicle and ovulation. The synthetic progestins are usually used medically because of the decreased effectiveness of progesterone when administered orally. The progestins are used in the treatment of amenorrhea, endometriosis, and functional uterine bleeding. Progestins are also used as oral contraceptives, either alone or in combination with an estrogen. Progestins also have many adverse reactions, including breakthrough bleeding, spotting, change in the menstrual flow, amenorrhea, breast tenderness, edema, weight increase or decrease, acne, chloasma or melasma, and mental depression.

◉ Estrogens and progestins are used combined as oral contraceptives. Contraceptive hormones provide health benefits not related to contraception, such as regulating the menstrual cycle and decreasing blood loss, iron deficiency anemia, and dysmenorrhea. When estrogen/progestin combinations are used as oral contraceptives, the adverse reactions of both may occur.

CASE STUDY

Judy Cowan, age 28 years, has been prescribed clomiphene to induce ovulation and pregnancy. Judy is very anxious and wants desperately to become pregnant. Her husband, Jim, has come to the clinic with her.

1. Before beginning treatment with clomiphene, the health care provider would want to determine if Judy has:
   a. liver disease
   b. ovarian cysts
   c. abnormal bleeding of unknown cause
   d. all of the above

2. What should Judy know before she begins drug therapy?
   a. there is a possibility she may experience nausea and vomiting with clomiphene use
   b. there is a possibility of birth defects with clomiphene use
   c. there is a possibility of hair loss with clomiphene use
   d. none of the above

3. Adverse reactions to clomiphene include:
   a. breast tenderness
   b. blurred vision
   c. nervousness
   d. all of the above

WEBSITE ACTIVITIES

1. Go to The National Institute on Drug Abuse website (http://www.steroidabuse.org) and find the online article "Community Drug Alert Bulletin—Anabolic Steroids." Read the information about the use of anabolic steroids among adolescents and write a paragraph summarizing that information.

2. Continuing in the same article, read about the practice of "stacking" with anabolic steroids. What potentially mistaken belief is this practice based on?

REVIEW QUESTIONS

1. What adverse reaction is most likely to occur in the early days of therapy in a patient taking a thyroid hormone?
   a. signs of congestive heart failure
   b. signs of hyperthyroidism
   c. signs of hypothyroidism
   d. signs of euthyroidism

2. The patient is informed that therapy with a thyroid hormone may not produce a full therapeutic response for:
   a. 24 hours
   b. 2 or 3 days
   c. several weeks or more
   d. 8 to 12 months

3. Which of the following adverse reactions would lead the health care provider to suspect cushingoid appearance in a patient taking a corticosteroid?
   a. moon face, hirsutism
   b. kyphosis, periorbital edema

c. pallor of the skin, acne

   d. exophthalmos

4. Which of the following statements made by a patient would indicate to the health care provider that the patient is experiencing an adverse reaction to radioactive iodine?

   a. "I am sleepy most of the day"

   b. "I am unable to sleep at night"

   c. "My throat hurts when I swallow"

   d. "My body aches all over"

5. When teaching the patient taking an oral contraceptive for the first time, the health care provider emphasizes the importance of taking:

   a. two tablets per day at the first sign of ovulation

   b. the drug with the evening meal or at bedtime

   c. the drug early in the morning before arising

   d. the drug each day for 20 days beginning on the first of the month

24 Drugs Acting on the Uterus

KEY TERMS

ergotism—an overdose of ergonovine
oxytocic drugs—used before birth to induce uterine contractions similar to those of
    normal labor
oxytocin—an endogenous hormone produced by the posterior pituitary gland
uterine atony—marked relaxation of the uterine muscle
uterine relaxants—drugs used to manage preterm labor by decreasing uterine activity

CHAPTER OBJECTIVES

On completion of this chapter, students will be able to:

1 Define the chapter's key terms.

2 Describe the general drug actions, uses, adverse reactions, contraindications, precautions and interactions of drugs acting on the uterus.

3 Discuss important points to keep in mind when educating the patient or family members about the use of drugs acting on the uterus.

Drug therapy is often beneficial during labor and delivery to promote the well being of a mother and her fetus. Depending on a patient's need, drugs may be used to stimulate, intensify, or inhibit uterine contractions. The two types of drugs discussed in this chapter for their effect on the uterus are the oxytocics and the uterine re-

laxants. Specific drugs are listed in the Summary Drug Table: Drugs Acting on the Uterus.

Oxytocic Drugs

Oxytocic drugs are used before birth to induce uterine contractions similar to those of normal labor. These drugs are desirable when early vaginal delivery is in the best interest of a mother and her fetus.

An oxytocic drug is one that stimulates the uterus. Included in this group of drugs are ergonovine (Ergotrate), methylergonovine (Methergine), and oxytocin (Pitocin).

Actions of Ergonovine and Methylergonovine

Ergonovine and methylergonovine increase the strength, duration, and frequency of uterine contractions and decrease the incidence of uterine bleeding.

SUMMARY DRUG TABLE   Drugs Acting on the Uterus

Generic Name	Trade Name*	Uses	Adverse Reactions	Dosage Ranges
Oxytocics ergonovine maleate *er-goe-noe'-veen*	Ergotrate, *generic*	Uterine atony and hemorrhage	Nausea, vomiting, elevated blood pressure, temporary chest pain, dizziness, headache	0.2 mg IM, IV q2–4h
methylergonovine maleate *meth-ill-er-goe noe'-veen*	Methergine	Routine management after delivery of the placenta uterine atony and hemorrhage	Nausea, vomiting, elevated blood pressure, transient chest pain, dizziness headache	0.2 mg IM, IV after delivery of the placenta; 0.2 mg PO TID, QID
oxytocin (parenteral) *ox-i-toe'-sin*	Pitocin, Syntocinon, *generic*	Antepartum: to initiate or improve uterine contractions; postpartum: to produce uterine contractions in third stage of labor, control of postpartum bleeding and hemorrhage	Nausea, vomiting, uterine hypertonicity or rupture, fetal bradycardia, water intoxication, cardiac arrhythmias, anaphylactic	Induction of labor: 1–2 mU/min IV infusion, gradually increase dosage by 1–2 mU/min with maximum dosage 20 mU/min; postpartum bleeding: IV infusion of 10–40 U in 1000 mL; 10 U IM
Uterine Relaxants ritodrine hydrochloride *ri'-toe-dreen*	Yutopar, *generic*	Preterm labor	Alterations in fetal and maternal heart rates and maternal blood pressure, palpitations, headache, nausea, vomiting	IV: 0.05–0.35 mg/min depending on patient response
terbutaline *ter-byoo'-ta-leen*	Brethaire, Brethine, *generic*	Preterm labor	Nervousness, restlessness, tremor, headache, anxiety, hypertension, palpitations, arrhythmias, hypokalemia, pulmonary edema	Preterm labor: IV 10 mcg/min q10 min up to 80 mcg/min; SQ: 250 mcg qh until contractions stop; PO: 2.5 mg q4–6h until delivery

*The term *generic* indicates the drug is available in generic form.

Uses of Ergonovine and Methylergonovine

Ergonovine and methylergonovine are given after the delivery of the placenta and are used to prevent postpartum and postabortal hemorrhage caused by **uterine atony** (marked relaxation of the uterine muscle).

Adverse Reactions of Ergonovine and Methylergonovine

The adverse reactions of ergonovine and methylergonovine include nausea, vomiting, elevated blood pressure, temporary chest pain, dizziness, water intoxication (fluid overload or fluid volume excess), and headache. Allergic reactions may also occur. In some instances, hypertension associated with seizure or

headache may occur. **Ergotism** (overdosage of ergonovine) is manifested by nausea, vomiting, abdominal pain, numbness, tingling of the extremities, and an increased blood pressure. In severe cases, these symptoms are followed by hypotension, respiratory depression, hypothermia, gangrene of the fingers and toes, convulsions, hallucinations, and coma.

Managing Adverse Reactions of Ergonovine and Methylergonovine

When ergonovine or methylergonovine is administered for uterine atony and hemorrhage, abdominal cramping can occur and is usually an indication of drug effectiveness. The uterus can be palpated in the lower abdomen as small, firm, and round. Persistent or severe cramping should be reported to the health care provider.

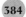

ALERT

Ergonovine and Calcium Deficiency

In some patients who are calcium-deficient, the uterus may not respond to ergonovine. The lack of response should immediately be reported to the health care provider. Administration of calcium by intravenous injection usually restores the drug response.

Although rare, ergotism or ergot poisoning can occur with the administration of excessive amounts of ergonovine or methylergonovine.

ALERT

Ergotism

Symptoms of ergotism that must be reported immediately include coolness, numbness, and tingling of the extremities, dyspnea, nausea, confusion, tachycardia or bradycardia, chest pain, hallucinations, and convulsions. If these reactions occur, then they must immediately be reported to the health care provider because use of the drug must be discontinued.

Contraindications, Precautions, and Interactions of Ergonovine and Methylergonovine

Ergonovine is contraindicated in those with a known hypersensitivity, patients with hypertension, and before the delivery of the placenta. Ergonovine is used cautiously in patients with heart disease, obliterative vascular disease, or liver or kidney disease, and in lactating women.

Methylergonovine is contraindicated in patients with a known hypersensitivity, hypertension, or preeclampsia. It should not be used to induce labor (pregnancy category C). Methylergonovine is used cautiously in patients with renal or hepatic impairment. When methylergonovine is administered concurrently with vasopressors or to patients who are heavy cigarette smokers, excessive vasoconstriction may occur.

Patient Management Issues with Ergonovine and Methylergonovine

When ergonovine and methylergonovine are administered after delivery, the patient's vital signs are monitored every 4 hours. The character and amount of vaginal bleeding are noted. The patient may report abdominal cramping with the use of these drugs. If cramping is moderately severe to severe, then the health care provider should be notified because it may be necessary to discontinue use of the drug.

Ergonovine is usually given during the third stage of labor after the placenta has been delivered. It is usually administered intramuscularly, but in emergencies when quicker response is needed, the drug may be administered intravenously.

Methylergonovine is usually given intramuscularly at the time of the delivery of the anterior shoulder or after the delivery of the placenta. The drug is not usually given intravenously because it may produce sudden hypertension and stroke. If the drug is given intravenously, then it is administered slowly over a period of 1 minute or more with close monitoring of the patient's blood pressure.

Actions of Oxytocin

Oxytocin is an endogenous hormone produced by the posterior pituitary gland (see Chapter 23). This hormone has uterine-stimulating properties, especially on a pregnant uterus. As pregnancy progresses, the sensitivity of the uterus to oxytocin increases, reaching a peak sensitivity immediately before the birth of the infant. This sensitivity enables oxytocic drugs to exert their full therapeutic effect on the uterus to produce the desired results. Oxytocin also has antidiuretic and vasopressor effects. The exact mechanism of oxytocin in normal labor and medically induced labor is not well understood.

Uses of Oxytocin

Oxytocin is administered intravenously for starting or improving labor contractions to obtain an early vaginal delivery of the fetus. An early vaginal delivery may be advisable when there are fetal or maternal problems; for example, a mother with diabetes and a large fetus, Rh blood-type problems, premature rupture of the membranes, uterine inertia, and eclampsia or preeclampsia. Oxytocin may also be used in the management of inevitable or incomplete abortion. Oxytocin is given intramuscularly during the third stage of labor (after the birth occurs and before the placenta is expelled) to produce uterine contractions and control postpartum bleeding and hemorrhage. It may also be used intranasally to stimulate the milk ejection (milk letdown) reflex.

Adverse Reactions of Oxytocin

Oxytocin may cause fetal bradycardia, uterine rupture, uterine hypertonicity (extreme tension of the uterine muscle), nausea, vomiting, cardiac arrhythmias, and anaphylactic reactions. Serious water intoxication may occur, particularly when the drug is administered by continuous infusion and a patient is receiving fluids by mouth. When used as a nasal spray, adverse reactions are rare.

Managing Adverse Reactions of Oxytocin

When oxytocin is administered, some adverse reactions must be tolerated or treated symptomatically until therapy is discontinued. For example, if the patient is nauseated, an emesis basin and perhaps a cool towel for the forehead are provided. If vomiting occurs, then the health care provider should be notified.

If contractions are frequent, prolonged, or excessive, then the infusion is stopped to prevent fetal anoxia or trauma to the uterus. Excessive stimulation of the uterus can cause uterine hypertonicity and possible uterine rupture. The patient is placed on her side and given supplemental oxygen. The effects of the drug diminish rapidly because oxytocin is short-acting.

When oxytocin is administered intravenously, there is a danger of a fluid volume excess (water intoxication), because oxytocin has an antidiuretic effect. Fluid intake and output are measured. In some instances, hourly measurements of the output are necessary. The patient is monitored for signs of fluid overload (see Chapter 32). If any of these signs or symptoms is noted, then the oxytocin infusion should be immediately discontinued.

Contraindications, Precautions, and Interactions of Oxytocin

Oxytocin is contraindicated in patients with known hypersensitivity, cephalopelvic disproportion (the fetal head is too large to travel through the mother's pelvis), an unfavorable fetal position or presentation, obstetric emergencies, fetal distress when delivery is not imminent, severe toxemia (preeclampsia, eclampsia), hypertonic uterus, or total placenta previa, or to induce labor when vaginal delivery is contraindicated. Oxytocin is not ordinarily a risk to the fetus when administered as indicated. When oxytocin is administered with a vasopressor, severe hypertension may occur.

Patient Management Issues with Oxytocin

The patient's blood pressure, pulse, and respiratory rate are measured every 5 to 10 minutes after the drug is administered. Excessive bleeding should be immediately reported to the health care provider.

ALERT

Oxytocin

All patients receiving intravenous oxytocin must be constantly observed to identify any complications. The health care provider should be immediately available at all times.

ALERT

Oxytocic Drugs and Hyperstimulation of the Uterus

Hyperstimulation of the uterus during labor may lead to uterine tetany (cramping) with marked impairment of the uteroplacental blood flow, uterine rupture, cervical rupture, amniotic fluid embolism, and trauma to the infant. Overstimulation of the uterus is dangerous to both the fetus and the mother and may occur in a uterus that is hypersensitive to oxytocin even when the drug is administered properly.

An electronic infusion device is used to control the infusion rate of oxytocin. The strength, frequency, and duration of contractions and the fetal heart rate are monitored closely.

When oxytocin is given intranasally to facilitate the letdown of milk, the patient is in an upright position, and the prescribed number of sprays is administered to one or both nostrils. The patient then waits a few minutes before breastfeeding the infant or pumping the breasts. If a breast pump is being used, then the amount of milk pumped from the breasts is recorded.

Educating the Patient and Family About Oxytocic Drugs

The treatment regimen is explained to the patient and family (when appropriate), and the patient is instructed to report any adverse reactions. If nasal spray is to be used, then the patient is taught its proper use.

Uterine Relaxants

Uterine relaxants are useful in the management of preterm labor. These drugs decrease uterine activity and prolong the pregnancy to allow the fetus to develop more fully, thereby promoting neonatal survival. Ritodrine (Yutopar) and terbutaline (Brethine) are two drugs currently used as uterine relaxants in the management of preterm (premature) labor.

Actions of Ritodrine

Ritodrine has an effect on β_2-adrenergic receptors, principally those that innervate the uterus. Stimulation of these β_2-adrenergic receptors inhibits uterine smooth muscle contractions. β_1-adrenergic receptors are located in the heart and are not stimulated by ritodrine when administered correctly.

Uses of Ritodrine

Ritodrine is used to manage preterm labor in pregnancies of greater than 20 weeks' gestation. Ritodrine administration requires hospitalization.

Adverse Reactions of Ritodrine

Alterations in fetal and maternal heart rates and maternal blood pressure frequently occur when ritodrine is administered intravenously. Additional frequent adverse reactions associated with intravenous administration include nausea, vomiting, headache, palpitations, nervousness, restlessness, and emotional upset. A rare but serious adverse reaction is pulmonary edema.

Contraindications, Precautions, and Interactions of Ritodrine

Ritodrine is contraindicated in patients with a known hypersensitivity and patients with antepartum hemorrhage, eclampsia or severe preeclampsia, cardiac disease, pulmonary hypertension, uncontrolled diabetes mellitus, or bronchial asthma (patients treated with betamimetics or steroids), and in pregnancies of less than 20 weeks' gestation or after intrauterine fetal death. Ritodrine is classified as a pregnancy category B drug and is given cautiously during pregnancy. Ritodrine is administered cautiously in patients with cardiac disease, migraine headaches, history of stroke, hyperthyroidism, or seizure disorders.

Ritodrine has decreased effectiveness when administered with a β-adrenergic blocking agent such as propranolol and an increased risk of pulmonary edema when administered with a corticosteroid. Co-administration of ritodrine with the sympathomimetics increases the effect of ritodrine. Cardiovascular effects (e.g., arrhythmias or hypotension) of ritodrine may increase when the drug is administered with diazoxide, general anesthetics, magnesium sulfate, or meperidine.

Actions of Terbutaline

Terbutaline (Brethine) is also classified as a β$_2$-adrenergic agonist (see Chapter 4). It decreases uterine activity and prolongs the pregnancy to allow the fetus to develop more fully, thereby promoting neonatal survival.

Uses of Terbutaline

Terbutaline is used primarily as a bronchodilator for patients with asthma and chronic obstructive pulmonary disease. The Food and Drug Administration has not approved terbutaline for treatment of preterm labor. Its use in the management of premature labor is investigational. However, many health care providers prefer terbutaline for the management of preterm labor, and it has proven to be highly effective for this purpose.

Adverse Reactions of Terbutaline

Adverse reactions of terbutaline include nervousness, restlessness, tremor, headache, anxiety, hypertension, hypokalemia (low serum potassium), arrhythmias, and palpitations. A serious but rare adverse reaction is pulmonary edema.

Contraindications, Precautions, and Interactions of Terbutaline

Terbutaline is contraindicated in patients with a known hypersensitivity, severe cardiac problems (tachyarrhythmias), digitalis toxicity, or hypertension. Terbutaline is classified as a pregnancy category B drug and is given

cautiously only after the 20th week of pregnancy. Terbutaline is administered cautiously in patients with cardiac disease, history of stroke, hyperthyroidism, or seizure disorders. When terbutaline is administered with the anesthetic halothane, there is an increased risk of cardiac arrhythmias. Additional information about terbutaline can be found in Chapter 12.

Patient Management Issues with Uterine Relaxants

Patient management with ritodrine and terbutaline is similar. An infusion pump is used to control the rate of flow. Terbutaline may be administered by the oral or subcutaneous route rather than via the intravenous route. A cardiac monitor is placed on the patient. To minimize hypotension, the patient is placed in a left lateral position unless the health care provider orders a different position.

The health care provider is kept informed of the patient's response to the drug because a dosage change may be necessary. The health care provider establishes guidelines for the regulation of the intravenous infusion rate, as well as determining the blood pressure and pulse ranges that require stopping the intravenous infusion.

Managing Adverse Reactions of Uterine Relaxants

Maternal and fetal vital signs are monitored every 15 minutes during administration of the drug. Uterine contractions are frequently monitored throughout the infusion.

ALERT

 Uterine Relaxants and Increased Pulse and Respiratory Rates

The health care provider should be notified of a pulse rate of 140 beats per minute, a persistently elevated pulse rate or irregular pulse, or an increase in respiratory rate of more than 20 breaths per minute. The patient is assessed for symptoms of pulmonary edema (e.g., dyspnea, tachycardia, increased respiratory rate, rales, and frothy sputum). These reactions could indicate pulmonary edema. The health care provider may decrease the dosage or discontinue the drug. The health care provider must be notified immediately if any of these symptoms occurs because use of the drug may be discontinued. After contractions cease, the dosage is tapered to the lowest effective dose by decreasing the infusion rate at regular intervals. The intravenous infusion is continued for at least 12 hours after uterine contractions have ceased. Because the duration of treatment is short, mild adverse reactions must be tolerated. If adverse reactions are severe, then the drug is discontinued or the dosage decreased.

Educating the Patient and Family About Uterine Relaxants

The health care provider usually discusses the expected outcome of treatment with the patient and answers any questions regarding therapy. Although the patient is monitored closely during therapy, the patient is instructed to notify the health care provider immediately if she experiences any of the following: nausea, vomiting, palpitations, or shortness of breath.

If oral terbutaline is prescribed for preterm labor, then the patient is instructed about the drug and the adverse reactions to report (excessive tremor, nervousness, drowsiness, headache, nausea, or dizziness). If contractions resume during oral therapy, then the patient is instructed to notify the health care provider if four to six contractions occur per hour.

KEY POINTS

○ Oxytocic drugs are used to induce uterine contractions similar to those of normal labor when early vaginal delivery is in the best interest of a mother and her fetus. Ergonovine and methylergonovine both increase the strength, duration, and frequency of uterine contractions and decrease the incidence of uterine bleeding. Adverse reactions include nausea, vomiting, elevated blood pressure, temporary chest pain, dizziness, water intoxication, and headache.

○ Oxytocin, an endogenous hormone produced by the posterior pituitary gland, has uterine-stimulating properties, especially on a pregnant uterus. Oxytocin is administered intravenously for starting or improving labor contractions to obtain an early vaginal delivery of the fetus. Oxytocin may cause fetal bradycardia, uterine rupture, uterine hypertonicity, nausea, vomiting, cardiac arrhythmias, anaphylactic reactions, and serious water intoxication. When oxytocin is administered, some adverse reactions must be tolerated or treated symptomatically until therapy is discontinued. When oxytocin is administered intravenously, there is a danger of a fluid volume excess (water intoxication). If contractions are frequent, prolonged, or excessive, the infusion is stopped to prevent fetal anoxia or trauma to the uterus.

○ Uterine relaxants are useful in the management of preterm labor. These drugs decrease uterine activity and prolong the pregnancy to allow the fetus to develop more fully. Ritodrine has an effect on β$_2$-adrenergic receptors, principally those that innervate the uterus, and may cause alterations in fetal and maternal heart rates and maternal blood pressure. Terbutaline is used primarily as a bronchodilator for patients with asthma and chronic obstructive pulmonary disease. Terbutaline is contraindicated in patients with a known hypersensitivity, severe cardiac problems (tachyarrhythmias), digitalis toxicity, or hypertension. It is classified as a pregnancy category B drug and is given cautiously only after the 20th week of pregnancy only, and is administered cautiously in patients with cardiac disease, history of stroke, hyperthyroidism, or seizure disorders.

CASE STUDY

Judith Watson, 28 years old, is admitted to the obstetric unit and is to receive oxytocin to induce labor. This is her first child, and she is extremely anxious.

1. What information should Ms. Watson's health care provider share with her?
   a. oxytocin is administered intravenously to start or improve labor contractions
   b. oxytocin is administered intramuscularly to speed up labor contractions
   c. oxytocin is administered to slow contractions
   d. it is not advisable to share any information with Ms. Watson regarding oxytocin

2. What patient management issues arise with oxytocin?
   a. patients receiving intravenous oxytocin must be under constant observation to watch for complications
   b. to minimize hypotension, the patient is placed in a left lateral position unless the health care provider orders a different position
   c. overstimulation of the uterus is healthy for both the fetus and the mother
   d. all of the above

3. Ms. Watson feels mild nausea as a result of the oxytocin. How should the health care provider respond?
   a. the drug should be immediately discontinued
   b. the dosage of oxytocin should be doubled
   c. ritodrine should be used instead of oxytocin
   d. reassure her that this is normal and that it will pass soon after the drug wears off

WEBSITE ACTIVITIES

1. Go to the Mayo Clinic website (www.mayoclinic.com) and click to do a drug search. Then search for ritodrine. Make a list of the most common and more common adverse reactions of this drug.

2. What additional adverse reactions are rare?

REVIEW QUESTIONS

1. When oxytocin is administered over a prolonged time, which of the following adverse reactions is most likely to occur?
   a. hyperglycemia
   b. renal impairment
   c. increased intracranial pressure
   d. water intoxication

2. Ritodrine is used:
   a. to manage preterm labor in pregnancies of more than 20 weeks' gestation
   b. to manage preterm labor in pregnancies of less than 20 weeks' gestation
   c. primarily as a bronchodilator
   d. primarily to treat obstructive pulmonary disease

3. Which of the following adverse reactions is most indicative of ergotism?
   a. numbness, tingling of the extremities
   b. headache, blurred vision
   c. tachycardia and cardiac arrhythmia
   d. diaphoresis, increased respiration

4. During administration of ritodrine, in what position would the patient most probably be placed?
   a. supine
   b. prone
   c. on the left side
   d. on the right side

25 Antibacterial Drugs

Sulfonamides
Actions of Sulfonamides
Uses of Sulfonamides
Adverse Reactions of Sulfonamides
> Managing Adverse Reactions of Sulfonamides

Contraindications, Precautions, and Interactions of
Sulfonamides
Patient Management Issues with Sulfonamides
> Managing Burns
> Maintaining Adequate Fluid Intake and Output

Educating the Patient and Family About Sulfonamides

Natural Remedies: Cranberry

Penicillins
Drug Resistance
Actions of Penicillins
> Identifying the Appropriate Penicillin

Uses of Penicillins
> Infectious Disease
> Prophylaxis

Adverse Reactions of Penicillins
> Hypersensitivity Reactions
> Superinfections
>> Candidiasis or Moniliasis

> Managing Adverse Reactions of Penicillins
>> Diarrhea
>> Impaired Skin Integrity
>> Impaired Oral Mucous Membranes
>> Fever

Contraindications, Precautions, and Interactions of
Penicillins
Patient Management Issues with Penicillins
Educating the Patient and Family About Penicillins

Natural Remedies: Goldenseal

Cephalosporins
Actions of Cephalosporins
Uses of Cephalosporins
Adverse Reactions of Cephalosporins
> Managing Adverse Reactions of Cephalosporins
>> Fever
>> Diarrhea
>> Impaired Skin Integrity

Contraindications, Precautions, and Interactions of
Cephalosporins
Patient Management Issues with Cephalosporins
> Oral Use of Cephalosporins

Educating the Patient and Family About Cephalosporins

Tetracyclines, Macrolides, and Lincosamides
Actions of Tetracyclines
Uses of Tetracyclines
Adverse Reactions of Tetracyclines
Contraindications, Precautions, and Interactions of
Tetracyclines
Actions of Macrolides
Uses of Macrolides
Adverse Reactions of Macrolides
Contraindications, Precautions, and Interactions of
Macrolides
Actions of Lincosamides
Uses of Lincosamides
Adverse Reactions of Lincosamides
Contraindications, Precautions, and Interactions of
Lincosamides
Patient Management Issues with Tetracyclines,
Macrolides, and Lincosamides
> Oral Use
>> Tetracyclines
>> Macrolides
>> Lincosamides

> Managing Adverse Drug Reactions of Tetracyclines,
Macrolides, and Lincosamides
>> Hyperthermia
>> Diarrhea

Educating the Patient and Family About Tetracyclines,
Macrolides, and Lincosamides

Fluoroquinolones and Aminoglycosides
Actions of Fluoroquinolones
Uses of Fluoroquinolones
Adverse Reactions of Fluoroquinolones
> Managing Adverse Drug Reactions of Fluoro-
quinolones

Contraindications, Precautions, and Interactions of
Fluoroquinolones
Actions of Aminoglycosides
Uses of Aminoglycosides
Adverse Reactions of Aminoglycosides
> Managing Adverse Drug Reactions of Aminoglyco-
sides
>> Neurotoxicity
>> Nephrotoxicity
>> Ototoxicity

Contraindications, Precautions, and Interactions of
Aminoglycosides
Patient Management Issues with Fluoroquinolones and
Aminoglycosides
> Fluoroquinolones

KEY TERMS

anaerobic—able to live without oxygen

anaphylactoid reaction—unusual or exaggerated allergic reaction

anaphylactic shock—a severe form of hypersensitivity reaction

antibacterial—active against bacteria

anti-infective—another word for antibacterial; drugs used to treat infections and bacteria

antitubercular drugs—drugs used to treat active cases of tuberculosis

bacterial resistance—ability of bacteria to produce substances that inactivate or destroy impact of a drug

bactericidal—an agent or drug that destroys bacteria

bacteriostatic—drugs that slow or retard the multiplication of bacteria

bowel prep—the use of drugs preoperatively to reduce the number of bacteria normally present in the intestine

cross-allergenicity—allergy to drugs in the same or related group

cross-sensitivity—synonymous with cross-allergenicity

culture and sensitivity tests—culturing performed to grow bacteria along with tests of their sensitivity to specific drugs

hypersensitivity—allergic

leprosy—a chronic, communicable disease spread by prolonged intimate contact with an infected person

Mycobacterium leprae—the bacteria that cause leprosy

Mycobacterium tuberculosis—the bacteria that cause tuberculosis

nonpathogenic—not disease causing

normal flora— nonpathogenic microorganisms within or on the body

penicillinase—an enzyme that inactivates penicillin

prophylaxis—prevention

pseudomembranous colitis—a common bacterial superinfection

Stevens-Johnson syndrome—serious allergic reaction to a drug, which initially exhibits reactions easily confused with less severe disorders

superinfection—an overgrowth of bacterial or fungal microorganisms not affected by the antibiotic being used for treatment

tuberculosis—a disease caused by *Mycobacterium tuberculosis*

CHAPTER OBJECTIVES

On completion of this chapter, students will be able to:

1 Define the chapter's key terms.

2 Describe the general drug actions, uses, adverse reactions, contraindications, precautions and interactions of antibacterial drugs.

3 Discuss important points to keep in mind when educating the patient or family members about the use of antibacterial drugs.

This chapter provides information on the sulfonamides, penicillins, cephalosporins, tetracyclines, macrolides, lincosamides, fluoroquinolones, aminoglycosides, antitubercular drugs, leprostatic drugs, and miscellaneous anti-infectives, all used for bacterial infections.

Sulfonamides

The sulfonamides (sulfa) drugs were the first antibiotic drugs developed that effectively treated infections. Although the use of sulfonamides has declined after the introduction of more effective anti-infectives, such as the penicillins and other antibiotics, these drugs still remain important for the treatment of certain types of infections.

Sulfonamides are **antibacterial** agents, meaning they are active against bacteria. Another term that may be used to describe the general action of these drugs is **anti-infective** because they are used to treat infections caused by certain bacteria. Sulfadiazine, sulfisoxazole, and sulfamethizole are examples of sulfonamide preparations.

Actions of Sulfonamides

Sulfonamides are primarily **bacteriostatic**, which means they slow or retard the multiplication of bacteria. This bacteriostatic activity is caused by sulfonamide antagonism to para-aminobenzoic acid, a substance that some, but not all, bacteria need to multiply. Once the rate of bacterial multiplication is slowed, the body's own defense mechanisms (white blood cells) are able to rid the body of the invading microorganisms and therefore control the infection.

SUMMARY DRUG TABLE   The Sulfonamides

Generic Name	Trade Name*	Uses	Adverse Reactions	Dosage Ranges
Single Agents				
sulfadiazine *sul-fa-dye´-a-zeen*	*generic*	Urinary tract infections caused by susceptible microorganisms, chancroid, acute otitis media, *Haemophilus influenzae* and meningococcal meningitis, rheumatic fever	Hematologic changes, Stevens-Johnson syndrome, nausea, vomiting, headache, diarrhea, chills, fever, anorexia, crystalluria, stomatitis, urticaria, pruritus	Loading dose: 2–4 g PO; maintenance dose: 2–4 g/d PO in 4–6 divided doses
sulfamethizole *sul-fa-meth´-i-zole*	Thiosulfil Forte	Urinary tract infections caused by susceptible microorganisms	Same as sulfadiazine	0.5–1 g PO tid, qid
sulfamethoxazole *sul-fa-meth-ox´-a-zole*	Gantanol, Urobak, *generic*	Urinary tract infections caused by susceptible microorganisms, meningococcal meningitis, acute otitis media	Same as sulfadiazine	Initial dose: 2 g PO; maintenance dose: 1 g PO bid, tid
sulfasalazine *sul-fa-sal´-a-zeen*	Azulfidine, Azulfidine EN-tabs, *generic*	Ulcerative colitis, rheumatoid arthritis	Same as sulfadiazine; may cause skin and urine to turn orange–yellow	Initial therapy: 1–4 g/d PO in divided doses; maintenance dose: 2 g/d in evenly spaced doses 500 mg qid
sulfisoxazole *sul-fi-sox´-a-zole*	*generic*	Same as sulfadiazine	Same as sulfadiazine	Loading dose: 2–4 g PO; maintenance dose: 4–8 g/d PO in 4–6 divided doses
Multiple Preparations				
trimethoprim (TMP) and sulfamethoxazole (SMZ) *trye-meth´-oh-prim; sul-fa-meth-ox´-a-zole*	Bactrim, Bactrim DS, Septra, Septra DS, *generic*	Urinary tract infections caused by susceptible microorganisms, acute otitis media, traveler's diarrhea caused by *Escherichia coli*	Gastrointestinal disturbances, allergic skin reactions, hematologic changes, Stevens-Johnson syndrome, headache	160 mg TMP/800 mg SMZ PO q12h; 8–10 mg/kg/d (based on TMP) IV in 2–4 divided doses
Miscellaneous Sulfonamide Preparations				
mafenide *Meph´-a-nide*	Sulfamylon	Second- and third-degree burns	Pain or burning sensation, rash, itching, facial edema	Apply to burned area 1–2 times/d
silver sulfadiazine *sil´-ver sul-fa-dye´-a-zeen*	Silvadene, Thermazene, SSD (cream)	Same as mafenide	Leukopenia, skin necrosis, skin discoloration, burning sensation	Same as mafenide

Uses of Sulfonamides

Sulfonamides are often used to control urinary tract infections caused by certain bacteria such as *Escherichia coli*, *Staphylococcus aureus*, and *Klebsiella enterobacter*. Mafenide (Sulfamylon) and silver sulfadiazine (Silvadene) are topical sulfonamides also used in the treatment of second- and third-degree burns. Additional uses of the sulfonamides are given in the Summary Drug Table: The Sulfonamides.

Adverse Reactions of Sulfonamides

Sulfonamides can cause a variety of adverse reactions. Some of these are serious or potentially serious; others are mild. The following hematologic changes may occur during sulfonamide therapy:

- agranulocytosis: decrease in or lack of granulocytes, a type of white blood cell
- thrombocytopenia: decrease in the number of platelets
- aplastic anemia: anemia caused by deficient red blood cell production in the bone marrow
- leukopenia: decrease in the number of white blood cells

These are examples of serious adverse reactions. If any of these occurs, then discontinuation of sulfonamide therapy may be required.

Anorexia (loss of appetite) is an example of a mild adverse reaction. Unless it becomes severe and pronounced weight loss occurs, it may not be necessary to discontinue sulfonamide therapy.

Various types of **hypersensitivity** (allergic) reactions may occur during sulfonamide therapy, including Stevens-Johnson syndrome, urticaria (hives), pruritus (itching), and generalized skin eruptions. **Stevens-Johnson** syndrome is manifested by fever, cough, muscular aches and pains, and headache, all of which are signs and symptoms of many other disorders. However, the appearance of lesions on the skin, mucous membranes, eyes, and other organs are diagnostically significant and may be the first conclusive signs of this syndrome. Any of these symptoms must be reported to the health care provider immediately.

Other adverse reactions that may occur during therapy include nausea, vomiting, diarrhea, abdominal pain, chills, fever, and stomatitis (inflammation of the mouth). In some instances, these may be mild. Other times they may cause serious problems requiring discontinuation of the drug. Sulfasalazine may cause the urine and skin to be an orange–yellow color; this is not abnormal.

Crystalluria (crystals in the urine) may occur during use of a sulfonamide, although this problem occurs less frequently with some of the newer sulfonamide preparations. Increasing fluid intake during sulfonamide therapy can often prevent this potentially serious problem.

The most frequent adverse reaction seen with the application of mafenide is a burning sensation or pain when the drug is applied to the skin. Other possible allergic reactions include rash, itching, edema, and urticaria. Burning, rash, and itching may also occur with silver sulfadiazine. It may be difficult to distinguish between an adverse reaction caused by the use of mafenide or silver sulfadiazine and reactions that may occur from the severe burn injury or from other agents used at the same time for the management of the burns.

Managing Adverse Reactions of Sulfonamides

The patient is observed for adverse reactions, especially an allergic reaction (see Chapter 1). If one or more adverse reactions should occur, then the next dose of the drug is withheld and the health care provider should be notified.

The patient is monitored for leukopenia and thrombocytopenia. Leukopenia may result in signs and symptoms of an infection, such as fever, sore throat, and cough. A patient with leukopenia should be protected from individuals who have an infection. With severe leukopenia, the patient may be placed in protective (reverse) isolation. Thrombocytopenia is manifested by easy bruising and unusual bleeding after moderate to slight trauma to the skin or mucous membranes. The extremities of a patient with thrombocytopenia must be handled with care to prevent bruising. Care is taken to prevent trauma when an immobile patient is moved. Skin is inspected daily for the extent of bruising and evidence of exacerbation of existing ecchymotic areas. The patient should be encouraged to use a soft-bristled toothbrush to prevent any trauma to the mucous membranes of the oral cavity. Any signs of leukopenia or thrombocytopenia should be reported immediately because this is an indication to stop drug therapy.

ALERT

Stevens–Johnson Syndrome

Stevens–Johnson syndrome is a serious and sometimes fatal hypersensitivity reaction. Lesions on the skin and mucous membranes are a diagnostically important symptom of this syndrome. The lesions appear as red wheals or blisters, often starting on the face, in the mouth, or on the lips, neck, and extremities. This syndrome, which also may occur with the use of other types of drugs, can be fatal. The health care provider must be alerted and the next dose of the drug withheld. In addition, care must be exercised to prevent injury to the involved areas.

Contraindications, Precautions, and Interactions of Sulfonamides

Sulfonamides are contraindicated in patients with known hypersensitivity, during lactation, and in children younger than 2 years old. Sulfonamides are not used near the end (at term) of pregnancy (pregnancy category D). If a sulfonamide is given near the end of pregnancy, then significant blood levels of the drug may occur, causing jaundice or hemolytic anemia in the neonate. Additionally, sulfonamides are not used for infections caused by group A beta-hemolytic streptococci because the sulfonamides have not been shown to be effective in preventing the complications of rheumatic fever or glomerulonephritis.

Sulfonamides are used with caution in patients with kidney or liver impairment or bronchial asthma. These drugs are given with caution to patients with allergies. Safety for use during pregnancy has not been established (pregnancy category C, except at term).

When a sulfonamide is taken with an oral anticoagulant, the action of the anticoagulant may be enhanced. The risk of bone marrow suppression may be increased when a sulfonamide is administered with methotrexate. When a sulfonamide is administered with a hydantoin, the serum hydantoin level may be increased.

Sulfonamides may inhibit the (hepatic) metabolism of the oral hypoglycemic drugs tolbutamide (Orinase) and chlorpropamide (Diabinese). This would increase the possibility of a hypoglycemic reaction.

Patient Management Issues with Sulfonamides

Temperature, pulse, respiratory rate, and blood pressure should be assessed every 4 hours or as ordered by the health care provider. If fever is present and the patient's temperature suddenly increases or if the temperature was normal and suddenly increases, then the health care provider should be contacted immediately.

Patients receiving sulfasalazine for ulcerative colitis should be observed for evidence of the relief or intensification of the symptoms of the disease.

When a sulfonamide is used for a burn, the burned areas are inspected every 1 to 2 hours because some treatment regimens require keeping the affected areas covered with the mafenide or silver sulfadiazine ointment at all times. Any adverse reactions should be reported immediately to the health care provider.

A patient receiving a sulfonamide drug almost always has an active infection. Some patients may be receiving one of these drugs to prevent an infection (prophylaxis) or as part of the management of a disease such as ulcerative colitis.

Unless the health care provider orders otherwise, sulfonamides are given to the patient when the stomach is empty, usually 1 hour before or 2 hours after meals. If gastrointestinal irritation occurs, then sulfasalazine may be given with food or immediately after meals. The patient should be instructed to drink a full glass of water when taking an oral sulfonamide and to drink at least eight large glasses of water each day until therapy is finished.

Managing Burns

When mafenide or silver sulfadiazine is used in the treatment of burns, the treatment regimen is outlined by the health care provider or the personnel in the burn treatment unit. There are various burn treatment regimens, such as debridement (removal of burned or dead tissue from the burned site), special dressings, and cleansing of the burned area. The use of a specific treatment regimen often depends on the extent of the burned area, the degree of the burns, and the physical condition and age of the patient. Other concurrent problems, such as lung damage caused by smoke or heat or physical injuries that occurred at the time of the burn injury, also may influence the treatment regimen.

The surface of the skin is cleaned and debris removed before each application of mafenide or silver sulfadiazine is applied with a sterile gloved hand. The drug is applied approximately one-sixteenth of an inch thick; thicker application is not recommended. The patient is kept away from any draft of air because even the slightest movement of air across the burned area can cause pain. The patient should be warned that stinging or burning might be felt during, and for a short time after, application of mafenide. Some burning also may be noted with the application of silver sulfadiazine.

Maintaining Adequate Fluid Intake and Output

Because one adverse reaction of the sulfonamide drugs is altered elimination patterns, the patient needs to maintain adequate fluid intake and output. Patients should be encouraged to increase fluid intake to 2000 mL or more per day to prevent crystalluria and stone formation in the genitourinary tract, as well as to aid in the removal of microorganisms from the urinary tract. The health care provider should be notified if the patient's urinary output decreases or the patient fails to increase his or her oral intake.

ALERT

Older Adults and Sulfonamides

Because kidney impairment is common in older adults, sulfonamides should be given with great caution. There is an increased danger of sulfonamides causing additional renal damage when renal impairment is already present. An increase of fluid intake up to 2000 mL (if the older adult can tolerate this amount) decreases the risk of crystals and stones forming in the urinary tract.

Educating the Patient and Family About Sulfonamides

When a sulfonamide is prescribed for an infection, some outpatients have a tendency to discontinue the drug once their symptoms have been relieved. The importance of completing the prescribed course of therapy to be sure all microorganisms causing the infection are eradicated is emphasized. Failure to complete a course

Health care providers have recommended the use of cranberry juice in combination with antibiotics for the long-term suppression of urinary tract infections. Cranberries are thought to act by preventing the bacteria from attaching to the walls of the urinary tract. The suggested amount is 6 ounces of the juice twice times daily. Extremely large doses can produce gastrointestinal disturbances such as diarrhea or abdominal cramping. Although cranberries may relieve symptoms or prevent the occurrence of a urinary tract infection, use will not cure a urinary tract infection. If a patient suspects a urinary tract infection, then medical attention is necessary.

Penicillins

The development of the sulfonamide antibiotics was a breakthrough in the treatment of bacterial infections. Since that time, there has been a quest to develop new and more effective antibiotic drugs. Sir Arthur Fleming discovered the antibacterial properties of natural penicillins in 1928 while he was performing research on influenza. Ten years later, British scientists studied the effects of natural penicillins on disease-causing microorganisms. After 1941, natural penicillins were used clinically for the treatment of infections. Although used for more than 50 years, the penicillins are still an important and effective group of antibiotics for the treatment of susceptible pathogens (disease-causing microorganisms).

There are four groups of penicillins: natural penicillins, penicillinase-resistant penicillins, aminopenicillins, and the extended-spectrum penicillins. See the Summary Drug Table: Penicillins for a more complete listing of the penicillins. Following are examples of the various groups.

- Natural penicillins: penicillin G and penicillin
- Penicillinase-resistant penicillin: cloxacillin, dicloxacillin, nafcillin
- Aminopenicillins: ampicillin, amoxicillin, bacampicillin
- Extended-spectrum penicillins: mezlocillin, piperacillin, ticarcillin

Drug Resistance

Because natural penicillins have been used for many years, drug-resistant strains of microorganisms have developed, making the natural penicillins less effective than some of the newer antibiotics for treating a broad range of infections. **Bacterial resistance** is the ability of bacteria to produce substances that inactivate or destroy penicillin. One example of bacterial resistance is the ability of certain bacteria to produce **penicillinase**, an enzyme that inactivates penicillin. Penicillinase-resistant penicillins were developed to combat this problem.

Key Points for Patients Taking Sulfonamides

❑ Take the drug as prescribed by your health care provider.

❑ Take the drug on an empty stomach either 1 hour before or 2 hours after a meal (exception: sulfasalazine is taken with food or immediately after a meal).

❑ Take the drug with a full glass of water. Do not increase or decrease the time between doses except as directed by your health care provider.

❑ Complete the full course of therapy. Do not discontinue this drug even though the symptoms of the infection have disappeared (unless advised to do so by your health care provider).

❑ Drink at least 8 to 10 8-oz glasses of fluid every day.

❑ Prolonged exposure to sunlight may result in skin reactions similar to a severe sunburn (photosensitivity reactions). When going outside, cover exposed areas of your skin or apply a protective sunscreen to exposed areas.

❑ Notify your health care provider immediately if you experience any of the following: fever, skin rash or other skin problems, nausea, vomiting, unusual bleeding or bruising, sore throat, or extreme fatigue.

❑ Keep all follow-up appointments to ensure your infection is controlled.

❑ When taking sulfasalazine, your skin or urine may turn an orange–yellow color; this is not abnormal. If you wear soft contact lenses, then a permanent yellow stain of the lenses may occur, so ask your eye doctor about wearing corrective lenses while taking this drug.

of therapy may result in a recurrence of the infection. Patient Education Box 25-1 includes key points about sulfonamides the patient and family members should know.

Natural Remedies: Cranberry

Cranberry, an herb, is commonly used preventively and as a treatment for the relief of symptoms of urinary tract infections. In the United States, cranberry is classified by the Food and Drug Administration (FDA) as a dietary supplement rather than a drug and is in the top 10 of best-selling herbal products. It is commercially available over the counter in the form of juice, tea, and capsules.

Urinary tract infections are a common form of infection, second only to respiratory infection in number of occurrences each year. Cranberry is believed to prevent bacteria from adhering to the walls of the urinary tract.

SUMMARY DRUG TABLE   Penicillins

Generic Name	Trade Name*	Uses	Adverse Reactions	Dosage Ranges
Natural Penicillins penicillin G (aqueous) *pen-i-sill'-in*	Pfizerpen, *generic*	Infections caused by susceptible microorganisms; syphilis, gonorrhea	Glossitis, stomatitis, gastritis, furry tongue, nausea, vomiting, diarrhea, rash, fever, pain at injection site, hypersensitivity reactions, hematopoietic changes	Up to 20–30 million U/d IV or IM; dosage may also be based on weight
penicillin G benzathine	Bicillin L-A, Permapen, *generic*	Infections caused by susceptible microorganisms, syphilis; prophylaxis of rheumatic fever or chorea	Same as penicillin G	Up to 2.4 million U/d IM
penicillin G procaine, IM	Wycillin	Infections caused by susceptible organisms	Same as penicillin G	600,000–2.4 million U/d IM
penicillin V	Beepen VK, Pen-Vee K, Veetids, *generic*	Infections caused by susceptible organisms	Same as penicillin G	125–500 mg PO q6h or q8h
Semisynthetic Penicillins **Penicillinase-Resistant Penicillins** cloxacillin sodium *klox-a-sill'-in*	Cloxapen, Tegopen, *generic*	Same as penicillin G	Same as penicillin G	250–500 mg PO q6h
dicloxacillin sodium *dye-klox-a-sill'-in*	Dynapen, Dycill, Pathocil, *generic*	Same as penicillin G	Same as penicillin G	125–250 mg PO q6h
nafcillin *naf-sill'-in*	Unipen, Nallpen	Same as penicillin G	Same as penicillin G	250 mg–1 g PO, 500 mg IM q4–6h; 3–6 g/d IV for 24–48 h only
oxacillin sodium *Ox-a-sill'-in*	Bactocill, *generic*	Same as penicillin G	Same as penicillin G	500 mg–1 g PO q4–6h; 250 mg–1 g q4–6h IM, IV
Aminopenicillins amoxicillin *a-mox-i-sill'-in*	Amoxil, Trimox, Wymox, *generic*	Same as penicillin G	Same as penicillin G	250–500 mg PO q8h or 875 mg PO BID
amoxicillin and clavulanate acid *a-mox-i-sill'-in/ klah-view-lan'-ate*	Augmentin	Same as penicillin G	Same as penicillin G	250–500 mg PO q8h or 875 mg q12h**
ampicillin, oral *am-pi-sill'-in*	Omnipen, Principen, Totacillin, *generic*	Same as penicillin G	Same as penicillin G	250–500 mg PO q6h
ampicillin sodium parenteral	Omnipen-N, *generic*	Same as penicillin G	Same as penicillin G	1–12 g/d IM, IV in divided doses q4–6h

Generic Name	Trade Name*	Uses	Adverse Reactions	Dosage Ranges
ampicillin/sulbactam *am-pi-sill'-in/ sull-bak'-tam*	Unasyn	Same as penicillin G	Same as penicillin G	0.5–1 g sulbactam with 1–2 g ampicillin IM or IV q6–8h
bacampicillin *bak'-am-pi-sill-in*	Spectrobid	Same as penicillin G	Same as penicillin G	400–800 mg PO q12h, may also be given based on weight
Extended-Spectrum Penicillins				
mezlocillin sodium *mez-loe-sill'-in*	Mezlin	Same as penicillin G	Same as penicillin G	200–300 mg/kg/d IV or IM in 4–6 divided doses; up to 350 mg/kg/d
piperacillin sodium and tazobactam sodium *pi-per-a-sill'-in/ tay-zoe-back'-tam*	Zosyn	Same as penicillin G	Same as penicillin G	12 mg/1.5 g IV given as 3.375 g q6h
piperacillin sodium *pi-per-a-sill'-in*	Pipracil	Same as penicillin G	Same as penicillin G	3–4 g q4–6h IV or IM; maximum dosage, 25 g/d
ticarcillin disodium *ty-kar-sill'-in*	Ticar	Same as penicillin G	Same as penicillin G	150–300 mg/kg/d IV q3, 4, or 6h; maximum dosage, 24 g/d; maximum dosage IM, 2 g/d
ticarcillin and clavulanate potassium *ty-kar-sill'-in*	Timentin	Same as penicillin G	Same as penicillin G	3.1 g IV q4–6h or 200–300 mg/kg/d IV in divided doses q4–6h

Natural penicillins also have a fairly narrow spectrum of activity, which means that they are effective against only a few strains of bacteria. Newer penicillins have been developed to combat this problem. These penicillins are a result of chemical treatment of a biologic precursor to penicillin. Because of their chemical modifications, they are more slowly excreted by the kidneys and, thus, have a somewhat wider spectrum of antibacterial activity. Penicillin β-lactamase inhibitor combinations are a type of penicillin that has a wider spectrum of antibacterial activity. Certain bacteria have developed the ability to produce enzymes called β-lactamases, which can destroy a component of the penicillin called the β-lactam ring. Fortunately, chemicals were discovered that inhibit the activity of these enzymes. Three examples of these β-lactamase inhibitors are clavulanic acid, sulbactam, and tazobactam. When these chemicals are used alone, they have little antimicrobial activity. However, when combined with certain penicillins, they extend the spectrum of penicillin's antibacterial activity. The β-lactamase inhibitors bind with penicillin and protect penicillin from destruction. See the Summary Drug Table: Penicillins for more information on these combinations.

Actions of Penicillins

Penicillins have the same type of action against bacteria. Penicillins prevent bacteria from using a substance that is necessary for the maintenance of the bacteria's outer cell wall. Unable to use this substance for cell wall maintenance, the bacteria swell, rupture, assume unusual shapes, and finally die (Fig. 25-1).

Penicillins may be bactericidal (destroy bacteria) or bacteriostatic (slow or retard the multiplication of bacteria). They are bactericidal against sensitive microorganisms (i.e., those microorganisms that will be affected by penicillin), provided there is an adequate

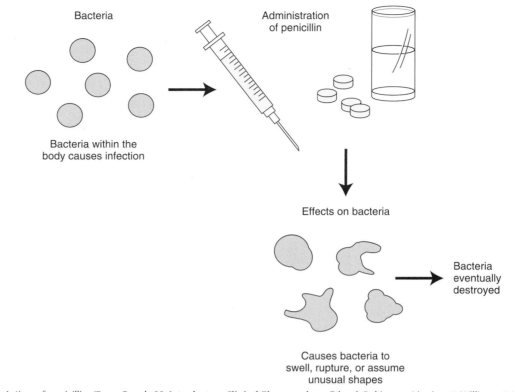

Bacteria

Bacteria within the
body causes infection

Administration
of penicillin

Effects on bacteria

Bacteria
eventually
destroyed

Causes bacteria to
swell, rupture, or assume
unusual shapes

FIGURE 25-1   Action of penicillin. (From Roach SS. *Introductory Clinical Pharmacology*, 7th ed. Baltimore: Lippincott Williams & Wilkins; 2004.)

concentration (blood level) of penicillin in the body. An inadequate concentration (or inadequate blood level) of penicillin may produce bacteriostatic activity, which may or may not control the infection.

Identifying the Appropriate Penicillin

To determine if a specific type of bacteria is sensitive to penicillin, **culture and sensitivity tests** are performed. A culture is performed by placing infectious material obtained from areas such as the skin, respiratory tract, and blood on a culture plate that contains a special growing medium. This growing medium is "food" for the bacteria. After a specified time, the bacteria are examined under a microscope and identified. The sensitivity test involves placing the infectious material on a separate culture plate and then placing small disks impregnated with various antibiotics over the area. After a specified time, the culture plate is examined. If there is little or no growth around a disk, then the bacteria are considered sensitive to that particular antibiotic. Therefore, this antibiotic will control the infection. (Fig. 25-2) If there is considerable growth around the disk, the bacteria are considered resistant to that particular antibiotic, and this antibiotic will not control the infection.

After a culture and sensitivity report is performed, the strain of microorganisms causing the infection is known, and the antibiotic to which these microorganisms are sensitive and resistant is identified. The health care provider then selects the antibiotic to which the microorganism is sensitive because that is the antibiotic that will be effective in the treatment of the infection.

Uses of Penicillins

Infectious Disease

Natural and semisynthetic penicillins are used in the treatment of bacterial infections caused by susceptible microorganisms. Penicillins may be used to treat infections such as urinary tract infections, septicemia, meningitis, intra-abdominal infection, gonorrhea, syphilis, pneumonia, and other respiratory infections. Examples of infectious microorganisms (bacteria) that may respond to penicillin therapy include gonococci, staphylococci, streptococci, and pneumococci. Culture and sensitivity tests are performed whenever possible to determine which penicillin will best control an infection caused by a specific strain of bacteria. A penicillinase-resistant penicillin is used as initial therapy for any suspected staphylococcal infection until culture and sensitivity results are known.

Prophylaxis

Penicillin is of no value in the treatment of viral or fungal infections. However, health care providers occasionally prescribe penicillin as **prophylaxis** (prevention) against a potential secondary bacterial infection that can occur in

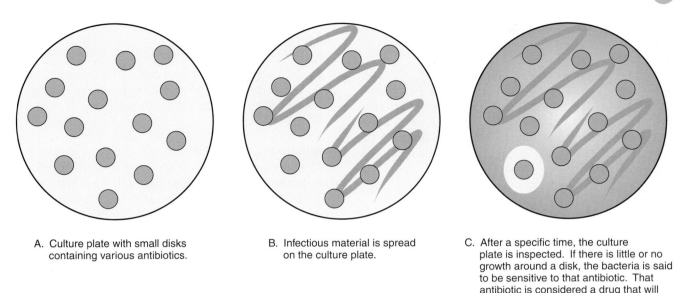

A. Culture plate with small disks containing various antibiotics.

B. Infectious material is spread on the culture plate.

C. After a specific time, the culture plate is inspected. If there is little or no growth around a disk, the bacteria is said to be sensitive to that antibiotic. That antibiotic is considered a drug that will control the infection.

FIGURE 25-2   Sensitivity testing. (From Roach SS. *Introductory Clinical Pharmacology*, 7th ed. Baltimore: Lippincott Williams & Wilkins; 2004.)

a patient with a viral infection. In these situations, the viral infection has weakened the body's defenses and the person is susceptible to other infections, particularly a bacterial infection. Penicillin also may be prescribed as prophylaxis for a potential infection in high-risk individuals, such as those with a history of rheumatic fever. Penicillin is taken several hours or, in some instances days, before and after an operative procedure, such as dental, oral, or upper respiratory tract procedures that can result in bacteria entering the bloodstream. Taking penicillin before and after the procedure will usually prevent a bacterial infection in these high-risk patients. Penicillin also may be given prophylactically on a continuing basis to those with rheumatic fever and chronic ear infections.

Adverse Reactions of Penicillins

Common adverse reactions include mild nausea, vomiting, diarrhea, sore tongue or mouth, fever, and pain at injection site. Penicillin can stimulate a hypersensitivity (allergic) reaction within the body. Another adverse reaction that may be seen with penicillin, as well as with almost all antibiotics, is a **superinfection** (a secondary infection that occurs during antibiotic treatment).

Other adverse reactions associated with penicillin are hematopoietic changes such as anemia, thrombocytopenia (low platelet count), leukopenia (low white blood cell count), and bone marrow depression. When penicillin is given orally, glossitis (inflammation of the tongue), stomatitis (inflammation of the mouth), dry mouth, gastritis, nausea, vomiting, and abdominal pain occur. When penicillin is given intramuscularly, there may be pain at the injection site. Irritation of the vein

and phlebitis (inflammation of a vein) may occur with intravenous use.

Hypersensitivity Reactions

A hypersensitivity (or allergic) reaction to a drug occurs in some patients, especially those with a history of allergy to many substances. Signs and symptoms of a hypersensitivity to penicillin are highlighted in Box 25-1.

Anaphylactic shock, which is a severe form of hypersensitivity reaction, also can occur (see Chapter 1). Anaphylactic shock occurs more frequently after parenteral use but can occur with oral use. This reaction is likely to be immediate and severe in susceptible patients. Signs of anaphylactic shock include severe

---

Box 25-1 Signs and Symptoms of Hypersensitivity to Penicillin

Skin rash
Urticaria (hives)
Sneezing
Wheezing
Pruritus (itching)
Bronchospasm (swelling the airway)
Laryngospasm (swelling of the larynx)
Angioedema (also called angioneurotic edema)—swelling of the skin and mucous membranes, especially around and in the mouth and throat
Hypotension—can progress to shock
Signs and symptoms resembling serum sickness—chills, fever, edema, joint and muscle pain, and malaise

hypotension, loss of consciousness, and acute respiratory distress. If not immediately treated, anaphylactic shock can be fatal.

Once a patient is allergic to one type of penicillin, he or she is most likely allergic to all penicillins. Those allergic to penicillin also have a higher incidence of allergy to the cephalosporins, which are discussed later in this chapter. Allergy to drugs in the same or related groups is called **cross-sensitivity** or **cross-allergenicity**.

Superinfections

Antibiotics can disrupt the **normal flora** (nonpathogenic microorganisms within the body), causing a superinfection. This new infection is "superimposed" on the original infection. The destruction of large numbers of **nonpathogenic** bacteria (normal flora) by the antibiotic alters the chemical environment. This allows uncontrolled growth of bacteria or fungal microorganisms, which are not affected by the antibiotic being used. A superinfection may occur with the use of any antibiotic, especially when these drugs are given for a long time or when repeated courses of therapy are necessary. A superinfection can develop rapidly and is potentially serious or life-threatening. Bacterial superinfections are commonly seen with the use of the oral penicillins and occur in the bowel. Symptoms of bacterial superinfection of the bowel include diarrhea or bloody diarrhea, rectal bleeding, fever, and abdominal cramping.

Fungal superinfections commonly occur in the vagina, mouth, and anal and genital areas. Symptoms include lesions of the mouth or tongue, vaginal discharge, and anal or vaginal itching. **Pseudomembranous colitis** is a common bacterial superinfection; candidiasis or moniliasis is a common type of fungal superinfection.

ALERT

Older Adults and Penicillin Use

Older adults who are debilitated, chronically ill, or taking penicillin for an extended period of time are more likely to have a superinfection. Pseudomembranous colitis is one type of a bacterial superinfection. This potentially life-threatening problem develops because of an overgrowth of the microorganism *Clostridium difficile*. This organism produces a toxin that affects the lining of the colon. Signs and symptoms include severe diarrhea with visible blood and mucus, fever, and abdominal cramps. This adverse reaction usually requires immediate discontinuation of the antibiotic. Mild cases may respond to drug discontinuation. Moderate to severe cases may require treatment with intravenous fluids and electrolytes, protein supplementation, and oral vancomycin (Vancocin).

ALERT

Pseudomembranous Colitis

Pseudomembranous colitis may occur after 4 to 9 days of treatment with penicillin or as long as 6 weeks after the drug is discontinued.

Candidiasis or Moniliasis. Another type of superinfection may occur because of an overgrowth of the yeast-like fungi that usually exist in small numbers in the vagina. The multiplication rate of these microorganisms is normally slowed and kept under control because of the presence of a strain of bacteria (Döderlein bacillus) in the vagina. If penicillin therapy destroys these normal microorganisms of the vagina, the fungi are now uncontrolled, multiply at a rapid rate, and cause symptoms of a fungal infection called candidiasis (or moniliasis). Symptoms include vaginal itching and discharge.

Candida fungal superinfections also occur in the mouth and around the anal and genital areas. Signs and symptoms include lesions in the mouth or anal/genital itching.

Managing Adverse Reactions of Penicillins

Treatment of minor hypersensitivity reactions may include use of an antihistamine such as Benadryl (for a rash or itching). Major hypersensitivity reactions, such as bronchospasm, laryngospasm, hypotension, and angioneurotic edema, require immediate treatment with drugs such as epinephrine, cortisone, or an intravenous antihistamine. When respiratory difficulty occurs, a tracheostomy may need to be performed.

ALERT

Intramuscular Use of Penicillin

A patient who has been given penicillin intramuscularly in the outpatient setting is asked to wait in the area for at least 30 minutes. Anaphylactic reactions are most likely to occur within 30 minutes after injection.

The patient should be closely observed for signs of a bacterial or fungal superinfection in the vaginal or anal area. Any signs and symptoms of a superinfection should be reported to the health care provider before the next dose of the drug is given. When symptoms are severe, additional treatment measures may be necessary, such as use of an antipyretic drug for fever or an antifungal drug.

Diarrhea. Diarrhea may be an indication of a superinfection of the gastrointestinal tract or pseudomembranous colitis. The patient's stools are inspected and the health care provider notified if diarrhea occurs because it may be necessary to stop the drug. If diarrhea does occur and there appears to be blood and mucus in the stool, then it is important to save a sample of the stool and test for occult blood using a test such as Hemoccult. If the stool tests positive for blood, then the sample is saved for possible further laboratory analysis.

Impaired Skin Integrity. Dermatologic reactions such as hives, rashes, and skin lesions can occur with the use of penicillin. In mild cases or when the benefit of the drug outweighs the discomfort of skin lesions, frequent skin care is given. Emollients, antipyretic creams, or a topical corticosteroid may be prescribed. An antihistamine may be prescribed. Harsh soaps and perfumed lotions are avoided. The patient is instructed to avoid rubbing the area and not to wear rough or irritating clothing. A rash or hives must be reported to the health care provider, because this may be a precursor to a severe anaphylactic reaction (see Hypersensitivity Reactions). In severe cases, the health care provider may discontinue penicillin therapy.

Impaired Oral Mucous Membranes. The use of oral penicillin may result in a fungal superinfection in the oral cavity. With impaired oral mucous membranes will be varying degrees of inflamed oral mucous membranes, swollen and red tongue, swollen gums, and pain in the mouth and throat. To detect this problem early, the patient's mouth is inspected daily for evidence of glossitis, sore tongue, ulceration, or a black, furry tongue. If the diet permits, yogurt, buttermilk, or acidophilus capsules may be taken to reduce the risk of fungal superinfection.

The mouth and gums are inspected often and frequent mouth care is given with a nonirritating solution. A soft bristled toothbrush is used when brushing is needed. A nonirritating soft diet may be required. Dietary intake is monitored to assure the patient is receiving adequate nutrition. Antifungal agents and/or local anesthetics are sometimes recommended to soothe the irritated membranes.

Fever. The patient's vital signs are taken every 4 hours or more often if necessary. Any increase in temperature should be reported to the health care provider because additional treatment measures, such as use of an antipyretic drug or change in the drug or dosage, may be necessary. An increase in body temperature several days after the start of therapy may indicate a secondary bacterial infection or failure of the drug to control the original infection. On occasion, the fever may be caused by an adverse reaction to the penicillin. In these cases, the fever can usually be managed by using an antipyretic drug.

Contraindications, Precautions, and Interactions of Penicillins

Penicillins are contraindicated in patients with a history of hypersensitivity to penicillin or cephalosporins.

Penicillins should be used cautiously in patients with renal disease, pregnancy (pregnancy category C), or lactation (may cause diarrhea or candidiasis in the infant), and in those with a history of allergies. Any indication of sensitivity is reason for caution. The drug is also used with caution in patients with asthma, renal disease, bleeding disorders, and gastrointestinal disease.

Some penicillins (ampicillin, bacampicillin, penicillin V) may interfere with the effectiveness of birth control pills that contain estrogen. There is a decreased effectiveness of the penicillin when it is administered with the tetracyclines. Large doses of penicillin can increase bleeding risks of patients taking anticoagulant agents. Some reports indicate that when oral penicillins are administered with beta-adrenergic blocking drugs (see Chapter 4), the patient may be at increased risk for an anaphylactic reaction. Absorption of most penicillins is affected by food. In general, penicillins should be given 1 hour before or 2 hours after meals.

Patient Management Issues with Penicillins

Before the first dose of penicillin, the patient's general health history is reviewed. The health history includes an allergy history, a history of all medical and surgical treatments, a drug history, and the current symptoms of the infection. If the patient has a history of allergy, particularly a drug allergy, then this must be explored to ensure the patient is not allergic to penicillin or a cephalosporin.

The patient's infected area is assessed when possible. Any signs and symptoms related to the patient's infection, such as color and type of drainage from a wound, pain, redness and inflammation, color of sputum, or presence of an odor are noted. A culture and sensitivity test is almost always ordered, and the results obtained before the first dose of penicillin is given.

The patient is monitored daily for a response to therapy, such as a decrease in temperature, the relief of symptoms caused by the infection (such as pain or discomfort), an increase in appetite, and a change in the appearance or amount of drainage (when originally present). Once an infection is controlled, patients often look better and even state that they feel better. The health care provider should be notified if signs and symptoms of the infection appear to worsen.

Additional culture and sensitivity tests may be performed during therapy because microorganisms causing the infection may become resistant to penicillin, or a superinfection may occur. A urinalysis, complete blood count, and renal and hepatic function tests also may be performed at intervals during therapy.

ALERT

Hypersensitivity Reaction

The patient should be closely observed for a hypersensitivity reaction, which may occur any time during therapy with the penicillins. If it should occur, then the health care provider should be contacted immediately and the drug withheld until the patient is seen by the health care provider.

The results of a culture and sensitivity test take several days because time is needed for the bacteria to grow on the culture media. However, infections are treated as soon as possible. In a few instances, the health care provider may determine that a penicillin is the treatment of choice until the results of the culture and sensitivity tests are known. In many instances, the health care provider selects a broad-spectrum antibiotic (i.e., an antibiotic that is effective against many types or strains of bacteria) for initial treatment because of the many penicillin-resistant strains of microorganisms.

Adequate blood levels of the drug must be maintained for the drug to be effective. Accidental omission or delay of a dose results in decreased blood levels, which will reduce the effectiveness of the antibiotic. Oral penicillins should be given on an empty stomach, 1 hour before or 2 hours after a meal. Bacampicillin (Spectrobid), penicillin V (Pen-Vee K), and amoxicillin (Amoxil) may be given without regard to meals.

When penicillin is administered intramuscularly, the patient may feel a stinging or burning sensation at the time the drug is injected into the muscle. Discomfort at the time of injection occurs because the drug is irritating to the tissues. Previous areas used for injection are checked for continued redness, soreness, or other problems. The health care provider should be informed if injection areas appear red or the patient reports pain in the area.

Educating the Patient and Family About Penicillins

Some patients do not adhere to the prescribed drug regimen for a variety of reasons, such as failure to comprehend the prescribed regimen or failure to understand the importance of continued and uninterrupted therapy. The drug regimen is carefully explained and the importance of continued and uninterrupted therapy is stressed when the patient is educated about their prescription. Patient Education Box 25-2 includes key points about penicillins the patient or family members should know.

PATIENT EDUCATION BOX 25-2

Key Points for Patients Taking Penicillins

PROPHYLAXIS (PREVENTION)
❑ Take the drug as prescribed until your health care provider discontinues therapy.

INFECTION
❑ Complete the full course of therapy. Do not stop taking the drug, even if your symptoms have disappeared, unless directed to do so by your health care provider.
❑ Take the drug at the prescribed times of day, because it is important to keep an adequate amount of the drug in your body throughout the entire 24 hours of each day.

PENICILLIN (ORAL)
❑ Take the drug on an empty stomach either 1 hour before or 2 hours after meals (exceptions: bacampicillin, penicillin V, amoxicillin).
❑ Take each dose with a full glass of water.
❑ To reduce the risk of superinfection, take yogurt, buttermilk, or acidophilus capsules.
❑ Notify your health care provider immediately if you experience any of the following: skin rash; hives (urticaria); severe diarrhea; vaginal or anal itching; sore mouth; black, furry tongue; sores in the mouth; swelling around the mouth or eyes; breathing difficulty; or gastrointestinal disturbances such as nausea, vomiting, and diarrhea. Do not take the next dose of the drug until you discuss the problem with your health care provider.

ORAL SUSPENSIONS
❑ Keep the container refrigerated (if so-labeled), shake the drug well before pouring (if so-labeled), and return the drug to the refrigerator immediately after pouring the dose. Drugs that are kept refrigerated lose their potency when kept at room temperature. A small amount of the drug may be left after the last dose is taken. Discard any remaining drug because the drug (in suspension form) begins to lose its potency after 7 to 14 days.
❑ Women prescribed ampicillin, bacampicillin, and penicillin V who take birth control pills containing estrogen should use additional contraception measures.
❑ Never give this drug to another individual, even if their symptoms appear the same as your symptoms.
❑ Notify your health care provider if the symptoms of your infection do not improve or if your condition becomes worse.
❑ If you are taking penicillin as prevention, you may feel well even though you need the long-term antibiotic therapy. Avoid any temptation to skip one or more doses or to stop taking drug for an extended time. Never skip doses or stop therapy unless told to do so by your health care provider.

Natural Remedies: Goldenseal

Goldenseal, also called *Hydrastis canadensis*, is an herb found growing in the certain areas of the northeastern United States. Goldenseal has long been used alone or in combination with echinacea for colds and influenza. However, there is no scientific evidence to support the use of goldenseal for cold and influenza or as a stimulant, as there is for the use of echinacea (see Chapter 27). Similarly, goldenseal is touted as an "herbal antibiotic," although there is no scientific evidence to support this use. Another myth surrounding goldenseal use is that taking the herb masks the presence of illicit drugs in the urine.

There are many traditional uses of the herb, such as an antiseptic for the skin, mouthwash for canker sores, wash for inflamed or infected eyes, and the treatment of sinus infections and digestive problems, such as peptic ulcers and gastritis. Some evidence supports the use of goldenseal to treat diarrhea caused by bacteria or intestinal parasites, such as Giardia. The herb is contraindicated during pregnancy and in patients with hypertension. Adverse reactions are rare when the herb is used as directed. However, this herb should not be taken for more than a few days to a week. Because of widespread use, destruction of its natural habitats, and renewed interest in its use as an herbal remedy, goldenseal was classified as an "endangered" plant in 1997 by the United States government.

Cephalosporins

The effectiveness of penicillin in the treatment of infections prompted research directed toward finding new antibiotics with a wider range of antibacterial activity. Cephalosporins are a valuable group of drugs that are effective in the treatment of almost all of the strains of bacteria affected by the penicillins, as well as some strains of bacteria that have become resistant to penicillin. Cephalosporins are structurally and chemically related to penicillin.

Cephalosporins are divided into first-, second-, and third-generation drugs. Particular cephalosporins also may be differentiated within each group according to the microorganisms that are sensitive to them. Generally, progression from the first-generation to the second-generation and then to the third-generation drugs shows an increase in the sensitivity of Gram-negative microorganisms and a decrease in the sensitivity of Gram-positive microorganisms. For example, a first-generation cephalosporin would have more use against Gram-positive microorganisms than would a third-generation cephalosporin. This scheme of classification is becoming less clearly defined as newer drugs are introduced. For a complete listing see the Summary Drug Table: Cephalosporins.

Actions of Cephalosporins

Cephalosporins affect the bacterial cell wall, making it defective and unstable. This action is similar to the action of penicillin. Cephalosporins are usually bactericidal (capable of destroying bacteria).

Uses of Cephalosporins

Cephalosporins are used in the treatment of infections caused by susceptible microorganisms. Examples of microorganisms that may be susceptible to cephalosporins include streptococci, staphylococci, citrobacters, gonococci, shigella, and clostridia. Culture and sensitivity tests are performed whenever possible to determine which antibiotic, including a cephalosporin, can best control an infection caused by a specific strain of bacteria. Pharyngitis, tonsillitis, otitis media, lower respiratory infections, urinary tract infections, septicemia, and gonorrhea are examples of the types of infections that may be treated with the cephalosporins.

Cephalosporins also may be used before, during, or after surgery to prevent infection in patients having surgery on a contaminated or potentially contaminated area, such as the gastrointestinal tract or vagina. In some instances, a specific drug may be recommended for postoperative prophylactic use only.

Adverse Reactions of Cephalosporins

The most common adverse reactions of cephalosporins are gastrointestinal disturbances, such as nausea, vomiting, and diarrhea.

Hypersensitivity (allergic) reactions may occur with use of the cephalosporins and range from mild to life-threatening. Mild hypersensitivity reactions include pruritus, urticaria, and skin rashes. More serious hypersensitivity reactions include Stevens-Johnson syndrome (fever, cough, muscular aches and pains, headache, and the appearance of lesions on the skin, mucous membranes, and eyes), liver or kidney dysfunction, aplastic anemia (anemia caused by deficient red blood cell production), and epidermal necrolysis (death of the epidermal layer of the skin).

Because of the close relation of the cephalosporins to penicillin, a patient allergic to penicillin also may be allergic to the cephalosporins.

Other adverse reactions that may be seen with cephalosporin use are headache, dizziness, nephrotoxicity (damage to the kidneys), malaise, heartburn, and fever. Intramuscular use often results in pain, tenderness, and inflammation at the injection site. Intravenous use has resulted in thrombophlebitis and phlebitis.

Therapy with cephalosporins may result in a bacterial or fungal superinfection. Diarrhea may be an indication of pseudomembranous colitis, which is one type of bacterial superinfection.

SUMMARY DRUG TABLE   Cephalosporins

Generic Name	Trade Name*	Uses	Adverse Reactions	Dosage Ranges
First-Generation Cephalosporins				
cefadroxil *saf-a-drox'-ill*	Duricef	Infection due to susceptible microorganisms	Nausea, vomiting, diarrhea, hypersensitivity reactions, superinfection, nephrotoxicity, headache, Stevens-Johnson syndrome, pseudomembranous colitis	1–2 g/d PO in divided doses
cefazolin sodium *sef-a'-zoe-lin*	Ancef, Kefzol, *generic*	Infections due to susceptible microorganisms; perioperative prophylaxis	Nausea, vomiting, diarrhea, hypersensitivity reactions, superinfection, nephrotoxicity, headache, Stevens-Johnson syndrome, pseudomembranous colitis	250 mg–1 g IM, IV 6–12h; perioperative, 0.5–1g IM, IV
cephalexin *sef'-a-lex-in*	Keflex, *generic*	Infections due to susceptible microorganisms	Same as cefadroxil	1–4 g/d PO in divided doses
Second-Generation Cephalosporins				
cefaclor *sef'-a-klor*	Ceclor	Treatment of infections due to susceptible organisms	Nausea, vomiting, diarrhea, hypersensitivity reactions, nephrotoxicity, headache, hematologic reactions	250 mg PO q8h
cefamandole *sef-a-man'-dole*	Mandol	Same as cefaclor	Same as cefaclor	500 mg to 1 g IM, IV q4–6h
cefotetan *sef-oh-tee'-tan*	Cefotan	Same as cefaclor; perioperative prophylaxis	Same as cefaclor	1–6 g IM, IV in equally divided doses; perioperative: 1–2 g IV
cefoxitin *sef-ox'-i-tin*	Mefoxin	Same as cefaclor; perioperative prophylaxis	Same as cefaclor	1–2 g IM q6–8h; 1–12 g/d IV in equally divided doses; perioperative, 1–2 g IV
cefpodoxime *sef-poed-ox'-eem*	Vantin	Same as cefaclor	Same as cefaclor	200–800 mg/d PO in equally divided doses
cefprozil *sef-proe'-zil*	Cefzil	Same as cefaclor	Same as cefaclor	250–500 mg PO q12h
cefuroxime *sef-yoor-ox'-eem*	Ceftin, Kefurox, Zinacef	Same as cefaclor; perioperative prophylaxis	Same as cefaclor	250 mg PO BID; 750 mg–1.5 g IM or IV q8h; perioperative, 1.5 g IV
loracarbef *lor-ah-kar'-bef*	Lorabid	Same as cefaclor	Same as cefaclor	200–400 mg PO q12h

Generic Name	Trade Name*	Uses	Adverse Reactions	Dosage Ranges
Third-Generation Cephalosporins				
cefdinir *sef'-din-er*	Omnicef	Same as cefaclor	Same as cefaclor	300 mg PO q12h or 600 mg q24h PO
cefepime hydrochloride *sef'-ah-pime*	Maxipime	Same as cefaclor	Same as cefaclor	0.5 mg–2 g IV, IM q12h
cefixime *sef-ix'-eem*	Suprax	Same as cefaclor	Same as cefaclor	400 mg/d as a single dose or divided doses
cefoperazone *sef-oh-per'-a-zone*	Cefobid	Same as cefaclor	Same as cefaclor	2–4 g/d IM, IV in equally divided doses
cefotaxime *sef-oh-taks'-eem*	Claforan	Same as cefaclor; perioperative prophylaxis	Same as cefaclor	2–8 g/d IM or IV in equally divided doses q6–8h; maximum 12 g/d
ceftazidime *sef-taz'-i-deem*	Fortaz, Tazidime, Ceptaz	Same as cefaclor	Same as cefaclor	250 mg–2 g IV, IM q8–12h
ceftibuten hydrochloride *sef-ta-byoo'-ten*	Cedax	Same as cefaclor	Same as cefaclor	400 mg/d for 10 days
ceftizoxime *sef-ti-zox'-eem*	Cefizox	Same as cefaclor	Same as cefaclor	1–2 g (range, 1–4 g) IM or IV q8–12h; maximum, 12 g/d
ceftriaxone *sef-try-ax'-on*	Rocephin	Same as cefaclor; perioperative prophylaxis; gonorrhea	Same as cefaclor	1–2 g/d IM, IV QID, BID; maximum, 4 g/d; perioperative, 1 g IV; gonorrhea, 250 mg IM as a single dose

*The term *generic* indicates the drug is available in generic form.

Managing Adverse Reactions of Cephalosporins

The patient is closely observed for any adverse drug reactions, particularly the signs and symptoms of a hypersensitivity reaction. A rash or hives should be reported to the health care provider because this may be a precursor to a severe anaphylactic reaction. In severe cases, the health care provider may discontinue the cephalosporin therapy. The patient is closely observed for signs and symptoms of a bacterial or fungal superinfection. If any occur, then the health care provider is notified before the next dose of the drug is due.

Rare cases of hemolytic anemia, including fatalities, have been reported with cephalosporins. The patient should be monitored for anemia. If a patient experiences anemia within 2 to 3 weeks after the start of cephalosporin therapy, then drug-induced anemia should be considered. If hemolytic anemia is suspected, then the health care provider will discontinue the drug therapy. The patient may require blood transfusions to correct the anemia. Frequent hematological studies may be required.

ALERT

Nephrotoxicity and Cephalosporins
Nephrotoxicity may occur with the use of these drugs. Early signs of this adverse reaction may become apparent by a decrease in urine output. Fluid intake and output are monitored and the health care provider notified if the output is less than 500 mL/day. Any changes in the fluid intake-to-output ratio or in the appearance of the urine may indicate nephrotoxicity. These findings should be reported to the health care provider promptly.

Fever. Vital signs are taken every 4 hours or as ordered by the health care provider. Any increase in temperature should be reported to the health care provider because additional treatment measures, such as use of an antipyretic drug or change in the drug or dosage, may be necessary.

Diarrhea. Frequent liquid stools may be an indication of a superinfection or pseudomembranous colitis. If pseudomembranous colitis occurs, it usually appears 4 to 10 days after treatment is started.

Each bowel movement is inspected, and the occurrence of diarrhea or loose stools containing blood and mucus is immediately reported to the health care provider, because it may be necessary to discontinue the drug use and institute treatment for diarrhea, a superinfection, or pseudomembranous colitis.

If there appears to be blood and mucus in the stool, then a sample of the stool is saved and tests for occult blood are performed using a test such as Hemoccult. If the stool tests positive for blood, then the sample is saved for possible laboratory testing for blood.

Impaired Skin Integrity. The patient's skin is inspected every 4 hours for redness, rash, or lesions that appear as red wheals or blisters. When a skin rash or irritation is present, frequent skin care is given. Emollients, antipyretic creams, or a topical corticosteroid may be prescribed. An antihistamine may be prescribed. Harsh soaps and perfumed lotions are avoided. The patient is instructed to avoid rubbing the area and not to wear rough or irritating clothing.

Contraindications, Precautions, and Interactions of Cephalosporins

Cephalosporins should not be used if the patient has a history of allergies to cephalosporins or penicillins.

Cephalosporins should be used cautiously in patients with renal or hepatic impairment and in patients with bleeding disorders. Safety of cephalosporin use has not been established in pregnancy or lactation; these drugs are assigned to pregnancy category B.

The risk of nephrotoxicity increases when cephalosporins are used with the aminoglycosides. The risk for bleeding increases when cephalosporins are taken with oral anticoagulants. A disulfiram-like reaction may occur if alcohol is consumed within 72 hours after cephalosporin use. Symptoms of a disulfiram-like reaction include flushing, throbbing in the head and neck, respiratory difficulty, vomiting, sweating, chest pain, and hypotension. Severe reactions may cause arrhythmias and unconsciousness. When cephalosporins are used with an aminoglycoside, the risk for nephrotoxicity increases.

Patient Management Issues with Cephalosporins

Patients with a history of an allergy to penicillin may also be allergic to a cephalosporin even though they have never received one of these drugs. If an allergy to either of these drug groups is suspected, then the health care provider is informed of this before the first dose of the drug is given. Liver and kidney function tests may be ordered.

The patient is monitored for a decrease in fever, the relief of symptoms caused by the infection (e.g., pain or discomfort), an increase in appetite, and a change in the appearance or amount of drainage (when originally present). The health care provider is notified if symptoms of the infection appear to worsen. The patient's skin is checked regularly for rash and the patient monitored for any loose stools or diarrhea.

Patients must be questioned about a possible allergy to cephalosporins or the penicillins before taking the first dose, even when an accurate drug history has been taken. If a patient has a history of possible cephalosporin or penicillin allergy, the health care provider is notified.

Oral Use of Cephalosporins

Cephalosporins are taken around the clock to provide adequate blood levels. Most cephalosporins may be taken with food to prevent gastric upset. Cefdinir may be taken without regard to food. The absorption of oral cefuroxime and cefpodoxime is increased when given with food. However, if the patient experiences gastrointestinal upset, the drug can be taken with food. Oral suspensions should be shaken well before taken.

Some cephalosporins are available as powder for a suspension and are reconstituted by a pharmacist or a nurse. This form of the drug is refrigerated until it is used.

Educating the Patient and Family About Cephalosporins

Patient Education Box 25-3 includes key points about cephalosporins the patient and family members should know.

Tetracyclines, Macrolides, and Lincosamides

This section discusses three groups of broad-spectrum antibiotics: the tetracyclines, the macrolides, and the lincosamides. Examples of the tetracyclines include doxycycline (Vibramycin), minocycline (Minocin), and tetracycline (Sumycin). Examples of the macrolides include azithromycin (Zithromax), clarithromycin (Biaxin), and erythromycin (E-Mycin). The lincosamides include clindamycin (Cleocin) and lincomycin (Lincocin). The Summary Drug Table: Tetracyclines, Macrolides, and Lincosamides describes these types of broad-spectrum antibiotics.

Actions of Tetracyclines

Tetracyclines are a group of anti-infectives composed of natural and semisynthetic compounds.

PATIENT EDUCATION BOX 25-3

Key Points for Patients Taking Cephalosporins

- ❑ Complete the full course of therapy. Do not stop the drug even if your symptoms disappear unless directed to do so by your health care provider.
- ❑ Take the drug at the prescribed times of day because it is important to keep an adequate amount of drug in your body at all times through each day.
- ❑ Take each dose with food or milk if you have stomach upset after taking the drug.
- ❑ Do not drink alcoholic beverages when taking the cephalosporins and for 3 days after completing the course of therapy because severe reactions may occur.
- ❑ Notify your health care provider immediately if you experience any of the following: vomiting, skin rash, hives (urticaria), severe diarrhea, vaginal or anal itching, sores in the mouth, swelling around the mouth or eyes, breathing difficulty, or stomach disturbances such as nausea, vomiting, and diarrhea. Do not take the next dose of the drug until you discuss the problem with your health care provider.
- ❑ Never give this drug to another person, even if their symptoms seem the same as yours.
- ❑ Notify your health care provider if the symptoms of your infection do not improve or if your condition becomes worse.

ORAL SUSPENSIONS

- ❑ Keep the container refrigerated (if so-labeled), shake the drug well before pouring (if so-labeled), and return the drug to the refrigerator immediately after pouring your

dose. Drugs that are kept refrigerated lose their potency when kept at room temperature. If a small amount of the drug is left after the last dose is taken, then discard it because the drug (in suspension form) begins to lose potency after a few weeks.

SIGNS OF SUPERINFECTION

- ❑ If you experience any of the following, report it immediately to your health care provider:
  - ❑ diarrhea, possibly severe with visible blood and mucus
  - ❑ fever
  - ❑ abdominal cramps
- ❑ A fungal superinfection commonly occurs in the mouth, vagina, and anogenital areas.
- ❑ If you experience any of the following symptoms, report it immediately to your health care provider:
  - ❑ scaly, reddened, papular rash commonly in the breast folds, at the axillae, groin, or umbilicus
  - ❑ white or yellow vaginal discharge
  - ❑ localized redness, inflammation, and excoriation, particularly inside the mouth, in the groin, or skin folds of the anogenital area
  - ❑ anal or vaginal itching
  - ❑ creamy white lace-like patches on the tongue, mouth, or throat
  - ❑ burning sensation in the mouth or throat

SUMMARY DRUG TABLE   Tetracyclines, Macrolides, and Lincosamides

Generic Name	Trade Name*	Uses	Adverse Reactions	Dosage Ranges
Tetracyclines demeclocycline *deh-meh-kloe- sye'-kleen*	Declomycin	Treatment of infections caused by susceptible microorganisms	Nausea, vomiting, diarrhea, hypersensitivity reactions, photosensitivity reactions, pseudomembranous colitis, hematologic changes, discoloration of teeth in fetus and young children	150 mg PO QID or 300 mg PO BID; gonorrhea: 600 mg PO initially then 300 mg PO q12h for 4 d
doxycycline *dox-i-sye'-kleen*	Doxychel Hyclate, Vibra-Tabs, Vibramycin, *generic*	Same as demeclocycline	Same as demeclocycline	100 mg PO q12h first day then 100–200 mg/d PO; gonorrhea: 200 mg PO immediately and 100 mg PO hs then 100 mg PO BID for 3 d; 200 mg IV first day then 100–200 mg/d IV
minocycline *min-oh-sye'-kleen*	Minocin, Minocin IV	Same as demeclocycline	Same as demeclocycline	200 mg PO initially then 100 mg IV q12h 100–200 mg initially then 50 mg PO QID
oxytetracycline *ox-i-tet-ra-sye'-kleen*	Terramycin, Terramycin IM, Uri-Tet	Same as demeclocycline	Nausea, vomiting, diarrhea, hypersensitivity reactions, photosensitivity reactions, pseudomembranous colitis, hematologic changes, discoloration of teeth in fetus and young children	1–2 g/d PO; 250 mg qd or 300 mg individual-ized doses q8–12h IM; 250–500 mg IV q12h
tetracycline *tet-ra-sye'-kleen*	Panmycin, Sumycin, Tetracap, *generic*	Same as demeclocycline	Same as demeclocycline	1–2 g/d PO in 2–4 divided doses
Macrolides azithromycin *ay-zi-thro-my'-cin*	Zithromax	Same as demeclocycline	Nausea, vomiting, diarrhea, abdominal pains, hypersensitivity reactions, pseudomembranous colitis	500 mg PO first day then 250 mg/d PO for 4 d
clarithromycin *klar-ith-ro-my'-cin*	Biaxin	Same as demeclocycline	Same as azithromycin	250–500 mg PO BID
dirithromycin *dir-ith-ro-my'-cin*	Dynabac	Same as demeclocycline	Nausea, vomiting, diarrhea, hypersensitivity reactions, photosensitivity reactions, pseudomembranous colitis, electrolyte imbalance	500 mg PO for 7–14 d
erythromycin base *er-ith-roe-my'-sin*	E-Mycin, Eryc, *generic*	Same as demeclocycline	Same as azithromycin	250 mg PO q6h or 333 mg q8h

Generic Name	Trade Name*	Uses	Adverse Reactions	Dosage Ranges
erythromycin ethylsuccinate	EryPed, E.E.S., *generic*	Same as demeclocycline	Same as azithromycin	400 mg PO q6h
erythromycin estolate	Ilosone, *generic*	Same as demeclocycline	Same as azithromycin	250 mg PO q6h
erythromycin IV	Ilotycin Glucepate, *generic*	Same as demeclocycline	Same as azithromycin	Up to 4 g/d IV in divided doses
troleandomycin	Tao	Same as demeclocycline	Same as clindamycin	250–500 mg QID PO
Lincosamides clindamycin *klin-da-my′-sin*	Cleocin, *generic*	Same as demeclocycline	Abdominal pain, esophagitis, nausea, vomiting, diarrhea, skin rash, blood dyscrasias, pseudomembranous colitis, hypersensitivity reactions	150–450 mg PO q6h; 600–2700 mg/d in 2–4 equal doses; up to 4.8 g/d IV, IM
lincomycin *lin-koe-my′-sin*	Lincocin, Lincorex	Same as demeclocycline	Same as clindamycin	500 mg PO q6–8h; 600 mg IM q12–24h; up to 8 g/d IV

*The term *generic* indicates the drug is available in generic form.

Tetracyclines exert their effect by inhibiting bacterial protein synthesis, which is a process necessary for reproduction of the microorganism. The ultimate effect of this action is that the bacteria are either destroyed or their multiplication rate is slowed. Tetracyclines are bacteriostatic (capable of slowing or retarding the multiplication of bacteria), whereas the macrolides and lincosamides may be bacteriostatic or **bactericidal** (capable of destroying bacteria).

Uses of Tetracyclines

Tectracyclines are useful in select infections when the organism shows sensitivity to them, such as in cholera, Rocky Mountain spotted fever, and typhus.

These antibiotics are effective in the treatment of infections caused by a wide range of Gram-negative and Gram-positive microorganisms. Tetracyclines are used for infections caused by Rickettsiae (Rocky Mountain spotted fever, typhus fever, and tick fevers). Tetracyclines are also used in situations in which penicillin is contraindicated, in the treatment of intestinal amebiasis, and in some skin and soft tissue infections. Oral tetracyclines are used in the treatment of uncomplicated urethral, endocervical, or rectal infections caused by *Chlamydia trachomatis* and as adjunctive treatment in severe acne. Tetracycline in combination with metronidazole and bismuth subsalicylate is useful in treating *Helicobacter pylori* (a bacteria in the stomach that can cause peptic ulcer).

Adverse Reactions of Tetracyclines

Gastrointestinal reactions that may occur during tetracycline use include nausea, vomiting, diarrhea, epigastric distress, stomatitis, and sore throat. Skin rashes also may occur. A photosensitivity (phototoxic) reaction may occur with these drugs, manifested by an exaggerated sunburn reaction when the skin is exposed to sunlight even for brief periods. Demeclocycline seems to cause the most serious photosensitivity reaction, whereas minocycline is least likely to cause this reaction.

Tetracyclines are not given to children younger than 9 years of age unless their use is absolutely necessary, because these drugs may cause permanent yellow–gray–brown discoloration of the teeth. The use of the tetracyclines, especially prolonged or repeated therapy, may result in bacterial or fungal overgrowth of nonsusceptible organisms.

Contraindications, Precautions, and Interactions of Tetracyclines

Tetracyclines are contraindicated if the patient is known to be hypersensitive. Tetracyclines also are contraindicated during pregnancy because of the possibility of toxic effects to the developing fetus. Tetracyclines are classified pregnancy category D drugs. These drugs also are contraindicated during lactation and in children younger than 9 years (may cause permanent discoloration of the teeth).

Tetracyclines are used cautiously in patients with renal function impairment. Larger doses can be extremely damaging to the liver.

Antacids containing aluminum, zinc, magnesium, or bismuth salts, or foods high in calcium impair absorption of tetracyclines. When taken with oral anticoagulants, an increase in the effects of the anticoagulant may occur. When tetracyclines are given to women using oral contraceptives, a decrease in the effect of the oral contraceptive may occur. This may result in breakthrough bleeding or pregnancy. When digoxin is used with a tetracycline, there is an increased risk for digitalis toxicity (see Chapter 14). The effects of this could last for months after tetracycline use is discontinued. Tetracyclines may reduce insulin requirements. Blood glucose levels should be monitored frequently during tetracycline therapy.

Actions of Macrolides

Macrolides are effective against a wide variety of pathogenic organisms, particularly infections of the respiratory and genital tract.

Macrolides are bacteriostatic or bactericidal in susceptible bacteria. The drugs act by binding to cell membranes and causing changes in protein function.

Uses of Macrolides

These antibiotics are effective in the treatment of infections caused by a wide range of Gram-negative and Gram-positive microorganisms. In addition, the drugs are used to treat acne vulgaris and skin infections, in conjunction with sulfonamides to treat upper respiratory infections caused by *Haemophilus influenzae*, and as prophylaxis before dental or other procedures in patients allergic to penicillin.

Adverse Reactions of Macrolides

Most of the adverse reactions seen with the use of azithromycin and clarithromycin are related to the gastrointestinal tract and include nausea, vomiting, diarrhea, and abdominal pain. Abdominal cramping, nausea, vomiting, diarrhea, and allergic reactions have been reported with the use of erythromycin. However, there appears to be a low incidence of adverse reactions associated with normal oral doses of erythromycin. As with almost all antibacterial drugs, pseudomembranous colitis may occur ranging in severity from mild to life-threatening.

Contraindications, Precautions, and Interactions of Macrolides

These drugs are contraindicated in patients with a hypersensitivity and patients with pre-existing liver disease.

These drugs are used cautiously during pregnancy and lactation. Azithromycin and erythromycin are pregnancy category B drugs, and clarithromycin, dirithromycin, and troleandomycin are pregnancy category C drugs. Because azithromycin, erythromycin, and troleandomycin are primarily eliminated from the body by the liver, these drugs should be used with great caution in patients with liver dysfunction. There is a decreased gastrointestinal absorption of the macrolides when administered with kaolin, aluminum salts, or magaldrate.

Use of macrolides increases serum levels of digoxin and increases the effects of anticoagulants. Use of antacids decreases the absorption of most macrolides. Macrolides should not be taken with clindamycin, lincomycin, or chloramphenicol; a decrease in the therapeutic activity of the macrolides can occur. Concurrent use of macrolides with theophylline may increase serum theophylline levels.

Actions of Lincosamides

Lincosamides, another group of anti-infectives, are effective against many Gram-positive organisms, such as streptococci and staphylococci.

Lincosamides act by inhibiting protein synthesis in susceptible bacteria, causing death.

Uses of Lincosamides

Because of their high potential for toxicity, lincosamides are usually used only for the treatment of serious infections in which penicillin or erythromycin (a macrolide) is not effective.

These antibiotics are effective in the treatment of infections caused by a wide range of Gram-negative and Gram-positive microorganisms. Lincosamides are used for the more serious infections. In serious infections, they may be used in conjunction with other antibiotics.

Adverse Reactions of Lincosamides

Abdominal pain, esophagitis, nausea, vomiting, diarrhea, skin rash, and blood dyscrasias may occur with the use of lincosamides. These drugs also can cause pseudomembranous colitis, which may range from mild to very severe. Discontinuing the drug may relieve mild symptoms of pseudomembranous colitis.

Contraindications, Precautions, and Interactions of Lincosamides

Lincosamides are contraindicated in patients with hypersensitivity, those with minor bacterial or viral infections, and during lactation and infancy.

These drugs are used with caution in patients with a history of gastrointestinal disorders, renal disease, or liver impairment. The neuromuscular blocking action of the lincosamides poses a danger to patients with myasthenia gravis (an autoimmune disease manifested by extreme weakness and exhaustion of the muscles).

When kaolin or aluminum is used with lincosamides, the absorption of the lincosamide is decreased. When lincosamides are used with the neuromuscular blocking drugs (drugs that are used as adjuncts to anesthetic drugs that cause paralysis of the respiratory system), the action of the neuromuscular blocking drug is enhanced, possibly leading to severe and profound respiratory depression.

Patient Management Issues with Tetracyclines, Macrolides, and Lincosamides

To help track the patient's progress, the patient's signs and symptoms of infection are identified and recorded before the drug is initially taken. Signs and symptoms may vary and often depend on the organ or system involved and whether the infection is external or internal. Examples of some of the signs and symptoms of an infection in various areas of the body are pain, drainage, redness, changes in the appearance of sputum, general malaise, chills and fever, cough, and swelling.

A thorough allergy history is taken, especially a history of drug allergies. Some antibiotics have a higher incidence of hypersensitivity reactions in those with a history of allergy to drugs or other substances.

The patient's vital signs are taken before the first dose of the antibiotic is given. The health care provider may order culture and sensitivity tests, and these should also be performed before the first dose of the drug is given. Other laboratory tests such as renal and hepatic function tests, complete blood count, and urinalysis may also be ordered.

When an antibiotic is ordered for the prevention of a secondary infection (prophylaxis), the patient is observed for signs and symptoms that may indicate the beginning of an infection despite the prophylactic use of the antibiotic. If signs and symptoms of an infection occur, then they must be reported to the health care provider.

Before therapy is begun, culture and sensitivity tests are performed to determine which antibiotic will best control the infection. These drugs are of no value in the treatment of infections caused by a virus or fungus, but a secondary bacterial infection may occur in a patient with a fungal or viral infection. The health care provider may then order one of the broad-spectrum antibiotics, but its purpose is for the prevention (prophylaxis) or treatment of a secondary bacterial infection that could potentially develop after the primary fungal or viral infection.

Oral Use

Tetracyclines. Tetracyclines are given on an empty stomach and should not be taken with dairy products (milk or cheese). The exceptions are doxycycline (Vibramycin) and minocycline (Minocin), which may be taken with dairy products or food. Troleandomycin and clarithromycin can be given without regard to meals. All tetracyclines should be given with a full glass of water (240 mL).

ALERT

Tetracyclines and Dairy Products

Tetracyclines should not be given along with dairy products (milk or cheese), antacids, laxatives, or products containing iron. When these drugs are prescribed, they are taken 2 hours before or after taking a tetracycline. Food or drugs containing calcium, magnesium, aluminum, or iron prevent the absorption of the tetracyclines if ingested concurrently.

Macrolides. Clarithromycin can be given without regard to meals. Clarithromycin may be taken with milk, if desired. Azithromycin tablets may be given without regard to meals. However, azithromycin suspension is taken 1 hour or more before a meal or 2 hours or more after a meal. Dirithromycin is taken with food or within 1 hour of eating. Erythromycin is taken on an empty stomach (1 hour before or 2 hours after meals) and with 180 to 240 mL of water.

Lincosamides. Food impairs the absorption of lincomycin. The patient should not eat for 1 to 2 hours before and after taking lincomycin. Clindamycin may be given without regard to food.

Managing Adverse Drug Reactions of Tetracyclines, Macrolides, and Lincosamides

The patient should be monitored at frequent intervals, especially during the first 48 hours of therapy. The occurrence of any adverse reaction should be reported to the health care provider before the next dose of the drug is due. Serious adverse reactions, such as a severe hypersensitivity reaction, respiratory difficulty, severe diarrhea, or a decided drop in blood pressure, must be reported to the health care provider immediately because a serious adverse reaction may require emergency intervention.

The patient is monitored for the signs and symptoms of a bacterial or fungal superinfection, such as vaginal or anal itching, sore throat, sores in the mouth, diarrhea, fever, chills, and sore throat. Any new signs and symptoms occurring during antibiotic therapy should be reported to the health care provider, who must then decide if these problems are part of the original infection or if a superinfection has occurred.

Hyperthermia. The patient's temperature is monitored at frequent intervals, usually every 4 hours unless the patient has an elevated temperature. When the patient has an elevated temperature, temperature, pulse, and respirations are monitored every hour until the temperature returns to normal.

Diarrhea. Diarrhea may be an indication of a superinfection or pseudomembranous colitis, both of which can be serious. All stools should be inspected for the presence of blood or mucus. If diarrhea does occur and there appears to be blood and mucus in the stool, then a sample of the stool is saved and tested for occult blood using a test such as Hemoccult. If the stool tests positive for blood, then the stool is saved for possible further laboratory analysis.

A patient with diarrhea should be encouraged to drink fluids to replace those lost with the diarrhea. An accurate intake and output record must be maintained to help determine fluid balance.

Educating the Patient and Family About Tetracyclines, Macrolides, and Lincosamides

The patient and family must understand the prescribed therapeutic regimen. Often patients stop taking a prescribed drug because they feel better.

In easy-to-understand terms, the adverse reactions associated with the specific prescribed antibiotic should be explained to the patient. The patient should be told to contact the health care provider if any potentially serious adverse reactions occur, such as hypersensitivity reactions, moderate to severe diarrhea, sudden onset of chills and fever, sore throat, or sores in the mouth.

Patient Education Box 25-4 includes key points about tetracycline, macrolides, and lincosamides the patient and family members should know.

Fluoroquinolones and Aminoglycosides

As various microorganisms became resistant to antibiotics, researchers sought to develop more powerful drugs that would be effective against these resistant pathogens. The fluoroquinolones and aminoglycosides are two groups of broad-spectrum antibiotics that resulted from this research. The Summary Drug Table: Fluoroquinolones and Aminoglycosides lists the fluoroquinolones and aminoglycosides discussed in this chapter.

PATIENT EDUCATION BOX 25-4

Key Points for Patients Taking Tetracyclines, Macrolides, and Lincosamides

❑ Take the drug at the prescribed time intervals. These time intervals are important because a certain amount of the drug must be in your body at all times for the infection to be controlled.

❑ Do not increase or skip a dose unless advised to do so by your health care provider.

❑ Complete the entire course of treatment. Never stop the drug, except on the advice of your health care provider, before the course of treatment is completed even if symptoms improve or disappear. Failure to complete the prescribed course of treatment may result in a return of the infection.

❑ Take each dose with a full glass of water. Follow the directions given by your pharmacist regarding taking the drug on an empty stomach or with food.

❑ Notify your health care provider if symptoms of your infection become worse or there is no improvement in the original symptoms after approximately 5 days.

❑ Do not drink alcoholic beverages during therapy unless approved by your health care provider.

❑ If taking a tetracycline, avoid exposure to the sun or any type of tanning lamp or bed. When exposure to direct sunlight is unavoidable, completely cover your arms and legs and wear a wide-brimmed hat to protect your face and neck. Application of a sunscreen may or may not be effec-

tive. Therefore, consult your health care provider before using a sunscreen to prevent a photosensitivity reaction.

❑ Although some drugs may be taken with food or milk to minimize the risk for gastrointestinal upset, most tetracyclines, when given with foods containing calcium, such as dairy products, are not absorbed as well as when they are taken on an empty stomach. If you are taking tetracycline at home, take the drug on an empty stomach, 1 hour before or 2 hours after a meal.

In addition, you should avoid the following foods before or after taking the drug:

❑ milk (whole, low–fat, skim, condensed, or evaporated)
❑ cream (half-and-half, heavy, light)
❑ sour cream
❑ coffee creamers
❑ creamy salad dressings
❑ eggnog
❑ milkshakes
❑ cheese (natural and processed)
❑ yogurt (regular, low-fat, or nonfat)
❑ cottage cheese
❑ ice cream
❑ frozen custard
❑ frozen yogurt
❑ ice milk

SUMMARY DRUG TABLE   Fluoroquinolones and Aminoglycosides

Generic Name	Trade Name*	Uses	Adverse Reactions	Dosage Ranges
Fluoroquinolones ciprofloxacin *si-proe-flox'-a-sin*	Cipro, Cipro IV	Treatment of infections caused by susceptible microorganisms	Nausea, diarrhea, headache, abdominal discomfort, photosensitivity, superinfections, hypersensitivity reactions	250–750 mg PO q12h; 200–400 mg IV q12h
enoxacin *en-ox'-a-sin*	Penetrex	Same as ciprofloxacin	Same as ciprofloxacin	200–400 mg PO q12h
gaitfloxacin *ga-tah-flox'-a-sin*	Tequin	Same as ciprofloxacin	Same as ciprofloxacin	200–400 mg qd PO or IV
levofloxacin *lee-voe-flox'-a-sin*	Levaquin	Same as ciprofloxacin	Same as ciprofloxacin	250–500 mg/d PO, IV
lomefloxacin *loh-meh-flox'-a-sin*	Maxaquin	Same as ciprofloxacin	Same as ciprofloxacin	400 mg PO once daily
moxifloxacin *mocks-ah-flox'-a- sin*	Avelox	Same as ciprofloxacin	Same as ciprofloxacin	400 mg qd PO
norfloxacin *nor- flox'-a-sin*	Noroxin	Same as ciprofloxacin, urinary tract infections, uncomplicated gonorrhea, prostatitis	Same as ciprofloxacin	400 mg PO q12h; 800 mg as single dose for gonorrhea
ofloxacin *oe-flox'-a-sin*	Floxin	Same as ciprofloxacin	Same as ciprofloxacin	200–400 mg PO, IV q12h
trovafloxacin *troh-va-flox'-a-sin* alatrofloxacin	Trovan Trovan IV	Same as ciprofloxacin	Same as ciprofloxacin, serious liver toxicity	100–200 mg/d PO, IV
Aminoglycosides amikacin *am-i-kay'-sin*	Amikin, Amikacin, *generic*	Treatment of serious infections caused by susceptible strains of microorganisms	Nausea, vomiting, diarrhea, rash, ototoxicity, nephrotoxicity, hypersensitivity reactions, neurotoxicity, superinfections, neuromuscular blockade	15 mg/kg IM, IV, in divided doses, not to exceed 1.5 g/d
gentamicin *jen-ta-mye'-sin*	Garamycin, *generic*	Same as amikacin	Same as amikacin	3 mg/kg/d q8h IM, IV, not to exceed 5 mg/ kg/d in divided doses
kanamycin *kan-a-mye'-sin*	Kantrex, *generic*	Same as amikacin; oral use for hepatic coma and for suppression of intestinal bacteria	Same as amikacin	7.5–15 mg/kg/d in divided doses IM; 15 mg/kg/d in divided doses IV; suppression of intestinal bacteria 1 g qh for 4h then 1 g q6h for 36–72 h PO; hepatic coma 8–12 g/d in divided doses PO

Generic Name	Trade Name*	Uses	Adverse Reactions	Dosage Ranges
neomycin *nee-o-mye'-sin*	Mycifradin, Neo-Tabs, *generic*	Same as amikacin, same as kanamycin	Same as amikacin	15 mg/kg/d q6h for 4 doses, then 300 mg IM bid, not to exceed 1 g/d; preoperative preparation of the bowel, see manu- facturer's recommenda- tions for complex 3-day regimen; hepatic coma 4–12 g/d
netilmicin *ne-til-mye'-sin*	Netromycin	Same as amikacin	Same as amikacin	Up to 6.5 mg/kg/d IV in divided doses
streptomycin *strep-toe-mye'-sin*	*Generic*	Same as amikacin, fourth drug in the treatment of TB	Same as amikacin	15 mg/kg/d IM or 25–30 mg/kg IM 2–3 times per week
tobramycin *toe-bra-mye'-sin*	Nebcin, *generic*	Same as amikacin	Same as amikacin	3–5 mg/kg/d IM, IV q8h

*The term *generic* indicates the drug is available in generic form.

Actions of Fluoroquinolones

Fluoroquinolones include ciprofloxacin (Cipro), enoxacin (Penetrex), gaitfloxacin (Tequin), lomefloxacin (Maxaquin), moxifloxacin (Avelox), ofloxacin (Floxin), and sparfloxacin (Zagam).

Fluoroquinolones exert their bactericidal (bacteria-destroying) effect by interfering with an enzyme (DNA gyrase) needed by bacteria for the synthesis of DNA. This interference prevents cell reproduction, leading to death of the bacteria.

Uses of Fluoroquinolones

Fluoroquinolones are used in the treatment of infections caused by susceptible microorganisms and are effective in the treatment of infections caused by Gram-positive and Gram-negative microorganisms. They are primarily used in the treatment of susceptible microorganisms in lower respiratory infections, infections of the skin, urinary tract infections, and sexually transmitted diseases. Ciprofloxacin, norfloxacin, and ofloxacin are available in ophthalmic forms for infections in the eyes.

Adverse Reactions of Fluoroquinolones

Bacterial or fungal superinfections and pseudomembranous colitis may occur with the use of these drugs. The use of any drug may result in a hypersensitivity reaction, which can range from mild to severe and in some cases can be life-threatening. Mild hypersensitivity reactions may only require discontinuing the drug, whereas the more serious reactions require immediate treatment. (Chapter 1 discusses hypersensitivity reactions.)

More common adverse effects of these drugs include nausea, diarrhea, headache, abdominal pain or discomfort, and dizziness. A more serious adverse reaction seen with use of the fluoroquinolones, especially lomefloxacin and sparfloxacin, is a photosensitivity reaction. This is manifested by an exaggerated sunburn reaction when the skin is exposed to the ultraviolet rays of sunlight or sunlamps.

Managing Adverse Drug Reactions of Fluoroquinolones

All fluoroquinolone drugs can cause pain, inflammation, or rupture of a tendon. The Achilles tendon is particularly vulnerable. This problem can be so severe that prolonged disability results, and, at times, surgical intervention may be necessary to correct the problem. In addition, the fluoroquinolone drugs, particularly sparfloxacin and lomefloxacin, cause dangerous photosensitivity reactions. Patients have experienced severe reactions even when sunscreens or sunblocks were used.

Contraindications, Precautions, and Interactions of Fluoroquinolones

Fluoroquinolones are contraindicated in patients with a history of hypersensitivity, in children younger than 18 years, and in pregnant women (pregnancy category C). These drugs also are contraindicated in patients whose lifestyles do not allow for adherence to the precautions regarding photosensitivity.

Fluoroquinolones are used cautiously in patients with renal impairment or a history of seizures, in geriatric patients, and in patients on dialysis.

Concurrent use of fluoroquinolones with theophylline causes an increase in serum theophylline levels. When used concurrently with cimetidine, cimetidine may interfere with the elimination of fluoroquinolones. Use of fluoroquinolones with an oral anticoagulant may cause an increase in the effects of the oral coagulant. Taking fluoroquinolones with antacids, iron salts, or zinc will decrease absorption of fluoroquinolones. There is a risk of seizures if fluoroquinolones are given with the nonsteroidal anti-inflammatory drugs. There is a risk of severe cardiac arrhythmias when the fluoroquinolones, gaitfloxacin and moxifloxacin, are used with drugs that increase the QT interval (e.g., quinidine, procainamide, amiodarone, and sotalol).

Actions of Aminoglycosides

Aminoglycosides include amikacin (Amikin), gentamicin (Garamycin), kanamycin (Kantrex), neomycin (Mycifradin), netilmicin (Netromycin), streptomycin, and tobramycin (Nebcin), which exert their bactericidal effect by blocking a step in protein synthesis necessary for bacterial multiplication. They disrupt the functional ability of the bacterial cell membrane, causing cell death.

Uses of Aminoglycosides

Aminoglycosides are used in the treatment of infections caused by susceptible microorganisms, and primarily in the treatment of infections caused by Gram-negative microorganisms.

Because oral aminoglycosides are poorly absorbed, they are useful for suppressing gastrointestinal bacteria. Oral aminoglycosides kanamycin (Kantrex) and neomycin (Mycifradin) are used preoperatively to reduce the number of bacteria normally present in the intestine (**bowel prep**). A reduction in intestinal bacteria is thought to lessen the possibility of abdominal infection that may occur after surgery on the bowel.

Kanamycin, neomycin, and paromomycin are used orally in the management of hepatic coma. In this disorder, liver failure results in an elevation of blood ammonia levels. By reducing the number of ammonia-forming bacteria in the intestines, blood ammonia levels may be lowered, thereby temporarily reducing some of the symptoms associated with this disorder.

Adverse Reactions of Aminoglycosides

Aminoglycosides may cause nephrotoxicity (damage to the kidneys) and ototoxicity (damage to the organs of hearing). Signs and symptoms of nephrotoxicity may include protein in the urine (proteinuria), hematuria (blood in the urine), an elevated blood urea nitrogen level, decreased urine output, and an increase in the serum creatinine concentration. Nephrotoxicity is usually reversible once the drug is discontinued. Signs and symptoms of ototoxicity include tinnitus, dizziness, roaring in the ears, vertigo, and a mild to severe loss of hearing. If hearing loss occurs, then it is most often permanent. Ototoxicity may occur during drug therapy or even after the drug is discontinued. The short-term use of kanamycin and neomycin as a preparation for bowel surgery rarely causes these two adverse reactions.

Neurotoxicity (damage to the nervous system by a toxic substance) may also occur with aminoglycosides. Signs and symptoms of neurotoxicity include numbness, skin tingling, circumoral (around the mouth) paresthesia, peripheral paresthesia, tremors, muscle twitching, convulsions, muscle weakness, and neuromuscular blockade (acute muscular paralysis and apnea).

Additional adverse reactions of aminoglycosides may include nausea, vomiting, anorexia, rash, and urticaria. When these drugs are given, individual drug references, such as the package insert, should be consulted for more specific adverse reactions.

As with the other anti-infectives, bacterial or fungal superinfections and pseudomembranous colitis may occur with the use of these drugs. The use of aminoglycosides may result in a hypersensitivity reaction, which can range from mild to severe and in some cases can be life threatening. Mild hypersensitivity reactions may only require discontinuing the drug, whereas more serious reactions require immediate treatment.

Managing Adverse Drug Reactions of Aminoglycosides

Aminoglycosides are potentially neurotoxic, nephrotoxic, and ototoxic and are capable of causing permanent damage to these organs and structures. The health care provider should be notified immediately when one or more signs and symptoms of these adverse reactions are suspected.

Neurotoxicity. Patients should be carefully observed for symptoms such as numbness or tingling of the skin, circumoral paresthesia, peripheral paresthesia (numbness or tingling in the extremities), tremors, and muscle twitching or weakness. Any symptom of neurotoxicity should be immediately reported to the health care provider. Convulsions can occur if the drug is not discontinued.

ALERT

 Respiratory Difficulties and Aminoglycosides

Neuromuscular blockade or respiratory paralysis may occur after aminoglycosides use. Therefore, any symptoms of respiratory difficulty must be reported immediately. If neuromuscular blockade occurs, then it may be reversed by the use of calcium salts, but mechanical ventilation may be required.

Nephrotoxicity. A patient taking an aminoglycoside is at risk for nephrotoxicity. Intake and output are measured and the health care provider is notified if the patient's output is less than 750 mL/day. A record is kept of the fluid intake and output as well as daily weight to assess hydration and renal function. Fluid intake is encouraged to 2000 mL/day (if the patient's condition permits). Any changes in the intake-to-output ratio or in the appearance of the urine may indicate nephrotoxicity. Such changes should be reported to the health care provider promptly. Daily laboratory tests (i.e., serum creatinine and blood urea nitrogen [BUN]) may be ordered to monitor renal function. Any elevation in the creatinine or BUN level is reported to the health care provider because an elevation may indicate renal dysfunction.

Ototoxicity. A patient taking aminoglycosides is at risk for ototoxicity. Auditory changes are irreversible, usually bilateral, and may be partial or total. The risk is greater in patients with renal impairment or those with pre-existing hearing loss. Any problems with hearing should be reported to the health care provider because continued use could lead to permanent hearing loss.

ALERT

Ototoxicity

To detect ototoxicity, the patient's symptoms or comments related to hearing are carefully evaluated, such as a ringing or buzzing in the ears or difficulty hearing. If hearing problems do occur, then this problem should be reported to the health care provider immediately. To monitor for damage to the eighth cranial nerve, an evaluation of hearing may be performed by audiometry before and throughout the course of therapy.

Contraindications, Precautions, and Interactions of Aminoglycosides

Aminoglycosides are contraindicated in patients with hypersensitivity, and should not be given to patients requiring long-term therapy because of the potential for ototoxicity and nephrotoxicity. One exception is the use of streptomycin for long-term management of tuberculosis. These drugs are contraindicated in patients with pre-existing hearing loss, myasthenia gravis, Parkinsonism, and during lactation or pregnancy. Neomycin, amikacin, gentamicin, kanamycin, netilmicin, and tobramycin are pregnancy category D drugs; the rest are category C.

Aminoglycosides are used cautiously in patients with renal failure (dosage adjustments may be necessary), in the elderly, and in patients with neuromuscular disorders.

Use of an aminoglycoside with a cephalosporin may increase the risks of nephrotoxicity. When an aminoglycoside is used with a loop diuretic, there is an increased risk of ototoxicity (irreversible hearing loss). There is an increased risk of neuromuscular blockage (paralysis of the respiratory muscles) if an aminoglycoside is given soon after general anesthetics (neuromuscular junction blockers).

Patient Management Issues with Fluoroquinolones and Aminoglycosides

The health care provider may order culture and sensitivity tests, and the culture is obtained before the first dose of the drug is given. When an aminoglycoside is to be given, laboratory tests such as renal and hepatic function tests, complete blood count, and urinalysis also may be ordered.

When kanamycin or neomycin is given for hepatic coma, the patient's level of consciousness and ability to swallow must be evaluated. A thorough allergy history, vital signs, and signs and symptoms of infection are also noted before giving the drug.

During drug therapy with the aminoglycosides or the fluoroquinolones, the patient's initial signs and symptoms of the infection are compared to current signs and symptoms. When kanamycin or neomycin is given for hepatic coma, the patient's general condition is noted daily.

The patient's vital signs are taken every 4 hours or as ordered by the health care provider, and if there are changes in the vital signs, such as a significant drop in blood pressure, an increase in the pulse or respiratory rate, or a sudden increase in temperature, then the health care provider should be notified.

When an aminoglycoside is being used, the patient's respiratory rate must be monitored because neuromuscular blockade can occur with these drugs. Any changes in the respiratory rate or rhythm are reported to the health care provider because immediate treatment may be necessary.

Fluoroquinolones

Patients who receive a fluoroquinolone are encouraged to increase their fluid intake. Norfloxacin and enoxacin are given on an empty stomach (e.g., 1 hour before or 2 hours after meals). Ciprofloxacin and lomefloxacin can be given without regard to meals. However, the manufacturer recommends that the drug be given 2 hours after a meal. Moxifloxacin is given once per day for the period prescribed. If the patient is taking an antacid, then moxifloxacin should be administered 4 hours before or 8 hours after the antacid.

Ciprofloxacin, gaitfloxacin, and ofloxacin are the only fluoroquinolones given intravenously. None of the fluoroquinolones is given intramuscularly.

Monitoring for Hyperthermia. The infectious process in a patient is usually accompanied by an elevated temperature. When the patient is being treated for infection, vital signs, particularly the body temperature, must be monitored. As the anti-infective works to rid the body of the infectious organism, the patient's body temperature should return to normal. Vital signs (temperature, pulse, and respiration) are taken frequently to monitor the drug's effectiveness in eradicating the infectious process. The health care provider should be notified if the patient's temperature is greater than 101° Fahrenheit.

Aminoglycosides

Oral aminoglycosides are usually given without regard to meals. With the exception of paromomycin, all of the aminoglycoside drugs can be given intramuscularly, and the health care provider is notified of any persistent localized reaction of pain, redness, or extreme tenderness. With the exception of paromomycin and streptomycin, all of the aminoglycoside drugs can be given intravenously.

Hepatic Coma. When the aminoglycosides kanamycin or neomycin are given orally as treatment for hepatic coma, care is needed. During the early stages of this disorder, various changes in the patient's level of consciousness may occur. At times, the patient may appear lethargic and respond poorly to commands. Because of these changes in the level of consciousness, the patient may have difficulty swallowing, and a danger of aspiration is present. If the patient appears to have difficulty taking an oral drug, then it is withheld and the health care provider is contacted.

Managing Adverse Drug Reactions of Fluoroquinolones or Aminoglycosides

A variety of adverse reactions can occur with the fluoroquinolones or aminoglycosides. The patient is observed, especially during the first 48 hours of therapy. Any adverse reaction should be reported to the health care provider before the next dose of the drug is due. If a serious adverse reaction such as a hypersensitivity reaction, respiratory difficulty, severe diarrhea, or a drop in blood pressure occurs, then the health care provider should be contacted immediately.

Any symptoms of the patient should be reported; certain symptoms may be an early sign of an adverse drug reaction. All changes in the patient's condition and any new problems that occur (e.g., nausea or diarrhea) should be reported as soon as possible. The health care provider will decide if these changes or problems are a part of the patient's infectious process or the result of an adverse drug reaction.

Diarrhea. Because superinfections and pseudomembranous colitis can occur during therapy with these drugs, the patient's stools are checked, and any incidence of diarrhea is reported immediately because this may indicate a superinfection or pseudomembranous colitis. If diarrhea does occur and blood and mucus appear in the stool, then a sample of the stool should be saved to be tested for occult blood using a test such as Hemoccult. If the stool tests positive for blood, then the sample should be saved for possible additional laboratory tests.

Educating the Patient and Family About Fluoroquinolones and Aminoglycosides

Carefully planned patient and family education is important to encourage compliance, relieve anxiety, and promote the desired result. The patient should be advised of the signs and symptoms of potentially serious adverse reactions, such as hypersensitivity reactions, moderate to severe diarrhea, sudden onset of chills and fever, sore throat, sores in the mouth, or extreme fatigue. The patient must understand the necessity of contacting the health care provider immediately if such symptoms occur. The patient should be cautioned against the use of alcoholic beverages during therapy unless approved by the health care provider. Patient Education Box 25-5 includes key points about fluoroquinolones and aminoglycosides the patient and family members should know.

Antitubercular Drugs

Tuberculosis is a major health problem throughout the world, infecting more than 8 million individuals each year. It is one of the world's leading causes of death from infectious disease. Individuals living in crowded conditions, those with compromised immune systems, and individuals with debilitative conditions are especially susceptible to tuberculosis.

Tuberculosis is an infectious disease caused by the *Mycobacterium tuberculosis* bacillus. The disease is transmitted from one person to another by droplets dispersed in the air when an infected person coughs or sneezes. These droplet nuclei are released into the air and inhaled by noninfected persons. Although tuberculosis primarily affects the lungs, other organs may also be affected. For example, if a person's immune system is poor, then the infection can spread from the lungs to other organs of the body. Extrapulmonary (outside of the lungs) tuberculosis is the term used to distinguish tuberculosis affecting the lungs from infection with the *M. tuberculosis* bacillus in other organs of the body. Organs that can be affected include the liver, kidneys, spleen, uterus, and bones. People with acquired immunodeficiency syndrome are at risk for tuberculosis because of their compromised immune systems. Tuberculosis responds well to long-term treatment with a combination of three or more antitubercular drugs.

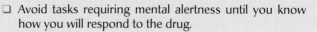

Key Points for Patients Taking Fluoroquinolones and Aminoglycosides

❑ Take the drug at the prescribed time intervals. These time intervals are important because a certain amount of the drug must be in your body at all times for the infection to be controlled.

❑ Drink six to eight large glasses of fluids while taking these drugs and take each dose with a full glass of water.

❑ Do not increase or omit the dose unless advised to do so by your health care provider.

❑ Complete the entire course of treatment. Do not stop the drug, except on the advice of your health care provider, before the course of treatment is complete even if your symptoms improve or disappear. Failure to complete the prescribed course of treatment may result in a return of the infection.

❑ Follow the directions supplied with the prescription regarding taking the drug with meals or on an empty stomach. With a drug that must be taken on an empty stomach, take it 1 hour before or 2 hours after a meal.

❑ Notify your health care provider if your symptoms of the infection become worse or do not improve after 5 to 7 days of drug therapy.

❑ Avoid any exposure to sunlight or ultraviolet light (tanning beds, sunlamps) while taking this drug and for several weeks after completing the course of therapy. Wear sunblock, sunglasses, and protective clothing when exposed to sunlight.

❑ Avoid tasks requiring mental alertness until you know how you will respond to the drug.

FLUOROQUINOLONES

❑ When taking a fluoroquinolone, report any signs of tendinitis, such as pain or soreness in your leg, shoulder, or back of your heel. Periodic applications of ice may help relieve the pain. Rest the involved area and avoid exercise.

❑ Do not take antacids or drugs containing iron or zinc because these drugs will decrease absorption of fluoroquinolones.

AMINOGLYCOSIDES

❑ Notify your health care provider if you experience any ringing in the ears or difficulty hearing, numbness or tingling around your mouth or in your extremities, or any change in your urinary pattern.

❑ When taking an aminoglycoside for preparation of the bowel before surgery, take the prescribed drug at the exact times indicated on the prescription container. Some bowel prep regimens are complex. For example, kanamycin prescribed for suppression of intestinal bacteria is taken orally every hour for 4 hours followed by 1 g every 6 hours for 36 to 72 hours.

Antitubercular drugs are used to treat active cases of tuberculosis and as a prophylactic to prevent the spread of tuberculosis. The drugs used to treat tuberculosis do not "cure" the disease, but they render the patient noninfectious to others. Antitubercular drugs are classified as primary and second-line drugs. Primary (first-line) drugs provide the foundation for treatment. Second-line or secondary drugs are less effective and more toxic than primary drugs. These drugs are used in various combinations to treat tuberculosis. Sensitivity testing may be performed to determine the most effective combination treatment, especially in areas of the country showing resistance. Second-line drugs are used to treat extrapulmonary tuberculosis or drug-resistant organisms. The primary antitubercular drugs are discussed in this section. Both primary and second-line antitubercular drugs are listed in the Summary Drug Table: Antitubercular Drugs. Certain fluoroquinolones such as ciprofloxacin, ofloxacin, levofloxacin, and sparfloxacin have proven effective against tuberculosis and are considered second-line drugs.

Actions of Antitubercular Drugs

Most antitubercular drugs are bacteriostatic (slow or retard the growth of bacteria) against the *M. tuberculosis* bacillus. These drugs usually act to inhibit bacterial cell wall synthesis, which slows the multiplication rate of the bacteria. Only isoniazid is bactericidal, with rifampin and streptomycin having some bactericidal activity.

Uses of Antitubercular Drugs

Antitubercular drugs are used in combination with other antitubercular drugs to treat active tuberculosis. Isoniazid is the only antitubercular drug used alone. Although isoniazid is used in combination with other drugs for the treatment of primary tuberculosis, a primary use is in preventive therapy (prophylaxis) against tuberculosis. For example, when a diagnosis of tuberculosis is present, family members of the infected individual must be given prophylactic treatment with isoniazid for 6 months to 1 year. Box 25-2 identifies prophylactic uses for isoniazid.

Resistance to Antitubercular Drugs

Of increasing concern is the development of mutant strains of tuberculosis that are resistant to many of the antitubercular drugs currently in use. Bacterial resistance develops, sometimes rapidly, with the use of antitubercular drugs. Treatment is individualized and based on laboratory studies identifying the drugs to which the organism is susceptible. To slow the development of

SUMMARY DRUG TABLE   Antitubercular Drugs

Generic Name	Trade Name*	Uses	Adverse Reactions	Dosage Ranges
Primary Drugs ethambutol *eth-am'-byoo-tole*	Myambutol	Pulmonary tuberculosis (TB)	Optic neuritis, fever, pruritis, headache, nausea, anorexia, dermatitis, hypersensitivity, psychic disturbances	15–25 mg/kg/d PO
isoniazid *eye-soe-nye'-a-zid*	INH, Laniazid, Nydrazid, *generic*	Active TB; prophylaxis for TB	Peripheral neuropathy, nausea, vomiting, epigastric distress, jaundice, hepatitis, pyridoxine deficiency, skin eruptions, hypersensitivity	Active TB: up to 300 mg/d PO or up to 300 mg/d IM, to 900 mg IM 2–3 times/wk; First-line treatment: 300 mg INH and 600 mg rifampin PO in single dose; TB prophylaxis: 30 mg/d PO
pyrazinamide *peer-a-zin'-a-mide*	*Generic*	Active TB	Hepatotoxicity, nausea, vomiting, diarrhea, myalgia, rashes	15–30 mg/kg/d maximum, 3 g/d PO; 50–70 mg/kg twice weekly PO
rifabutin *rif-ah-byou'-tin*	Mycobutin	Active TB	Nausea, vomiting, diarrhea, rash, discolored urine	300 mg PO as a single dose or BID
rifampin *rif-am'-pin*	Rifadin, Rimactane, *generic*	Active TB	Heartburn, drowsiness, fatigue, dizziness, epigastric distress, hematologic changes, renal insufficiency, rash	600 mg PO, IV
streptomycin *strep-toe-mye'-sin*	*Generic*	TB; infections caused by susceptible microorganisms	Nephrotoxicity, ototoxicity, numbness, tingling, paresthesia of the face, nausea, dizziness	Up to 1 g/d IM
isoniazid (150 mg) and rifampin 300 mg	Rifamate	TB	See individual drugs	1–2 tablets daily PO
Second-line Drugs aminosalicylate *a-meen-oh-sal'-sa-late* (p-aminosalicylic acid; 4-aminosalicylic acid)	Paser	TB	Nausea, vomiting, diarrhea, abdominal pain, hypersensitivity reactions	4 g (1 packet) PO TID
capreomycin sulfate *kap-ree-oh-mye'-sin*	Capastat Sulfate	TB	Hypersensitivity reactions, nephrotoxicity, hepatic impairment, pain and induration at injection site, ototoxicity	I g/d (maximum, 20 mg/kg/d) IM
cycloserine *sye-kloe-ser'-een*	Seromycin Pulvules	TB	Convulsions, somnolence, confusion, renal impairment, sudden development of congestive heart failure, psychoses	500 mg to 1 g PO in divided doses

*The term *generic* indicates the drug is available in generic form.

Box 25-2 **Prophylactic Uses for Isoniazid**

Isoniazid may be used in the following situations:
- Household members and other close associates of those with tuberculosis recently diagnosed
- Those whose tuberculin skin test has become positive in the past 2 years
- Those with positive skin tests whose radiographic findings indicate nonprogressive, healed, or quiescent (causing no symptoms) tubercular lesions
- Those at risk for tuberculosis (e.g., those with Hodgkin disease, severe diabetes mellitus, leukemia, and other serious illnesses and those receiving corticosteroids or drug therapy for a malignancy)
- All patients younger than 35 years (primarily children to age 7) who have a positive skin test
- Persons with acquired immunodeficiency syndrome or those who are positive for the human immunodeficiency virus and have a positive tuberculosis skin test or a negative tuberculosis skin test but a history of a previous significant reaction to purified protein derivative (a skin test for tuberculosis)

bacterial resistance, the Centers for Disease Control recommends the use of three or more drugs in initial therapy and retreatment. Using a combination of drugs slows the development of bacterial resistance.

Tuberculosis caused by drug-resistant organisms should be considered in patients who have no response to therapy and in patients who have been treated in the past.

Standard Treatment

The standard treatment of tuberculosis is divided into two phases: the initial phase followed by a continuing phase. During the initial phase, drugs are used to kill the rapidly multiplying *M. tuberculosis* and to prevent drug resistance. The initial phase lasts approximately 2 months and the continuing phase approximately 4 months, with the total treatment regimen lasting for 6 to 9 months, depending on the patient's response to therapy.

The initial phase must contain three or more of the following drugs: isoniazid, rifampin, and pyrazinamide, along with either ethambutol or streptomycin. The Centers for Disease Control recommends treatment to begin as soon as possible after the diagnosis of tuberculosis. The treatment recommendation regimen is for the use of rifampin, isoniazid, and pyrazinamide for a minimum of 2 months (8 weeks), followed by rifampin and isoniazid for 4 months (16 weeks) in areas with a low incidence of tuberculosis. In areas of high incidence of tuberculosis, the Centers for Disease Control recommends the addition of streptomycin or ethambutol for the first 2 months.

Retreatment

At times treatment fails because of noncompliance with the drug regimen or because of inadequate initial drug treatment. When treatment fails, retreatment is necessary. Retreatment generally includes the use of four or more antitubercular drugs. Retreatment drug regimens most often consist of the secondary drugs ethionamide, aminosalicylic acid, cycloserine, and capreomycin. Ofloxacin and ciprofloxacin may also be used in retreatment. At times during retreatment, as many as seven or more drugs may be used, with the ineffective drugs discontinued when susceptibility test results are available.

Adverse Reactions of Ethambutol

Optic neuritis (a decrease in visual acuity and changes in color perception), which appears to be related to the dose given and the duration of treatment, has occurred in some patients receiving ethambutol. Usually, this adverse reaction disappears when the drug is discontinued. Other adverse reactions are dermatitis, pruritus, **anaphylactoid reaction** (an unusual or exaggerated allergic reaction), joint pain, anorexia, nausea, and vomiting.

Any changes in visual acuity or any visual changes should be promptly reported to the health care provider. Vision changes are usually reversible if the drug is discontinued as soon as symptoms appear. The patient may need help walking and with self-care activities if visual disturbances occur. Psychic disturbances may occur. If the patient appears depressed, withdrawn, noncommunicative, or has other personality changes, then the problem must be reported to the health care provider.

Contraindications, Precautions, and Interactions of Ethambutol

Ethambutol is contraindicated in patients with a history of hypersensitivity. Ethambutol is not recommended for children younger than 13 years. The drug is used with caution during lactation, in patients with hepatic and renal impairment, and during pregnancy (category B). Because of the danger of optic neuritis, the drug is used cautiously in patients with diabetic retinopathy or cataracts.

Adverse Reactions of Isoniazid

The incidence of adverse reactions appears to be higher when larger doses of isoniazid are prescribed. Adverse reactions include hypersensitivity reactions, hematologic changes, jaundice, fever, skin eruptions, nausea, vomiting, and epigastric distress. Severe, and sometimes fatal, hepatitis has been associated with isoniazid therapy and may appear after many months of treatment. Peripheral neuropathy (numbness and tingling of the extremities) is the most common symptom of toxicity.

Because of the risk of hepatitis, patients must be carefully monitored at least monthly for any evidence of liver dysfunction. Patients should be told to report any of the following symptoms: anorexia, nausea, vomiting, fatigue, weakness, yellowing of the skin or eyes, darkening of the urine, or numbness in the hands and feet.

ALERT

‼ Older Adults and Antitubercular Drug Use

Older adults are particularly susceptible to a potentially fatal hepatitis when taking isoniazid, especially if they consume alcohol on a regular basis. Two other antitubercular drugs, rifampin and pyrazinamide, can cause liver dysfunction in older adults. Careful observation and monitoring for signs of liver impairment are necessary (e.g., increased serum aspartate transaminase, increased serum alanine transferase, increased serum bilirubin, and jaundice).

Contraindications, Precautions, and Interactions of Isoniazid

Isoniazid is contraindicated in patients with a history of hypersensitivity. The drug is used with caution during lactation, in patients with liver or kidney impairment, and during pregnancy (category C). Daily consumption of alcohol when taking isoniazid may result in a higher incidence of drug-related hepatitis. Aluminum salts may reduce the oral absorption of isoniazid. The action of the anticoagulants may be enhanced when taken with isoniazid. There is a possibility of increased serum levels of phenytoin with concurrent use of isoniazid. When isoniazid is taken with foods containing tyramine, such as aged cheese and meats, bananas, yeast products, and alcohol, an exaggerated sympathetic-type response can occur (e.g., hypertension, increased heart rate, palpitations).

Adverse Reactions of Pyrazinamide

Hepatotoxicity is the principal adverse reaction of pyrazinamide use. Symptoms of hepatotoxicity may range from none (except for slightly abnormal hepatic function tests) to a more severe reaction such as jaundice. Nausea, vomiting, diarrhea, myalgia, and rashes also may occur.

Patients should have baseline liver functions tests to use as a comparison when monitoring liver function during pyrazinamide therapy. The patient should be closely monitored for symptoms of a decline in hepatic functioning (i.e., yellowing of the skin, malaise, liver tenderness, anorexia, or nausea). The health care provider may order periodic liver function tests. Hepatotoxicity appears to be dose related and may appear at any time during therapy.

Contraindications, Precautions, and Interactions of Pyrazinamide

Pyrazinamide is contraindicated in patients with a history of hypersensitivity. The drug is also contraindicated in patients with acute gout (a metabolic disorder resulting in increased levels of uric acid) and those with severe hepatic damage. The drug is used with caution during lactation, in patients with liver or kidney renal impairment, and during pregnancy (category C). Pyrazinamide is used cautiously in patients infected with human immunodeficiency virus, who may require longer treatment, and in patients with diabetes mellitus, in whom management is more difficult. Pyrazinamide decreases the effects of allopurinol, colchicines, and probenecid.

Adverse Reactions of Rifampin

Nausea, vomiting, epigastric distress, heartburn, fatigue, dizziness, rash, hematologic changes, and renal insufficiency may occur with rifampin. Rifampin may also cause a red–orange discoloration of body fluids, including urine, tears, saliva, sweat, and sputum. The patient is advised not to wear soft contact lenses during therapy because they may be permanently stained.

Contraindications, Precautions, and Interactions of Rifampin

Rifampin is contraindicated in patients with a history of hypersensitivity. The drug is used with caution during lactation, in patients with hepatic and renal impairment, and during pregnancy. Serum concentrations of digoxin may be decreased by rifampin. Isoniazid and rifampin used concurrently may result in a higher risk of hepatotoxicity than when either drug is used alone. The use of rifampin with an oral anticoagulant or oral hypoglycemic may decrease the effects of the anticoagulant or hypoglycemic drug. There is a decrease in the effect of the oral contraceptives, chloramphenicol, phenytoin, and verapamil when these agents are used concurrently with rifampin.

Adverse Reactions of Streptomycin

Nephrotoxicity (damage to the kidneys), ototoxicity (damage to the organs of hearing by a toxic substance), numbness, tingling, tinnitus (ringing in the ears), nausea, vomiting, vertigo (dizziness), and circumoral (around the mouth) paresthesia may occur with streptomycin. Soreness at the injection site may also be noted, especially when the drug is given for a long time.

This drug may cause ototoxicity, resulting in hearing loss. Any signs of hearing loss, including tinnitus, and vertigo should be reported. Patients may have their hearing checked by audiometry before beginning therapy and periodically during therapy. Tinnitus, roaring noises, or a sense of fullness in the ears indicates the need for audiometric examination or termination of the drug. Hearing loss occurs most often for high-frequency sounds. These drugs must be discontinued if the patient reports any hearing loss or if tinnitus occurs. Prompt action is critical for preventing permanent hearing loss.

Contraindications, Precautions, and Interactions of Streptomycin

Streptomycin is contraindicated in patients with a history of hypersensitivity to the drug or any other aminoglycosides. Streptomycin is a pregnancy category D drug and can cause fetal harm when given to a pregnant woman. This drug is used cautiously in patients with pre-existing hearing difficulty or tinnitus and in patients with renal insufficiency. The ototoxic effects of streptomycin are potentiated when taken with ethacrynic acid, furosemide, or mannitol.

Patient Management Issues with Antitubercular Drugs

Once the diagnosis of tuberculosis is confirmed, the health care provider selects the drug that will best control the spread of the disease and make the patient noninfectious to others. Many laboratory and diagnostic tests may be necessary before starting antitubercular therapy, including radiographic studies, culture and sensitivity tests, and various types of laboratory tests, such as a complete blood count. A family history and a history of contacts are included in the assessment if the patient has active tuberculosis.

Directly Observed Therapy

Because the antitubercular drugs must be taken for prolonged periods, compliance with the treatment regimen becomes a problem and increases the risk of the development of resistant strains of tuberculosis. To help prevent the problem of noncompliance, the patient makes periodic visits to the office of the health care provider or the health clinic, where the drug is taken in the presence of a health care worker. The patient is observed swallowing each dose of the medication regimen. In some cases, the antitubercular drug is given under observation in the patient's home, place of employment, or school. Directly observed therapy may occur daily or two to three times weekly, depending on the patient's health care regimen.

Treatment Regimens

Ethambutol. Ethambutol is given once every 24 hours at the same time each day with food to prevent gastric upset. The patient should be told that

the urine, feces, saliva, sputum, sweat, and tears may be colored red–orange or brown–orange and that this is normal.

Isoniazid. Isoniazid is given to the patient whose stomach is empty, at least 1 hour before or 2 hours after meals. If gastrointestinal upset occurs, then the patient can take the drug with food. The patient is reminded to minimize alcohol consumption because of the increased risk of hepatitis.

Pyrazinamide. This drug is given once per day with food to prevent gastric upset. An alternative dosing regimen of twice-weekly dosing has been developed to promote patient compliance on an outpatient basis.

Rifampin. Rifampin is taken once daily on an empty stomach, at least 1 hour before or 2 hours after meals. Patients should be told that their urine, feces, saliva, sputum, sweat, and tears may be colored red–orange and that this is normal.

Streptomycin. Streptomycin is usually given daily as a single intramuscular injection. In patients 60 years of age or older, the dosage is reduced because of the risk of increased toxicity.

Educating the Patient and Family About Antitubercular Drugs

Antitubercular drugs are given for a long time, and careful patient and family education and close medical supervision are necessary. Noncompliance can be a problem whenever a disease or disorder requires long-term treatment. For this reason, the directly observed therapy method is preferred. The patient and family must understand that short-term therapy is of no value in treating this disease. Any statements the patient or family makes that suggest the patient may not be compliant should be reported to the health care provider.

The dosage schedule and adverse reactions associated with the prescribed antitubercular drug are reviewed with the patient and family. Patient Education Box 25-6 includes key points the patient and family members should know.

Leprostatic Drugs

Leprosy is a chronic, communicable disease spread by prolonged, intimate contact with an infected person. Peripheral nerves and skin are affected. Lesions may be confined to a few isolated areas or may be fairly widespread over the entire body. Leprostatic drugs generally control the disease and prevent complications.

Leprosy, also referred to as Hansen disease, is caused by the bacterium *Mycobacterium leprae*. Although rare in colder climates, this disease may occur in tropical and

Key Points for Patients Taking Antitubercular Drugs

❑ The results of your antitubercular therapy must be monitored at periodic intervals. Laboratory and diagnostic tests and visits to your health care provider's office or clinic are necessary.

❑ Take these drugs exactly as directed on the prescription container. Do not skip, increase, or decrease a dose unless advised to do so by your health care provider.

❑ Do not use nonprescription drugs, especially those containing aspirin, unless use is approved by your health care provider.

❑ Discuss alcoholic beverages with your health care provider. A limited amount of alcohol may be allowed, but excessive intake usually must be avoided.

ETHAMBUTOL

❑ Take this drug once per day at the same time each day. If you miss a dose, do not double the dose the next day. Notify your health care provider if you experience any changes in vision or a skin rash.

ISONIAZID

❑ Take this drug 1 hour before or 2 hours after meals. However, if you experience gastric upset, take isoniazid with food.

❑ Notify your health care provider if you experience weakness, yellowing of your skin, loss of appetite, darkening of your urine, skin rashes, or numbness or tingling of your hands or feet.

❑ Avoid tyramine-containing foods, such as coffee, tea, colas, red wine, and certain dairy products; ask your health care provider for a list of foods not to eat.

❑ To prevent pyridoxine (vitamin B6) deficiency, 6 to 50 mg of pyridoxine daily may be prescribed.

PYRAZINAMIDE

❑ Notify your health care provider if you experience any of the following: nausea, vomiting, loss of appetite, fever, malaise, visual changes, yellow discoloration of your skin, or severe pain in your knees, feet, or wrists.

RIFAMPIN

❑ Take the drug once daily on an empty stomach (1 hour before or 2 hours after meals).

❑ A red–brown or red–orange discoloration of tears, sputum, urine, or sweat may occur.

❑ Soft contact lenses may be permanently stained if you wear them while taking the drug. Talk to your eye doctor about wearing glasses during this time.

❑ Notify your health care provider if you experience any yellow discoloration of your skin, fever, chills, unusual bleeding or bruising, and skin rash or itching.

❑ If you are taking an oral contraceptive, check with your ealth care provider because reliability of the contraceptive may be affected.

---

subtropical zones. Dapsone and clofazimine (Lamprene) are the two drugs currently used to treat leprosy. They are described in the Summary Drug Table: Leprostatic Drugs.

Actions and Uses of Clofazimine

Clofazimine is primarily bactericidal against *M. leprae*. The exact mode of action of this drug is unknown. Clofazimine is used to treat leprosy.

Adverse Reactions of Clofazimine

Clofazimine may cause pigmentation of the skin, abdominal pain, diarrhea, nausea, and vomiting.

Contraindications, Precautions, and Interactions of Clofazimine

Clofazimine is used cautiously in patients with gastrointestinal disorders, diarrhea, and during pregnancy (pregnancy category C) and lactation. If clofazimine is

SUMMARY DRUG TABLE   Leprostatic Drugs

Generic Name	Trade Name*	Uses	Adverse Reactions	Dosage Ranges
clofazimine *kloe-fazz-ih-meen*	Lamprene	Leprosy	Skin pigmentation (pink to brown–black), skin dryness, rash, abdominal/epigastric pain, nausea, dryness, burning, or itching of the eyes	100–200 mg/d PO
dapsone *dap'-sone*	*Generic*	Leprosy; dermatitis herpetiformis	Blood cell hemolysis, anemia, peripheral neuropathy, headache, insomnia, phototoxicity, nausea, vomiting, anorexia, blurred vision	50–300 mg/d PO

*The term *generic* indicates the drug is available in generic form.

used during pregnancy, then the infant may be born with pigmented skin. No significant drug–drug interactions are associated with the use of clofazimine.

Actions and Uses of Dapsone

Dapsone is bactericidal and bacteriostatic against *M. leprae*. The drug is used to treat leprosy. Dapsone may also be used in the treatment of dermatitis herpetiformis, a chronic, inflammatory skin disease.

Adverse Reactions of Dapsone

Use of dapsone may result in hemolysis (destruction of red blood cells), nausea, vomiting, anorexia, and blurred vision.

Contraindications, Precautions, and Interactions of Dapsone

Dapsone is used with caution in patients with anemia, severe cardiopulmonary disease, hepatic dysfunction, and during pregnancy (pregnancy category C). Dapsone is contraindicated during lactation. Substantial amounts of dapsone are excreted in breast milk and can cause hemolytic reactions in neonates. No significant drug–drug interactions are associated with the use of dapsone.

Patient Management Issues with Leprostatic Drugs

These drugs are often given on an outpatient basis. Treatment with a leprostatic drug may require many years. These patients are faced with long-term medical and drug therapy and possibly severe disfigurement.

Leprostatic drugs are given orally and with food to minimize gastric upset. Antitubercular drugs, such as rifampin, can be given concurrently during initial therapy to minimize bacterial resistance to the leprostatic drug.

Educating the Patient and Family About Leprostatic Drugs

Compliance can be a problem with the long-term treatment regimen. Depression or indifference may indicate treatment noncompliance. Patient education emphasizes the treatment regimen, the dosage schedule, possible adverse effects, and the importance of scheduled follow-up visits.

The patient should be told that changes in skin pigmentation might occur, ranging from red to brown–black. Skin discoloration may take months to years to reverse after use of the drug is discontinued.

Miscellaneous Anti-Infectives

The anti-infectives discussed in this section are singular drugs; that is, they are not related to each other and do not belong to any one of the drug groups discussed earlier in the chapter. Some of these drugs are used only for the treatment of one type of infection, whereas others may be limited to the treatment of serious infections not treatable by other anti-infectives (see Summary Drug Table: Miscellaneous Anti-Infectives).

Actions and Uses of Chloramphenicol

Chloramphenicol (Chloromycetin) interferes with or inhibits protein synthesis, a process necessary for the growth and multiplication of microorganisms. This is a potentially dangerous drug (see below), and therefore its use is limited to serious infections when less potentially dangerous drugs are ineffective or contraindicated.

Adverse Reactions of Chloramphenicol

Serious and sometimes fatal blood dyscrasias (a pathologic disorder of cellular elements of blood) are the chief adverse reaction seen with the use of chloramphenicol. In addition, superinfection, hypersensitivity reactions, nausea, vomiting, and headache may occur. Patients receiving oral chloramphenicol are often hospitalized so that frequent blood studies can be performed during treatment with this drug.

Contraindications, Precautions, and Interactions of Chloramphenicol

Chloramphenicol is contraindicated in patients with known hypersensitivity. This drug is used cautiously in patients with severe liver or kidney disease, in geriatric patients, in individuals with glucose-6-phosphate dehydrogenase deficiency, and during pregnancy (category C) or lactation. Newborns are at increased risk for experiencing adverse reactions because of their inability to metabolize and excrete chloramphenicol.

The effects of oral hypoglycemic drugs, oral anticoagulants, and phenytoin may be increased when taken with chloramphenicol. Phenobarbital or rifampin may decrease chloramphenicol blood levels.

Actions and Uses of Linezolid

Linezolid (Zyvox) is the first of a new classification, an oxazolidinone, that acts by binding to a site on a specific ribosomal RNA and preventing the formation of a component necessary for the bacteria to replicate. It is both bacteriostatic (to enterococci and staphylococci)

SUMMARY DRUG TABLE   Miscellaneous Anti-Infectives

Generic Name	Trade Name*	Uses	Adverse Reactions	Dosage Ranges
chloramphenicol *klor-am-fen'-i-kole*	Chloromycetin, *generic*	Serious, susceptible infections in which other less potentially dangerous drugs are ineffective or contraindicated	Serious to fatal blood dyscrasias, superinfections, hypersensitivity, nausea, vomiting, headache	50 mg/kg/d PO, IV in divided doses
linezolid *lah-nez'-oh-lid*	Zyvox	Infections caused by vancomycin-resistant *Enterococcus faecium*; pneumonia caused by *Staphylococcus aureus* and penicillin-susceptible *Streptococcus pneumoniae*; skin and skin structure infections	Nausea, diarrhea, headache, insomnia, pseudomembranous colitis	600 mg PO or IV q12h
meropenem *meh-row-pen'-em*	Merrem IV	Intra-abdominal and soft tissue infections caused by multiresistant Gram-negative organisms	Headache, diarrhea, abdominal pain, nausea, pain and inflammation at injection site, pseudomembranous colitis	1 g IV q8h
metronidazole *me-troe-nid'-uh- zole*	Flagyl, Protostat, *generic*	Infections caused by susceptible anaerobic microorganisms, amebiasis, trichomonas	Nausea, diarrhea, anorexia, seizures, numbness, hyper-sensitivity reactions, disulfiram-like reactions with alcohol ingestion	7.5–15 mg/kg IV q6h; 7.5 mg/kg PO q6h
pentamidine isethionate *pen-tam'-ih-deen ice-uh-thigh'-uh-nate*	NebuPent, Pentam 300	*Pneumocystis carinii* pneumonia (PCP) (IM, IV); prevention of PCP (inhalation)	Nausea, anxiety, anorexia, headache, metallic taste in mouth, chills, severe hypotension, leukopenia, hypoglycemia, thrombocytopenia	4 mg/kg IM, IV once per day; 300 mg once every 4 wk by nebulizer
spectinomycin *spek-tin-oe-mye'-cin*	Trobicin	Gonorrhea	Soreness at injection site, urticaria, dizziness, rash, chills, fever, hypersensitivity reactions	2 g IM as single dose; up to 4 g IM
vancomycin *van-koe-mye'-cin*	Vancocin, Vancoled, *generic*	Serious susceptible Gram-positive infections not responding to treatment with other antibiotics	Nephrotoxicity, ototoxicity, nausea, chills, fever, urticaria, sudden fall in blood pressure, redness on face, neck, arms, and back	500 mg to 2 g/d PO in divided doses; 500 mg IV q6h or 1 g IV q8–12h

*The term *generic* indicates the drug is available in generic form.

and bacteriocidal (against streptococci). The drug is used in the treatment of vancomycin-resistant enterococcus, nosocomial (hospital-acquired) and community-acquired pneumonia, and skin and skin structure infections, including those caused by methicillin-resistant *Staphylococcus aureus*.

Adverse Reactions of Linezolid

The most common adverse reactions include nausea, vomiting, diarrhea, headache, and insomnia. The drug may also cause fatigue, depression, nervousness, and photosensitivity. Pseudomembranous colitis and thrombocytopenia are the more serious adverse reactions caused by linezolid.

Contraindications, Precautions, and Interactions of Linezolid

The drug is contraindicated in those allergic to it, in pregnancy (category C) and lactation, and in those with phenylketonuria (oral form only). Linezolid is used cautiously in patients with bone marrow depression, hepatic dysfunction, renal impairment, hypertension, or hyperthyroidism.

When linezolid is used with antiplatelet drugs such as aspirin or nonsteroidal anti-inflammatory drugs, there is an increased risk of bleeding and thrombocytopenia. When administered with the monoamine oxidase inhibitors (see Chapter 10), the effects of the monoamine oxidase inhibitors are decreased. There is a risk of severe hypertension if linezolid is combined with large amounts of food containing tyramine (e.g., aged cheese, caffeinated beverages, yogurt, chocolate, red wine, beer, pepperoni).

Actions and Uses of Meropenem

Meropenem (Merrem IV) inhibits synthesis of the bacterial cell wall and causes the death of susceptible cells. This drug is used for intra-abdominal infections caused by *Pseudomonas aeruginosa, Escherichia coli, Klebsiella pneumoniae,* and other susceptible organisms. Meropenem also is effective against bacterial meningitis caused by *Neisseria meningitidis, Streptococcus pneumoniae,* and *Haemophilus influenzae*.

Adverse Reactions of Meropenem

The most common adverse reactions of meropenem include headache, nausea, vomiting, diarrhea, anorexia, abdominal pain, generalized pain, flatulence, rash, and superinfections. This drug also can cause an abscess or phlebitis at the injection site.

Contraindications, Precautions, and Interactions of Meropenem

Meropenem is contraindicated in patients who are allergic to cephalosporins and penicillins and in patients with renal failure. This drug is not recommended in children younger than 3 months or for women during pregnancy (category B) or lactation. Meropenem is used cautiously in patients with central nervous system disorders, seizure disorders, or kidney or liver failure. When taken with probenecid, the excretion of meropenem is inhibited.

Actions and Uses of Metronidazole

The action of metronidazole (Flagyl) is not well-understood, but it is thought to disrupt DNA and protein synthesis in susceptible organisms. This drug may be used in the treatment of serious infections, such as intra-abdominal, bone, soft tissue, lower respiratory, gynecologic, and central nervous system infections caused by susceptible **anaerobic** (able to live without oxygen) microorganisms. It is also used for amebiasis and trichomonas.

Adverse Reactions of Metronidazole

The most common adverse reactions are related to the gastrointestinal tract and may include nausea, anorexia, and occasionally vomiting and diarrhea. The most serious adverse reactions involve the central nervous system and include seizures and numbness of the extremities. Hypersensitivity reactions also may be seen. Thrombophlebitis may occur with intravenous use of the drug.

Contraindications, Precautions, and Interactions of Metronidazole

This drug is contraindicated in patients with known hypersensitivity and during the first trimester of pregnancy (category B). This drug is used cautiously in patients with blood dyscrasias, seizure disorders, or liver dysfunction. Safety in children (other than orally for amebiasis) has not been established.

The metabolism of metronidazole may decrease when used with cimetidine. When used with phenobarbital, the effectiveness of metronidazole may decrease. When metronidazole is taken with warfarin, the effectiveness of the warfarin is increased.

Actions and Uses of Pentamidine Isethionate

Pentamidine isethionate (Pentam 300, the parenteral form; NebuPent, the aerosol form) is used in the treatment (parenteral form) or prevention (aerosol form) of *Pneumocystis carinii* pneumonia, which occurs in those with AIDS. The action of this drug is not fully understood.

Adverse Reactions of Pentamidine Isethionate

More than half of the patients receiving this drug by the parenteral route experience some adverse reaction. Severe and sometimes life-threatening reactions include leukopenia (low white blood cell count), hypoglycemia (low blood sugar), thrombocytopenia (low platelet count), and hypotension (low blood pressure). Moderate or less severe reactions include changes in some laboratory tests, such as the serum creatinine and liver function tests. Other adverse reactions include anxiety, headache, hypotension, chills, nausea, and anorexia. Aerosol use may result in fatigue, a metallic taste in the mouth, shortness of breath, and anorexia.

Contraindications, Precautions, and Interactions of Pentamidine Isethionate

This drug is contraindicated in individuals with hypersensitivity. Pentamidine isethionate is used cautiously in patients with hypertension, hypotension, hyperglycemia, renal impairment, diabetes mellitus, liver impairment, bone marrow depression, pregnancy (category C), or lactation.

An additive nephrotoxicity develops when pentamidine isethionate is used with other nephrotoxic drugs (e.g., aminoglycosides, vancomycin, or amphotericin B). An additive bone marrow depression occurs when the drug is used with antineoplastic drugs or when the patient has received radiation therapy recently.

Actions and Uses of Spectinomycin

Spectinomycin (Trobicin) is chemically related to but different from the aminoglycosides. This drug exerts its action by interfering with bacterial protein synthesis. Spectinomycin is used for the treatment of gonorrhea.

Adverse Reactions of Spectinomycin

Soreness at the injection site, urticaria, dizziness, rash, chills, fever, and hypersensitivity reactions may occur with this drug.

Contraindications, Precautions, and Interactions of Spectinomycin

This drug is contraindicated in known cases of hypersensitivity and in infants. If another sexually transmitted disease is present with gonorrhea, then additional anti-infectives may be needed to eradicate the infectious processes. Safe use during pregnancy (category B) or lactation and in children has not been established.

No known significant drug or food interactions for spectinomycin are known.

Actions and Uses of Vancomycin

Vancomycin (Vancocin) acts against susceptible Gram-positive bacteria by inhibiting bacterial cell wall synthesis and increasing cell wall permeability. This drug is used in the treatment of serious Gram-positive infections that do not respond to treatment with other anti-infectives. It also may be used in treating anti-infective–associated pseudomembranous colitis caused by *Clostridium difficile*.

Adverse Reactions of Vancomycin

Nephrotoxicity (damage to the kidneys) and ototoxicity (damage to the organs of hearing) may occur with this drug. Additional adverse reactions include nausea, chills, fever, urticaria, sudden fall in blood pressure with parenteral use, and skin rashes.

Contraindications, Precautions, and Interactions of Vancomycin

This drug is contraindicated in patients with known hypersensitivity. Vancomycin is used cautiously in patients with renal or hearing impairment and during pregnancy (category C) and lactation.

When used with other ototoxic and nephrotoxic drugs, additive effects may occur.

Patient Management Issues with Miscellaneous Anti-Infectives

Before beginning use of these drugs, the patient's vital signs are taken. A thorough allergy history is taken, especially a history of drug allergies. When culture and sensitivity tests are ordered, these procedures must be performed before the first dose of the drug is given. Other laboratory tests such as renal and hepatic function tests, complete blood count, and urinalysis also may be ordered before and during drug therapy for early detection of toxic reactions.

The patient's vital signs are monitored every 4 hours or as ordered by the health care provider, who should be notified if there are changes in the vital signs, such as a significant drop in blood pressure, an increase in the pulse or respiratory rate, or a sudden increase in temperature.

The patient is monitored at frequent intervals, especially during the first 48 hours of therapy. Any adverse reaction should be reported to the health care provider before the next dose of the drug is due.

Chloramphenicol

The oral drug is given when the patient's stomach is empty, 1 hour before or 2 hours after meals. If gastrointestinal distress occurs, then it is acceptable to give the drug with food.

Linezolid

The drug is given orally or intravenously. When the drug is taken orally, it is taken every 12 hours and may be taken with or without food. If nausea develops, then the drug may be taken with food. Foods high in tyramine (see Chapter 5) are avoided because of the risk of hypertension. The patient's platelet count must be monitored regularly, particularly if the drug is used for longer than 2 weeks.

Meropenem

This drug is used only by the intravenous route.

Metronidazole

The oral form is given with meals to avoid gastrointestinal upset. The patient is informed that an unpleasant metallic taste may be noted. The patient should be advised to avoid alcoholic beverages during and for at least 1 day after treatment. When metronidazole is mixed with alcohol, the patient may experience flushing, nausea, vomiting, headache, and abdominal cramping.

Patients being treated for gynecologic infections, such as trichomoniasis, should be told that sexual contact with infected partners may lead to reinfection, so sexual partners must be treated concurrently.

Pentamidine Isethionate

This drug may be given by aerosol, and the nebulizer should be explained or demonstrated to the patient. Blood pressure is monitored frequently during use because sudden, severe hypotension may occur. Because hypotension can occur after a single dose, the patient should be lying down when the drug is given. The patient is monitored for signs of hypoglycemia (weakness, diaphoresis, cool skin, shakiness) and hyperglycemia (flushed dry skin, fruity breath odor, increased thirst, and increased urination).

Spectinomycin

The patient is told the importance of following the health care provider's recommendation regarding a follow-up examination to determine if the infection has been eliminated. All sexual contacts need to receive treatment.

Vancomycin

Vancomycin can be taken orally or by intermittent intravenous infusion.

Managing Adverse Reactions of Miscellaneous Anti-Infectives

Diarrhea. Diarrhea may be a sign of a superinfection or pseudomembranous colitis, both of which are adverse reactions that may be seen with the use of any anti-infective. Each stool is checked, and any changes in color or consistency are reported. When vancomycin is given as part of the treatment for pseudomembranous colitis, it is important that the color and consistency of each stool is recorded to determine the effectiveness of therapy.

Pain. Pain at the injection site may occur when these drugs are given intramuscularly. The patient is warned that discomfort may be felt when it is injected and that additional discomfort may be experienced for a brief time afterward. A warm moist compress placed over the injection site helps alleviate the discomfort.

Nephrotoxicity and Ototoxicity

Nephrotoxicity must be monitored. Any changes in the patient's intake and output ratio or in the appearance of the urine must be reported immediately because these may indicate nephrotoxicity.

Ototoxicity is also closely monitored in all patients receiving an anti-infective. Any ringing in the ears, difficulty hearing, or dizziness should be reported to the health care provider. Changes in hearing may not be noticed initially by the patient, but when changes occur they usually progress from difficulty in hearing high-pitched sounds to problems hearing low-pitched sounds.

Educating the Patient and Family About Miscellaneous Anti-Infectives

When pentamidine is prescribed for aerosol use at home, the use of the special nebulizer is explained, as well as directions for cleaning and maintaining the nebulizer equipment.

When metronidazole is prescribed, the patient is advised to avoid the use of alcoholic beverages because a severe reaction may occur.

Patient Education Box 25-7 includes key points about miscellaneous anti-infective drugs that the patient and family members should know.

KEY POINTS

⬤ Sulfonamides are primarily bacteriostatic. They are used to control urinary tract infections and to treat second- and third-degree burns. Hematologic changes may occur during sulfonamide therapy, including agranulocytosis, thrombocytopenia, aplastic anemia, and leukopenia. Sulfonamides are contraindicated in patients with known hypersensitivity, during lactation, and in children younger than 2 years old.

⬤ Penicillins may be used to treat infections such as urinary tract infections, septicemia, meningitis, intraabdominal infection, gonorrhea, syphilis, pneumonia, and other respiratory infections. Health care providers occasionally prescribe penicillin as prophylaxis against a potential secondary bacterial infection that can occur in a patient with a viral infection. Common adverse reactions include mild nausea, vomiting, diarrhea, sore tongue or mouth, fever, and pain at injection site. Penicillins are contraindicated in patients with a history of hypersensitivity to penicillin or cephalosporins, and should be used cautiously in patients with renal disease, during pregnancy (pregnancy category C) and lactation (may cause diarrhea or candidiasis in the infant), and in those with a history of allergies.

⬤ Cephalosporins are effective in the treatment of almost all of the strains of bacteria affected by the penicillins, as well as some strains of bacteria that have become resistant to penicillin. Cephalosporins are usually bactericidal and are used to treat infections caused by susceptible microorganisms, including streptococci, staphylococci, citrobacters, gonococci, shigella, and clostridia. The most common adverse reactions of cephalosporins are gastrointestinal disturbances, such as nausea, vomiting, and diarrhea. Cephalosporins should not be used if the patient has a history of allergies to cephalosporins or penicillins, and should be used cautiously in patients with renal or hepatic impairment and in patients with bleeding disorders.

⬤ Tetracyclines are used in select infections when the organism shows sensitivity to them, such as in cholera, Rocky Mountain spotted fever, and typhus. Gastrointestinal reactions that may occur during tetracycline use include nausea, vomiting, diarrhea, epigastric distress, stomatitis, and sore throat. Skin rashes also may occur. Tetracyclines are contraindicated if the patient is known to be hypersensitive and during pregnancy.

⬤ Macrolides are effective against a wide variety of pathogenic organisms, particularly infections of the respiratory and genital tract. Adverse reactions of azithromycin and clarithromycin are related to the gastrointestinal tract and include nausea, vomiting, diarrhea, and abdominal pain. These drugs are contraindicated in patients with hypersensitivity and patients with pre-existing liver disease.

⬤ Lincosamides, another group of anti-infectives, are effective against many Gram-positive organisms, such as streptococci and staphylococci. Because of their high potential for toxicity, lincosamides are usually used only for the treatment of serious infections in which penicillin or erythromycin (a macrolide) is not effective. Abdominal pain, esophagitis, nausea, vomiting, diarrhea, skin rash, and blood dyscrasias may occur with lincosamides. Lincosamides are contraindicated in patients with hypersensitivity, those with minor bacterial or viral infections, and during lactation and infancy.

⬤ Fluoroquinolones are primarily used in the treatment of susceptible microorganisms in lower respiratory infections, infections of the skin, urinary tract infections, and sexually transmitted diseases. Bacterial or fungal superinfections and pseudomembranous colitis may occur with the use of both of these drugs. Fluoroquinolones are contraindicated in patients with a history of hypersensitivity, in children younger than 18 years, and in pregnant women (pregnancy category C). Aminoglycosides are used in the treatment of infections caused by susceptible microorganisms, primarily Gramnegative microorganisms. Aminoglycosides may cause nephrotoxicity or ototoxicity. Aminoglycosides are contraindicated in patients with hypersensitivity and should not be given to patients requiring long-term therapy because of the potential for ototoxicity and nephrotoxicity. One exception is the use of streptomycin for long-term management of tuberculosis.

◉ Antitubercular drugs are used in combination with other antitubercular drugs to treat active tuberculosis. Optic neuritis, which appears to be related to the dose given and the duration of treatment, has occurred in some patients receiving ethambutol. Ethambutol is contraindicated in patients with a history of hypersensitivity. Ethambutol is not recommended for children younger than 13 years. With isoniazid use, the incidence of adverse reactions appears to be higher when larger doses are prescribed. Adverse reactions include hypersensitivity reactions, hematologic changes, jaundice, fever, skin eruptions, nausea, vomiting, and epigastric distress. Isoniazid is contraindicated in patients with a history of hypersensitivity. Hepatotoxicity is the principal adverse reaction seen with pyrazinamide use. Pyrazinamide is contraindicated in patients with a history

of hypersensitivity or acute gout. Nausea, vomiting, epigastric distress, heartburn, fatigue, dizziness, rash, hematologic changes, and renal insufficiency may occur with rifampin. Rifampin is contraindicated in patients with a history of hypersensitivity. The drug is used with caution during lactation, in patients with hepatic and renal impairment, and during pregnancy. Streptomycin may cause ototoxicity, resulting in hearing loss. Streptomycin is contraindicated in patients with a history of hypersensitivity to the drug or any other aminoglycosides.

◉ Clofazimine and dapsone is used to treat leprosy and may cause pigmentation of the skin, abdominal pain, diarrhea, nausea, and vomiting. Clofazimine is used cautiously in patients with gastrointestinal disorders, diarrhea, and during pregnancy (pregnancy category C) and lactation. Use of dapsone may result in hemolysis, nausea, vomiting, anorexia, and blurred vision. Dapsone is used with caution in patients with anemia, severe cardiopulmonary disease, or hepatic dysfunction, and during pregnancy (pregnancy category C).

◉ Miscellaneous anti-infectives include chloramphenicol, linezolid, meropenem, metronidazole, pentamidine isethionate, spectinomycin, and vancomycin. Some of these drugs are used only for the treatment of one type of infection, whereas others may be limited to the treatment of serious infections not treatable by other anti-infectives. Headache, nausea, and vomiting are common shared adverse reactions to miscellaneous anti-infectives. All of the miscellaneous anti-infectives are contraindicated in patients with known hypersensitivity.

CASE STUDY

Ms. Bartlett, age 80, has been prescribed a sulfonamide (Gantanol) for a urinary tract infection and is to take the drug for 10 days. You note that Ms. Bartlett seems forgetful and at times confused.

1. Ms. Bartlett's forgetfulness could be important to her drug regimen because:
    a. taking a sulfonamide with a full glass of water is an important part of treatment
    b. the drug should not be discontinued until the full course of therapy is complete
    c. the drug should be taken either 1 hour before or 2 hours after a meal
    d. all of the above

2. Ms. Bartlett is interested in whether there are potential adverse reactions with this drug. You tell her:
    a. she will sleep much more than normal
    b. her skin will burn quickly in the sun
    c. she will likely be hungrier than usual
    d. she may have allergic reactions

3. Ms. Bartlett holds is taking other medications, including an anticoagulant. Her health care provider may adjust her dosage because:
    a. Gantanol may enhance the action of the anticoagulant
    b. Gantanol may diminish the action of the anticoagulant
    c. the anticoagulant may enhance the action of Gantanol
    d. the anticoagulant may diminish the action of Gantanol

WEBSITE ACTIVITIES

1. Go to the MEDLINEplus website (http:/medlineplus.gov/) and click on "Drug Information." Search for information on tetracycline. (The site uses the term "MED Master" for the main entry on the drug.) What nine types of questions does the site answer about tetracycline?

1. _____

2. _____

3. _____

4. _____

5. _____

6. _____

7. _____

8. _____

9. _____

2. What important warning does this page make about tetracycline?

REVIEW QUESTIONS

1. Mr. Thomas, who is receiving oral penicillin, reports he has a sore mouth and shows you his bright red oral mucous membranes. The health care provider should be notified immediately because these symptoms may be caused by:
   a. a vitamin C deficiency
   b. a superinfection
   c. dehydration
   d. poor oral hygiene

2. Common adverse reactions to cephalosporin include:
   a. hypotension, dizziness, urticaria
   b. nausea, vomiting, diarrhea
   c. skin rash, constipation, headache
   d. bradycardia, pruritus, insomnia

3. A patient asks why her health care provider prescribed an antibiotic when she was told that she has a viral infection. The most correct response is that the antibiotic may be used to prevent a:
   a. primary fungal infection
   b. repeat viral infection
   c. secondary bacterial infection
   d. breakdown of the immune system

4. Patients taking a fluoroquinolone are encouraged to:
   a. nap 1 to 2 hours daily while taking the drug
   b. eat a high-protein diet

c. increase their fluid intake

   d. avoid foods high in carbohydrates

5. When being given spectinomycin for gonorrhea, Mr. Jackson is advised to:

   a. return for a follow-up examination

   b. limit his fluid intake to 1200 mL per day while taking the drug

   c. return the next day for a second injection

   d. avoid drinking alcohol for the next 10 days

6. Which of the following drugs is the only antitubercular drug to be prescribed alone?

   a. rifampin

   b. pyrazinamide

   c. streptomycin

   d. isoniazid

7. Which of the following hematologic changes may result from the use of dapsone?

   a. hemolysis

   b. leukopenia

   c. decreased platelets

   d. increase in the hematocrit

26 Other Anti-Infective Drugs

KEY TERMS

amebiasis—invasion of the body by the ameba *Entamoeba histolytica*
anthelmintic—drugs with actions against helminths
cinchonism—a group of symptoms associated with quinine, including tinnitus, dizziness, headache, gastrointestinal disturbances, and visual disturbances
fungicidal—able to destroy fungi
fungistatic—able to slow or retard the multiplication of fungi
fungus—a colorless plant that lacks chlorophyll
helminthiasis—invasion of the body by helminths (worms)
helminths—worms
mycotic infection—a superficial or deep infection caused by a fungi disease in humans that may be yeast-like or mold-like
onychomycosis—nail fungus condition
parasite—an organism that lives in or on another organism (the host) without contributing to the survival or well-being of the host
tinea corporis—ringworm
tinea cruris—jock itch
tinea pedis—athlete's foot

CHAPTER OBJECTIVES

On completion of this chapter, students will be able to:

1 Define the chapter's key terms.

2 Describe the general drug actions, uses, adverse reactions, contraindications, precautions and interactions of antiviral, antifungal, and antiparasitic drugs.

3 Discuss important points to keep in mind when educating the patient or family members about the use of antiviral, antifungal, and antiparasitic drugs.

Viruses, fungi, and parasites can cause infection in humans. This chapter discusses antiviral, antifungal, and antiparasitic drugs.

Antiviral Drugs

More than 200 viruses have been identified that cause disease. Acute viruses, such as the common cold, have a rapid onset and quick recovery. Chronic viral infections, such as acquired immunodeficiency syndrome (AIDS), have recurrent episodes of exacerbations (increases in severity of symptoms of the disease) and remissions (periods of partial or complete disappearance of the signs and symptoms). Box 26-1 describes the viruses discussed in this chapter.

Although viral infections are common, for many years only a limited number of drugs were available for their treatment. Over the past decade, the number of antiviral drugs has increased significantly. Several of the antiviral

(text continued on page 439)

Box 26-1 **Viral Infections**

Cytomegalovirus (CMV)

• CMV, a virus of the herpes family, is a common viral infection. Healthy individuals may become infected but have no symptoms. However, immunocompromised patients (such as those with HIV or cancer) may have the infection. Symptoms include malaise, fever, pneumonia, and superinfection. Infants may acquire the virus from the mother while in the uterus, resulting in learning disabilities and mental retardation. CMV can infect the eye, causing retinitis. Symptoms of CMV retinitis are blurred vision and decreased visual acuity. Visual impairment is irreversible and can lead to blindness if untreated.

Herpes Simplex Virus (HSV)

• HSV has two types: HSV-1, which causes oral, ocular, or facial infections, and HSV-2, which causes genital infection. However, either type can cause disease at either body site. HSV-1 causes painful vesicular lesions in the oral mucosa, face, or around the eyes. HSV-2, also called genital herpes, is usually transmitted by sexual contact and causes painful vesicular lesions on the mucous membranes of the genitalia. Vaginal lesions may appear as mucous patches with gray ulcerations. The patient may appear irritable, lethargic, and jaundiced, and may have difficulty breathing or experience seizures. The lesions usually heal within 2 weeks. A severe systemic disease may develop in immunosuppressed patients.

Herpes Zoster

• Herpes zoster (shingles) is caused by the varicella (chickenpox) virus. It is highly contagious. The virus causes chickenpox in children and is easily spread via the respiratory system. Recovery from childhood chickenpox results in the infection lying dormant in the nerve cells. The virus may become reactivated later in life as the older adult's immune system weakens or the individual becomes ill with other disorders. The lesions of herpes zoster appear as pustules along a sensory nerve route. Pain often continues for several months after the lesions have healed.

Human Immunodeficiency Virus (HIV)

• HIV, which causes AIDS, is a type of viral infection transmitted through an infected person's bodily secretions, such as blood or semen. HIV destroys the immune system, causing the body to develop opportunistic infections such as Kaposi sarcoma, *Pneumocystis carinii* pneumonia, or tuberculosis. Symptoms include chills and fever, night sweats, dry productive cough, dyspnea, lethargy, malaise, fatigue, weight loss, and diarrhea.

Influenza

• Influenza, commonly called the flu, is an acute respiratory illness caused by influenza viruses A and B. Symptoms include fever, cough, sore throat, runny or stuffy nose, headache, muscle aches, and extreme fatigue. Most people recover within 1 to 2 weeks. Influenza may cause severe complications such as pneumonia in children, the elderly, and other vulnerable groups. The viruses causing influenza continually change over time, which enables them to evade the immune system of the host.

• These rapid changes in the most commonly circulating types of influenza virus necessitate annual changes in the composition of the "flu" vaccine.

Respiratory Syncytial Virus (RSV)

• RSV infection is highly contagious and infects mostly children, causing bronchiolitis and pneumonia. Infants younger than 6 months are the most severely affected. In adults, RSV causes colds and bronchitis, with fever, cough, and nasal congestion. When RSV affects immunocompromised patients, the consequences can be severe and sometimes fatal.

SUMMARY DRUG TABLE   Antiviral Drugs

Generic Name	Trade Name*	Uses	Adverse Reactions	Dosage Ranges
abacavir sulfate *ab-ah-kav'-ear*	Ziagen	HIV infection	Nausea, vomiting, diarrhea, anorexia, liver dysfunction	300 mg BID
acyclovir *ay-sye'-kloe-ver*	Zovirax	Herpes simplex, herpes zoster	Nausea, vomiting, diarrhea, headache, dizziness, lethargy, confusion, rashes, crystalluria, phlebitis	Oral, 200 mg q4h while awake for a total of 5 capsules/d; IV, 5–10 mg/kg q8h; topical, apply to lesions q3h
amantadine *a-man'-ta-deen*	Symmetrel, *generic*	Prevention and treatment of influenza A; Parkinson disease	Nausea, vomiting, diarrhea, dizziness, hypotension, blurred vision, psychosis, urinary retention	200 mg/d PO or 100 mg PO BID; up to 400 mg/d
amprenavir *am-prenn'-ah-veer*	Agenerase	HIV infection, in combination with other antivirals	Asthenia, peripheral and circumoral paresthesias, nausea, vomiting, diarrhea, anorexia, abdominal pain, rash, hyperglycemia, hypertriglyceridemia	1200 mg PO BID
cidofovir *si-doh'-foh-vir*	Vistide	Retinitis in patients with AIDS	Headache, nausea, vomiting, diarrhea, anorexia, dyspnea, alopecia, rash, neutropenia, nephrotoxicity	5 mg/kg IV once per wk for 2 wk, then once every 2 wk for maintenance
delavirdine *dell-ah-vur'-den*	Rescriptor	Same as amprenavir	Headache, asthenia, malaise, paresthesia, nausea, diarrhea, rash	400 mg PO TID
didanosine *dye-dan'-oh-sin*	Videx	HIV infection	Headache, rhinitis, cough, nausea, rash, vomiting, anorexia, hepatotoxicity, pancreatitis, peripheral neuropathy	For patients with creatinine clearance (Ccr) ≥60 mL/min and weighing ≥60 kg, 400 mg/d or 200 mg BID; weighing <60 kg, 250 mg/d or 125 mg BID; weighing ≥60 kg, 250 mg BID in buffered powder; weighing <60 kg, 167 mg BID in in buffered powder
docosanol *doe-koe-zah-nole*	Abreva	HSV types 1 and 2	Headache, skin irritation	Apply to lesions 5 times/d
efavirenz *ef-ah-vi'-renz*	Sustiva	HIV infection	Erythema, pruritus, dizziness, fatigue, nausea, vomiting	200–600 mg/d PO

Generic Name	Trade Name*	Uses	Adverse Reactions	Dosage Ranges
famciclovir *fam-sye'-kloe-vir*	Famvir	Acute herpes zoster, HSV type 2	Fatigue, fever, nausea, vomiting, diarrhea, sinusitis, constipation, headache	Herpes zoster: 500 mg PO q8h for 7 d; HSV-2: 125 mg PO BID for 5 d
foscarnet *foss-kar'-net*	Foscavir	cytomegalovirus (CMV) retinitis; acyclovir-resistant HSV types 1 and 2	Headache, seizures, nausea, vomiting, diarrhea, anemia, abnormal renal function tests	CMV retinitis: 60 mg/kg IV q8h for 2–3 wk; maintenance dose, 90–120 mg/kg IV; HSV: 40 mg/kg IV q8–12h
ganciclovir *gan-sye'-kloe-vir*	Cytovene, Vitrasert	CMV retinitis	Hematologic changes, fever, rash, anemia	5 mg/kg IV q12h for 14–21 d, then QD
imiquimod *im-ee'-kwee-mod*	Aldara	External genitalia and perianal warts	Local skin irritation, itching, excoriation/flaking	Apply externally 3 times/wk
indinavir *in-din'-ah-ver*	Crixivan	HIV infection	Headache, nausea, vomiting, diarrhea, hyperbilirubinemia, cough, dysuria, acne	800 mg PO q8h
lamivudine *la-ah-vew'-den*	3TC, Epivir	HIV infection (combined with zidovudine)	Headache, asthenia, nausea, diarrhea, agranulocytopenia, nasal congestion, cough, fever, rash, pancreatitis, hepatomegaly	150 mg PO BID
lopinavir/ritonavir *low-pin'-ah-veer/ rih-ton'-ah-veer*	Kaletra	Same as amprenavir	Same as amprenavir	400 mg lopinavir/100 mg ritonavir PO BID; 533 mg lopinavir/133 mg ritonavir PO BID
nelfinavir *nell-fin'-a-veer*	Viracept	Same as amprenavir	Diarrhea, nausea, GI pain, rash, dermatitis	750–1250 mg PO BID
nevirapine *neh-vear'-ah-peen*	Viramune	Same as amprenavir	Rash, fever, headache, nausea, stomatitis, liver dysfunction, paresthesia	200 mg PO QD or BID
oseltamivir *oh-sell-tam'-ih-veer*	Tamiflu	Treatment of influenza A and B	Nausea, vomiting, diarrhea, abdominal pain, dizziness, headache, cough	75–150 mg/d PO
penciclovir *pen-sye'-kloe-ver*	Denavir	HSV types 1 and 2	No significant adverse reactions reported; headache, taste perversion	Apply q2h while awake for 4 d
ribavirin *rye-ba-vye'-rin*	Virazole	Severe lower respiratory tract infections (infants and young children)	Worsening of pulmonary status, bacterial pneumonia, hypotension	Administered by aerosol with special aerosol generator
rimantadine HCL *ri-man'-ta-deen*	Flumadine	Influenza A virus	Light-headedness, dizziness, insomnia, nausea, anorexia	100 mg/d PO BID

Generic Name	Trade Name*	Uses	Adverse Reactions	Dosage Ranges
ritonavir *ri-ton'-ah-ver*	Norvir	HIV infection	Peripheral and circumoral paresthesias, nausea, vomiting, diarrhea, anorexia, dysuria	600 mg PO BID
saquinavir, saquinavir mesylate *sa-kwen'-a-veer*	Fortovase, Invirase	HIV infection in combination with other drugs	Headache, nausea, GI pain, diarrhea, asthenia, elevated CPK	Fortovase: Six 200-mg capsules PO TID; Invirase: Three 200-mg capsules PO TID
stavudine *stay-vew'-den*	Zerit	HIV infection	Headache, nausea, diarrhea, fever, agranulocytopenia	40 mg PO q12h
valacyclovir *val-ah-sye'-kloe-ver*	Valtrex	HSV type 2; herpes zoster	Nausea, dizziness, headache, vomiting, anorexia, diarrhea	HSV type 2: 500 mg PO BID for 5 d; herpes zoster: 1 g PO TID for 7 d
valganciclovir *val-gan-si'-klo-veer*	Valcyte	CMV retinitis	Headache, insomnia, diarrhea, nausea, vomiting, neutropenia, fever	900 mg PO BID
vidarabine *vy-dare'-ah-been*	Ara-A, Vira-A	Keratitis, keratocon-junctivitis caused by HSV types 1 and 2	Burning, itching, irritation, tearing, sensitivity to light	Ophthalmic ointment: 0.5 inch into lower conjunctival sac 2–5 times daily
zalcitabine *zal-cye'-tay-been*	Hivid	Combination therapy with zidovudine in advanced HIV	Nausea, vomiting, oral ulcers, peripheral neuropathy, headache, diarrhea, congestive heart failure	0.75 mg with 200 mg zidovudine q8h
zanamivir *zan-am'-ah-ver*	Relenza	Influenza virus	Nausea, headache, diarrhea, anorexia, rhinitis, flulike symptoms, rash, bronchospasm	2 inhalations BID q12h
zidovudine (AZT) *zid-o-vew'-den*	Retrovir	HIV infection	Asthenia, malaise, weakness, headache, anorexia, diarrhea, nausea, abdominal pain, dizziness, insomnia, anemia, agranulocytosis	100 mg q4h PO; 1–2 mg/kg IV q4h

*The term *generic* indicates the drug is available in generic form.

drugs are discussed here in greater detail than others. These include acyclovir (Zovirax), amantadine (Symmetrel), didanosine (Videx), ribavirin (Virazole), zanamivir (Relenza), and zidovudine (AZT, Retrovir). The Summary Drug Table: Antiviral Drugs presents a more complete listing of the antiviral drugs currently in use.

Actions of Antiviral Drugs

Viruses can reproduce only within a living cell. A virus consists of either DNA or RNA surrounded by a protein shell. The virus can reproduce only when it uses the body's cellular material (Fig. 26-1). Most antiviral drugs act by inhibiting viral DNA or RNA replication in the virus, causing viral death.

Uses of Antiviral Drugs

Although infections caused by a virus are common, antiviral drugs have limited use because they are effective against only a small number of specific viral infections. General uses of the antiviral drugs include the treatment of:

- initial and recurrent mucosal and cutaneous herpes simplex virus 1 and 2 infections in immunocompromised patients, encephalitis, and herpes zoster
- human immunodeficiency virus (combined with other drugs)
- cytomegalovirus retinitis (inflammation of the retina of the eye)
- genital herpes
- influenza A respiratory tract illness
- respiratory syncytial virus, a severe lower respiratory tract infection
- viral herpes infections

Specific uses for the antiviral drugs are listed in the Summary Drug Table: Antiviral Drugs.

Unlabeled Uses of Antiviral Drugs

Because there are a limited number of antiviral drugs and more than 200 viral diseases, the health care provider may prescribe an antiviral drug for some other use even though documentation of its effectiveness for that use is lacking. Approval by the Food and Drug Administration (FDA) is necessary for a drug to be prescribed. On occasion, the use of a drug for a specific disorder or condition may be under investigation or may be approved for use in another country. In this instance, the health care provider may prescribe the drug for the condition under investigation. The use of the drug for a specific disorder or condition that is not officially approved by the FDA is called an "unlabeled use." Examples of unlabeled uses of the antiviral drugs include treatment of cytomegalovirus and initial and recurrent mucosal and cutaneous herpes simplex virus 1 and 2 infections after transplant and varicella pneumonia; the treatment of cytomegalovirus retinitis in immunocompromised patients; and the use of ribavirin for influenza A and B (aerosol form), acute and chronic hepatitis, herpes genitalis, and measles (oral form).

General Adverse Reactions of Antiviral Drugs

Antiviral drugs are given systemically or as topical drugs. When used systemically, these drugs may be administered orally or intravenously. Rapid intravenous administration can result in crystalluria (presence of crystals in the urine). The most common adverse reactions when these drugs are administered systemically are gastroin-

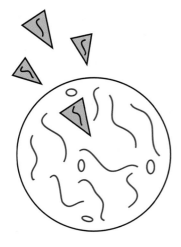 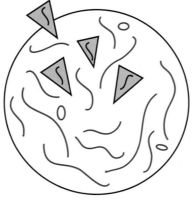 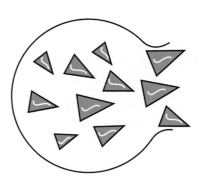

1. Viral cells attack and enter a living cell.

2. Genetic material from the virus attacks the cell and replicates, using material within the cell.

3. New viral cells are released from the cell to attack other cells.

FIGURE 26-1   1. Viral cells attack and enter a living cell. 2. Genetic material from the virus attacks the cell and replicates, using material within the cell. 3. New viral cells are released from the cell to attack other cells. (From Roach SS. *Introductory Clinical Pharmacology*, 7th ed. Baltimore: Lippincott Williams & Wilkins; 2004.)

testinal disturbances, such as nausea, vomiting, diarrhea, and anorexia. When administered topically, the antiviral drugs can cause transient burning, stinging, and pruritus at the application site. Other adverse reactions for specific drugs are listed in the Summary Drug Table: Antiviral Drugs.

General Contraindications, Precautions, and Interactions of Antiviral Drugs

All antiviral drugs are contraindicated in patients with previous hypersensitivity. The antiviral drugs are also contraindicated in patients with congestive heart failure, seizures, or renal disease, and during lactation. The antiviral drugs are given with caution in patients with renal impairment. Antivirals are used with caution in children, during pregnancy (except ribavirin, a pregnancy category X drug), and during lactation. Other contraindications, precautions, and interactions are listed for specific drugs. Numerous interactions are possible with the antiviral drugs. Only the most significant interactions are listed for selected drugs.

General Patient Management Issues with Antiviral Drugs

Patients taking antiviral drugs may have a serious infection that causes a decrease in their natural defenses against disease. The patient's general state of health and resistance to infection are evaluated before using an antiviral drug.

The antiviral drugs may cause anorexia, nausea, or vomiting. These effects range from mild to severe. The patient may be able to tolerate small, frequent meals with soft, nonirritating foods if nausea is mild. Frequent sips of carbonated beverages or hot tea may be helpful for others. If the patient has severe nausea or is vomiting, then the health care provider should be notified.

Skin lesions are carefully monitored for worsening or improvement. Should the lesions not improve, the health care provider should be informed. When an antiviral drug is applied topically, gloves are used when applying it to avoid spreading the infection. These drugs may also cause a rash as an adverse reaction. Any rash should be reported to the health care provider. Depending on the patient's symptoms, vital signs may be monitored every 4 hours or as ordered by the health care provider.

Some patients with a viral infection are acutely ill. Others may experience fatigue, lethargy, dizziness, or weakness as an adverse reaction to the antiviral agent. These patients must be carefully monitored. Call lights are placed in a convenient place for the patient and are answered promptly. If fatigue, dizziness, or weakness is present, the patient may require help with walking or the activities of daily living. Activities should be planned so as to provide adequate rest periods.

When patients are immunosuppressed, they are at increased risk for bacterial or other infection. The patient should be protected from individuals with upper respiratory infections. All caregivers should use good handwashing technique.

ALERT

Antivirals for Human Immunodeficiency Virus

Patients receiving antiviral drugs for human immunodeficiency infections may continue to have opportunistic infections and other complications associated with the virus. All patients should be closely monitored for signs of infection such as fever (even low-grade fever), malaise, sore throat, or lethargy.

Acyclovir

Adverse Reactions of Acyclovir

Acyclovir is used orally, topically, and parenterally (intravenously). When given intravenously, acyclovir can cause phlebitis, lethargy, confusion, tremors, skin rashes, nausea, and crystalluria. Adverse reactions when given orally include nausea, vomiting, diarrhea, headache, dizziness, and skin rashes. Topical use may cause transient burning, stinging, and pruritus.

When given intravenously, adequate hydration to prevent crystalluria should be maintained by encouraging the patient to drink 2000 to 3000 mL of fluid each day (if the disease condition permits). In addition, the patient's mental status is monitored.

Contraindications, Precautions, and Interactions of Acyclovir

This drug is used cautiously in patients with preexisting neurologic, kidney, liver, respiratory, or fluid and electrolyte abnormalities. The drug is given with caution to patients with a history of seizures. Acyclovir is a pregnancy category C drug and is used cautiously during pregnancy and lactation. Incidences of extreme drowsiness have occurred when acyclovir is given with zidovudine. There is an increased risk of nephrotoxicity when acyclovir is administered with other nephrotoxic drugs. When administered with amphotericin B, the risk of nephrotoxicity is increased. Administration with probenecid causes a decrease in the renal excretion of acyclovir, prolonging the effects of acyclovir and increasing the risk of drug toxicity.

Patient Management Issues with Acyclovir

Treatment with acyclovir is begun as soon as symptoms of herpes simplex appear. The drug may be given topically, orally, or intravenously. The drug may be given orally, without regard to food. If gastrointestinal upset occurs, then acyclovir is given with food. Patients with a history of congestive heart failure may not be able to tolerate an increase in fluids, so they must be monitored closely to prevent fluid overload. Neurologic symptoms such as seizures may occur with the use of acyclovir. When used topically, a finger cot or glove is used to prevent spread of infection.

Amantadine

Adverse Reactions of Amantadine

Adverse reactions of amantadine include gastrointestinal upset with nausea and vomiting, anorexia, asthenia (weakness, loss of strength), constipation, depression, visual disturbances, psychosis, urinary retention, and orthostatic hypotension.

The patient should be monitored for the occurrence of drowsiness, dizziness, light-headedness, or mood changes (irritability or mood change).

Contraindications, Precautions, and Interactions of Amantadine

Amantadine is used cautiously in patients with seizure disorders, psychiatric problems, kidney impairment, or cardiac disease. Amantadine is a pregnancy category B drug and is used cautiously during pregnancy and lactation. Concurrent use of antihistamines, phenothiazines, tricyclic antidepressants, disopyramide, and quinidine may increase the anticholinergic effects (dry mouth, blurred vision, constipation) of amantadine.

Patient Management Issues with Amantadine

This drug is used for the prevention or treatment of respiratory tract illness caused by influenza A virus. Some patients are prescribed this drug to manage extrapyramidal effects caused by drugs used to treat parkinsonism (see Chapters 5 and 6). The capsules must be protected from moisture to prevent deterioration.

Didanosine

Adverse Reactions of Didanosine

Adverse reactions reported with didanosine include headache, peripheral neuropathy, rhinitis, cough, diarrhea, nausea, vomiting, anorexia, hepatotoxicity, and pancreatitis.

Although rare, pancreatitis and peripheral neuropathy are possible adverse reactions seen with didano-sine. It is important to remain alert for symptoms of pancreatitis (nausea, vomiting, abdominal pain, jaundice, and elevated enzymes) and for signs of peripheral neuropathy (numbness, tingling, or pain in the feet or hands), and to report any symptoms immediately to the health care provider.

Contraindications, Precautions, and Interactions of Didanosine

This drug is used cautiously in patients with peripheral vascular disease, neuropathy, chronic pancreatitis, or impaired liver function. Didanosine is a pregnancy category B drug and is used cautiously during pregnancy and lactation. There may be a decrease in the effectiveness of dapsone in preventing *Pneumocystis carinii* pneumonia when didanosine is administered with dapsone. Use of didanosine with zalcitabine may cause additive neuropathy. Absorption of didanosine is decreased when it is administered with food.

Patient Management Issues with Didanosine

For patients with human immunodeficiency virus infection who cannot tolerate zidovudine or who have exhibited decreased therapeutic effect with zidovudine, didanosine should be taken on an empty stomach (at least 1 hour before or 2 hours after meals). The tablets are not swallowed whole but should be chewed or crushed and mixed thoroughly with at least 1 oz of water.

Ribavirin

Adverse Reactions of Ribavirin

Ribavirin is given by inhalation and can cause worsening of respiratory status, hypotension, and ocular irritation, including erythema (redness of skin), conjunctivitis, and blurred vision. Respiratory function should be monitored closely throughout therapy. Any worsening of respiratory function should be reported to the health care provider.

Contraindications, Precautions, and Interactions of Ribavirin

Ribavirin may be teratogenic and embryotoxic (pregnancy category X) and is contraindicated during pregnancy, in patients with chronic obstructive pulmonary disease, and during lactation. Ribavirin is used cautiously at all times during administration of the drug. Ribavirin may antagonize the antiviral action of zidovudine and potentiate the hematologic toxic effects of zidovudine. When ribavirin is used concurrently with digitalis, the risk of digitalis toxicity increases.

Patient Management Issues with Ribavirin

Ribavirin is taken by inhalation using a small-particle aerosol generator (SPAG-2 aerosol generator).

Zanamivir

Adverse Reactions of Zanamivir

Common adverse effects include headache, nausea, diarrhea, anorexia, rhinitis, and flu-like symptoms. The most serious adverse reactions are related to respiratory effects and include severe bronchospasm that may lead to death. The risk is higher in patients with asthma or chronic obstructive pulmonary disease. A fast-acting bronchodilator should be on hand in case bronchospasm occurs. Zanamivir use should be discontinued and the health care provider notified promptly if respiratory symptoms worsen.

Contraindications, Precautions, and Interactions of Zanamivir

Zanamivir is used cautiously with pregnancy (category C), lactation, asthma, chronic obstructive pulmonary disease, or other underlying respiratory diseases. No significant drug interactions have been reported with the use of zanamivir.

Patient Management Issues with Zanamivir

This drug is available as a powder blister for inhalation. The drug should be started within 2 days of onset of flu symptoms.

Zidovudine

Adverse Reactions of Zidovudine

Adverse reactions of zidovudine include headache, weakness, malaise, nausea, abdominal pain, and diarrhea. Hematologic changes include anemia and granulocytopenia (low levels of granulocytes, a type of white blood cell, in the blood). With zidovudine, bone marrow depression may occur, making the patient susceptible to infection and easy bruising. The patient should be protected from individuals with upper respiratory infection. All caregivers should use good handwashing technique. Care is taken to prevent trauma, because even slight trauma can result in bruising if the platelet count is low.

Contraindications, Precautions, and Interactions of Zidovudine

This drug is used cautiously in patients with bone marrow depression or severe liver or kidney impairment. Zidovudine is a pregnancy category C drug and is used cautiously during pregnancy and lactation. There is an increased risk of bone marrow depression when zidovudine is taken with antineoplastic drugs, other drugs causing bone marrow depression, and in patients undergoing or who have recently undergone radiation therapy. An additive neurotoxicity may occur when zidovudine is taken with acyclovir. Clarithromycin decreases blood levels of zidovudine. The blood levels of zidovudine are increased when it is given with lamivudine.

Patient Management Issues with Zidovudine

The patient is assessed for an increase in severity of symptoms of human immunodeficiency virus (HIV) and for symptoms of opportunistic infections.

Educating the Patient and Family About Antiviral Drugs

When an antiviral drug is given orally, the dosage regimen is explained to the patient and family. The patient is instructed to take the drug exactly as directed and for the full course of therapy. If a dose is missed, then the patient should take it as soon as remembered but should not double the dose at the next dosage time. Any adverse reactions should be reported to the health care provider. The patient must understand that these drugs do not cure viral infections but should decrease symptoms and increase feelings of well-being.

Patients should report any symptoms of infection such as an elevated temperature (even a slight elevation), sore throat, difficulty breathing, weakness, or lethargy. The patient must be aware of possible signs of pancreatitis (nausea, vomiting, abdominal pain, jaundice [yellow discoloration of the skin or eyes]) and peripheral neuritis (tingling, burning, numbness, or pain in the hands or feet). Any indication of pancreatitis or peripheral neuritis should be reported at once.

Patient Education Box 26-1 includes key points about antiviral drugs that the patient and family members should know.

PATIENT EDUCATION BOX 26-1

Key Points for Patients Taking Antiviral Drugs

ACYCLOVIR
- ❑ This drug is not a cure for herpes simplex, but it will shorten the course of the disease and promote healing of the lesions.
- ❑ The drug will not prevent the spread of the disease to others.
- ❑ Do not apply the topical form more often than prescribed. Apply this drug with a finger cot or gloves and cover all lesions.
- ❑ Do not have sexual contact while lesions are present.
- ❑ Notify your health care provider if you experience burning, stinging, or itching, or if your rash worsens or becomes pronounced.

Key Points for Patients Taking Antiviral Drugs (continued)

AMANTADINE

❏ Do not drive a car or perform work for which mental alertness is necessary until the effect of the drug is apparent, because your vision and coordination can be affected.

❏ Rise slowly from a prone to a sitting position to decrease the possibility of light-headedness.

❏ Report changes such as nervousness, tremors, slurred speech, or depression. If you are on an alternate dosage schedule, then mark your calendar to designate the days the drug is to be taken.

DIDANOSINE

❏ Take this drug on an empty stomach because food decreases absorption.

❏ Follow the instructions for use carefully. Crush the drug and mix it with water.

❏ Discontinue use of the drug and notify your health care provider if you experience any numbness or tingling of the extremities.

❏ Report any signs of abdominal pain, nausea, or vomiting.

❏ Didanosine is not a cure for acquired immunodeficiency syndrome and does not prevent the spread of the disease, but it may decrease the symptoms.

RIBAVIRIN

❏ This drug is taken through a small-particle aerosol generator. Report any worsening of your respiratory function, dizziness, confusion, or shortness of breath to your health care provider.

❏ Because this drug is a pregnancy category X drug, women of childbearing age should take care not to inhale the drug. When a child is taking the drug, the mother and other females of childbearing age in direct contact with the child should observe respiratory precautions.

ZANAMIVIR

❏ This drug is taken every 12 hours for 5 days using a Diskhaler delivery system. If you are also using a bronchodilator, then use the bronchodilator before the zanamivir if both are prescribed at the same time. The drug may cause dizziness. You should use caution if driving an automobile or operating dangerous machinery. Treatment with this drug does not decrease the risk of transmission of the "flu" to others.

ZIDOVUDINE

❏ This drug may cause dizziness.

❏ Avoid activities requiring alertness until you know how you will respond to the drug.

❏ This drug does not cure AIDS and does not prevent transmission of HIV to others. Notify your health care provider if you experience fever, sore throat, or signs of infection. Your health care provider may prescribe frequent blood tests to monitor for a decrease in the immune response that indicates the need to decrease the dosage or to discontinue use of the drug for a period of time.

Natural Remedies: Lemon Balm

Lemon balm is a perennial herb with heart-shaped leaves that has been used for hundreds of years. Its scientific name is *Melissa officinalis*. Traditionally, the herb has been used for Graves disease and as a sedative, antispasmodic, and an antiviral agent. When used topically, lemon balm has antiviral activity against herpes simplex virus. No adverse reactions have been reported when lemon balm is used topically.

Antifungal Drugs

A **fungus** is a colorless plant that lacks chlorophyll. Fungi that cause disease in humans may be yeast-like or mold-like; the resulting infections are called **mycotic infections** or fungal infections. Fungal infections range from superficial skin infections to life-threatening systemic infections. Systemic fungal infections are serious infections that occur when fungi gain entrance into the interior of the body.

Mycotic (fungal) infections may be one of two types:

1. Superficial mycotic infections
2. Deep (systemic) mycotic infections

The superficial mycotic infections occur on the surface of, or just below, the skin or nails. Superficial infections include **tinea pedis** (athlete's foot), **tinea cruris** (jock itch), **tinea corporis** (ringworm), **onychomycosis** (nail fungus), and yeast infections, such as those caused by *Candida albicans*. Yeast infections or those caused by *C. albicans* affect women in the vulvovaginal area and can be difficult to control. Women who are at increased risk for vulvovaginal yeast infections include those who have diabetes, are pregnant, or are taking oral contraceptives, antibiotics, or corticosteroids.

Deep mycotic infections develop inside the body, such as in the lungs. Treatment for deep mycotic infections is often difficult and prolonged. The Summary

SUMMARY DRUG TABLE   Antifungal Drugs

Generic Name	Trade Name*	Uses	Adverse Reactions	Dosage Ranges
amphotericin B desoxycholate *am-foe-ter'-i-sin*	Amphocin, Fungizone IV, *generic*	Systemic fungal infections	Headache, hypotension, fever, shaking, chills, malaise, nausea, vomiting, diarrhea, abnormal renal function, joint and muscle pain	Desoxycholate: 0.25 mg/kg/d IV
amphotericin B, lipid-based	Abelcet, AmBisome, Amphotec			Lipid-based: 3–6 mg/kg/d IV
caspofungin acetate *kass-poe-fun-jin*	Cancidas	Invasive aspergillosis, hepatic insufficiency	Headache, rash, nausea, vomiting, abdominal pain, hematologic changes, fever	70 mg loading dose IV, followed by 50 mg/d IV
fluconazole *floo-kon'-a-zole*	Diflucan	Oropharyngeal and esophageal candidiasis, vaginal candidiasis, cryptococcal meningitis	Headache, nausea, vomiting, diarrhea, skin rash	50–400 mg/d PO, IV
flucytosine (5-FC) *floo-sye'-toe-seen*	Ancobon	Systemic fungal infections	Nausea, diarrhea, rash, anemia, leukopenia, thrombocytopenia, renal insufficiency	50–150 mg/kg/d PO q6h
griseofulvin microsize *griz-ee-oh-full'-vin*	Fulvicin V/F, Grifulvin V, Grisactin	Ringworm infections of the skin, hair, nails	Nausea, vomiting, diarrhea, oral thrush, headache, rash, urticaria	Microsize: 30–50 lb, 125–250 mg/d; >50 lb, 250–500 mg/d PO
griseofulvin ultramicrosize	Fulvicin P/G, Gris-PEG			Ultramicrosize: 30–50 lb, 82.5–165 mg/d; >50 lb, 165–330 mg/d in divided doses PO; Microsize: 500 mg–1g PO; Ultramicrosize: 330–750 mg PO
itraconazole *eye-tra-kon'-a-zole*	Sporanox	Capsules or parenteral: fungal infections; oral solution: oral or esophageal candidiasis	Nausea, vomiting, diarrhea, rash, abdominal pain, edema	200–400 mg/d PO, IV as a single or divided dose
ketoconazole *kee-toe-koe'-na-zole*	Nizoral, *generic*	Treatment of fungal infections	Nausea, vomiting, abdominal pain, headache, pruritus	200 mg/d PO; may increase to 400 mg/d PO
nystatin, oral *nye-stat'-in*	*Generic*	Nonesophageal membrane GI candidiasis	Rash, diarrhea, nausea, vomiting	500,000–1,000,000 U TID

*The term *generic* indicates the drug is available in generic form.

Drug Table: Antifungal Drugs identifies drugs that are used to combat fungal infections.

Actions of Antifungal Drugs

Antifungal drugs may be **fungicidal** (able to destroy fungi) or **fungistatic** (able to slow or retard the multiplication of fungi). Amphotericin B (Fungizone IV), miconazole (Monistat), nystatin (Mycostatin), and ketoconazole (Nizoral) are thought to have an effect on the cell membrane of the fungus, resulting in a fungicidal or fungistatic effect. The fungicidal or fungistatic effect of these drugs appears to be related to their concentration in body tissues. Fluconazole (Diflucan) has fungistatic activity that appears to result from the depletion of sterols (a group of substances related to fats) in the fungus cells.

Griseofulvin (Grisactin) exerts its effect by being deposited in keratin precursor cells, which are then gradually lost (because of the constant shedding of top skin cells) and replaced by new, noninfected cells. The mode of action of flucytosine (Ancobon) is not clearly understood. Clotrimazole (Lotrimin, Mycelex) binds with phospholipids in the fungal cell membrane, increasing permeability of the cell and resulting in loss of intracellular components.

Uses of Antifungal Drugs

Antifungal drugs are used to treat superficial and deep fungal infections. The antifungal drugs specifically discussed in this chapter are: amphotericin B (Fungizone), fluconazole (Diflucan), flucytosine (Ancobon), griseofulvin (Grisactin), ketoconazole (Nizoral), and miconazole (Monistat). The specific uses of antifungal drugs are given in the Summary Drug Table: Antifungal Drugs. Miconazole is an antifungal drug used to treat vulvovaginal "yeast" infections and is representative of all of the vaginal antifungal agents. Fungal infections of the skin or mucous membranes may be treated with topical or vaginal preparations. A listing of the topical antifungal drugs appears in Table 26-1, and the vulvovaginal antifungal agents are listed in Table 26-2.

General Adverse Reactions of Antifungal Drugs

When topical antifungal drugs, such as clotrimazole, are applied to the skin or mucous membranes, few adverse reactions occur. On occasion, a local reaction, such as irritation or burning, may occur with topical use. The vulvovaginal antifungal drugs may cause local irritation, redness, stinging, or abdominal pain. Few adverse reactions occur with the use of the vulvovaginal antifungal drugs.

TABLE 26-1 Topical Antifungal Drugs

Generic Name (Form)	Trade Names	Uses
amphotericin B (cream or lotion)	Fungizone	Mycotic infections
butenafine HCL (Cream)	Mentax	Mycotic infections
ciclopirox (cream, lotion)	Loprox, Penlac Nail Lacquer	Tinea pedis, tinea cruris, tinea corporis, mild to moderate onychomycosis of fingernails and toenails
clioquinol (cream)	generic	Tinea pedis, tinea cruris, and other ringworm infections
clotrimazole (Cream, solution, lotion)	Lotrimin, generic	Tinea pedis, tinea cruris, tinea corporis
econazole (cream)	Spectazole	Tinea pedis, tinea cruris, tinea corporis
gentian violet (solution)	generic	Abrasions, minor cuts, surface injuries, and superficial fungus infections
haloprogin	Halotex	Tinea pedis, tinea cruris, tinea corporis
miconazole nitrate (cream, solution, spray)	Fungoid Tincture, Lotrimin, Micatin, Monistat	Tinea pedis, tinea cruris, tinea corporis
naftifine (cream, gel)	Naftin	Cutaneous or mucocutaneous mycotic infections
oxiconazole nitrate (cream, lotion)	Oxistat	Tinea pedis, tinea cruris, tinea corporis
sulconazole nitrate (cream, solution)	Exelderm	Tinea pedis, tinea cruris, tinea corporis
tolnaftate (cream, solution, gel, spray)	Aftate, Genaspor, Tinactin, Ting, generic	Tinea pedis, tinea cruris, tinea corporis
triacetin (solution, cream, spray)	Fungoid, Ony-Clear Nail	Tinea pedis, tinea cruris, tinea corporis
undecylenic acid (ointment, cream, powder)	Cruex, Desenex	Tinea pedis; relief and prevention of diaper rash, itching, burning and chafing, prickly heat; tinea cruris; excessive perspiration, irritation of the groin area

TABLE 26-2 Vaginal Antifungal Drugs

Generic Name	Select Trade Name(S)
butoconazole nitrate *Byoo-toe-koe'-nuh-zole*	Femstat 3, Gynazole-1, Mycelex-3
clotrimazole *Kloe-trye'-ma-zole*	Lotrimin 3, Mycelex-7, *generic*
miconazole nitrate *mi-kon'-a-zole*	Monistat 3, Monistat 7, Monistat Dual Pak, M-Zole 3 Combination Pack, *generic*
nystatin *nye-stat'-in*	*Generic*
terconazole *ter-kon'-a-zole*	Terazol 7, Terazol 3
tioconazole *tee-o-kon'-a-zole*	Monistat 1, Vagistat-1

General Patient Management Issues with Antifungal Drugs

Careful observation of the patient is required every 2 to 4 hours for adverse drug reactions when the antifungal drug is given by the oral or parenteral route. When these drugs are applied topically to the skin, the area is inspected at the time of each application for localized skin reactions. When these drugs are administered vaginally, the patient is asked about any discomfort or other sensations experienced after insertion of the antifungal preparation. The patient's response to therapy should be monitored daily.

Superficial and deep fungal infections respond slowly to antifungal therapy. Many patients experience anxiety and depression over the fact that therapy must continue for a prolonged time. The patient and family should be helped to understand that therapy must be continued until the infection is under control. In some cases, therapy may take weeks or months.

When the patient is taking a drug that is potentially toxic to the kidneys, fluid intake and output must be carefully monitored. In some instances, hourly measurements of the urinary output may be required. Periodic laboratory tests are usually ordered to monitor the patient's response to therapy and to detect toxic drug reactions. Serum creatinine levels and blood urea nitrogen levels are checked frequently during the course of therapy to monitor kidney function. If the blood urea nitrogen or the serum creatinine levels are excessive, then the health care provider may discontinue the drug therapy or reduce the dosage until kidney function improves.

Many fungal infections are associated with lesions that are at risk for infection. The patient's temperature, pulse, respiration, and blood pressure are monitored every 4 hours or more often if needed. The patient is inspected for superficial fungal infections of the skin or skin structures (e.g., hair and nails). Any skin lesions, such as rough itchy patches, cracks between the toes, and sore and reddened areas are noted. The skin is checked for localized signs of infection (i.e., increased redness or swelling). Skin lesions are monitored daily. Gloves should be used when caring for open lesions to minimize autoinoculation or transmission of the disease.

Amphotericin B

Adverse Reactions of Amphotericin B

Amphotericin B is the most effective drug available for the treatment of most systemic fungal infections. Use often results in serious reactions, including fever, shaking, chills, headache, malaise, anorexia, joint and muscle pain, abnormal renal function or kidney damage, nausea, vomiting, and anemia. This drug is given parenterally, usually for a period of several months. Its use is reserved for serious and potentially life-threatening fungal infections. Some of these adverse reactions may be lessened by use of aspirin, antihistamines, or antiemetics.

Managing Adverse Reactions of Amphotericin B. Fever (sometimes with shaking chills) may occur within 15 to 20 minutes after administration of the drug. The patient's vital signs must be carefully monitored during the first 30 to 60 minutes, and thereafter 2 to 4 hours during therapy, depending on the patient's condition.

Fluid intake and output must be carefully monitored because this drug may be nephrotoxic (harmful to the kidneys). In some instances, hourly measurements of urinary output may be necessary. Periodic laboratory tests are usually ordered to monitor the patient's response to therapy and detect toxic drug reactions.

A L E R T

Renal Damage and Amphotericin B

Kidney damage is the most serious adverse reaction of amphotericin B. Renal impairment usually improves with modification of dosage regimen (reduction of dosage or increasing time between dosages). Serum creatinine levels and blood urea nitrogen levels are checked frequently during the course of therapy to monitor kidney function.

Contraindications, Precautions, and Interactions of Amphotericin B

Amphotericin B is contraindicated in patients with a known hypersensitivity and during lactation. It is used cautiously in patients with renal dysfunction or electrolyte imbalances, and in combination with antineoplastic drugs (because it can cause severe bone marrow suppression). This drug is a pregnancy category B drug and is used during pregnancy only when the situation is life-threatening. When given with the corticosteroids, severe hypokalemia may occur. There may be an increased risk of digitalis toxicity if digoxin is administered concurrently with amphotericin B. Use with nephrotoxic drugs (e.g., aminoglycosides or cyclosporine) may increase the risk of nephrotoxicity in patients also taking amphotericin B. Amphotericin B decreases the effects of miconazole. Amphotericin B is given only under close supervision in the hospital setting.

Patient Management Issues with Amphotericin B

Amphotericin B is taken daily or every other day over several months. The patient is often acutely ill with a life-threatening deep fungal infection. The intravenous infusion rate and the infusion site are checked frequently during use of the drug. This is especially important if the patient is restless or confused.

On occasion, amphotericin B may be given as an oral solution for oral candidiasis. The patient is instructed to swish and hold the solution in the mouth for several minutes (or as long as possible) before swallowing.

Fluconazole

Adverse Reactions of Fluconazole

Use may result in nausea, vomiting, headache, diarrhea, abdominal pain, and skin rash. Abnormal liver function tests may occur and may require follow-up tests to determine if liver function has been affected.

Managing Adverse Reactions of Fluconazole. Because older adults are more likely to have decreased renal function, they are at increased risk for further renal impairment or renal failure.

ALERT

  Older Adults and Fluconazole

Before an older patient or one that has renal impairment uses this drug, the health care provider may order a creatinine clearance test.

Contraindications, Precautions, and Interactions of Fluconazole

Fluconazole is contraindicated in patients with known hypersensitivity. The drug is used cautiously in patients with renal impairment and during pregnancy (category C) and lactation. The drug is given during pregnancy only if the benefit of the drug clearly outweighs any possible risk to the infant. When fluconazole is taken with an oral hypoglycemic, there is an increased effect of the oral hypoglycemic. Fluconazole may decrease the metabolism of phenytoin and warfarin.

Patient Management Issues with Fluconazole

The drug may be taken orally or intravenously.

Flucytosine

Adverse Reactions of Flucytosine

Use may result in nausea, vomiting, diarrhea, rash, anemia, leukopenia, and thrombocytopenia. Signs of renal impairment include elevated blood urea nitrogen and serum creatinine levels. Periodic renal function tests are usually performed during therapy.

Managing Adverse Reactions of Flucytosine. Before therapy is begun, electrolytes, hematological status, and renal status are determined. Renal impairment can cause accumulation of the drug. To reduce the incidence of gastrointestinal distress, the capsules may be taken one or two at a time during a 15-minute period. If gastrointestinal distress still occurs, then the health care provider should be notified.

Contraindications, Precautions, and Interactions of Flucytosine

Flucytosine is contraindicated in patients with known hypersensitivity. Flucytosine is used cautiously in patients with bone marrow depression and with extreme caution in those with renal impairment. The drug is also used cautiously during pregnancy (category C) and lactation. When flucytosine and amphotericin B are taken concurrently, the risk of flucytosine toxicity is increased.

Patient Management Issues with Flucytosine

Flucytosine is given orally. To decrease or prevent nausea and vomiting, the capsules may be taken a few at a time during a 15-minute period.

Griseofulvin

Adverse Reactions of Griseofulvin

Use may result in a hypersensitivity-like reaction that includes rash and urticaria. Nausea, vomiting, oral thrush, diarrhea, and headache also may occur.

Contraindications, Precautions, and Interactions of Griseofulvin

Griseofulvin is contraindicated in patients with known hypersensitivity and in those with severe liver disease. This drug is used cautiously during pregnancy (category C) and lactation. It is used with caution when given concurrently with penicillin because of the possibility of cross-sensitivity. When griseofulvin is given with warfarin, the anticoagulant effect may be decreased. When used with a barbiturate, the effect of griseofulvin may be decreased. A decrease in the effects of an oral contraceptive may occur with griseofulvin therapy, causing breakthrough bleeding, pregnancy, or amenorrhea. Blood salicylate concentrations may be decreased when a salicylate is administered with griseofulvin.

Patient Management Issues with Griseofulvin

This drug is given orally. Prolonged therapy is usually needed to eliminate the fungus.

Itraconazole

Adverse Reactions of Itraconazole

The most common adverse reactions are nausea, vomiting, and diarrhea. On occasion, severe hypokalemia (low potassium level) has occurred in patients receiving the drug on a daily basis. Hepatotoxicity is a possibility with itraconazole use.

Managing Adverse Reactions of Itraconazole. Although rare, hepatitis may develop during itraconazole use. The patient is closely monitored for signs of hepatitis, including anorexia, abdominal pain, unusual tiredness, jaundice, and dark urine. The health care provider may order periodic liver function tests.

Contraindications, Precautions, and Interactions of Itraconazole

Itraconazole is contraindicated in patients with a known hypersensitivity. The drug is used cautiously in patients with hepatitis, human immunodeficiency virus, or impaired liver function, and in pregnant women (pregnancy category C). In patients with hypochlorhydria, the absorption of itraconazole is decreased. Multiple drug interactions occur with itraconazole. Itraconazole elevates blood concentrations of digoxin and cyclosporine. Phenytoin decreases blood levels of itraconazole and alters the metabolism of phenytoin. Histamine antagonists, isoniazid, and rifampin decrease plasma levels of itraconazole. There is an increased anticoagulant effect when warfarin is used concurrently with itraconazole.

Patient Management Issues with Itraconazole

This drug is given orally with food to increase absorption. When used intravenously, it is not diluted with any other diluent.

Ketoconazole

Adverse Reactions of Ketoconazole

This drug is usually well-tolerated, but nausea, vomiting, headache, dizziness, abdominal pain, and pruritus may occur. Most adverse reactions are mild and transient. On rare occasions, hepatic toxicity may occur, in which case the drug must be discontinued immediately. Periodic hepatic function tests are used to monitor for hepatic toxicity.

Contraindications, Precautions, and Interactions of Ketoconazole

Ketoconazole is contraindicated in patients with known hypersensitivity. Ketoconazole is used cautiously in patients with liver impairment and during pregnancy (category C) and lactation. The absorption of ketoconazole is impaired when the drug is taken with histamine antagonists and antacids. Ketoconazole enhances the anticoagulant effect of warfarin and causes an additive hepatotoxicity when given with other hepatotoxic drugs and alcohol. Use of ketoconazole with rifampin or isoniazid may decrease the blood levels of ketoconazole.

Patient Management Issues with Ketoconazole

This drug is given with food to minimize gastrointestinal irritation. Antacids, anticholinergics, or histamine blockers should not be used until at least 2 hours after ketoconazole is given.

Miconazole

Adverse Reactions of Miconazole

Use of miconazole for a vulvovaginal fungal infection may cause irritation, sensitization, or vulvovaginal burning. Skin irritation may result in redness, itching, burning, or skin fissures. Other adverse reactions with miconazole include cramping, nausea, and headache. Adverse reactions associated with topical use are usually not severe.

Contraindications, Precautions, and Interactions of Miconazole

Miconazole is contraindicated in patients with known hypersensitivity. The drug is given cautiously in cases of chronic or recurrent candidiasis. Recurrent or chronic candidiasis requires an evaluation for diabetes. The drug is used cautiously during pregnancy (category C). If used during pregnancy, then a vaginal applicator may be contraindicated and manual insertion of the vaginal tablets preferred. Because small amounts of these drugs may be absorbed from the vagina, the drug is used during the first trimester only when essential.

Patient Management Issues with Miconazole

This drug is self-administered on an outpatient basis.

Educating the Patient and Family About Antifungal Drugs

Patient Education Box 26-2 includes key points about antifungal drugs that the patient and family members should know.

Natural Remedies: Antifungal Herbs

Researchers have identified several antifungal herbs that are effective against tinea pedis (athlete's foot), such as tea tree oil (*Melaleuca alternifolia*) and garlic (*Allium sativum*). Tea tree oil comes from an evergreen tree native to Australia. The herb has been used as a nonirritating antimicrobial for cuts, stings, wounds, burns, and

---

PATIENT EDUCATION BOX 26-2

Key Points for Patients Taking Antifungal Drugs

❑ Clean the involved area and apply the ointment or cream to your skin as directed by your health care provider.

❑ Do not increase or decrease the amount you use or how often you use the ointment or cream unless directed to do so by your health care provider.

❑ During treatment for a ringworm infection, keep your towels and facecloths separate from those of other family members to avoid the spread of the infection. Keep the affected area clean and dry.

FLUCYTOSINE

❑ You may experience nausea or vomiting with this drug. Reduce or eliminate these effects by taking a few capsules at a time during a 15-minute period. If your nausea, vomiting, or diarrhea persists, then notify your health care provider as soon as possible.

GRISEOFULVIN

❑ Although you may not notice the beneficial effects for some time, take the drug for the full course of therapy. Avoid exposure to sunlight and sunlamps because an exaggerated skin reaction (which is similar to severe sunburn) may occur even after a brief exposure to ultraviolet light. Notify your health care provider if you experience fever, soar throat, or skin rash.

KETOCONAZOLE

❑ Complete the full course of therapy as prescribed by your health care provider. Do not take this drug with an antacid. In addition, avoid the use of nonprescription drugs unless use of a specific drug is approved by

your health care provider. This drug may produce headache, dizziness, and drowsiness. If you experience drowsiness or dizziness, then be cautious while driving or performing other hazardous tasks. Notify your health care provider if your abdominal pain, fever, or diarrhea becomes pronounced.

ITRACONAZOLE

❑ Take this drug with food. Therapy will continue for at least 3 months until the infection is controlled. Report unusual fatigue, yellow skin, darkened urine, anorexia, nausea, or vomiting to your health care provider.

MICONAZOLE

❑ If you use the drug (cream or tablet) vaginally, then insert the drug high in the vagina using the applicator provided with the product. Wear a sanitary napkin after insertion of the drug to prevent staining of your clothing and bed linen.

❑ Continue taking the drug during your menstrual period if you are using the vaginal route.

❑ Do not have intercourse while taking this drug, or advise your partner to use a condom to avoid reinfection.

❑ To prevent recurrent infections, avoid nylon and tight-fitting garments. If you have no improvement in 5 to 7 days, then stop using the drug and consult your health care provider because a more serious infection may be present.

❑ If you experience abdominal pain, pelvic pain, rash, fever, or offensive-smelling vaginal discharge, then do not use the drug but notify your health care provider.

---

acne. It can be found in shampoos, soaps, and lotions. Tea tree oil should not be ingested orally but is effective when used topically for minor cuts and stings. Tea tree oil is used as an antifungal to relieve and control the symptoms of tinea pedis. Topical application is most effective when used in a cream with at least 10% tea tree oil. Several commercially prepared ointments are available. The cream is applied to affected areas twice daily for several weeks.

Garlic is used as an antifungal. A cream of 0.4% ajoene (the antifungal component of garlic) has been found to relieve symptoms of athlete's foot and, like tea tree oil, is applied twice daily.

Antiparasitic Drugs

A **parasite** is an organism that lives in or on another organism (the host) without contributing to the survival or well-being of the host. **Helminthiasis** (invasion of the body by **helminths** [worms]), malaria (an infectious disease caused by a protozoan and usually transmitted to humans through a bite from an infected mosquito),

and **amebiasis** (invasion of the body by the ameba *Entamoeba histolytica*) are worldwide health problems caused by parasites.

Pinworm is a helminth infection that is common everywhere, whereas most other helminth infections are predominantly found in countries or areas of the world that lack proper sanitary facilities. Malaria is rare in the United States but sometimes occurs in individuals who have traveled to or lived in areas where this disease is a health problem. The first antimalarial drug, quinine, is derived from the bark of the cinchona tree. Amebiasis is seen throughout the world but is less common in developed countries where sanitary facilities prevent the spread of the causative organism.

Anthelmintic Drugs

Anthelmintic (against helminths) drugs are used to treat helminthiasis. Roundworms, pinworms, whipworms, hookworms, and tapeworms are examples of helminths. Table 26-3 lists the organisms that cause helminth infections. The anthelmintic drugs are listed in the Summary Drug Table: Anthelmintic Drugs.

TABLE 26-3 Common Names and Causative Organisms or Parasitic Infections

Common Name	Causative Organism
Roundworm	*Ascaris lumbricoides*
Pinworm	*Enterobius vermicularis*
Whipworm	*Trichuris trichiura*
Threadworm	*Strongyloides stercoralis*
Hookworm	*Ancylostoma duodenale, Necator americanus*
Beef tapeworm	*Taenia saginata*
Pork tapeworm	*Taenia solium*
Fish tapeworm	*Diphyllobothrium latum*

Although the actions of anthelmintic drugs vary, their prime purpose is to kill the parasite. Adverse reactions of the anthelmintic drugs, if they do occur, are usually mild when the drug is used in the recommended dosage.

Actions, Uses, and Adverse Reactions of Albendazole

Albendazole (Albenza) interferes with the synthesis of the parasite's microtubules, resulting in death of susceptible larva. This drug is used to treat larval forms of pork tapeworm and to treat liver, lung, and peritoneum disease caused by the dog tapeworm.

Contraindications, Precautions, and Interactions of Albendazole

Albendazole is contraindicated in patients with known hypersensitivity and during pregnancy (category C). The drug has caused embryotoxic and teratogenic effects in experimental animals. Albendazole is used cautiously in patients with hepatic impairment and during lactation. The effects of albendazole are increased with dexamethasone and cimetidine.

Actions, Uses, and Adverse Reactions of Mebendazole

Mebendazole (Vermox) blocks the uptake of glucose by the helminth, resulting in a depletion of the helminth's own glycogen. Glycogen depletion results in a decreased formation of adenosine triphosphate, which is required by helminths for reproduction and survival. This drug is used to treat whipworm, pinworm, roundworm, American hookworm, and the common hookworm. Treatment with mebendazole may cause transient abdominal pain and diarrhea.

SUMMARY DRUG TABLE   Anthelmintic Drugs

Generic Name	Trade Name*	Uses	Adverse Reactions	Dosage Ranges
albendazole *al-ben'-dah-zohl*	Albenza	Parenchymal neurocysticercosis caused by pork tapeworms, hydatid disease (caused by the larval form of the dog tapeworm)	Abnormal liver function tests, abdominal pain, nausea, vomiting, headache, dizziness	≥60 kg: 400 mg BID; <60 kg: 15 mg/kg/d
mebendazole *me-ben'-dah-zole*	Vermox, *generic*	Treatment of whipworm, pinworm, roundworm, common and American hookworm	Transient abdominal pain, diarrhea	100 mg PO morning and evening for 3 consecutive d; pinworm: 100 mg PO as a single dose
pyrantel *pi-ran'-tel*	Antiminth, Reese's Pinworm	Treatment of pinworm and roundworm	Anorexia, nausea, vomiting, abdominal cramps, diarrhea, rash	11 mg/kg PO as a single dose
thiabendazole *thye-a-ben'-da-zole*	Mintezol	Treatment of threadworm	Hypersensitivity reactions, drowsiness, dizziness	<150 lb: 10 mg/lb per dose PO; >150 lb: 1.5 g/dose PO Maximum daily dose, 3g

*The term *generic* indicates the drug is available in generic form.

Contraindications, Precautions, and Interactions of Mebendazole

Mebendazole is contraindicated in patients with known hypersensitivity. Mebendazole is also contraindicated during pregnancy (category C). The drug, like albendazole, has caused embryotoxic and teratogenic effects in experimental animals. Use of mebendazole with the hydantoins and carbamazepine may reduce plasma levels of mebendazole.

Actions, Uses, and Adverse Reactions of Pyrantel

The activity of pyrantel (Antiminth) is probably caused by its ability to paralyze helminths. Paralysis causes the helminth to release its grip on the intestinal wall; it is then excreted in the feces. Pyrantel is used to treat roundworm and pinworm. Some patients receiving pyrantel may experience gastrointestinal side effects, such as nausea, vomiting, abdominal cramps, or diarrhea.

Contraindications, Precautions, and Interactions of Pyrantel

Pyrantel is contraindicated in patients with known hypersensitivity. Pyrantel is used with caution in individuals with liver dysfunction, malnutrition, or anemia. Pyrantel is a pregnancy category C drug and is used during pregnancy only if the potential benefit outweighs the risk to the fetus. Pyrantel and piperazine are antagonists and should not be given together.

Actions, Uses, and Adverse Reactions of Thiabendazole

The exact mechanism of action of thiabendazole (Mintezol) is unknown. This drug appears to suppress egg or larval production and therefore may interrupt the lifecycle of the helminth. Thiabendazole is used to treat threadworm. Thiabendazole may cause hypersensitivity reactions, drowsiness, and dizziness.

Contraindications, Precautions, and Interactions of Thiabendazole

Thiabendazole is contraindicated in patients with known hypersensitivity. Thiabendazole is used with caution in patients with liver or kidney disease. Thiabendazole is a pregnancy category C drug and is used during pregnancy only if the potential benefit outweighs the risk to the fetus. When thiabendazole is administered with the xanthine derivatives, the plasma level of the xanthine may increase to toxic levels. Xanthine plasma levels must be monitored closely in case a dosage reduction is necessary.

Patient Management Issues with Anthelmintic Drugs

The diagnosis of a helminth infection is made by examination of the stool for ova and all or part of the helminth. Several stool specimens may be necessary before the helminth is seen and identified. The patient history also may lead to a suspicion of a helminth infection, but some patients have no symptoms. When a pinworm infection is suspected, a specimen is taken from the anal area.

Patients with massive helminth infections may or may not be acutely ill. Acutely ill patients require hospitalization, but many individuals with helminth infections can be treated on an outpatient basis.

Depending on hospital policy, as well as the type of helminth infection, linen precautions may be necessary. Gloves are worn when changing bed linens, emptying bedpans, or obtaining or handling stool specimens, and thorough handwashing is required after removing the gloves. Patients should wash their hands thoroughly after personal care and using a bedpan.

All stools that are passed after the drug is given should be saved. Each stool is inspected for passage of the helminth. If stool specimens are to be saved for laboratory examination, then hospital procedure should be followed for saving the stool and transporting it to the laboratory. If the patient is acutely ill or has a massive infection, then vital signs are monitored every 4 hours, and fluid intake and output is measured. The patient is observed for adverse drug reactions, as well as severe episodes of diarrhea. The health care provider should be informed if these occur.

With mebendazole, the patient may chew, swallow whole, or mix the tablets with food. The patient should take this drug with foods high in fat to increase absorption. A complete blood count is obtained before therapy and periodically during therapy because mebendazole can cause leukopenia or thrombocytopenia.

Patients can take pyrantel anytime without regard to meal or time of day. Patients may take the drug with milk or fruit juices.

Patient should take thiabendazole with food to minimize gastrointestinal upset and distress.

Managing Adverse Reactions of Anthelmintic Drugs. Gastrointestinal upset may occur, causing nausea, vomiting, abdominal pain, and diarrhea. Taking the drug with food often helps to alleviate the nausea. Patients may require frequent, small meals of easily digested food. If the patient vomits, then the health care provider may prescribe an antiemetic or a different anthelmintic agent. If the patient has diarrhea, then the health care provider should be notified because a change in the drug regimen may be needed. The number, consistency, color, and frequency of the patient's stools are recorded. Fluid intake and output is monitored.

Educating the Patient and Family About Anthelmintic Drugs

When an anthelmintic is prescribed on an outpatient basis, the patient or a family member is given complete instructions about household precautions to follow until the helminth is eliminated from the intestine. Patient Education Box 26-3 includes key points about anthelmintic drugs that the patient and family members should know.

Antimalarial Drugs

Malaria is transmitted from person to person by a certain species of the *Anopheles* mosquito. The four different protozoans causing malaria are *Plasmodium falciparum, P. malariae, P. ovale,* and *P. vivax.* Drugs used to treat or prevent malaria are called antimalarial drugs. Three antimalarial drugs are discussed here: chloroquine, doxycycline, and quinine sulfate. Other antimalarial drugs in use today are listed in the Summary Drug Table: Antimalarial Drugs.

Actions of Antimalarial Drugs

The plasmodium that causes malaria must enter the mosquito to develop, reproduce, and be transmitted. When the mosquito bites a person infected with malaria, it ingests the male and female forms (gametocytes) of the plasmodium. The gametocytes mate in the mosquito's stomach and ultimately form sporozoites (an animal reproductive cell) that make their way to the salivary glands of the mosquito. When the mosquito bites a noninfected person, the sporozoites enter the person's bloodstream and lodge in the liver and other tissues. The sporozoites then undergo asexual cell division and reproduction and form merozoites. The merozoites then divide asexually and enter the red blood cells of the person, where they form the male and female forms of the plasmodium. The symptoms of malaria (shaking, chills, and fever) appear when the merozoites enter the individual's red blood cells.

Antimalarial drugs interfere with the lifecycle of the plasmodium, primarily when it is present in red blood cells. Destruction at this stage of the plasmodium lifecycle prevents the development of the male and female forms of the plasmodium. This in turn keeps the mosquito (when the mosquito bites an infected individual) from ingesting the male and female forms of the plasmodium, thus effectively ending the plasmodium lifecycle (Fig. 26-2).

Uses of Antimalarial Drugs

Two terms are used when discussing the uses of antimalarial drugs:

1. Suppression: the prevention of malaria
2. Treatment: the management of a malarial attack

Not all antimalarial drugs are effective in suppressing or treating all four of the plasmodium species that cause malaria. In addition, strains have developed that are resistant to some antimalarial drugs. The health care provider must select the antimalarial drug that reportedly is effective, at present, for the type of malaria the individual either has (for treatment) or could be exposed to (for prevention) in a specific area of the world.

Chloroquine (Aralen) is also used in the treatment of extraintestinal amebiasis (see following section on amebicides). Doxycycline is also used to treat infections caused by *Neisseria gonorrhoeae, Treponema pallidum, Listeria monocytogenes, Clostridium,* and *Bacillus anthracis* when penicillin is contraindicated. Quinine also may be used for the prevention or treatment of nocturnal leg cramps.

Adverse Reactions and Contraindications, Precautions, and Interactions of Antimalarial Drugs

Adverse Reactions of Chloroquine. The adverse reactions of chloroquine (Aralen HCl and phosphate) and hydroxychloroquine include hypotension, electrocardiographic changes, visual disturbances, headache, nausea, vomiting, anorexia, diarrhea, and abdominal cramps.

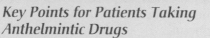

PATIENT EDUCATION BOX 26-3

Key Points for Patients Taking Anthelmintic Drugs

- ❑ Report any symptoms of infection (low-grade fever or sore throat) or thrombocytopenia (easy bruising or bleeding).
- ❑ Follow the dosage schedule exactly as printed on the prescription container. It is absolutely necessary to follow the directions for taking the drug to eliminate the helminth.
- ❑ Follow-up stool specimens will be necessary, because this is the only way to determine the success of drug therapy.
- ❑ To prevent reinfection and the infection of others in the household, change and launder your bed linens and undergarments daily, separately from those of other members of your family.
- ❑ Daily bathing (showering is best) is recommended. Disinfect toilet facilities daily, and disinfect the bathtub or shower stall immediately after bathing. Use the disinfectant recommended by your health care provider or use a chlorine bleach solution. Scrub the surfaces thoroughly and allow the disinfectant to remain in contact with the surfaces for several minutes.
- ❑ Wash your hands thoroughly after urinating or defecating and before preparing and eating food.
- ❑ Clean under your fingernails daily and avoid putting your fingers in your mouth or biting your nails.

ALBENDAZOLE
- ❑ This drug can cause serious harm to a developing fetus. Use a barrier contraceptive during the course of therapy and for 1 month after discontinuing the therapy.

SUMMARY DRUG TABLE   Antimalarial Drugs

Generic Name	Trade Name*	Uses	Adverse Reactions	Dosage Ranges
atovaquone and proguanil HCl *uh-toe'-vuh-kwone*	Malarone	Prevention and treatment of malaria	Headache, fever, myalgia, abdominal pain, diarrhea	Prevention: 1–2 d before travel; 1 tablet PO per day during period of exposure and for 7 days after exposure. Treatment: 4 tablets PO daily for 3 d
chloroquine *klor'-oh-kwin*	Aralen	Treatment and prevention of malaria	Hypotension, electrocardiographic changes, headache, nausea, vomiting, anorexia, diarrhea, abdominal cramps, visual disturbances	Treatment: *Dose expressed as base.* 160–200 mg (4–5 mL) IM and repeat in 6 h if necessary. Prevention: 300 mg PO weekly; treatment: initially 600 mg PO and 300 mg PO 6 h later, then 300 mg/d PO for 2 d
doxycycline *dox-i-sye'-kleen*	Monodox, Vibramycin, Vibra-Tabs *generic*	Short-term prevention of malaria	Photosensitivity, anorexia, nausea, vomiting, diarrhea, superinfection, rash	100 mg PO QD
halofantrine *hay'-low-fan-trin*	Halfan	Treatment of malaria	Abdominal pain, nausea, vomiting, anorexia, diarrhea, dizziness	500 mg PO q6h for 3 doses, repeat dose regimen in 7 d
hydroxychloroquine sulfate *hye-drox-ee-klor'-oh- kwin*	Plaquenil Sulfate	Prevention and treatment of malaria	Same as chloroquine	*Dose expressed as base.* Prevention: 310 mg PO weekly; treatment: initially 620 mg PO, and 310 mg 6 h later, then 310 mg/d PO for 2 d
mefloquine hydrochloride *me'-flow-kwin*	Lariam	Prevention and treatment of malaria	Vomiting, dizziness, disturbed sense of balance, nausea, fever, headache, visual disturbances	Prevention: 250 mg/wk PO for 4 wk, then 250 mg PO every other week; treatment: 5 tablets PO as a single dose
primaquine phosphate *prim'-a-kween*	*Generic*	Treatment of malaria	Nausea, vomiting, epigastric distress, abdominal cramps	*Dose expressed as base.* 15 mg/d PO for 14 d
pyrimethamine *peer-i-meth'-a-mine*	Daraprim	Prevention and treatment of malaria	Nausea, vomiting, hematologic changes, anorexia	Prevention: 25 mg PO once weekly; treatment: 50 mg/d for 2 days
quinine sulfate *kwi'-nine*	*Generic*	Treatment of malaria	Cinchonism, vertigo, hematologic changes, skin rash, visual disturbances	260–650 mg TID for 6–12 d
sulfadoxine and pyrimethamine *sul-fa-dox'-een peer-i-meth'-a-meen*	Fansidar	Prevention and treatment of malaria	Hematologic changes, nausea, emesis, headache, hypersensitivity reactions, Stevens-Johnson syndrome	Prevention: 1 tablet PO weekly or 2 tablets every 2 wk; treatment: 2–3 tablets PO as a single dose

*The term *generic* indicates the drug is available in generic form.

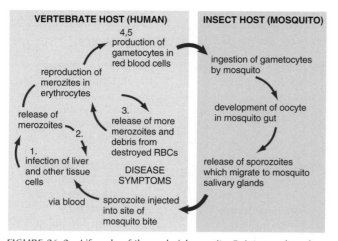

FIGURE 26-2 Lifecycle of the malarial parasite. Points numbered on the illustration indicate the location of the malarial lifecycle where specific drugs might be effective. (1) Chlorguanide, pyrimethamine, and primaquine used for causal prophylaxis. (2) Primaquine used to prevent relapses. (3) Drugs against the erythrocytic phase: potent action—chloroquine, amodiaquine, quinine; limited action—primaquine and chlorguanide. (4) Gametocidal drugs: primaquine. (5) Gametocyte-sterilizing drugs; chlorguanide, pyrimethamine. (From Roach SS. *Introductory Clinical Pharmacology*, 7th ed. Baltimore: Lippincott Williams & Wilkins; 2004.)

Contraindications, Precautions, and Interactions of Chloroquine. Chloroquine is contraindicated in patients with known hypersensitivity. Chloroquine is used cautiously in patients with liver disease or bone marrow depression and during pregnancy. The drug should be used with extreme caution in children.

Because the effects of chloroquine during pregnancy (pregnancy category C) are unknown, this drug is given only when clearly needed and the potential benefits outweigh potential hazards to the fetus. There is an increased risk of hepatotoxicity when chloroquine is taken with other hepatotoxic drugs.

Foods that acidify the urine (cranberries, plums, prunes, meats, cheeses, eggs, fish, and grains) may increase excretion and decrease the effectiveness of chloroquine.

Adverse Reactions of Doxycycline. Doxycycline (Vibramycin) is an antibiotic belonging to the tetracycline group of antibiotics. The adverse reactions associated with this drug are discussed in Chapter 25 and include photosensitivity, anorexia, nausea, and vomiting.

Contraindications, Precautions, and Interactions of Doxycycline. Doxycycline is contraindicated in patients with known hypersensitivity. Because the effects of doxycycline during pregnancy are unknown, this drug is contraindicated during pregnancy (category D). The drug is used cautiously in patients with kidney or liver impairment and during lactation. Absorption of the drug is decreased when it is taken with antacids or iron. There is a decrease of the therapeutic effects of doxycycline when the drug is taken with barbiturates, pheny-

toins, and carbamazepine. There is an increased risk of digoxin toxicity when digoxin is taken with doxycycline.

Adverse Reactions of Quinine. The use of quinine can cause cinchonism at full therapeutic doses. **Cinchonism** is a group of symptoms associated with quinine, including tinnitus, dizziness, headache, gastrointestinal disturbances, and visual disturbances. These symptoms usually disappear when the dosage is reduced. Other adverse reactions include hematologic changes, vertigo, and skin rash.

Contraindications, Precautions, and Interactions of Quinine. Quinine is contraindicated in patients with known hypersensitivity. The drug is also contraindicated in pregnant women (pregnancy category X) and in patients with myasthenia gravis (may cause respiratory distress and dysphagia). Quinine absorption is delayed when taken with antacids containing aluminum. Plasma digitalis levels may increase when digitalis preparations and quinine are given concurrently. Plasma levels of warfarin are increased when taken with quinine.

Patient Management Issues with Antimalarial Drugs

If the patient is hospitalized with malaria, then vital signs are taken every 4 hours or as ordered by the health care provider. The patient is observed every 1 to 2 hours for the symptoms of malaria (headache, nausea, muscle aching, and high fever). Improvement or exacerbation of signs and symptoms of malaria is documented and reported to the health care provider. Antipyretics may be ordered for fever. If the patient is acutely ill, then fluid intake and output are measured. In some instances, intravenous fluids may be required.

When an antimalarial drug such as chloroquine is used for prophylaxis (prevention), therapy should begin 2 weeks before exposure and continue for 6 to 8 weeks after the client leaves the area where malaria is prevalent. The initial treatment with quinine may be given parenterally. Parenteral injection of chloroquine is avoided because the drug can cause respiratory distress, shock, and cardiovascular collapse when given intramuscularly or intravenously. If chloroquine must be given parenterally, then the route should be changed to oral as soon as possible.

Managing Adverse Reactions of Antimalarial Drugs. Adverse reactions associated with the antimalarial drugs, such as dizziness, hypotension, and visual disturbances are monitored. Other adverse reactions are listed in the Summary Drug Table: Antimalarial Drugs.

Patients receiving an antimalarial drug may also experience nausea. Good nutrition is essential in the healing process. Several small meals may be preferable to three large meals.

Some patients experience dizziness and hypotensive episodes when taking antimalarial drugs. The blood pressure should be monitored frequently if the patient is hospitalized. If dizziness occurs, the patient may need help with walking and self-care activities. The patient is instructed to rise slowly from a reclining position, sit a few minutes before standing, and stand a few minutes before beginning to walk. A patient taking these drugs on an outpatient basis is told to avoid driving or performing hazardous tasks if dizziness occurs.

The patient taking chloroquine may experience a number of visual disturbances, such as disturbed color vision, blurred vision, night blindness, diminished visual fields, or optic atrophy.

ALERT

Chloroquine and Visual Disturbances

Any visual disturbance in patients taking chloroquine should be reported to the health care provider. Irreversible retinal damage has occurred in patients on long-term therapy with these drugs.

Frequent ophthalmic examinations are necessary for patients receiving long-term or high-dose regimens of chloroquine. When vision is affected, the patient is assessed for the extent of visual impairment. Outpatients should be told not to drive until assessed by an ophthalmologist. Furniture should be positioned out of walkways, scatter rugs removed, items frequently used placed in convenient places, and grab bars placed to help the patient maintain balance. The patient may need help walking and with other activities.

Educating the Patient and Family About Antimalarial Drugs

When an antimalarial drug is prescribed for the prevention (suppression) of malaria, the drug regimen is carefully reviewed with the patient. When the drug is to be taken once per week, patients should select a day of the week that will best remind them to take the drug. The importance of taking the drug exactly as prescribed is emphasized, because failure to take the drug on an exact schedule will not give protection against malaria.

When an antimalarial drug is used for prevention of malaria and taken once per week, the patient must take the drug on the same day each week. The program of prevention is usually started 2 weeks before departure to an area where malaria is prevalent.

Patient Education Box 26-4 includes key points about antimalarial drugs the patient and family members should know.

Amebicides

Amebicides (drugs that kill amebas) are used to treat amebiasis caused by the parasite *E. histolytica*. An ameba is a one-celled organism found in soil and water. Exam-

---

PATIENT EDUCATION BOX 26-4

Key Points for Patients Taking Antimalarial Drugs

CHLOROQUINE

❑ Take this drug with food or milk. Avoid foods that acidify urine (cranberries, plums, prunes, meats, cheeses, eggs, fish, and grains).

❑ This drug may cause diarrhea, loss of appetite, nausea, stomach pain, or vomiting. Notify your health care provider if your symptoms become pronounced.

❑ Chloroquine may cause a yellow or brown discoloration to your urine; this is normal and will go away when the drug therapy is discontinued.

❑ Notify the health care provider if you experience any of the following:
  ❑ visual changes
  ❑ ringing in your ears
  ❑ difficulty in hearing
  ❑ fever
  ❑ sore throat
  ❑ unusual bleeding or bruising
  ❑ unusual color (blue–black) of the skin
  ❑ skin rash
  ❑ unusual muscle weakness

DOXYCYCLINE

❑ This drug can cause photosensitivity. Even relatively brief exposure to sunlight may cause sunburn. Avoid exposure to the sun by wearing protective clothing (e.g., long-sleeved shirts and wide-brimmed hats) and by using a sunscreen.

QUININE

❑ Take this drug with food or immediately after a meal.

❑ Do not drive or perform other hazardous tasks requiring alertness if you experience blurred vision or dizziness.

❑ Do not chew the tablet or open the capsule because the drug is irritating to the stomach.

❑ If you experience itching, rash, fever, difficulty breathing, or vision problems, then stop taking the drug and notify your health care provider.

---

ples of amebicides are listed in the Summary Drug Table: Amebicides.

Actions and Uses of Amebicides

Amebicides are drugs that kill amebas. The two types of amebiasis are intestinal and extraintestinal. In the intestinal form, the ameba is confined to the intestine. In the extraintestinal form, the ameba is found outside of the intestine, such as in the liver. The extraintestinal form of amebiasis is more difficult to treat.

Iodoquinol (Yodoxin) and metronidazole (Flagyl) are used to treat intestinal amebiasis. Metronidazole is also used to treat infections caused by susceptible

SUMMARY DRUG TABLE   Amebicides

Generic Name	Trade Name*	Uses	Adverse Reactions	Dosage Ranges
chloroquine hydrochloride *klor'-oh-kwin*	Aralen	Extraintestinal amebiasis when oral therapy not feasible	Hypotension, electrocardiographic (ECG) changes, headache, nausea, vomiting, anorexia, diarrhea, abdominal cramps, psychic stimulation, visual disturbances	*Dose expressed as base.* 160–200 mg/d IM for 10–12 d
chloroquine phosphate *klor'-oh-kwin*	Aralen Phosphate, *generic*	Extraintestinal amebiasis when oral therapy not feasible	Hypotension, ECG changes, headache, nausea, vomiting, anorexia, diarrhea, abdominal cramps, psychic stimulation	1 g (600 mg base)/d for 2 d, then 500 mg (300 mg base)/d for 2–3 wk
iodoquinol *eye-oh-doe-kwin'-ole*	Yodoxin	Treatment of intestinal amebiasis	Skin eruptions, nausea vomiting, fever, chills, abdominal cramps, vertigo, diarrhea	650 mg PO TID after meals for 20 d
metronidazole *me-troe-ni'-da-zole*	Flagyl, *generic*	Treatment of intestinal amebiasis	Headache, nausea, peripheral neuropathy, disulfiram-like interaction with alcohol	750 mg PO TID for 5–10 d
paromomycin *par-oh-moe-mye'-sin*	Humatin	Treatment of intestinal amebiasis	Nausea, vomiting, diarrhea	25–35 mg/kg/d in 3 divided doses with meals for 5–10 d

*The term *generic* indicates the drug is available in generic form.

microorganisms and is discussed in Chapter 25. Paromomycin is an aminoglycoside with amebicidal activity and is used to treat intestinal amebiasis. Chloroquine hydrochloride (Aralen) is used to treat extraintestinal amebiasis.

Adverse Reactions and Contraindications, Precautions, and Interactions of Amebicides

Adverse Reactions of Chloroquine. Hypotension, electrocardiographic changes, headache, nausea, vomiting, anorexia, diarrhea, abdominal cramps, and psychic stimulation can occur with the use of chloroquine hydrochloride or phosphate.

Contraindications, Precautions, and Interactions of Chloroquine. Chloroquine is contraindicated in patients with known hypersensitivity. Precautions and interactions for chloroquine are listed in the previous section on Antimalarial Drugs.

Adverse Reactions of Iodoquinol. Various types of skin eruptions, nausea, vomiting, fever, chills, abdominal cramps, vertigo, and diarrhea can occur with iodoquinol use.

Contraindications, Precautions, and Interactions of Iodoquinol. Iodoquinol is contraindicated in patients with known hypersensitivity. Iodoquinol is used with caution in patients with thyroid disease and during pregnancy and lactation. Iodoquinol may interfere with the results of thyroid function tests. This interference may last as long as 6 months after iodoquinol therapy is discontinued.

Adverse Reactions of Metronidazole. Convulsive seizures, headache, nausea, and peripheral neuropathy (numbness and tingling of the extremities) have been reported with the use of metronidazole.

Contraindications, Precautions, and Interactions of Metronidazole. Metronidazole is contraindicated in patients with known hypersensitivity. Metronidazole is contraindicated during the first trimester of pregnancy (category B) but is given during the second and third trimesters of pregnancy. Metronidazole is used cautiously in patients with blood dyscrasias, seizure disorders, and severe liver impairment. The patient must avoid alcohol while taking metronidazole.

When metronidazole is used with cimetidine, the metabolism of metronidazole is decreased; when it is used with phenobarbital, the metabolism is increased, possibly causing a decrease in the effectiveness of metronidazole. Metronidazole increases the effects of warfarin.

Adverse Reactions of Paromomycin. This drug has relatively few adverse reactions. The most common include nausea, vomiting, and diarrhea. More serious adverse reactions, although rare, are nephrotoxicity and ototoxicity.

Contraindications, Precautions, and Interactions of Paromomycin. Paromomycin is contraindicated in patients with known hypersensitivity. Paromomycin is given with caution during pregnancy. Paromomycin is used with caution in patients with bowel disease. High doses and prolonged therapy are avoided because the drug may be absorbed in large amounts by patients with bowel disease, causing ototoxicity and kidney impairment.

Patient Management Issues with Amebicides

Diagnosis of amebiasis is made by examining the stool and considering the patient's symptoms. Once the patient has received a diagnosis of amebiasis, local health department regulations often require investigation into the source of infection. A history of foreign travel is necessary. If the patient has not traveled to a foreign country, then further investigation of the patient's lifestyle, such as local travel, use of restaurants, and the local water supply (especially well water) may be necessary to identify the source of the infection. In addition, it is common practice to test immediate family members for amebiasis.

If the patient is acutely ill or has vomiting and diarrhea, then fluid intake and output are measured and the patient is closely monitored for signs of dehydration. If dehydration is apparent, then the health care provider should be notified. If the patient is or becomes dehydrated, then oral or intravenous fluid and electrolyte replacement may be necessary. Vital signs are taken every 4 hours or as ordered by the health care provider.

Patients with amebiasis may or may not be acutely ill. Isolation is usually not necessary, but hospital policy may require isolation procedures. Stool precautions are usually necessary. Thorough handwashing is required after all patient care and handling of stool specimens.

Managing Adverse Reactions of Amebicides. The patient is monitored for adverse reactions associated with the amebicides such as diarrhea and gastrointestinal upsets. Other adverse reactions are listed on the Summary Drug Table: Amebicides.

The number, character, and color of the patient's stools are closely monitored. Daily stool specimens may be ordered to be sent to the laboratory for examination. All stool specimens saved are immediately delivered for examination to the laboratory because the organisms die (and then cannot be seen microscopically) when the specimen cools. Laboratory personnel are informed that the patient has amebiasis because the specimen must be kept at or near body temperature until examined under a microscope.

A patient with severe or frequent episodes of diarrhea is monitored for symptoms of dehydration. The health care provider is notified if signs of dehydration become apparent because intravenous fluids may be necessary.

Because most amebicides cause gastrointestinal upset, particularly nausea, maintaining adequate nutrition is important. The patient's body weight is monitored daily to identify any changes (increase or decrease). Small frequent meals (five to six daily) may be more appealing than three large meals.

Educating the Patient and Family About Amebicides

The importance of completing the full course of treatment must be stressed. Patient Education Box 26-5 includes key points about amebicides that the patient and family members should know.

PATIENT EDUCATION BOX 26-5

Key Points for Patients Taking Amebicides

- ❑ Follow directions to take the drug exactly as prescribed. Complete the full course of therapy to eradicate the ameba. Failure to complete treatment may result in a return of the infection.
- ❑ Follow measures to control the spread of infection. Wash your hands immediately before eating or preparing food and after defecation.
- ❑ Food handlers should not resume work until after completing the full course of treatment and stools do not contain the ameba.

CHLOROQUINE

- ❑ Notify your health care provider if you experience any of the following: ringing in your ears, difficulty hearing, visual changes, fever, sore throat, or unusual bleeding or bruising.

IODOQUINOL

- ❑ Notify your health care provider if you experience nausea, vomiting, or other gastrointestinal distress that becomes severe.

METRONIDAZOLE

- ❑ This drug may cause gastric upset.
- ❑ Take this drug with food or meals.
- ❑ Do not drink alcohol in any form until your course of treatment is completed. Alcohol may cause a mild or severe reaction, with symptoms of severe vomiting, headache, nausea, abdominal cramps, flushing, and sweating. These symptoms may be so severe that hospitalization may be required.

PAROMOMYCIN

- ❑ Take this drug 3 times per day with meals.
- ❑ Report any ringing in your ears, dizziness, severe gastrointestinal upset, decrease in urinary output, or other urinary difficulties.

KEY POINTS

○ Most antiviral drugs act by inhibiting viral DNA or RNA replication in the virus, causing viral death. Although infections caused by a virus are common, antiviral drugs have limited use because they are effective against only a small number of specific viral infections. The health care provider may prescribe an antiviral drug for an unlabeled use even though documentation of its effectiveness is lacking. The most common adverse reactions when these drugs are used systemically are gastrointestinal disturbances, such as nausea, vomiting, diarrhea, and anorexia. When administered topically, the antiviral drugs can cause transient burning, stinging, and pruritus. Antiviral drugs are contraindicated in patients with congestive heart failure, seizures, kidney disease, and during lactation, and are given with caution in patients with kidney impairment and require dosage adjustments.

○ Superficial mycotic (fungal) infections occur on the surface of, or just below, the skin or nails. Deep mycotic infections develop inside the body, such as in the lungs. Treatment for deep mycotic infections is often difficult and prolonged. When topical antifungal drugs are applied to the skin or mucous membranes, few adverse reactions occur. The vulvovaginal antifungal drugs may cause local irritation, redness, stinging, or abdominal pain. Few adverse reactions occur with the vulvovaginal antifungal drugs. The most effective systemic antifungals often cause serious reactions, including fever, shaking, chills, headache, malaise, anorexia, joint and muscle pain, abnormal renal function, nausea, vomiting, and anemia.

○ Antiparasitic drugs are used to treat parasites, organisms that live in or on another organism (the host) without contributing to the survival or well being of the host. Invasion of the body by helminths, malaria, and amebiasis are problems caused by parasites. Anthelmintics are used to kill parasites. Adverse reactions are mild when the drug is used in the recommended dosage. Contraindications, precautions, and interactions are drug-specific. Antimalarial drugs interfere with the lifecycle of the plasmodium and are used for both suppression and treatment. Adverse reactions to antimalarials include nausea, anorexia, and vomiting. Amebicides are used to treat amebiasis. Adverse reactions of amebicides include nausea, vomiting, anorexia, abdominal cramps, and headache.

CASE STUDY

Ms. Jenkins, age 77 years, has herpes zoster. Her health care provider prescribes acyclovir 200 mg every 4 hours while awake.

1. Ms. Jenkins would like to know more about the adverse reactions associated with acyclovir. She should be told:
   a. urinary retention is the primary adverse reaction
   b. psychosis is an adverse reaction to acyclovir
   c. headache, nausea, and rashes are known adverse reactions
   d. all of the above

2. Ms. Jenkins is especially concerned about possible stomach upset. She can be told that if the acyclovir causes nausea, she should:
   a. take the medicine with food
   b. take the medicine on an empty stomach
   c. take lots of antacids
   d. none of the above

3. Ms. Jenkins would not have been prescribed acyclovir if she had pre-existing:
   a. electrolyte abnormalities
   b. kidney abnormalities
   c. respiratory abnormalities
   d. any of the above

WEBSITE ACTIVITIES

1. Go to the Center for Disease Control Travel's Health website (http://www.cdc.gov/travel/) and click on "Diseases" in the Contents listing. Follow through to see the description and

transmission information about malaria. What are the three ways malaria may be transmitted?

1. _____

2. _____

3. _____

2. Return to the CDC Traveler's Health starting page. Make a list of the types of information available at this web site.

REVIEW QUESTIONS

1. Patients receiving antiviral drugs for human immunodeficiency infections should be closely monitored for signs of infection such as:
   a. fever
   b. malaise
   c. sore throat
   d. all of the above

2. Didanosine is properly taken when:
   a. tablets are crushed and mixed thoroughly with water to be drunk
   b. the drug is given only by subcutaneous injection
   c. the oral drug is given with meals
   d. the oral drug is given mixed with orange juice or apple juice

3. Mr. Carr is receiving amphotericin B for a systemic fungal infection. Which of the following would most likely indicate that Mr. Carr is experiencing an adverse reaction to amphotericin B?
   a. fever and chills
   b. back pain
   c. drowsiness
   d. flushing of the skin

4. Griseofulvin would not be given to a patient if the patient has:
   a. anemia
   b. respiratory disease
   c. a recent myocardial infarction
   d. severe liver disease

5. A patient asks how antimalarial drugs prevent or treat malaria. The correct response is that this group of drugs:
   a. kills the mosquito that carries the protozoa
   b. interferes with the lifecycle of the protozoa causing malaria
   c. ruptures the red blood cells that contain merozoites
   d. increases the body's natural immune response to the protozoa

6. When a patient is instructed how to take chloroquine for the prevention of malaria, the patient is told:
   a. to take the drug on an empty stomach
   b. to protect the skin from the sun because the drug can cause a severe sunburn
   c. therapy should begin 2 weeks before possible exposure
   d. to take the drug with a citrus drink to enhance absorption

KEY TERMS

active immunity—the reaction of the body when exposed to certain infectious
microorganisms (antigens) of forming antibodies to the invading microorganism

antibody—a globulin (protein) produced by the B lymphocytes as a defense against an
antigen

antigen—a substance, usually a protein, that stimulates the body to produce antibodies

antigen–antibody response—the reaction of specific circulating antibodies to a specific
antigen

antivenin—an antitoxin specific for an animal or insect venom

attenuated—weakened, as in the antigen strain used for vaccine development

booster—the administration of an additional dose of the vaccine to "boost" the
production of antibodies to a level that will maintain the desired immunity

cell-mediated immunity—the process of T lymphocytes and macrophages (large cells that
surround, engulf, and digest microorganisms and cellular debris) working together to
destroy an antigen

globulin—proteins present in blood serum or plasma that contain antibodies

humoral immunity—based on the antigen–antibody response, special lymphocytes
(white blood cells) produce circulating antibodies to act against a foreign substance

immune globulin—solutions obtained from human blood containing antibodies that
have been formed by the body to specific antigens

immunity—the ability of the body to identify and resist microorganisms that are
potentially harmful

passive immunity—a type of immunity occurring from the administration of ready-made
antibodies from another individual or animal

toxin—a poisonous substance produced by some bacteria

toxoid—a toxin that is weakened but still capable of stimulating the formation of
antitoxins

vaccine—artificial active immunity created with killed or weakened antigens for the
purpose of creating resistance to disease

CHAPTER OBJECTIVES

On completion of this chapter, students will be able to:

1 Define the chapter's key terms.

2 Describe the general drug actions, uses, adverse reactions, contraindications, precautions, and interactions of immunologic agents.

3 Discuss important points to keep in mind when educating the patient or family members about the use of immunologic agents.

Immunity is the ability of the body to identify and resist microorganisms that are potentially harmful. This ability enables the body to fight or prevent infectious disease and inhibit tissue and organ damage. The immune system is not confined to any one part of the body. Immune stem cells, formed in the bone marrow, may remain in the bone marrow until maturation or migrate to different body sites for maturation. After maturation, most immune cells circulate in the body and exert specific effects. The immune system has two distinct, but overlapping, mechanisms with which to fight invading organisms:

- cell-mediated defenses (cellular immunity)
- antibody-mediated defenses (humoral immunity)

Cell-Mediated Immunity

Cell-mediated immunity is the result of the activity of many leukocyte actions, reactions, and interactions that range from simple to complex. This type of immunity depends on the actions of the T lymphocytes, which are responsible for a delayed type of immune response. The T lymphocyte becomes sensitized by its first contact with a specific antigen. Subsequent exposure to an antigen stimulates multiple reactions aimed at destroying or inactivating the offending antigen. T lymphocytes and macrophages (large cells that surround, engulf, and digest microorganisms and cellular debris) work together in cell-mediated immunity to destroy the antigen. T lymphocytes attack the antigens directly, rather than produce antibodies (as is performed in humoral immunity). Cellular reactions may also occur without macrophages. Several T lymphocytes (T cells) are involved in cell-mediated immunity:

- helper T4 cells: function within the bloodstream identifying and destroying antigens
- helper T1 cells: increase B lymphocyte antibody production
- helper T2 cells: increase activity of cytotoxic (killer) T cells, which attack the cell directly by altering the cell membrane and causing cell lysis (destruction)
- suppressor T cells: suppress the immune response

- memory T lymphocytes: recognize previous contact with antigens and activate an immune response

T lymphocytes defend against viral infections, fungal infections, and some bacterial infections. If cell-mediated immunity is lost, as in the case of acquired immunodeficiency syndrome, then the body is unable to protect itself against many viral, bacterial, and fungal infections.

Humoral Immunity

In **humoral immunity** special lymphocytes (white blood cells), called B lymphocytes, produce circulating antibodies to act against a foreign substance. This type of immunity is based on the antigen–antibody response. An **antigen** is a substance, usually a protein, that stimulates the body to produce antibodies. An **antibody** is a globulin (protein) produced by the B lymphocytes as a defense against an antigen. Humoral immunity protects the body against bacterial and viral infections.

Specific antibodies are formed for a specific antigen; for example, chickenpox antibodies are formed when the person is exposed to the chickenpox virus (the antigen). This is called an **antigen–antibody response**. Once manufactured, antibodies circulate in the bloodstream, sometimes for only a short time and at other times for the life of the person. When an antigen enters the body, specific antibodies neutralize the specific invading antigen; this is called immunity. Therefore, the individual with specific circulating antibodies is immune (or has immunity) to a specific antigen. Immunity is the resistance that an individual has against disease.

Cell-mediated and humoral immunity are interdependent. Cell-mediated immunity influences the function of the B lymphocytes, and humoral immunity influences the function of the T lymphocytes.

Active and Passive Immunity

Active and passive immunity involve the use of agents that stimulate antibody formation (active immunity) or the injection of ready-made antibodies found in the serum of immune individuals or animals (passive immunity).

Active Immunity

When a person is exposed to certain infectious microorganisms (antigens), the body begins to form antibodies (or build an immunity) to the invading microorganism. This is called **active immunity**. The two types of active immunity are naturally acquired active immunity and artificially acquired active immunity. The Summary Drug Table: Agents for Active Immunization identifies agents that produce active immunity.

(text continued on page 466)

SUMMARY DRUG TABLE   Agents for Active Immunization

Generic Drug	Trade Name*	Uses	Adverse Reactions	Dosage Ranges
Vaccines, Bacterial bcg vaccine *bee-see-gee-vak'-seen*	Tice BCG	Infants and children with negative tuberculin skin test who are at high risk for intimate and prolonged exposure to pulmonary tuberculosis	Rare; minor local reactions such as local tenderness, pain at injection site, malaise, nausea, diarrhea, headache, fever	0.2–0.3 mL percutaneous
cholera vaccine *kol'-er-ah-vak'-seen*	*Generic*	Immunization against cholera in individuals traveling to or living in countries where cholera is endemic or epidemic	Same as for BCG vaccine	0.2–0.3 mL SC, IM with a booster of 0.5 mL at 10 y
Haemophilus influenzae type b conjugate and hepatitis B vaccine *he'-maw-fil-us in-flu-en'-zah kon-jew'-gate hep-ah-tie'-tus bee-vak'-seen*	ActHIB, Comvax, HibTITER Vaccine, PedvaxHIB	Routine immunization of children	Same as for BCG vaccine	0.5 mL IM
lyme disease vaccine (recombinant OspA) *lime-vak'-seen*	LYMErix	Active immunization against Lyme disease in individuals 15–70 years of age who are at risk of contracting the disease	Same as for BCG vaccine	30 mcg IM, SC at 0, 1, and 12 mo
meningococcal polysaccharide vaccine *men-in-jo'-kok'-al po-ly-sack'-a-ride vak'-seen*	Menomune A/C/Y/W-135	Active immunization against invasive meningococcal disease	Same as for BCG vaccine	0.5 mL SC only
pneumococcal vaccine, polyvalent *new-mo-kok'-kal vak'-seen*	Pneumovax 23, Pnu-Imune 23	Immunization against pneumococcal pneumonia and bacteremia caused by the types of pneumococci included in the vaccine	Same as for BCG vaccine	0.5 mL SC or IM
pneumococcal 7-valent conjugate vaccine (diphtheria CRM197 protein) *new-mo-kok'-kal-vak'-seen*	Prevnar	Active immunization against *Streptococcus pneumoniae* for infants and toddlers	Rare; minor local reactions such as local tenderness, pain at injection site, decreased appetite, irritability, drowsiness, malaise, nausea, diarrhea, fever	0.5 mL IM

Generic Drug	Trade Name*	Uses	Adverse Reactions	Dosage Ranges
typhoid vaccine *tye'-foid-vak'-seen*	Typhim Vi, Vivotif Berna, *generic*	Immunization against typhoid	Same as for BCG vaccine	Oral: One capsule on alternate days 1h before a meal for a total of 4 capsules; Parenteral: Adults and children 10 years and older, 2 doses of 0.5 mL SC; children younger than 10 years, 2 doses of 0.25 mL SC; Booster: 0.1–0.5 mL intradermally
Vaccines, Viral measles virus vaccine, live, attenuated *me'-zuls-vak'-seen*	Attenuvax	Active immunization against measles	Same as for BCG vaccine	0.5 mL SC
rubella virus vaccine, live *ru-bell'-a-vi'-rus-vak'-seen*	Meruvax II	Selective active immunization against rubella	Same as for BCG vaccine	Total volume of reconstituted vial SC
mumps virus vaccine, live *mumps-vi'-rus-vak'-seen*	Mumpsvax	Selective active immunization against mumps	Same as for BCG vaccine	0.5 mL SC (total volume of reconstituted vaccine)
rubella and mumps virus vaccine, live *ru-bell'-a-and mumps-vi'-rus-vak'-seen*	Biavax-II	Active immunization against rubella and mumps	Same as for BCG vaccine	0.5 mL SC
measles (rubeola) and rubella virus vaccine, live *me'-zuls-ru-be'-o-la and ru-bell'-ah*	M-R-Vax II	Active immunization against rubeola and rubella	Same as for BCG vaccine	0.5 mL SC
poliovirus vaccine, live, oral, trivalent (OPV; TOPV; Sabin) *po-lee'-o-vi'-rus-live*	Orimune	Active immunization against poliovirus	Rare; malaise, nausea, diarrhea, fever	Three doses 0.5 mL PO at specified intervals
poliovirus vaccine, inactivated (IPV) *po-lee'-o-vi'-rus vak'-seen*	IPOL	Active immunizations for the poliovirus	Same as for BCG vaccine	Three doses of 0.5 mL SC at 2 months, 4 mo, and 12–15 mo; children receive a booster dose before entering school
influenza virus vaccine *in-flu'-en-za-vi'-rus vak'-seen*	FluShield, Fluvirin, Fluzone	Active immunization against the specific influenza virus strains contained in the formulation	Same as for BCG vaccine	One or two doses of 0.25–0.5 mL IM

Generic Drug	Trade Name*	Uses	Adverse Reactions	Dosage Ranges
Japanese encephalitis virus vaccine *en-ceph'-ah-lie-tis vak'-seen*	JE-VAX	For active immunization against Japanese encephalitis for individuals older than 1 y	Same as for BCG vaccine	Three doses given to adults and children >3 y: 1 mL SC on days 0, 7, and 30; children 1–3 years: 0.5 mL SC on days 0, 7, and 30
rotavirus vaccine *row'-ta-vi'-rus-vak'-seen*	RotaShield	Prevention of gastroenteritis caused by rotavirus serotypes contained in the vaccines	Fever, decreased appetite, abdominal cramping, irritability, and decreased activity	Three 2.5-mL doses given orally
yellow fever vaccine	YF-Vax	Active immunity against yellow fever virus, primarily among travelers to yellow fever endemic areas	Malaise, usually appearing 7–14 d after administration, myalgia, and headache	0.5 mL SC; booster dose suggested q10 y
hepatitis B vaccine, recombinant *hep-ah-tie'-tis-B-vak'-seen*	Engerix-B, Recombivax HB	Immunization against infections caused by all known subtypes of hepatitis B virus	Headache, light-headedness, vertigo, dizziness, paresthesia, insomnia, disturbed sleep, pruritus, rash, urticaria, erythema, nausea, vomiting, abdominal pain, dyspepsia, constipation, anorexia, diarrhea, hypersensitivity, local pain and soreness at injection site, swelling, induration, or tenderness at injection site, arthralgia, influenza-like symptoms, fatigue, tinnitus, earache	3–4 doses of 0.5–2 mL
hepatitis A vaccine, inactivated *hep-ah-tie'-tis A vak'-seen*	Havrix, Vaqta	Active immunization of individuals 2 mo of age and older against disease caused by hepatitis A virus (HAV)	Headache, hypertonic episode, insomnia, photophobia, vertigo, pruritus, rash, urticaria, erythema, dermatitis, anorexia, nausea, abdominal pain, diarrhea, vomiting, arthralgia, pharyngitis, cough, fatigue, fever, and malaise; soreness, pain, tenderness, induration, redness, swelling, or rash at injection site	Administered IM; dosage varies with product. See package insert for specific dosages.
hepatitis A, inactivated and hepatitis B, recombinant vaccine *hep-ah-tie'-tis A in-ac'-ti-va-ted hep-ah-tie'-tis B vak'-seen*	Twinrix	Active immunization against hepatitis A and B viruses	Same as for hepatitis A, inactivated	Administered IM in single-dose vial and single-dose prefilled syringes. See package insert for recommended dose.

Generic Drug	Trade Name*	Uses	Adverse Reactions	Dosage Ranges
varicella virus vaccine *var-i-sel-a-vak'-seen*	Varivax	Vaccination against varicella in people older than 1 y	Children: Upper respiratory illness, cough, irritability, nervousness, fatigue, disturbed sleep, diarrhea, loss of appetite, vomiting, otitis, diaper rash, headache, teething, malaise; Adults: fever; injection site complaints of soreness, erythema, swelling, induration and numbness, varicella-like rash; upper respiratory illness; headache; fatigue; cough; myalgia; disturbed sleep; nausea; diarrhea; stiff neck; irritability; nervousness; constipation	Children 1–12 y: one dose 0.5 mL SC; Adults: 0.5 mL; SC two doses
rabies vaccine *ray'-bees-vak'-seen*	Imovax Rabies I.D. Vaccine (human diploid cell), Imovax Rabies Vaccine (human diploid cell), RabAvert, Rabies Vaccine Adsorbed	Pre-exposure: immunization of people with greater than usual risk of exposure to rabies virus by reason of occupation (e.g., veterinarians, laboratory workers, animal handlers, forest rangers, people staying >1 mo in countries where rabies is a constant threat); postexposure prophylaxis: bite by a carrier animal that is unprovoked and rabies is present in the area	Transient pain, erythema, swelling or itching at the injection site, headache, nausea, abdominal pain, muscle aches, and dizziness	Pre-exposure prophylaxis: on days 0, 7, 21 to 28 and then q2–5 years based on antibody titers 1 mL IM (Imovax Rabies Vaccine or Rabies Vaccine Adsorbed) or 0.1 mL I.D. (Imovax Rabies I.D.) Postexposure: Do not give intradermally, only IM, 20 IU/kg as soon as possible after exposure, followed by IM vaccine doses on days 0, 3, 7, 14 and 28
Toxoids tetanus toxoid *tet'-ah-nus-toks'-oyd*	Tetanus Toxoid, Adsorbed Tetanus Toxoid, Fluid	Active immunization of children older than 6 wk and adults against tetanus	Cochlear lesion, brachial plexus neuropathies, paralysis of the radial nerve, accommodation paresis, EEG disturbances, urticaria, rash, malaise, fever, chills, pain, hypotension, nausea, and local redness, warmth, edema, induration and sterile abscess at injection site	0.5 mL IM
diphtheria and tetanus toxoids, combined (DT;Td) *dip-ther'-ee-ah-tet'-ah-nus-toks'-oyds*	Diphtheria and Tetanus Toxoids, adsorbed (for pediatric use), Diphtheria and Tetanus Toxoids, adsorbed (for adult use)	Immunization against diphtheria and tetanus	See adverse reactions for both diphtheria and tetanus toxoids.	See package inserts for specific dosage.

Generic Drug	Trade Name*	Uses	Adverse Reactions	Dosage Ranges
diphtheria and tetanus toxoids and acellular pertussis vaccine, adsorbed (DTaP) *dip-ther'-ee-ah-tet'-ah-nu-toks'-oyds-a-sell'-u-lar-per-tuss'-us*	Certiva, Infanrix, Tripedia	Active immunization against diphtheria, tetanus, and pertussis simultaneously	See adverse reactions for diphtheria and tetanus toxoids, and pertussis vaccine	Follow package instructions for preparation and IM administration
diphtheria and tetanus toxoids, acellular pertussis and *Haemophilus influenzae* type B	TriHIBit	Active immunization against diphtheria, tetanus, and pertussis and *Haemophilus influenzae* type B	See adverse reactions for diphtheria and tetanus toxoids, pertussis, and *Haemophilus influenzae* type B	See package insert for specific dosages; For IM administration only, usual dose is 0.5 mL
Vaccine diphtheria and tetanus toxoids and a cellular pertussis adsorbed, hepatitis B (recombinant) and inactivated poliovirus combined	Pediatrix	Active immunization against diphtheria, tetanus, pertussis and all known subtypes of hepatitis B virus, and poliomyelitis immunization	See adverse reactions against individual vaccines	Primary immunization series: 3 doses of 0.5 mL at 6-to 8-wk intervals IM (first dose is 2 mo of age, but may be given as early as 6 wk of age)

*The term *generic* indicates the drug is available in generic form.

Naturally acquired active immunity occurs when a person is exposed to a disease, experiences the disease, and the body manufactures antibodies to provide future immunity to the disease. It is called active immunity because the antibodies were produced by the person who had the disease (Fig. 27-1). Thus, having the disease produces immunity.

Artificially acquired active immunity occurs when an individual is given a killed or weakened antigen, which stimulates the formation of antibodies against the antigen. The antigen does not cause the disease, but the individual will still manufacture specific antibodies against the disease. When a vaccine containing an **attenuated** (weakened) antigen is given, the individual may experience a few minor symptoms of the disease or even a mild form of the disease, but the symptoms are almost always milder and usually last for a short time.

The decision to use an attenuated, rather than a killed, virus as a vaccine to provide immunity is based

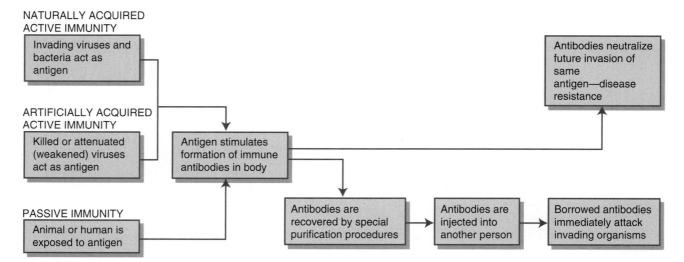

FIGURE 27-1 Active and passive immunity. (From Roach SS. *Introductory Clinical Pharmacology*, 7th ed. Baltimore: Lippincott Williams & Wilkins; 2004.)

on research. For example, many antigens, when killed, cause a poor antibody response, whereas when the antigen is merely weakened, a good antibody response occurs. Immunization against a specific disease provides artificially acquired active immunity.

Artificially acquired immunity against some diseases may require periodic booster injections to keep an adequate antibody level (or antibody titer) circulating in the blood. A **booster** injection is the administration of an additional dose of the vaccine to "boost" the production of antibodies to a level that will maintain the desired immunity. The booster is given months or years after the initial vaccine and may be needed because the life of some antibodies is short.

The measles vaccine is considered an immunization. Immunization is a form of artificial active immunity and an important method of controlling some infectious diseases that can cause serious and sometimes fatal consequences. Currently, many infectious diseases may be prevented by **vaccine** (artificial active immunity), including the following diseases:

- cholera
- diphtheria
- *Haemophilus influenzae* type B
- hepatitis A
- hepatitis B
- influenza
- Japanese encephalitis
- Lyme disease
- mumps
- measles
- pertussis
- pneumococcal disease
- poliomyelitis
- rubella
- tetanus
- typhoid
- varicella
- yellow fever

Passive Immunity

Passive immunity is obtained from the administration of immune globulins or antivenins. This type of immunity provides the individual with ready-made antibodies from another human or an animal. Passive immunity provides immediate immunity to the invading antigen, but lasts for only a short time. The Summary Drug Table: Agents for Passive Immunity Identifies agents for passive immunizations. An example of passive immunity is the administration of immune globulins, such as hepatitis B immune globulin. Administration of this vaccine is an attempt to prevent hepatitis B after the individual has been exposed to the virus.

Immunologic Agents

Some immunologic agents capitalize on the body's natural defenses by stimulating the immune response, thereby creating within the body protection to a specific disease. Other immunologic agents supply ready-made antibodies to provide passive immunity. Examples of immunologic agents include vaccines, toxoids, and immune globulins.

Vaccines and Toxoids

Actions of Vaccines and Toxoids

Antibody-producing tissues cannot distinguish between an antigen that is capable of causing disease (a live antigen), an attenuated antigen, or a killed antigen. Because of this phenomenon, vaccines, which contain either an attenuated or a killed antigen, have been developed to create immunity to certain diseases. The live antigens are either killed or weakened during the manufacturing process. Although the vaccine contains weakened or killed antigens, they do not have sufficient strength to cause disease. Although rare, vaccination with any vaccine may not result in a protective antibody response in all individuals given the vaccine.

A **toxin** is a poisonous substance produced by some bacteria, such as *Clostridium tetani*, the bacteria that cause tetanus. A toxin is capable of stimulating the body to produce antitoxins, which are substances that act in the same manner as antibodies. Toxins are powerful substances and, like other antigens, they can be attenuated. A toxin that is attenuated (or weakened) but still capable of stimulating the formation of antitoxins is called a **toxoid**.

Uses of Vaccines and Toxoids

An example of passive immunity is the administration of immune globulins (see Summary Drug Table: Agents for Passive Immunity), such as hepatitis B immune globulin. Administration of this vaccine is an attempt to prevent hepatitis B after the individual has been exposed to the virus.

Both vaccines and toxoids are administered to stimulate the immune response within the body to specific antigens or toxins. These agents must be administered before exposure to the pathogenic organism. The initiation of the immune response, in turn, produces resistance to a specific infectious disease. The immunity produced in this manner is active immunity. Uses of vaccines and toxoids include:

- routine immunization of infants and children
- immunization of adults against tetanus
- adults at high risk for certain diseases (e.g., pneumococcal and influenza vaccines for individuals with serious respiratory disorders)
- children or adults at risk for exposure to a particular disease (e.g., hepatitis B for health care providers)
- immunization of prepubertal girls or nonpregnant women of childbearing age against rubella

SUMMARY DRUG TABLE   Agents for Passive Immunity

Generic Name	Trade Name*	Uses	Adverse Reactions	Dosage Ranges
Immune Globulins				
cytomegalovirus immune globulin intravenous, human (CMV-IGIV) *sy-toe'-meg-a-lo-vi'-rus em-une'-glob'-u-lin*	CytoGam	Prophylaxis of CMV associated with organ transplant (kidney)	Flushing, chills, muscle cramps, back pain, fever, nausea, vomiting, wheezing, decrease in blood pressure	15 mg/kg IV over 30 min, increase to 30 mg/kg for 30 min, then 60 mg/kg to a maximum of 150 mg/kg
hepatitis B immune globulin (human) (HBIG) *hep-ah-ti'-tus-em-une'-glob'-u-lin*	BayHep B, Nabi-HB	Postexposure prophylaxis to blood containing HBsAg, perinatal exposure of infants born to HBsAg-positive mothers, sexual exposure to an HBsAg-positive person, household exposure to people with acute HBV infections	Local tenderness, pain, muscle stiffness at injection site, urticaria, angioedema, malaise, nausea, diarrhea, headache, chills, and fever	0.06 mL/kg (3–5 mL) IM
immune globulin (human) (IG; IGIM; gamma globulin; IgG) *em-une'-glob'-u-lin*	BayGam	Prophylaxis after exposure to hepatitis A, prevention or modification of measles in one who has not been vaccinated or has not had measles previously, immunoglobulin deficiency, passive immunity against varicella, and rubella	Same as HBIG	0.02 mL/kg (0.1 mL/lb)–1.2 mL/kg IM
immune globulin intravenous (IGIV) *em-une'-glob'-u-lin*	Gamimune N, Gammagard S/D, Gammar-P I.V., Iveegam, Polygam S/D, Sandoglobulin, Venoglobulin	Immunodeficiency syndrome, idiopathic thrombocytopenic purpura, B-cell chronic lymphocytic leukemia (Gammagard S/D, Polygam SID), bone marrow transplantation (Gamimune N only), pediatric HIV (Gamimune N only)	Same as HBIG	100–400 mg/kg IV; dosage varies, see package insert
lymphocyte immune globulin, antithymocyte globulin (equine) *lymph'-o-site-em-une'-glob'-u-lin*	Atgam	Renal transplantation, aplastic anemia	Same as HBIG	Adults: 10–30 mg/kg/d; Children: 5–25 mg/kg/d IV
rabies immune globulin, human (RIG) *ray'-bees-em-une'-glob'-u-lin*	Bay Rab, Imogam	Immunization for those suspected of exposure to rabies	Same as HBIG	20 IU/kg IM

Generic Name	Trade Name*	Uses	Adverse Reactions	Dosage Ranges
Rh (D) immune globulin (RH [D] IGIM) *R-h-d-em-une' glob'-u-lin*	Gamulin Rh, RhoGAM	Prevention of Rh hemolytic disease	Same as HBIG	300 mcg (1 vial) IM within 72 h of delivery
Rh (D) immune globulin IV (human) (Rh [D] IGIV) *R-h-d-em-une'-glob'-u-lin*	WinRho SDF	Suppression of Rh isoimmunization in nonsensitized Rh (D)-negative women, immune thrombocytopenic purpura, transfusion to suppress Rh isoimmunization in Rh (D)-negative female children and female adults in their childbearing years	Same as HBIG	300–1200 mcg IM or IV
Rh (D) immune globulin microdose (Rh [D] IG) *r-h-d-em-une'-glob'-u-lin*	BayRho-D Mini Dose, MICRhoGAM	Prevent isoimmunization of Rh (D)-negative women at the time of spontaneous or induced abortion	Local tenderness, pain, muscle stiffness at injection site, urticaria	50 mcg (1 vial) IM
respiratory syncytial virus immune globulin IV (human) (RSV-IGIV) *sin-sish'-al-vi'-rus em-une'-glob'-u-lin*	RespiGam	Respiratory syncytial virus (RSV)	Same as HBIG	1.5–6 mL/kg/h IV to a total monthly infusion of 750 mg/kg
tetanus immune globulin (human) (TIG) *tet'-ah-nus-em-une'-glob'-u-lin*	BayTet	Tetanus prophylaxis after injury in patients whose immunization is incomplete or uncertain	Same as HBIG	250 units IM
varicella-zoster immune globulin (human) (VZIG) *var'-i-sel-a-zos-ter'-em-une'-glob'-u-lin*	*Generic*	Passive immunization of exposed, susceptible individuals who are at greater risk of complications from varicella than are healthy individuals	Same as HBIG	125–625 units IM (dosage varies depending on weight); See package insert for exact dosage
Antivenins crotalidae polyvalent immune Fab (ovine origin) *kro-tal'-i-day pol-ee-va-lent em-une'-fab*	CRO Fab	For treatment of mild to moderate North American rattlesnake bites	Same as HBIG	4–6 vials, depending on severity of symptoms, dilute each vial with 10 mL sterile water, then with 250 mL 0.9% sodium chloride; give each 250 mL over 60 min
antivenin *(micrurus fulvius)* *an-tee'-ven-in*	*Generic*	Passive transient protection for toxic effects of venoms of coral snake in U.S.	Same as HBIG	30–50 mL slow IV injection; flush with IV fluids after antivenin has been infused; may require up to 100 mL

*The term *generic* indicates the drug is available in generic form.

Adverse Reactions of Vaccines and Toxoids

Adverse reactions from the administration of vaccines or toxoids are usually mild. Chills, fever, muscular aches and pains, rash, and lethargy may be present. Pain and tenderness at the injection site may also occur. Although rare, a hypersensitivity reaction may occur. The Summary Drug Table: Agents for Active Immunization provides a listing of the more rare, but serious, adverse reactions.

Minor adverse reactions, such as fever, rashes, and aching of the joints, are possible with the administration of a vaccine. In most cases, these reactions subside within 48 hours.

ALERT

 Serious Adverse Reactions from Immunization

In most cases, the risk of serious adverse reactions from an immunization is much smaller than the risk of contracting the disease for which the immunizing agent is given.

Contraindications, Precautions, and Interactions of Vaccines and Toxoids

Immunologic agents are contraindicated in patients with a known hypersensitivity to the agent or any component of it. The measles, mumps, rubella, and varicella vaccines are contraindicated in patients who have ever had an allergic reaction to gelatin, neomycin, or a

previous dose of one of the vaccines. The measles, mumps, rubella, and varicella vaccines are contraindicated during pregnancy, especially during the first trimester, because of the danger of birth defects. Women are instructed to wait at least 3 months before getting pregnant after receiving these vaccines. Vaccines and toxoids are contraindicated during acute febrile illnesses, leukemia, lymphoma, immunosuppressive illness or drug therapy, and nonlocalized cancer. See Box 27-1 for additional information on the contraindications for immunologic agents.

The immunologic agents are used with extreme caution in individuals with a history of allergies. Sensitivity testing may be performed in individuals with a history of allergies. No adequate studies have been conducted in pregnant women, and it is not known whether these agents are excreted in breast milk. Thus, the immunologic agents (pregnancy category C) are used with caution in pregnant women and during lactation.

Vaccinations containing live organisms are not administered within 3 months of immune globulin administration because antibodies in the globulin preparation may interfere with the immune response to the vaccination. Corticosteroids, antineoplastic drugs, and radiation therapy depress the immune system to such a degree that insufficient numbers of antibodies are produced to prevent the disease. When the salicylates are administered with the varicella vaccination, there is an increased risk of Reye syndrome.

Immune Globulins and Antivenins

Actions of Globulins and Antivenins

Globulins are proteins present in blood serum or plasma that contain antibodies. **Immune globulins** are solutions obtained from human blood containing antibodies that have been formed by the body to specific antigens. Because they contain ready-made antibodies, they are given for passive immunity against disease. An **antivenin** is an antitoxin specific for an animal or insect venom.

Uses of Globulins and Antivenins

The immune globulins are administered to provide passive immunization to one or more infectious diseases. Those receiving immune globulins receive antibodies only to the diseases to which the donor blood is immune. The onset of protection is rapid but of short duration (1 to 3 months).

Antivenins are used for passive, transient protection from the toxic effects of bites by spiders (black widow and similar spiders) and snakes (rattlesnakes, copperhead and cottonmouth, and coral). The most effective response is obtained when the drug is administered within 4 hours after exposure.

Box 27-1 Contraindications for Immunization

- Moderate or severe illness, with or without fever
- Anaphylactoid reactions (e.g., hives, swelling of the mouth and throat, difficulty breathing, hypotension, and shock)
- Known allergy to vaccine or vaccine constituents, particularly gelatin, eggs, or neomycin
- Individuals with an immunologic deficiency should not receive a vaccine (virus is transmissible to the immunocompromised individual).
- Immunizations are postponed during the administration of steroids, radiation therapy, and antineoplastic (anticancer) drug therapy
- Virus vaccines against measles, rubella, and mumps should not be given to pregnant women
- Patients who experience severe systemic or neurologic reactions after a previous dose of the vaccine should not be given any additional doses

Adverse Reactions of Immune Globulins and Antivenins

Adverse reactions to immune globulins are rare. However, local tenderness and pain at the injection site may occur. The most common adverse reactions include urticaria, angioedema, erythema, malaise, nausea, diarrhea, headache, chills, and fever. Adverse reactions, if they occur, usually last for several hours. Systemic reactions are extremely rare.

The antivenins may cause various reactions, with hypersensitivity being the most severe. Some antivenins are prepared from horse serum, and if a patient is sensitive to horse serum, serious reactions and death may result. The immediate reactions usually occur within 30 minutes after administration of the antivenin. Symptoms include apprehension; flushing; itching; urticaria (hives); edema of the face, tongue, and throat; cough; dyspnea; vomiting; cyanosis (blue coloration of the skin); and collapse. Other adverse reactions are included in the Summary Drug Table: Agents for Passive Immunity.

Contraindications, Precautions, and Interactions of Immune Globulins and Antivenins

The immune globulins are contraindicated in patients with a history of allergic reactions after administration of human immunoglobulin preparations and individuals with isolated immunoglobulin A deficiency (individuals could have an anaphylactic reaction to subsequent administration of blood products that contain immunoglobulin A).

ALERT

Human Immune Globulin Intravenous Products

Human immune globulin intravenous products have been associated with renal impairment, acute renal failure, osmotic nephrosis, and death. Individuals with a predisposition to acute renal failure, such as those with preexisting kidney disease, diabetes mellitus, individuals older than 65 years, or patients receiving nephrotoxic drugs should not be given human immune globulin intravenous products.

The antivenins are contraindicated in patients with hypersensitivity to horse serum or any other component of the serum.

The immune globulins and antivenins are administered cautiously during pregnancy (pregnancy category C) and lactation and in children.

Antibodies in the immune globulin preparations may interfere with the immune response to live virus vaccines, particularly measles, but also others, such as mumps and rubella. Live virus vaccines should be administered 14 to 30 days before or 6 to 12 weeks after administration of immune globulins. No known interactions have been reported with antivenins.

Patient Management Issues with Immunologic Agents

Before the administration of any vaccine, an allergy history is taken. If a patient is known or thought to have allergies of any kind, then the health care provider must be informed before the vaccine is given. Some vaccines contain antibodies obtained from animals, whereas other vaccines may contain proteins or preservatives to which the individual may be allergic. A highly allergic person may have an allergic reaction that could be serious and even fatal. If the patient has an allergy history, then the health care provider may decide to perform skin tests for allergy to one or more of the components or proteins in the vaccine. It must also be determined whether the patient has any conditions that contraindicate the administration of the agent (e.g., cancer, leukemia, lymphoma, immunosuppressive drug therapy).

A patient is usually not hospitalized after administration of an immunologic agent. However, a patient may be asked to stay in the clinic or office for observation for approximately 30 minutes after the injection to observe for any signs of hypersensitivity (e.g., laryngeal edema, hives, pruritus, angioneurotic edema, and severe dyspnea). Emergency resuscitation equipment should be available in the event of a severe hypersensitivity reaction.

On occasion, it may be necessary to postpone the regular immunization schedule, particularly for children. This is of special concern to parents. The decision to delay immunization because of illness or for other reasons must be discussed with the health care provider. However, the decision to administer or delay vaccination because of febrile illness (illness causing a fever) depends on the severity of the symptoms and the specific disorder. In general, all vaccines can be administered to those with minor illness, such as a cold virus or a low-grade fever. However, moderate or severe febrile illness is a contraindication. In instances of moderate or severe febrile illness, vaccination is performed as soon as the acute phase of the illness is over.

It may be beneficial to increase the fluids in the diet, allow for adequate rest, and keep the atmosphere quiet and nonstimulating. The health care provider may prescribe acetaminophen every 4 hours to control these reactions. Local irritation at the injection site may be treated with warm or cool compresses, depending on the patient's preference. A lump may be felt at the injection site after a diphtheria, pertussis, or tetanus injection or other immunization. This is not abnormal and will resolve itself within several days to several months.

Vaccine Adverse Event Reporting System

The Vaccine Adverse Event Reporting System is a national vaccine safety surveillance program co-sponsored by the Centers for Disease Control and Prevention and the Food and Drug Administration. The Vaccine Adverse Event Reporting System collects and analyzes information from reports of adverse reactions after immunization. Anyone can report to the Vaccine Adverse Event Reporting System, and reports are sent in by vaccine manufacturers, health care providers, and vaccine recipients and their parents or guardians.

Educating the Patient and Family About Immunologic Agents

Because of the effectiveness of various types of vaccines in the prevention of disease, parents are encouraged to have infants and young children receive the immunizations suggested by the health care provider.

Those traveling to a foreign country are urged to contact their health care provider or local health department well in advance of their departure date for information about other immunizations that will be needed. Immunizations should be given well in advance of departure because it may take several weeks to produce adequate immunity.

When an adult or child is receiving a vaccine for immunization, the health care provider explains to the patient or a family member the possible reactions that may occur, such as soreness at the injection site or fever.

Serious viral infections of the central nervous system and fatalities have occurred with the use of some vaccines. Although the number of these incidents is small, a risk factor still remains when some vaccines are given. Parents should understand that a risk is also associated with not receiving immunization against some infectious diseases. That risk may be higher and just as serious as the risk associated with the use of vaccines. When a large segment of the population is immunized, the small number of those not immunized are less likely to be exposed to and infected with the disease-producing microorganism. However, when large numbers of the population are not immunized, there is a great increase in the chances of exposure to the infectious disease and a significant increase in the probability that the individual will experience the disease.

Parents or guardians are encouraged to report to their health care provider any adverse reactions or serious adverse events occurring after administration of a vaccine, or to report the event to Vaccine Adverse Event Reporting System.

Patient Education Box 27-1 includes key points about immunologic agents the patient and family members should know when a child is to receive a vaccination.

PATIENT EDUCATION BOX 27-1

Key Points for Patients Taking Immunologic Agents

If your child is receiving a vaccination:

❑ The risks of contracting vaccine-preventable diseases is much higher than the adverse reactions associated with immunization.

❑ Bring all of your child's immunization records to all visits with your health care provider.

❑ Ask your health care provider to provide you with the date for return for your child's next vaccination.

❑ Certain adverse reactions (e.g., fever, soreness at the injection site) are common. In general, these reactions are short-lived. Acetaminophen and warm compresses will help to ease these reactions.

❑ Report any unusual or severe adverse reactions after the administration of a vaccination to your health care provider.

Natural Remedies

Shiitake

Lentinan, a derivative of the shiitake mushroom, is proving to be valuable in boosting the body's immune system and may prolong the survival time of patients with cancer by supporting immunity. In Japan, lentinan is commonly used to treat cancer. Additional possible benefits of this herb are to lower cholesterol levels by increasing the rate at which cholesterol is excreted from the body. Under no circumstances should shiitake or lentinan be used for cancer or any serious illness without consulting a health care provider.

The shiitake mushroom is an edible variety of mushroom and is not associated with severe adverse reactions. Mild side effects such as skin rashes or gastrointestinal upsets have been reported. Shiitake mushroom is available in fresh, capsule, and liquid form. For general health maintenance, the dosage guidelines are three to four fresh shiitake mushrooms, one to five capsules, or 1 dropper three to four times daily.

Echinacea

Echinacea, a frequently used herb, is taken to stimulate the immune system function by increasing the number and activity of immune cells and to stimulate phagocytosis (ingestion and destruction of bacteria and other harmful substances). It appears to shorten the duration of colds and influenza, although a study reported in the *Journal of the American Medical Association* suggests that echinacea is not effective in young children for the treatment and prevention of colds. The researchers reported that use of echinacea from the onset of symptoms did not lessen the number of days the colds lasted or the severity of symptoms.

Echinacea is available in pill, tincture, and tea form. Most herbalists recommend that echinacea should be taken at the initial signs of infection, when symptoms first become apparent. Small repeated doses throughout the day may be better than taking larger doses less frequently. The herb should not be taken for more than 8 consecutive weeks. The standard recommendation is 7 to 14 days of treatment.

Although rare, adverse reactions such as nausea and other mild gastrointestinal effects may occur. Individuals with allergies to daisy-type plants are more susceptible to reactions, and if a patient has lupus, rheumatoid arthritis, multiple sclerosis, tuberculosis, or HIV, then echinacea intake should be limited.

KEY POINTS

⦾ The immune system has two distinct but overlapping mechanisms with which to fight invading organisms: cell-mediated defenses (cellular immunity) and antibody-mediated defenses (humoral immunity). Cell-mediated immunity and humoral immunity are interdependent: cell-mediated immunity influences the function of the B lymphocytes, and humoral immunity influences the function of the T lymphocytes.

⦾ Active and passive immunity involve the use of agents that stimulate antibody formation (active immunity) or the injection of ready-made antibodies found in the serum of immune individuals or animals (passive immunity). Immunization is a form of artificial active immunity and an important method of controlling some of the infectious diseases that are capable of caus-

ing serious and sometimes fatal consequences. Passive immunity provides the individual with ready-made antibodies from another human or an animal.

⦾ Some immunologic agents stimulate the immune response, thereby creating within the body protection to a specific disease. Other immunologic agents supply ready-made antibodies to provide passive immunity. Examples of immunologic agents include vaccines, toxoids, and immune globulins.

⦾ A toxin that is attenuated (or weakened) but still capable of stimulating the formation of antitoxins is called a toxoid. Both vaccines and toxoids are administered to stimulate the immune response within the body to specific antigens or toxins. These agents must be administered before exposure to the pathogenic organism. The initiation of the immune response, in turn, produces resistance to a specific infectious disease. Adverse reactions from the administration of vaccines or toxoids are usually mild. Chills, fever, muscular aches and pains, rash, and lethargy may occur, along with pain and tenderness at the injection site. The immunologic agents are used with extreme caution in individuals with a history of allergies.

⦾ Immune globulins are solutions obtained from human blood containing antibodies that have been formed by the body to specific antigens. Because they contain ready-made antibodies, they are given for passive immunity against disease. The immune globulins are administered to provide passive immunization to one or more infectious diseases. Those receiving immune globulins receive antibodies only to the diseases to which the donor blood is immune. Adverse reactions to immune globulins are rare but may include urticaria, angioedema, erythema, malaise, nausea, diarrhea, headache, chills, and fever.

CASE STUDY

Ms. Wilson has brought her 2-month-old daughter, Michelle, to the clinic for the first of her polio vaccine immunizations (OPV). Ms. Wilson is nervous about the immunization, and she wonders whether the process is necessary for her daughter's health at such a young age.

1. Ms. Wilson should be told:
   a. it is acceptable to postpone the series until her daughter is 1 year old if it will help Ms. Wilson relax
   b. the risk of not having the immunization is greater than the risk of any problem from receiving the vaccine
   c. the vaccine is optional; polio is rare, and the immunization was more critical in earlier generations
   d. none of the above

2. Ms. Wilson wants to know whether she can expect her daughter to have an adverse reaction to the vaccination. She should be told:
   a. there are no adverse reactions associated with the polio vaccine
   b. mild symptoms may occur, but they are rare
   c. possible adverse reactions include bleeding and skin rashes
   d. none of the above

3. Ms. Wilson mentions that her daughter seems to have a slight cold. She wonders whether the immunization should be postponed. She should be told:
   a. immunization will help to prevent her daughter from becoming ill with polio, and as long as her cold symptoms are mild, it is acceptable to immunize her
   b. immunization can be performed even with high fevers
   c. if any signs of a cold or other virus are present, then the immunization should be postponed
   d. none of the above

WEBSITE ACTIVITIES

1. Go to the Vaccine Adverse Event Reporting System website (http://www.vaers.org) and click on "Frequently Asked Questions." Search for information about who can report to the Vaccine Adverse Event Reporting System. Write a brief list about the percentages of reports from different groups of people.

2. From the starting page of this website, click on "VAERS Data." Search for information about the limitations of the Vaccine Adverse Event Reporting System, and write a brief statement outlining this information.

REVIEW QUESTIONS

1. When discussing the possibility of adverse reactions after receiving a vaccine, the parents of a young child are told that:
   a. adverse reactions may be severe, and the child should be monitored closely for 24 hours
   b. adverse reactions are usually mild
   c. the child will likely experience a hypersensitivity reaction
   d. the most common adverse reaction is a severe headache

2. Which of the following food allergies would alert the health care provider to a possibility of an allergy to the measles vaccine?
   a. Jell-O gelatin
   b. peanut butter
   c. sugar
   d. corn

3. What type of immunity does an immune globulin produce?
   a. artificially acquired active immunity
   b. naturally acquired active immunity
   c. passive immunity
   d. cell-mediated immunity

4. What type of immunity will be produced by the hepatitis B vaccine recombinant?
   a. artificially acquired active immunity
   b. naturally acquired active immunity
   c. passive immunity
   d. cell-mediated immunity

28 Antineoplastic Drugs

KEY TERMS

alopecia—the loss of hair
anemia—decrease in red blood cells
anorexia—loss of appetite
antineoplastic drugs—drugs used for cure, control, or palliative (relief of symptoms) treatment of malignancies
bone marrow suppression—a potentially dangerous adverse reaction to antineoplastic drugs resulting in decreased production of blood cells
chemotherapy—drug therapy with antineoplastic drugs
extravasation—escape of fluid from a blood vessel into surrounding tissues
leukopenia—a decrease in the white blood cells or leukocytes; a symptom of bone marrow suppression
oral mucositis—inflammation of the oral mucous membranes
stomatitis—inflammation of the mouth
thrombocytopenia—a decrease in the thrombocytes; a symptom of bone marrow suppression
vesicant—an adverse drug reaction resulting in tissue necrosis, which is caused by the infiltration or extravasation of the drug out of a blood vessel and into soft tissue

CHAPTER OBJECTIVES

On completion of this chapter, students will be able to:

1 Define the chapter's key terms.

2 Describe the general drug actions, uses, adverse reactions, contraindications, precautions and interactions of antineoplastic drugs.

3 Discuss important points to keep in mind when educating the patient and family members about the use of antineoplastic drugs.

Antineoplastic drugs are used in the treatment of malignant diseases (cancer). These drugs can be used for cure, control, or palliative (relief of symptoms) therapy. Although these drugs may not always lead to a complete cure of the malignancy, they often slow the rate of tumor growth and delay metastasis (spreading of the cancer to other sites) (Fig. 28-1). Use of these drugs is one of the tools in the treatment of cancer. The term **chemotherapy** is often used to refer to therapy with antineoplastic drugs.

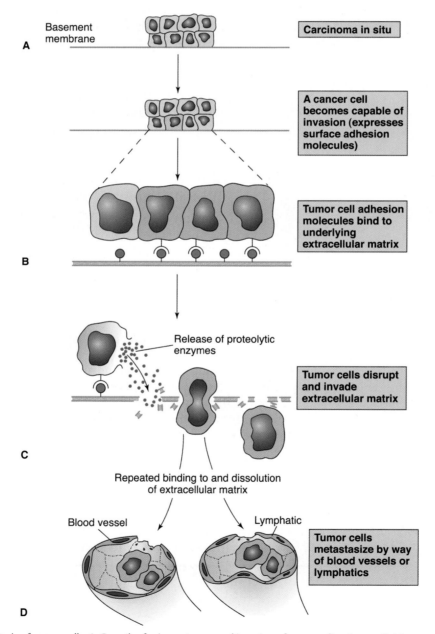

FIGURE 28-1 Metastasis of cancer cells. A, Growth of primary tumor and invasion of surrounding tissues. B, Movement of tumor cells into the endothelium and basement membrane of the surrounding capillary. C, Shed tumor cells in lungs, brain, and liver become trapped and penetrate the capillary wall to establish themselves in this new environment. D, Proliferation at the new site, which requires a conducive environment with blood supply and nutrition.

Many antineoplastic drugs are available to treat malignancies. The antineoplastic drugs covered in this chapter include the alkylating drugs, antibiotics, antimetabolites, hormones, mitotic inhibitors, and selected miscellaneous drugs. Antineoplastic drugs not specifically discussed in this chapter are listed in the Summary Drug Table: Antineoplastic Drugs.

Actions of Antineoplastic Drugs

Generally, most antineoplastic drugs affect cells that rapidly proliferate (divide and reproduce). Malignant neoplasms or cancerous tumors usually consist of rapidly proliferating aberrant (abnormal) cells. Cancer cells have no biological feedback controls that stop their aberrant growth or proliferation. Cancer cells are more sensitive to antineoplastic drugs when the cells are in the process of growing and dividing. Chemotherapy is administered at the time the cell population is dividing as part of a strategy to optimize cell death.

However, the normal cells that line the mouth and gastrointestinal tract, and cells of the gonads, bone marrow, hair follicles, and lymph tissue are also rapidly dividing cells and are usually affected by these drugs. Thus, antineoplastic drugs may affect normal as well as malignant (cancerous) cells.

text continued on page 483.

SUMMARY DRUG TABLE   Antineoplastic Drugs

Generic Name	Trade Name*	Uses	Adverse Reactions	Dosage Ranges
Alkylating Drugs busulfan *byoo-sul'-fan*	Busulfex, Myleran	Chronic myelogenous leukemia	Leukopenia, anemia, cataracts, anxiety, skin rash, thrombocytopenia, fever, anorexia, nausea, vomiting, diarrhea, stomatitis, constipation, tachycardia, hypertension, insomnia, dizziness	1–12 mg/d PO; 0.8 mg/kg IV
chlorambucil *klor-am'-byoo-sill*	Leukeran	Chronic lymphocytic leukemia, malignant lymphomas, Hodgkin disease	Bone marrow depression, hyperuricemia, nausea, vomiting, diarrhea, hepatotoxicity, tremors	0.03–0.2 mg/kg/d PO
cyclophosphamide *sye-klo-foss'-fam- ide*	Cytoxan, Neosar	Malignant lymphomas, Hodgkin disease, multiple myeloma, leukemia, carcinoma of the ovary and breast, neuroblastoma, retinoblastoma	Leukopenia, thrombocytopenia, anemia, anorexia, nausea, vomiting, diarrhea, cystitis, alopecia	Initial dose: 40–50 mg/kg IV; maintenance doses: 1–5 mg/kg/d PO; 3–15 mg/kg IV
ifosfamide *eye-fos'-fam-ide*	Ifex	Testicular cancer	Hemorrhagic cystitis, mental confusion, coma, alopecia, nausea, vomiting, anorexia, diarrhea, hematuria	1.2 g/m²/d IV
iomustine *loe-mus'-teen*	CeeNU	Brain tumors, Hodgkin disease	Nausea, vomiting, diarrhea, thrombocytopenia, leukopenia, alopecia, anemia, stomatitis	100–300 mg/m² PO
mechlorethamine *me-klor-eth'-a-meen*	Mustargen	Hodgkin disease, lymphosarcoma, bronchogenic carcinoma, leukemia, mycosis fungoides	Nausea, vomiting, jaundice, alopecia, lymphocytopenia, granulocytopenia, thrombocytopenia, skin rash, diarrhea	0.4 mg/kg IV as a total dose for a course of therapy, which may be given as a single dose or divided dose
melphalan *mel'-fa-lan*	Alkeran	Multiple myeloma, carcinoma of the ovary	Nausea, vomiting, bone marrow depression, skin rash, alopecia, diarrhea	6 mg/d PO; 16 mg/m² IV

Generic Name	Trade Name*	Uses	Adverse Reactions	Dosage Ranges
thiotepa *thye-oh-tep'-a*	Thioplex, *generic*	Carcinoma of the breast, ovary, bladder, Hodgkin disease, lymphosarcomas, intracavity effusions caused by localized metastatic disease	Nausea, vomiting, pain at injection site, bone marrow depression, dermatitis, dysuria	0.3–0.4 mg/kg IV; dosage is higher for intracavity or intratumoral administration; bladder instillation: 60 mg retained for 2 h
Antibiotics bleomycin sulfate *blee-oh-my'-sin*	Blenoxane	Carcinoma of the head and neck, lymphomas, testicular carcinoma	Pneumonitis, pulmonary fibrosis, erythema, rash, fever, chills, vomiting	0.25–0.5 U/kg IV, IM, SC
dactinomycin *dak-ti-no-my'-sin*	Cosmegen	Wilms tumor, choriocarcinoma, Ewing sarcoma, testicular carcinoma	Anorexia, alopecia, bone marrow depression, nausea, vomiting	Up to 15 mcg/kg/d IV; may also be given by isolation perfusion at 0.035–0.05 mg/kg
daunorubicin citrate liposomal *daw-noe-roo'-bi-sin*	DaunoXome	Kaposi sarcoma	Fatigue, headache, diarrhea, nausea, cough, fever	40 mg/m² IV
daunorubicin HCl *daw-noe-roo'-bi-sin*	*Generic*	Leukemia	Bone marrow depression, alopecia, acute nausea and vomiting, fever, chills	25–45 mg/m²/d IV
doxorubicin HCl *dox-oh-roo'-by-sin*	Adriamycin, Rubex	Acute leukemia, neuroblastoma, soft tissue and bone sarcomas, carcinomas of the breast, ovary, bladder, lymphomas, Wilms tumor	Alopecia, acute nausea and vomiting, mucositis, chills, bone marrow depression, fever	25–75 mg/m²/d IV
epirubicin *ep-ee-roo'-by-sin*	Ellence	Breast cancer	Alopecia, local toxicity, rash, itching, amenorrhea, hot flashes, nausea, vomiting, mucositis, leukopenia, neutropenia, anemia, thrombocytopenia, infection, lethargy, conjunctivitis	100–120 mg/m² IV
idarubicin HCl *eye-da-roo'-by-sin*	Idamycin	Leukemia	Congestive heart failure, arrhythmias, chest pain, myocardial infarction, nausea, vomiting, alopecia	12 mg/m² daily × 3 d IV
mitomycin *mye-toe-my'-sin*	Mutamycin	Adenocarcinoma of the stomach, pancreas	Bone marrow depression, anorexia, nausea, vomiting, headache, blurred vision, fever	10–20 mg/m²/d IV
plicamycin *plye-ka-my'-sin*	Mithracin	Malignant tumors of the testes, hypercalcemia, and hypercalciuria associated with neoplasms	Hemorrhagic syndrome (epistaxis, hematemesis, widespread hemorrhage in the GI tract, generalized advanced bleeding), vomiting, diarrhea, anorexia, nausea, stomatitis	Testicular tumors: 25–30 mcg/kg/d IV; hypercalcemia, hypercalciuria: 25 mcg/ kg/d IV for 3–4 d

Generic Name	Trade Name*	Uses	Adverse Reactions	Dosage Ranges
valrubicin *val-roo'-by-sin*	Valstar	Bladder cancer	Bladder discomfort, dysuria, urinary frequency, urinary tract infection	800 mg intravesically weekly for 6 wk
Antimetabolites capecitabine *kap-ah-seat'-ah-bean*	Xeloda	Breast cancer	Dermatitis, diarrhea, nausea, vomiting, leukopenia, granulocytopenia, thrombocytopenia, hand and foot syndrome, stomatitis, abdominal pain, constipation, dyspnea, anemia, hyperbilirubinemia, fatigue, weakness, anorexia	2500 mg/m^2/d PO
cladribine *kla'-dri-bean*	Leustatin	Hairy cell leukemia	Neutropenia, fever, infection, fatigue, nausea, headache, rash, injection site reactions, nephrotoxicity, neurotoxicity	0.09 mg/kg/d IV
cytarabine *sye-tare'-a-bean*	Cytosar-U, *generic*	Acute myelocytic or lymphocytic leukemia	Bone marrow depression, nausea, vomiting, diarrhea, anorexia	100–200 mg/m^2/d IV, SC
fludarabine *floo-dar'-a-bean*	Fludara	Chronic lymphocytic leukemia	Bone marrow depression, fever, chills, infection, nausea, vomiting, rash, diarrhea	25 mg/m^2 IV
fluorouracil (5-FU) *flure-oh-yoor'-a-sill*	Adrucil, *generic*	Carcinoma of the breast, stomach, pancreas, colon, and rectum	Diarrhea, anorexia, nausea, vomiting, alopecia, bone marrow depression, angina, stomatitis	3–12 mg/kg/d IV
gemcitabine HCl *jem-site'-ah-ben*	Gemzar	Pancreatic cancer, non–small-cell lung cancer	Anemia, proteinuria, nausea, vomiting, fever, rash, leukopenia, neutropenia, thrombocytopenia, diarrhea, constipation, alopecia	1000–1250 mg/m^2 IV
mercaptopurine (6-mercaptopurine, 6-MP) *mer-kap-toe- pyoor'-een*	Purinethol	Acute lymphatic leukemia, acute or chronic myelogenous leukemia	Bone marrow depression, hyperuricemia, hepatotoxicity, skin rash	2.5–5 mg/kg/d PO; do not exceed 5 mg/kg/d
methotrexate *meth-o-trex'-ate*	Rheumatrex, *generic*, Dose Pack	Lymphosarcoma, severe psoriasis, cancer of the head, neck, breast, lung, rheumatoid arthritis (RA)	Ulcerative stomatitis, nausea, rash, pruritus, renal failure, bone marrow depression, fatigue, fever, chills	Antineoplastic dosages vary widely depending on type of tumor; psoriasis: 10–50 mg/wk IV, IM, PO; RA: dose pack directed
pentostatin *pen'-toe-stat-in*	Nipent	Alpha-interferon refractory hairy cell leukemia	Bone marrow depression, anemia, nausea, vomiting, diarrhea, rash, fever	4 mg/m^2 IV every other week
thioguanine (TG) *thye-oh-gwon'-een*	*Generic*	Acute leukemias	Bone marrow depression, hepatic toxicity, nausea, vomiting, stomatitis, hyperuricemia	2–3 mg/kg/d PO

Generic Name	Trade Name*	Uses	Adverse Reactions	Dosage Ranges
Mitotic Inhibitors (Antimitotic Agents)				
docetaxel *dohs-eh-tax'-el*	Taxotere	Breast cancer, non–small-cell lung cancer	Nausea, skin rash, pruritus, stomatitis, vomiting, anemia, leukopenia, neutropenia, arthralgia, alopecia, asthenia, fever, infections	60–100 mg/m² IV
paclitaxel *pass-leh-tax'-ell*	Taxol	Ovarian cancer, breast cancer, AIDS-related Kaposi sarcoma	Diarrhea, nausea, vomiting, flushing, myalgia, arthralgia, fever, peripheral neuropathy, opportunistic infections	135–175 mg/m² IV
vinblastine sulfate (VLB; LCR) *vin-blas'-teen*	Velban, *generic*	Hodgkin disease, lymphocytic lymphoma, histiocytic lymphoma, mycosis fungoides, testicular cancer, Kaposi sarcoma, breast cancer	Leukopenia, nausea, vomiting, paresthesias, malaise, weakness, mental depression, headache, hypertension, alopecia, diarrhea, constipation	3.7–18.4 mg/m² IV
vincristine sulfate (VCR; LRC) *vin-kris'-teen*	Oncovin, Vincasar PFS, *generic*	Acute leukemia, combination therapy for various cancers	Same as vinblastine	1.4 mg/m² IV
Hormones *Androgens* testolactone *tess-toe-lak'-tone*	Teslac	Palliative treatment of advanced disseminated metastatic breast carcinoma in postmenopausal women and premenopausal women whose ovarian function has been terminated	Paresthesia, glossitis, anorexia, nausea, vomiting, maculopapular erythema, aches, edema of the extremities, nail growth disturbances, increase in blood pressure, virilization	250 mg QID PO
Antiandrogens bicalutamide *bye-cal-loo'-ta- mide*	Casodex	Prostate cancer	Hot flushes, hypertension, dizziness, paresthesia, insomnia, rash, constipation, nausea, diarrhea, nocturia, hematuria, peripheral edema, bone pain, dyspnea, general pain, back pain, asthenia, infection	50 mg once daily PO
flutamide *flu'-ta-mide*	Eulexin	Early stage and metastatic prostate cancer	Hot flashes, loss of libido, impotence, diarrhea, nausea, vomiting, gynecomastia	125 mg PO TID at 8-h intervals PO (up to 750 mg/d)
nilutamide *nah-loo'-ta-mide*	Nilandron	Metastatic prostate cancer	Pain, headache, asthenia, abdominal pain, chest pain, flu symptoms, fever, liver toxicity, insomnia, nausea, constipation, testicular atrophy, dyspnea, pain, asthenia	150–300 mg/d PO

Generic Name	Trade Name*	Uses	Adverse Reactions	Dosage Ranges
Progestins medroxyproges- terone *me-drox'-ee-proe- jess'-te-rone*	Depo-Provera	Endometrial or renal cancer	Breakthrough bleeding, spotting, change in menstrual flow, amenorrhea, rash with or without pruritus, acne, fluid retention, edema, increase or decrease in weight, sudden, partial, or complete loss of vision, migraine, nausea	400–1000 mg IM per wk; if disease stabilizes 400 mg/mo IM
megestrol acetate *me-jess'-trole*	Megace, *generic*	Breast or endometrial cancer	Same as medroxyprogesterone	Breast cancer: 160 mg/d PO; endometrial cancer: 40–320 mg/d in divided doses PO
Estrogens diethylstilbestrol diphosphate *dye-eth-il-stil-bess'- trole*	Stilphostrol	Inoperable prostatic carcinoma	Headache, dizziness, intolerance to contact lens, edema, thromboembolism, hypertension, nausea, weight changes, testicular atrophy, acne, breast tenderness, gynecomastia	Oral: 50–200 mg TID PO (not to exceed 1 g/d); Parenteral: 0.5–1 g/d IV
estramustine phosphate sodium estradiol and nitrogen mustard *ess-tra-muss'-teen*	Emcyt	Metastic or progressive prostatic carcinoma	Same as diethylstilbestrol and diarrhea, vomiting, decreased libido, sodium and water retention, skin rash	10–16 mg/kg/d PO in 3–4 divided doses
Antiestrogens tamoxifen citrate *ta-mox'-i-fen*	Nolvadex, *generic*	Breast cancer in menopausal women, preventative therapy for women at high risk for breast cancer	Fluid retention, vaginal discharge, nausea, vomiting, hypercalcemia, ophthalmic changes, hot flashes, vaginal bleeding and discharge	20–40 mg/d
toremifene citrate *tore-em'-ah-feen*	Fareston	Breast cancer	Hot flushes, nausea, vomiting, vaginal bleeding, vaginal discharge, menstrual irregularities, skin rash	60 mg once daily PO
Gonadotropin-Releasing Hormone Analogs goserelin acetate *goe'-se-rel-in*	Zoladex	Prostate cancer, end- ometriosis, advanced breast cancer, endometrial thinning	Lethargy, dizziness, insomnia, anorexia, nausea, sexual dysfunction, headache, emotional lability, depression, sweating, acne, breast atrophy, peripheral edema, lower urinary tract symptoms, hot flashes, pain, edema, upper respiratory tract infection, rash	3.6 mg SC q28d or 10.8 mg q3 mo into the upper abdominal wall

Generic Name	Trade Name*	Uses	Adverse Reactions	Dosage Ranges
leuprolide acetate *loo-proe'-lide*	Lupron, Lupron Depot	Advanced prostatic carcinoma, endometriosis, central precocious puberty, uterine leiomyomata	Edema, headache, dizziness, bone pain, nausea, vomiting, anorexia, ECG changes, hypertension	1 mg SC daily; Depot: 7.5–30 mg IM; endometriosis: Depot, 3.75 IM monthly; uterine leiomyomata: 3.75 IM monthly
triptorelin pamoate *trip-toe-rell'-in*	Trelstar Depot	Advanced prostate cancer	Hot flushes, skeletal pain, injection site pain, hypertension, headache, insomnia, dizziness, vomiting, diarrhea, impotence	3.75 mg IM
Aromatase Inhibitors anastrazole *an-ahs'-troh-zol*	Arimidex	Advanced breast cancer	Vasodilation, headache, dizziness, insomnia, GI disturbances, nausea, constipation, diarrhea, cough, increased dyspnea, hot flushes, asthenia, pain, back pain, peripheral edema, bone pain	1 mg once daily
exemestane *ex-ah'-mess-tane*	Aromasin	Advanced breast cancer	Depression, insomnia, anxiety, dizziness, nausea, vomiting, abdominal pain, anorexia, constipation, diarrhea, dyspnea, fatigue, hot flashes, pain, peripheral edema	25 mg/d PO
letrozole *le'-tro-zol*	Femara	Advanced breast cancer	Same as for anastrazole	2.5 mg once daily PO
Miscellaneous Anticancer Drugs ***Epipodophyllotoxins*** etoposide *e-toe-poe'-side*	Toposar, VePesid, *generic*	Testicular cancer, small-cell lung cancer	Nausea, vomiting, anorexia, diarrhea, constipation, alopecia, granulocytopenia	Testicular cancer: 50–100 mg/m^2/d IV; small-cell lung cancer: 35–50 mg/m^2/d IV (oral dose is 2 times the IV dose rounded to the nearest 50 mg)
teniposide (VM-26) *teh-nip-oh-side*	Vumon	Leukemia	Nausea, vomiting, anorexia, diarrhea, constipation, alopecia, rash, leukopenia, thrombocytopenia, anemia	165–250 mg/m^2 IV
Enzymes asparaginase *a-spare'-a-gi-nase*	Elspar	Leukemia	Hypersensitivity reactions (rash, urticaria, arthralgia, respiratory distress, acute anaphylaxis), depression, somnolence, fatigue, coma, anorexia, nausea, vomiting	200–1000 IU/kg/d IV; 6000 IU/m^2/d IM
pegaspargase (PEG-asparaginase) *peg-ass-par'-jase*	Oncaspar	Acute lymphoblastic leukemia	Nausea, vomiting, fever, malaise, dyspnea, diarrhea, hypotension	2500 mg/m^2 IM or IV

Generic Name	Trade Name*	Uses	Adverse Reactions	Dosage Ranges
Platinum Coordination Complex				
carboplatin *kar'-boe-pla-tin*	Paraplatin	Advanced ovarian cancer	Peripheral neuritis; vomiting; nausea; abdominal pain; diarrhea; constipation; decreased serum sodium, magnesium, calcium, and potassium; increased blood urea nitrogen; visual disturbances; ototoxicity	360 mg/m^2 IV
cisplatin *sis'-pla-tin*	Platinol-AQ	Metastatic testicular tumors, advanced bladder cancer, ovarian tumors	Ototoxicity, peripheral neuropathies, nausea, vomiting, anorexia, bone marrow suppression, nephrotoxicity	$20–70 \text{ mg/m}^2$ IV
Anthracenedione				
mitoxantrone HCl *mye-toe-zan'-trone*	Novantrone	Acute leukemias, bone pain in advanced prostatic cancer	Nausea, vomiting, diarrhea, headache, seizures, abdomina pain, mucositis, congestive heart failure, bone marrow depression	12 mg/m^2 IV
Substituted Ureas				
hydroxyurea *hye-drox-ee- yoor-ee'-ah*	Droxia, Hydrea	Melanoma, chronic myelocytic leukemia, ovarian cancer	Headache, dizziness, stomatitis, anorexia, nausea, vomiting, diarrhea, constipation, bone marrow depression, impaired renal tubular function, rash, mucositis, fever, chills, malaise	$20–80 \text{ mg/kg}$ PO
Methylhydrazine Derivatives				
procarbazine HCl *proe-kar'-ba-zeen*	Matulane	Hodgkin disease	Leukopenia, anemia, nausea, vomiting, anorexia, thrombocytopenia	$1–6 \text{ mg/kg}$ PO
Cytoprotective Agents				
amifostine *am-ih-foss'-teen*	Ethyol	Renal toxicity associated with repeated administration of cisplatin in patients with advanced ovarian cancer	Nausea, vomiting, hypotension, fever, chills, dyspnea, skin rash, urticaria	910 mg/m^2 IV QID
dexrazoxane *dex-ray-zox'-ane*	Zinecard	Cardiomyopathy associated with doxorubicin administration in women with metastatic breast cancer	Alopecia, nausea, vomiting, fatigue, malaise, anorexia, stomatitis, fever, infection, diarrhea, neurotoxicity	500 mg/m^2 IV
DNA Topoisomerase Inhibitors				
irinotecan HCl *eh-rin-oh'-te-kan*	Camptosar	Metastatic carcinoma of the colon or rectum	Dizziness, somnolence, confusion, vasodilation, hypotension, thrombophlebitis, diarrhea, nausea, vomiting, abdominal pain, anorexia, constipation, mucositis, dyspnea, asthenia, pain, fever	125 mg/m^2 IV

Generic Name	Trade Name*	Uses	Adverse Reactions	Dosage Ranges
topotecan HCl *toe-poh'-te-kan*	Hycamtin	Ovarian cancer, small-cell lung cancer	Alopecia, rash, nausea, vomiting, diarrhea, constipation, abdominal pain, stomatitis, anorexia, dyspnea, headache, fatigue, fever, pain, asthenia, bone marrow depression	1.5 mg/m^2 IV
Biological Response Modifiers aldesleukin *al-dess-loo'-kin* (interleukin-2; IL-2)	Proleukin	Metastatic renal-cell carcinoma	Nausea, diarrhea, stomatitis, hypotension, anorexia, bone marrow depression, pulmonary congestion, dyspnea, oliguria	600,000 IU/kg IV q8h
BCG, intravesical	Pacis, TheraCys, TICE BCG	Carcinoma in situ of the bladder	Dysuria, urinary frequency, cystitis, hematuria, urinary incontinence	120 mg instilled in the bladder once per week for 6 wk
denileukin diftitox *deh-nih-loo'-kin diff'-tih-tox*	Ontak	Cutaneous T-cell lymphoma	Hypotension, vasodilation, tachycardia, dizziness, paresthesia, rash, pruritus, nausea, vomiting, anorexia, diarrhea	9–18 g/kg/d IV
levamisole (HCl) *lev-am'-ih-sole*	Ergamisol	Combination therapy in patients with Dukes stage C colon cancer	Nausea, vomiting, diarrhea, stomatitis, anorexia	50 mg q8h PO
Retinoids tretinoin *tret'-i-noyn*	Vesanoid	Acute promyelocytic leukemia	Headache, fever, weakness, fatigue, skin/mucous membrane dryness, increased sweating, visual disturbances, ocular disturbances, alopecia, bone pain	45 mg/m^2/d PO
Rexinoids bexarotene *bex-air'-oh-teen*	Targretin	Cutaneous T-cell lymphoma	Elevated blood lipids, hypothyroidism, headache, asthenia, rash, leukopenia, anemia, nausea, infection, peripheral edema, abdominal pain, dry skin	300 mg/m^2/d PO
Monoclonal Antibodies alemtuzumab *ay-lem-tuh'-zoo-mab*	Campath	B-cell chronic lymphocytic leukemia	Hypotension, headache, dizziness, rash, bone marrow suppression, fever, chills, asthenia, nausea, vomiting, diarrhea, stomatitis, fatigue	3–30 mg IV
gemtuzumab ozogamicin *gem-too'-zoo-mab oh-zoh-gam'-ih-sin* rituximab *rih-tuck-sih-mab*	Mylotarg Rituxan	Acute myeloid leukemia Non-Hodgkin lymphoma	Chills, fever, nausea, vomiting, headache, hypotension, hypertension hypoxia, dyspnea, bone marrow depression, infusion reactions, hypotension, dizziness, anxiety, night sweats, rash, pruritus, nausea, diarrhea, vomiting, bone marrow depression	9 mg/m^2 IV 375 mg/m^2 IV

Generic Name	Trade Name*	Uses	Adverse Reactions	Dosage Ranges
ibritumomab tiuxetan *ib-ri-tu'-moe-mab tie-ux-eh'-tan*	Zevalin	Non-Hodgkin lymphoma	Infections, allergic reactions (bronchospasms and angioedema), bone marrow depression, hemorrhage, anemia, nausea, vomiting, abdominal pain, diarrhea, increased cough, dyspnea, dizziness, arthralgia, anorexia, ecchymosis	250 mg/m² IV
trastuzumab *trass-to-zoo'-mab*	Herceptin	Breast cancer	Anemia, leukopenia, diarrhea, infection, nausea, vomiting, pain, headache, dizziness, dyspnea, hypotension, rash, asthenia, infusion reactions, pulmonary adverse effects	2–4 mg/kg IV
Unclassified Antineoplastics imatinib mesylate *eh-mat'-eh-nib*	Gleevec	Chronic myeloid leukemia, gastrointestinal stromal tumors, acute lymphocytic leukemia	Gastric irritation, arthralgia, muscle cramps, hemorrhage, pyrexia, weakness, epistaxis, fatigue, ecchymosis, fluid retention, night sweats	400–800 mg/d PO
porfimer sodium *poor-fi'-mer*	Photofrin	Esophageal cancer	Atrial fibrillation, insomnia, constipation, nausea, abdominal pain, vomiting, pleural effusion, dyspnea, pneumonia, pharyngitis, anemia, fever, chest pain, pain, photosensitivity	2 mg/kg IV
mitotane *mye'-toe-tane*	Lysodren	Adrenal cortical carcinoma	Leukocytosis, GI symptoms (nausea, vomiting, diarrhea, abdominal pain), fatigue, edema, hyperglycemia, dyspnea, cough, rash, or itching, headaches, dizziness	2–16 g/d PO

*The term *generic* indicates the drug is available in generic form.

Chemotherapy is administered in a series of cycles to allow for recovery of the normal cells and to destroy more of the malignant cells (Fig. 28-2). According to cell kill theory, a drug regimen is intended to kill 90% of the cancer cells during the first course of treatment. The second course, according to this theory, targets the remaining cancer cells and reduces those cells by 90%. Further courses of chemotherapy continue to reduce the number of cancer cells, until all cells are killed. This theory is the rationale for using repeated doses of chemotherapy with several antineoplastic drugs. Every malignant cell must be destroyed for the cancer to be cured. Each cycle of treatment with the antineoplastic drugs kills some, but by no means all, of the malignant cells. Therefore, repeated courses of chemotherapy are used to kill more and more of the malignant cells, until theoretically none is left.

Actions of Alkylating Drugs

Alkylating drugs interfere with the process of cell division of malignant and normal cells. The drug binds with DNA, causing breaks and preventing DNA replication. Malignant cells appear to be more susceptible to the effects of alkylating drugs. Examples of alkylating drugs include busulfan (Myleran, Busulfex) and chlorambucil (Leukeran).

Actions of Antineoplastic Antibiotics

The antineoplastic antibiotics, unlike their anti-infection antibiotic relatives, do not have anti-infective (against infection) ability. Their action is similar to the alkylating drugs. Antineoplastic antibiotics appear to interfere with DNA and RNA synthesis and therefore delay

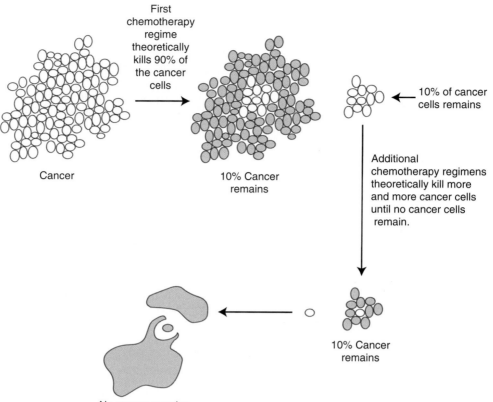

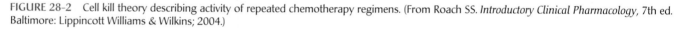

FIGURE 28–2 Cell kill theory describing activity of repeated chemotherapy regimens. (From Roach SS. *Introductory Clinical Pharmacology*, 7th ed. Baltimore: Lippincott Williams & Wilkins; 2004.)

or inhibit cell division, including the reproducing ability of malignant cells. Examples of antineoplastic antibiotics include bleomycin (Blenoxane), doxorubicin (Adriamycin), and plicamycin (Mithracin).

Actions of Antimetabolites

The antimetabolites interfere with various metabolic functions of cells, thereby disrupting normal cell functions. They inactivate enzymes or alter the structure of DNA, changing the ability of DNA to replicate. These drugs are most effective in the treatment of rapidly dividing neoplastic cells. Examples of the antimetabolites include methotrexate and fluorouracil (Adrucil).

Actions of Hormones

The exact method of antineoplastic action of hormones is unclear. These drugs also appear to counteract the effect of male or female hormones in hormone-dependent tumors (see Chapter 23). They appear to alter the hormonal environment of the cell. Examples of hormones used as neoplastic drugs include the androgen testolactone (Teslac), conjugate estrogens (see Chapter 23), and the progestin megestrol (Megace).

Gonadotropin-releasing hormone analogs, for example, goserelin (Zoladex), appear to act by inhibiting the anterior pituitary secretion of gonadotropins, thus suppressing the release of pituitary gonadotropins. These drugs primarily decrease serum testosterone levels and therefore are used in the treatment of advanced prostatic carcinomas.

Actions of Mitotic Inhibitors

Mitotic inhibitors (antimitotics) interfere with or stop cell division. Examples of mitotic inhibitors include paclitaxel (Taxol) and vincristine (Oncovin).

Actions of Miscellaneous Antineoplastic Drugs

The mechanisms of action of these unrelated drugs are not entirely clear. Examples of miscellaneous antineoplastics include cisplatin (Platinol) and hydroxyurea (Hydrea).

Uses of Antineoplastic Drugs

Antineoplastic drugs may be given alone or in combination with other antineoplastic drugs. In many instances, a combination of these drugs produces better results than the use of a single antineoplastic drug.

Although many antineoplastic drugs share a similar activity (i.e., they interfere in some way with cell division), their uses are not necessarily similar. The more common uses of specific antineoplastic drugs are given in the Summary Drug Table.

Adverse Reactions of Antineoplastic Drugs

Antineoplastic drugs often produce a wide variety of adverse reactions. Some of these reactions are dose-dependent; that is, their occurrence is more common or their intensity is more severe with higher doses. Other adverse reactions occur primarily because of the effect the drug has on many cells of the body. Because the antineoplastic drugs affect cancer cells and rapidly proliferating normal cells (e.g., cells in the bone marrow, gastrointestinal tract, reproductive tract, and the hair follicles), adverse reactions occur as the result of the action on these cells. Adverse reactions common to many of the antineoplastic drugs include bone marrow suppression, nausea, vomiting, stomatitis, diarrhea, and hair loss.

Some adverse reactions are desirable; for example, the depressing effect of certain antineoplastic drugs on the bone marrow, because this adverse drug reaction is essential in the treatment of the leukemias. Other adverse reactions are not desirable, such as severe vomiting or diarrhea.

Antineoplastic drugs are potentially toxic and often cause many serious adverse reactions. Some of these adverse effects must be accepted because the only alternative is to stop treatment of the malignancy. A treatment plan is developed that will prevent, lessen, or treat most or all of the symptoms of a specific adverse reaction. An example of prevention is giving an antiemetic before administering an antineoplastic drug known to cause severe nausea and vomiting.

Adverse reactions occurring with the administration of these drugs may range from very mild to life-threatening. Some of these reactions, such as the loss of hair (**alopecia**), may have little effect on the physical status of the patient but may affect the patient's mental health.

Common adverse reactions of antineoplastic drugs are listed in the Summary Drug Table: Antineoplastic Drugs.

Managing Adverse Reactions of Antineoplastic Drugs

Not all patients respond the same to antineoplastic drugs. For example, although an antineoplastic drug may cause vomiting, the amount of fluid and electrolytes the patient loses through vomiting may vary. One patient may require only sips of water once nausea and vomiting have subsided, whereas another may require intravenous fluid and electrolyte replacement.

Because a hemorrhagic syndrome may occur with plicamycin, assessments for hemorrhage are planned. Hyperuricemia (elevated blood uric acid levels) may occur with some drugs, such as melphalan (Alkeran) or mercaptopurine (Purinethol), so fluid intake and output measurements are planned. Because other antineoplastic drugs are nephrotoxic, blood urea nitrogen levels and serum creatinine are monitored closely during therapy.

ALERT

Older Patients and Adverse Reactions to Antineoplastic Drugs

Older adults are at increased risk for adverse reactions from the antineoplastic drugs because of their higher incidence of chronic disease, particularly kidney impairment and cardiovascular disease. A lower dosage of an antineoplastic may be used for patients with renal impairment. Creatinine clearance is used to monitor renal function in older adults.

Alopecia

Alopecia (loss of hair) is a common adverse reaction of some antineoplastic drugs. Some drugs cause severe hair loss, whereas others cause gradual thinning. Drugs causing severe hair loss include doxorubicin and vinblastine. Methotrexate, bleomycin, vincristine, and etoposide cause gradual hair loss.

A patient given these drugs should be informed that hair loss may occur. This problem occurs 10 to 21 days after the treatment cycle is completed. Hair loss is temporary, and hair will grow again when the drug therapy is completed.

Anorexia

Anorexia (loss of appetite resulting in an inability to eat) is common with antineoplastic drugs. Patients often report alterations in their sense of taste during the course of chemotherapy. Small, frequent meals (5 to 6 meals daily) are usually better-tolerated than three large meals. Breakfast is often the best-tolerated meal of the day. The patient is taught the importance of eating meals high in nutritive value, particularly protein (e.g., eggs, milk products, tuna, beans, peas, and lentils). Some patients can eat high-protein finger foods such as cheese or peanut butter and crackers. Nutritional supplements may also be prescribed. The patient's body weight is monitored at least weekly and any weight loss is reported. If the patient continues to lose weight, then a feeding tube may be used to administer a nutritionally complete liquid. Although this is not ideal, a hospitalized patient who is malnourished and weak may benefit from this intervention.

Bone Marrow Suppression

Bone marrow suppression is a potentially dangerous adverse reaction of decreased production of blood cells. Bone marrow suppression is manifested by abnormal laboratory test results and clinical evidence of leukopenia, thrombocytopenia, or anemia. For example, there is a decrease in the white blood cells or leukocytes (**leukopenia**), a decrease in the thrombocytes (**thrombocytopenia**), and a decrease in the red blood cells, resulting in anemia. Patients with leukopenia have a lower resistance to infection and must be monitored closely for any signs of infection.

ALERT

Signs of Infection

Any of the following signs of infection should be reported to the health care provider immediately: a temperature of 100.4°Fahrenheit or higher, cough, sore throat, chills, frequent urination, or a low white blood cell count.

Thrombocytopenia is characterized by a decrease in the platelet count. Patients with thrombocytopenia are monitored for bleeding tendencies, and precautions are taken to prevent bleeding. The patient should not use razors, nail trimmers, dental floss, firm toothbrushes, or any sharp objects. The patient is monitored closely for easy bruising, skin lesions, and bleeding from any orifice (opening) of the body.

ALERT

Symptoms of Thrombocytopenia

Any of the following should be reported to the health care provider immediately: bleeding gums, easy bruising, petechiae (pinpoint hemorrhages), increased menstrual bleeding, tarry stools, bloody urine, or coffee-ground emesis.

Anemia occurs as the result of a decreased production of red blood cells in the bone marrow and is characterized by fatigue, dizziness, shortness of breath, and palpitations. Blood transfusions may sometimes be necessary to correct the anemia.

Nausea and Vomiting

Nausea and vomiting are common adverse reactions of antineoplastic drugs. The health care provider may order an antiemetic approximately 30 minutes before treatment begins and continue the antiemetic for several days after administration of the chemotherapy. Small, frequent meals are provided as the patient can tolerate food. Greasy or fatty foods and unpleasant sights, smells, and tastes should be avoided. Cold foods, dry foods, and salty foods may be better-tolerated.

Stomatitis

Because the cells in the mouth grow rapidly, they are particularly sensitive to the effects of antineoplastic drugs. **Stomatitis** (inflammation of the mouth) or **oral mucositis** (inflammation of the oral mucous membranes) may occur 5 to 7 days after chemotherapy and continue up to 10 days after therapy. This adverse reaction can also affect the patient's nutrition. The patient must avoid any foods or products that are irritating to the mouth, such as alcoholic beverages, spices, strong mouthwashes, or toothpaste. Soft or liquid foods high in nutritive value should be given. Any white patches on the tongue, throat, or gums; any burning sensation; and bleeding from the mouth or gums should be reported to the health care provider. The health care provider may order a topical viscous anesthetic, such as lidocaine viscous, before meals to decrease discomfort when eating.

Diarrhea

Measures to manage diarrhea include a low-residue diet while the bowel rests. Electrolytes are monitored and supplemented as needed. Adequate hydration must be maintained; intravenous fluids may be necessary. If diarrhea is severe, then therapy may be delayed or stopped, or the dose decreased.

Tissue Integrity

Some antineoplastic drugs are **vesicants** (i.e., they cause tissue necrosis if they infiltrate or extravasate out of the blood vessel and into the soft tissue). If **extravasation** occurs, then underlying tissue is damaged. The damage can be severe, causing physical deformity or loss of vascularity or tendon function. Examples of vesicant drugs are daunorubicin, doxorubicin, and vinblastine.

ALERT

Extravasation and At-Risk Patients

Patients at risk for extravasation are those unable to communicate pain they feel with extravasation, the elderly, debilitated or confused patients, and any patient with fragile veins.

When the patient is receiving a vesicant, the intravenous site should be monitored continuously. Extravasation may occur without warning, or signs may be detected. The earlier the extravasation is detected, the less likely soft-tissue damage will occur. If an extravasation is suspected, then the infusion is stopped immediately and the extravasation reported to the health care provider.

ALERT

Signs of Extravasation

Signs of an extravasation include:

- swelling (most common)
- stinging, burning, or pain at the injection site (not always present)
- redness
- lack of blood return (if this is the only symptom, then the intravenous administration should be re-evaluated)

Anxiety

Patients and family members are usually devastated by the diagnosis of a malignancy. Patients undergoing chemotherapy require a great deal of emotional support from all members of the medical team. Kindness and gentleness in giving care and an understanding of the strain placed on the patient and the family may help reduce some of the fear and anxiety experienced during treatment.

Contraindications, Precautions, and Interactions of Antineoplastic Drugs

The information provided here is general, and the contraindications, precautions, and interactions for each antineoplastic drug vary. Antineoplastic drugs are contraindicated in patients with leukopenia, thrombocytopenia, anemia, serious infections, serious renal disease, or known hypersensitivity to the drug and during pregnancy (see Box 28-1 for pregnancy classifications of selected antineoplastic drugs).

Box 28-1 Pregnancy Classification for Selected Antineoplastic Drugs

Pregnancy Category C

cyclophosphamide	asparaginase	pegaspargase
levamisole	dacarbazine	dactinomycin

Pregnancy Category D

busulfan	idarubicin	vincristine
cladribine	mitomycin	anastrozole
chlorambucil	fluorouracil	mitoxantrone
cisplatin	toremifene	pentostatin
ifosfamide	hydroxyurea	teniposide
mechlorethamine	mercaptopurine	vinblastine
melphalan	thioguanine	bleomycin
procarbazine	mitoxantrone	epirubicin
thiotepa	flutamide	doxorubicin
daunorubicin	megestrol	teniposide
tamoxifen	etoposide	

Pregnancy Category X

diethylstilbestrol	bicalutamide	goserelin
methotrexate	plicamycin	triptorelin

Antineoplastic drugs are used cautiously in patients with renal or hepatic impairment, active infection, or other debilitating illnesses, or in those who have recently completed treatment with other antineoplastic drugs or radiation therapy.

Contraindications, Precautions, and Interactions of Alkylating Drugs

The alkylating drugs may antagonize the effects of antigout drugs by increasing serum uric acid levels. Dosage adjustment of the antigout drug may be needed. If cisplatin is used concurrently with aminoglycosides, then there may be an increase in nephrotoxicity and ototoxicity. When cisplatin is used concurrently with loop diuretics, there is an increased risk of ototoxicity. Administering live viral vaccines with cyclophosphamide may decrease the antibody response of the vaccine.

Contraindications, Precautions, and Interactions of Antineoplastic Antibiotics

Plasma digoxin levels may decrease when the drug is administered with bleomycin. When bleomycin is used with cisplatin, there is an increased risk of bleomycin toxicity. Pulmonary toxicity may occur when bleomycin is administered with other antineoplastic drugs. Plicamycin, mitomycin, mitoxantrone, and dactinomycin have an additive bone marrow depressant effect when administered with other antineoplastic drugs. Mitomycin, mitoxantrone, and dactinomycin decrease antibody response to live virus vaccines. Dactinomycin potentiates or reactivates skin or gastrointestinal reactions of radiation therapy. There is an increased risk of bleeding when plicamycin is administered with aspirin, warfarin, heparin, or a nonsteroidal anti-inflammatory drug.

Contraindications, Precautions, and Interactions of Antimetabolite Drugs

Antimetabolite drugs may antagonize the effects of antigout drugs by increasing serum uric acid concentration. Toxicity from methotrexate may be increased by other nephrotoxic drugs. When the antimetabolites are administered with other antineoplastic drugs, bone marrow suppression is additive. Vitamin preparations containing folic acid may decrease the effects of methotrexate. Alcohol ingestion while taking methotrexate may increase the risk of hepatotoxicity. Concurrent use of methotrexate and a nonsteroidal anti-inflammatory drug may cause severe methotrexate toxicity. Fluorouracil is not compatible with diazepam, doxorubicin, and methotrexate. Food decreases the absorption of fluorouracil. Live viral vaccines should not be administered if a patient is receiving fluorouracil, because a decrease in antibody production may occur, causing the vaccine to be ineffective. Severe cardiomyopathy with left ventricular failure has occurred when fluorouracil and cisplatin are given together.

Contraindications, Precautions, and Interactions of Hormones

Bicalutamide may increase the effect of oral anticoagulants. Flutamide enhances the action of leuprolide. Additive antineoplastic effects may occur when leuprolide is administered with megestrol or flutamide. Estrogens decrease the effectiveness of tamoxifen.

Contraindications, Precautions, and Interactions of Mitotic Inhibitors

Additive bone marrow depressive effects occur when a mitotic inhibitor drug is administered with another antineoplastic drug or radiation therapy. Administration of vincristine with digoxin results in a decreased therapeutic effect of the digoxin and decreased plasma digoxin levels. There is a decrease in serum concentrations of phenytoin when administered with vinblastine.

Contraindications, Precautions, and Interactions of Miscellaneous Antineoplastic Drugs

When asparaginase is administered to a patient with diabetes, the risk for hyperglycemia is increased; a dosage adjustment of the oral antidiabetic drug may be necessary. Glucocorticoids decrease the effectiveness of aldesleukin. When aldesleukin is administered with an antihypertensive drug, there is an additive hypotensive effect. Etoposide may decrease the immune response to live viral vaccines.

There is an increased risk for bone marrow suppression when levamisole or hydroxyurea is administered with another antineoplastic drug. Use of levamisole with phenytoin increases the risk of phenytoin toxicity. Pegaspargase may alter drug response of anticoagulants. When procarbazine is administered with other central nervous system depressants, such as alcohol, antidepressants, antihistamines, opiates, or the sedatives, an additive central nervous system effect may occur. Procarbazine may potentiate hypoglycemia when administered with insulin or oral antidiabetic drugs.

Patient Management Issues with Antineoplastic Drugs

After the administration of an antineoplastic drug, the patient assessment is based on the following:

• general condition
• the individual response to the drug
• adverse reactions that may occur

• guidelines established by the primary health care provider or hospital
• results of periodic laboratory tests

A complete blood count may be used to determine the response of the bone marrow to an antineoplastic drug. Liver function tests may be used to detect liver toxicity, which may be an adverse reaction that can be seen with the administration of some of these drugs.

If laboratory tests indicate a severe depressant effect on the bone marrow or other test abnormalities, then the health care provider may reduce the next drug dose or temporarily stop chemotherapy to allow the affected body systems to recover.

Administration of Antineoplastic Drugs

Antineoplastic drugs such as melphalan, busulfan, and chlorambucil are usually given orally. (Melphalan and busulfan are also available as injectable products for specific indications.) Most oral drugs are taken by the patient at home. The section on Educating the Patient and Family provides information to include in helping the patient and family members understand the treatment.

Although some of these drugs are given orally, others are given by the parenteral route. Goserelin (Zoladex), a hormonal antineoplastic drug used to treat breast cancer, is administered subcutaneously in an unusual way. The drug is contained in a dry pellet that is implanted in the soft tissue of the abdomen, where it is gradually absorbed over 1 to 3 months. After a local anesthetic, such as lidocaine, is administered, a large needle (usually 16 gauge) is used to insert the pellet.

The intravenous route of drug delivery is the most common and most reliable method of drug delivery.

Educating the Patient and Family About Antineoplastic Drugs

When the patient is hospitalized, all treatments and possible adverse effects are explained to the patient before the initiation of therapy.

Some of these drugs are taken orally at home. Some hospitals or health care providers give printed instructions to the patient. The patient has a right to know the dangers associated with these drugs and what adverse reactions may occur.

Some patients are given antineoplastic drugs in the medical office or outpatient clinic. Again, the treatment regimen is explained thoroughly to the patient and family members. In some instances, a drug to prevent nausea may be taken before administration of the drugs in the medical office or clinic. Most patients are compliant with therapy, although some patients might decide to skip a dose to feel better temporarily. The importance of maintaining the dosing schedule exactly as prescribed must be emphasized. A calendar marked with the doses to take, the dates the drug is to be taken, and space to record each dose may help the patient. One course of therapy is generally prescribed at a time to avoid inadvertent overdosing that could be life-threatening.

Patient Education Box 28-1 includes key points about antineoplastic drugs the patient and family members should know.

Natural Remedies: Green Tea

Green tea and black tea come from the same plant. The difference is in the processing. Green tea is simply dried tea leaves, whereas black tea is fermented, giving

it the dark color, the stronger flavor, and the lowest amount of tannins and polyphenols. The beneficial effects of green tea lie in the polyphenols, or flavonoids, that have antioxidant properties. Antioxidants are thought to play a major role in preventing disease (e.g., colon cancer) and reducing the effects of aging. Green tea polyphenols are powerful antioxidants. The polyphenols are thought to act by inhibiting the reactions of free radicals within the body thought to play a role in aging. The benefits of green tea include an overall sense of well-being, cancer prevention, dental health, and maintenance of heart and liver health. Green tea used as directed is safe and well tolerated. It contains as much as 50 mg of caffeine per cup. Decaffeinated green tea retains all of the polyphenol content. The recommended dosage is 2 to 5 cups per day. Standardized green tea extracts vary in strength, so dosages may need to be adjusted. Because green tea contains caffeine, nervousness, restlessness, insomnia, and gastrointestinal upset may occur. Green tea should be avoided during pregnancy because of its caffeine content. Patients with hypertension, cardiac conditions, anxiety, insomnia, diabetes, and ulcers should use green tea with caution.

KEY POINTS

● Antineoplastic drugs may be given alone or in combination with other antineoplastic drugs. Although many antineoplastic drugs share a similar activity (i.e., they interfere in some way with cell division), their uses are not necessarily similar.

● Alkylating drugs interfere with the process of cell division of malignant and normal cells. The alkylating drugs may antagonize the effects of antigout drugs by increasing serum uric acid levels.

● The antineoplastic antibiotics include bleomycin (Blenoxane), doxorubicin (Adriamycin), and plicamycin (Mithracin). Contraindications of the antineoplastic antibiotics include a decrease in plasma digoxin levels, pulmonary toxicity, an additive bone marrow depressant effect, a decreased antibody response to live virus vaccines, and an increased risk of bleeding. Adverse reactions and contraindication are drug-specific.

● The antimetabolites interfere with various metabolic functions of cells, thereby disrupting normal cell functions. These drugs are most effective in the treatment of rapidly dividing neoplastic cells. Antimetabolite drugs may antagonize the effects of antigout drugs by increasing the serum uric acid concentration. When the antimetabolites are administered with other antineoplastic drugs, bone marrow suppression is additive.

● The exact method of antineoplastic action of hormones is unclear. These drugs also appear to counteract the effect of male or female hormones in hormone-dependent tumors. Examples of hormones used as neoplastic drugs include the androgen testolactone (Teslac), conjugate estrogens, and the progestin megestrol (Megace).

○ Mitotic inhibitors (antimitotics) interfere with or stop cell division. Examples of mitotic inhibitors include paclitaxel (Taxol) and vincristine (Oncovin). Additive bone marrow depressive effects occur when the mitotic inhibitor drugs are administered with other antineoplastic drugs or radiation therapy.

○ Because the antineoplastic drugs affect cancer cells and rapidly proliferating normal cells (i.e., cells in the bone marrow, gastrointestinal tract, reproductive tract, and the hair follicles), adverse reactions occur as the result of the action on these cells. Adverse reactions common to many of the antineoplastic drugs include bone marrow suppression, nausea, vomiting, stomatitis, diarrhea, and hair loss.

CASE STUDY

Dennis, age 10 years, has leukemia and is to begin chemotherapy with chlorambucil (Leukeran). His parents are anxious about the treatment and have many questions.

1. One question they have involves potential adverse reactions to Leukeran. They should be told:
   a. bone marrow depression, nausea, diarrhea, and alopecia are possible
   b. bone marrow depression, nausea, diarrhea, and tremors are possible
   c. bone marrow depression, nausea, diarrhea, and cystitis are possible
   d. none of the above

2. Dennis's parents wonder if Dennis will lose his appetite. They should be told:
   a. it is not uncommon for patients to experience alterations in their sense of taste
   b. small, frequent meals are usually better tolerated than two or three big meals
   c. it is important that Dennis eat foods with high nutritional quality
   d. all of the above

3. Dennis seems upset but uncommunicative. His parents are worried that he has questions that he may be afraid to ask. They should be told that:
   a. everyone on the health care team will help to support him emotionally throughout the course of his treatment
   b. the health care provider is the sole resource for addressing his emotional well-being
   c. in the interest of time, they should answer any questions he may have because the health care team will be busy managing his physical well-being
   d. if Dennis has questions, it is up to him to ask the questions when he is ready

WEBSITE ACTIVITIES

1. Go to the National Comprehensive Cancer Network website (http://www.nccn.org) and click on "About NCCN." Read about the mission of NCCN, when it was established, and the types of organizations that comprise its membership.

2. Return to the starting page and click on "Network Hospitals." Select the member hospital nearest your area and read the opening section in its profile. Write a brief statement about the focus of that cancer center.

REVIEW QUESTIONS

1. Which of the following findings would be most indicative that the patient has thrombocytopenia?
   a. nausea
   b. blurred vision
   c. headaches
   d. easy bruising

2. Which of the following is the most common symptom of extravasation?
   a. swelling around the injection site
   b. redness along the vein and around the injection site
   c. pain at the injection site
   d. tenderness along the path of the vein

3. Which of the following adverse reactions to the antineoplastic drugs is most likely to affect the patient's mental health and self-esteem?
   a. hematuria
   b. alopecia
   c. nausea
   d. diarrhea

4. When assessing a patient for leukopenia, the health care provider:
   a. checks the patient every 8 hours for hematuria
   b. monitors the patient for fever, sore throat, chills
   c. checks female patients for increased menstrual bleeding
   d. asks about frequency of skin rashes

5. Which of the following interventions would be most helpful for a patient with stomatitis?
   a. avoiding foods that irritate the mouth
   b. eating soft or liquid foods
   c. avoiding alcohol and strong mouthwashes
   d. all of the above

29 Drugs That Affect the Musculoskeletal System

KEY TERMS

chrysiasis—grey to blue pigmentation of the skin that may occur from gold deposits in
    tissues
corticosteroids—hormones secreted from the adrenal cortex that contain potent anti-
    inflammatory action
gout—a form of arthritis in which uric acid accumulates in increased amounts in the
    blood and often is deposited in the joints
musculoskeletal—the bone and muscular structure of the body
osteoarthritis—a noninflammatory joint disease resulting in degeneration of the articular
    cartilage and changes in the synovial membrane
rheumatoid arthritis—a chronic disease characterized by inflammatory changes within
    the body's connective tissue

CHAPTER OBJECTIVES

On completion of this chapter, students will be able to:

1 Define the chapter's key terms.

2 Describe the general drug actions, uses, adverse reactions, contraindications, precautions, and interactions of drugs that affect the musculoskeletal system.

3 Discuss important points to keep in mind when educating the patient or family members about the use of drugs that affect the musculoskeletal system.

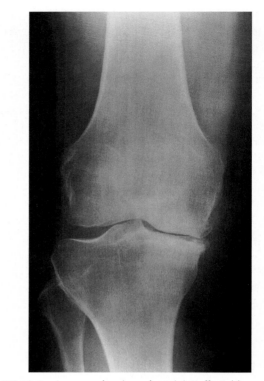

A variety of drugs are used in the treatment of **musculoskeletal** (bone and muscle) disorders. Examples of the musculoskeletal disorders discussed in this chapter include osteoarthritis (Fig. 29-1), rheumatoid arthritis, gout, and Paget disease. These and other musculoskeletal disorders are described in Table 29-1. The drug selected is based on the musculoskeletal disorder being treated, the severity of the disorder, and the patient's positive or negative response to past therapy. For example, early cases of **rheumatoid arthritis** (a chronic disease characterized by inflammatory changes within the body's connective tissue) may respond well to the salicylates, whereas advanced rheumatoid arthritis not responding to other drug therapies may require the use of one of the gold compounds.

FIGURE 29-1 An x-ray showing a knee joint affected by severe osteoarthritis. (With permission from Koval KJ, Zuckerman JD. Atlas of Orthopaedic Surgery: A Multimedia Reference. Philadelphia: Lippincott Williams & Wilkins; 2004.)

TABLE 29-1   Selected Musculoskeletal Disorders

Disorder	Description
Synovitis	.Synovitis is an inflammation of the synovial membrane of a joint resulting in pain, swelling, and inflammation. It occurs in disorders such as rheumatic fever, rheumatoid arthritis, and gout.
Arthritis	Arthritis is the inflammation of a joint. The term is frequently used to refer to any disease involving pain or stiffness of the musculoskeletal system.
Osteoarthritis or degenerative joint disease (DJD)	Osteoarthritis is a noninflammatory degenerative joint disease marked by degeneration of the articular cartilage, changes in the synovial membrane, and hypertrophy of the bone at the margins.
Rheumatoid arthritis (RA)	RA is a chronic systemic disease that produces inflammatory changes throughout the connective tissue in the body. It affects joints and other organ systems of the body. Destruction of articular cartilage occurs, affecting joint structure and mobility. RA primarily affects individuals between 20 and 40 years of age.
Gout	Gout is a form of arthritis in which uric acid accumulates in increased amounts in the blood and often is deposited in the joints. The deposit or collection of urate crystals in the joints causes the symptoms (pain, redness, swelling, joint deformity).
Osteoporosis	Osteoporosis is a loss of bone density occurring when the loss of bone substance exceeds the rate of bone formation. Bones become porous, brittle, and fragile. Compression fractures of the vertebrae are common. This disorder occurs most often in postmenopausal women, but can occur in men as well.
Paget disease (osteitis deformans)	Paget disease is a chronic bone disorder characterized by abnormal bone remodeling. The disease disrupts the growth of new bone tissue causing the bone to thicken and become soft. This weakens the bone, which increases susceptibility of fracture even with slight trauma or collapse of the bone (e.g., the vertebrae).

The salicylates and nonsteroidal anti-inflammatory drugs are important in the treatment of arthritic conditions. For example, the salicylates and nonsteroidal anti-inflammatory drugs are used in the treatment of rheumatoid arthritis and **osteoarthritis** (a noninflammatory joint disease resulting in degeneration of the articular cartilage and changes in the synovial membrane), as well as relief of pain or discomfort resulting from musculoskeletal injuries such as sprains. Chapter 10 discusses these drugs in detail.

Gold Compounds

Gold suppresses or prevents, but does not cure, arthritis and synovitis (inflammation of the joints). The therapeutic effects from gold compounds occur slowly. Early improvement is often limited to reduction in morning stiffness. The full effects of gold therapy do not occur for 6 to 8 weeks or in some cases after 6 months of therapy.

Actions of Gold Compounds

The exact mechanism of action of the gold compounds (for example, gold sodium thiomalate, aurothioglucose, and auranofin) in the suppression or prevention of inflammation is unknown. Gold compounds decrease synovial inflammation and retard cartilage and bone destruction. Gold decreases the concentration of rheumatoid factor and immunoglobulins.

Uses of Gold Compounds

Gold compounds are used to treat active juvenile and adult rheumatoid arthritis not controlled by other anti-inflammatory drugs. When cartilage and bone damage has already occurred, however, gold cannot reverse structural changes to the joints. The greatest benefit appears to occur in patients in the early stages of disease.

Adverse Reactions of Gold Compounds

Adverse reactions to the gold compounds may occur any time during therapy, as well as many months after therapy has been discontinued. Dermatitis (inflammation of the skin) and stomatitis (inflammation of mucosa of the mouth, gums, and possibly the tongue) are the most common adverse reactions. Pruritus (itching) often occurs before the skin eruption becomes apparent. Photosensitivity reactions (exaggerated sunburn reaction when the skin is exposed to sunlight or ultraviolet light) may also occur. **Chrysiasis** (grey to blue pigmentation of the skin) may occur and is caused by gold deposits in tissues. Gold dermatitis is exacerbated by exposure to sunlight.

Managing Adverse Reactions of Gold Compounds

The patient is closely observed for evidence of dermatitis. Itching may occur before a skin reaction and should be reported to the health care provider immediately. If itching occurs, then a soothing lotion or an antiseptic cream may be used. The environment should be kept free of irritants that aggravate itching, such as rough fabrics, excessive warmth, or excessive dryness.

The patient's mouth should be inspected daily for ulceration of mucous membranes. A metallic taste may occur before stomatitis becomes evident. The patient should inform the health care provider if a metallic taste occurs. Good oral care is necessary. Teeth should be brushed after each meal and the mouth rinsed with plain water to remove food particles. Mouthwash may also be used, but excessive use may result in oral infections caused by the destruction of the normal bacteria present in the mouth.

ALERT

Older Adults and Gold Compounds
Gold compounds are given cautiously to older adults. Tolerance for gold therapy decreases with advancing age.

While taking gold compounds, the patient is monitored closely for thrombocytopenia (abnormally low numbers of platelets in the blood). The health care provider orders frequent blood studies (usually once per month or more frequently).

ALERT

Symptoms of Thrombocytopenia
If the patient experiences signs and symptoms of thrombocytopenia (e.g., easy bruising, bleeding gums, epistaxis, melena), then the health care provider should be notified immediately.

Contraindications, Precautions, and Interactions of Gold Compounds

The gold compounds are contraindicated in patients with a known hypersensitivity. Parenteral administration is contraindicated in patients with uncontrolled diabetes, hepatic disease, uncontrolled hypertension, uncontrolled congestive heart failure, systemic lupus erythematosus, or blood dyscrasias and in those having recent radiotherapy. Oral administration is contraindicated in patients with necrotizing enterocolitis, pulmonary fibrosis, or hematologic disorders and during pregnancy (category C) and lactation.

The gold compounds are used cautiously in patients with a history of hypersensitivity to other drugs, previous kidney or liver disease, diabetes, or hypertension.

Concurrent administration of auranofin with phenytoin may increase phenytoin blood levels.

Drugs Used in the Treatment of Gout

Gout is a form of arthritis in which uric acid accumulates in increased amounts in the blood and often is deposited in the joints. The deposit or collection of urate crystals in the joints causes the symptoms (pain, redness, swelling, joint deformity) of gout (Fig. 29-2).

Actions of Drugs Used for Gout

Allopurinol (Zyloprim) reduces the production of uric acid, thus decreasing serum uric acid levels and the deposit of urate crystals in joints. The exact mechanism of action of colchicine is unknown, but it does reduce the inflammation associated with the deposit of urate crystals in the joints. This probably accounts for its ability to relieve the severe pain of acute gout. Colchicine has no effect on uric acid metabolism.

In those with gout, the serum uric acid level is usually elevated. Sulfinpyrazone increases the excretion of uric acid by the kidneys, which lowers serum uric acid levels and consequently retards the deposit of urate crystals in the joints. Probenecid (Benemid) works in the same manner and may be given alone or with colchicine as combination therapy when the patient has frequent, recurrent attacks of gout. Probenecid also has been used to prolong the plasma levels of the penicillins and cephalosporins.

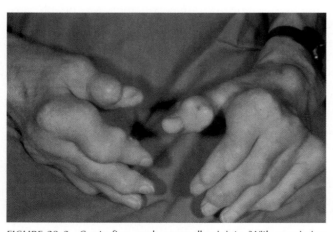

FIGURE 29-2   Gout often produces swollen joints. (With permission from Rubin E, Farber JL. Pathology, 3rd ed. Philadelphia: Lippincott Williams & Wilkins; 1999.)

Uses of Drugs for Gout

Drugs indicated for treatment of gout may be used to manage acute attacks of gout or in preventing acute attacks of gout (prophylaxis).

Adverse Reactions of Drugs for Gout

One adverse reaction associated with allopurinol is skin rash, which in some cases has been followed by serious hypersensitivity reactions such as exfoliative dermatitis and Stevens-Johnson syndrome (see Chapter 25 for a description of this syndrome). Other adverse reactions include nausea, vomiting, diarrhea, abdominal pain, and hematologic changes.

Colchicine administration may result in nausea, vomiting, diarrhea, abdominal pain, and bone marrow depression. When this drug is given to patients with an acute attack of gout, the health care provider may order the drug given at frequent intervals until gastrointestinal symptoms occur. Probenecid administration may cause headache, gastrointestinal symptoms, urinary frequency, and hypersensitivity reactions. Upper gastrointestinal disturbances may be seen with the administration of sulfinpyrazone. Even when the drug is given with food, milk, or antacids, gastrointestinal distress may persist and the drug therapy may need to be discontinued. The adverse reactions seen with other agents used in the treatment of gout are listed in the Summary Drug Table: Drugs Used to Treat Musculoskeletal Disorders.

Managing Adverse Reactions of Drugs for Gout

A liberal fluid intake is encouraged, and the patient's intake and output should be measured. The daily urine output should be at least 2 L. An increased urinary output is necessary to excrete the urates (uric acid) and prevent uratic acid stone formation in the genitourinary tract.

The patient should be reminded frequently of the importance of increasing fluid intake. If the patient fails to increase the oral intake, then the health care provider should be notified. In some instances, it may be necessary to administer intravenous fluids to supplement the oral intake when the patient fails to drink approximately 3000 mL of fluid per day.

Allopurinol may cause a skin rash. This rash may precede a serious adverse reaction, Stevens-Johnson syndrome (see Chapter 25). The presence of any rash should immediately be reported to the health care provider.

Contraindications, Precautions, and Interactions of Drugs for Gout

The drugs used for gout are contraindicated in patients with known hypersensitivity. Probenecid is contraindicated in patients with blood dyscrasias or uric acid

SUMMARY DRUG TABLE   Drugs Used to Treat Musculoskeletal Disorders

Generic Name	Trade Name*	Uses	Adverse Reactions	Dosage Ranges
Drugs Used to Treat Osteoporosis **Bisphosphonates** alendronate sodium *ah-len'-drew-nate*	Fosamax	Treatment and prevention of postmenopausal osteoporosis; glucocorticoid-induced osteoporosis; osteoporosis in men; Paget disease	Headache, abdominal pain, arthralgia, recurrent bone pain, nausea, diarrhea, esophageal ulceration, dysphagia	Postmenopausal osteoporosis, osteoporosis in men: 35–70 mg/wk or 10 mg/d PO; in glucocorticoid-induced osteoporosis: 5–10 mg/d PO; Paget disease: 40 mg/d PO
etidronate *e-tid'-ro-nate*	Didronel, Didronel IV	Paget disease, postoperative treatment after total hip replacement	Headache, abdominal pain, arthralgia, recurrent bone pain, nausea, diarrhea	5–10 mg/kg/d PO (not to exceed 6 mo) or 11 mg/d PO, if retreatment is necessary wait at least 90 d; 7.5 mg/kg/d IV; postoperative total hip replacement: 20 mg/kg/d PO
risedronate sodium *rah-sed'-dro-nate*	Actonel	Treatment and prevention of postmenopausal osteoporosis, glucocorticoid-induced osteoporosis, Paget disease	Headache, abdominal pain, arthralgia, recurrent bone pain, nausea, diarrhea	Osteoporosis: 5 mg/d PO; Paget disease: 30 mg/d PO for 2 mos
Gold Compounds auranofin *au-rane'-oh-fin*	Ridaura	Rheumatoid arthritis	Dermatitis, stomatitis, photosensitivity, pruritus, hematologic changes, nausea, vomiting, anorexia, rash, urticaria, metallic taste	6–9 mg/d PO (may give 3 mg BID or 6 mg QD)
aurothioglucose *aur-oh-thye-oh-gloo'-kose*	Solganal	Rheumatoid arthritis	Dermatitis, stomatitis, photosensitivity, pruritus, hematologic changes, nausea, vomiting, anorexia, rash, urticaria, metallic taste	10–50 mg IM; initial dose: 10 mg IM; 2nd & 3rd doses, 25 mg IM; 4th & subsequent doses, 50 mg IM until 0.8–1 g is given; dosage may be continued at 50 mg IM q3–4wk
gold sodium thiomalate *thi-oh-ma'-late*	Aurolate, *generic*	Rheumatoid arthritis	Dermatitis, stomatitis, photosensitivity, pruritus, hematologic changes, nausea, vomiting, anorexia, rash, urticaria, metallic taste	10–50 mg IM; initial dose: 10 mg IM; dosage increased weekly until 1 g is reached; dose may be continued at 25–50 mg IM every other wk for 2–20 wk

Generic Name	Trade Name*	Uses	Adverse Reactions	Dosage Ranges
Drugs Used to Treat Gout				
allopurinol *al-oh-pure'-i-nole*	Zyloprim, *generic*	Management of symptoms of gout	Rash, exfoliative dermatitis, Stevens-Johnson syndrome, nausea, vomiting, diarrhea, abdominal pain, hematologic changes	100–800 mg/d PO
colchicine *kol'-chi-seen*	*generic*	Relief of acute attacks of gout, prevention of gout attacks	Nausea, vomiting, diarrhea, abdominal pain, bone marrow depression	Acute attack: Initial dose 0.5–1.2 mg PO or 2 mg IV then 0.5–1.2 mg PO q1–2h or 0.5 mg IV q6h until attack aborted or adverse effects occur; prophylaxis: 0.5–0.6 mg/d PO
probenecid *proe-ben'-e-sid*	Benemid, *generic*	Treatment of hyperuricemia of gout and gouty arthritis	Headache, anorexia, nausea, vomiting, urinary frequency, flushing, dizziness	0.25 mg PO BID for 1 wk then 0.5 mg PO BID
sulfinpyrazone *sul-fin-peer'-a-zone*	*generic*	Treatment of gouty arthritis	Upper GI disturbances, rash, blood dyscrasias	200–400 mg/d PO in 2 divided doses
Skeletal Muscle Relaxants				
baclofen *bak'-loe-fen*	Lioresal, *generic*	Spasticity due to multiple sclerosis, spinal cord injuries	Drowsiness, dizziness, nausea, urinary frequency, weakness, rash, hypotension, headache, confusion	15–80 mg/d PO in divided doses
carisoprodol *ker-eye-soe-proe'-dol*	Soma, *generic*	Relief of discomfort due to acute, painful musculoskeletal conditions	Dizziness, drowsiness, tachycardia, nausea, vomiting	350 mg PO TID, QID
chlorphenesin carbamate *klor-fen'-e-sin*	Maolate	Discomfort due to musculoskeletal disorders	Drowsiness, dizziness, light-headedness, confusion, headache rash, blurred vision, GI upset	400–800 mg PO in divided doses
chlorzoxazone *klor-zox'-a-zone*	Paraflex, Parafon Forte DSC, *generic*	Relief of discomfort due to acute, painful musculoskeletal condition	GI disturbances, drowsiness, dizziness, rash	250–750 mg PO TID, QID
cyclobenzaprine hydrochloride *sye-kloe-ben'-za-preen*	Flexeril, *generic*	Relief of discomfort due to acute, painful musculoskeletal conditions	Drowsiness, dizziness, dry mouth, nausea, constipation	10–60 mg/d PO in divided doses

Generic Name	Trade Name*	Uses	Adverse Reactions	Dosage Ranges
dantrolene sodium *dan'-troe-leen*	Dantrium	Spasticity due to spinal cord injury, stroke, cerebral palsy, multiple sclerosis	Drowsiness, dizziness, weakness, constipation, tachycardia, malaise	Initial dose: 25 mg/d PO then 50–400 mg/d PO in divided doses
diazepam *dye-az'-e-pam*	Valium, *generic*	Relief of skeletal muscle spasm, spasticity due to cerebral palsy, epilepsy, paraplegia, anxiety	Drowsiness, sedation, sleepiness, lethargy, constipation, diarrhea, bradycardia, tachycardia, rash	2–10 mg PO BID–QID; 2–20 mg IM, IV; sustained release, 15–30 mg qd PO
methocarbamol *meth-oh-kar'-ba-mol*	Robaxin, *generic*	Discomfort due to musculoskeletal disorders	Drowsiness, dizziness, light-headedness, confusion, headache, rash, blurred vision, GI upset	1–1.5 g QID PO; up to 3 g/d IM, IV
orphenadrine citrate *or-fen'-a-dreen*	Banflex, Flexoject, Flexon, Norflex *generic*	Discomfort due to musculoskeletal disorders	Drowsiness, dizziness, light-headedness, confusion, headache, rash, blurred vision, GI upset	100 mg BID PO; 60 mg IV or IM q12h
Corticosteroids prednisolone *pred-niss'-oh-lone*	Delta-Cortef, *generic*	Ankylosing spondylitis, bursitis, acute gouty arthritis, rheumatoid arthritis	See Chapter 23	5–60 mg/d PO
prednisone *pred'-ni-sone*	Deltasone, Orasone, *generic*	Ankylosing spondylitis, bursitis, acute gouty arthritis, rheumatoid arthritis	See Chapter 23	5–60 mg/d PO
Miscellaneous Drugs etanercept *ee-tah-ner'-sept*	Enbrel	Rheumatoid arthritis	Congestion, abdominal pain, dyspepsia, irritation at injection site, increased risk of infections, optic neuritis, pancytopenia	25 mg SC twice weekly
hylan G-F 20 (hyaluronic acid derivatives)	Synvisc, Hyalgan	Treatment of osteoarthritic knee pain in patients with no response to other treatment	Temporary pain, swelling and/or fluid accumulation in the injected knee, nausea, rash	2 mL by intra-articular injections once weekly for 3 wk

Generic Name	Trade Name*	Uses	Adverse Reactions	Dosage Ranges
hydroxychloro-quine sulfate *hye-drox-ee-klor'-oh-kwin*	Plaquenil Sulfate, *generic*	Rheumatoid arthritis-antimalarial	Irritability, nervousness, retinal and corneal changes, anorexia, nausea, vomiting, hematologic effects	200–600 mg/d PO
leflunomide *le-flu'-no-mide*	Arava	Rheumatoid arthritis	Hypertension, alopecia, rash, nausea	Initial dose: 100 mg for 3d; maintenance dose: 20 mg/d
methotrexate *meth-oh-trex'-ate*	Rheumatrex Dose Pak, *generic*	Rheumatoid arthritis, antineoplastic	Nausea, vomiting, anorexia, severe bone marrow depression, nephrotoxicity, leukopenia, stomatitis, blurred vision	7.5 mg PO once per wk or 2.5 mg at 12-h intervals for 3 doses once per wk
penicillamine *pen-I-sill'-a-meen*	Cuprimine, Depen	Rheumatoid arthritis	Pruritus, rash, anorexia, nausea, vomiting, epigastric pain, bone marrow depression, proteinuria, hematuria, increased skin friability, tinnitus	Initial dose: 125–250 mg/d PO and increased to obtain remission. Maximum daily dose is 1.0 g PO
sulfasalazine *sul-fa-sal'-a-zeen*	Azulfidine, *generic*	Rheumatoid arthritis, ulcerative colitis	Nausea, emesis, abdominal pains, crystalluria, hematuria, Stevens-Johnson syndrome, rash, headache, drowsiness, diarrhea	2–4 g/d PO in divided doses

*The term *generic* indicates the drug is available in generic form.

kidney stones and in children younger than 2 years. Sulfinpyrazone is contraindicated in patients with peptic ulcer disease and gastrointestinal inflammation. Colchicine is contraindicated in patients with serious gastrointestinal, renal, hepatic, or cardiac disorders and those with blood dyscrasias.

Allopurinol is used cautiously in patients with liver and renal impairment and during pregnancy (pregnancy category C) and lactation. Probenecid is used cautiously in patients with renal impairment, previous hypersensitivity to sulfa drugs, peptic ulcer disease, and those who are pregnant (pregnancy category B). Sulfinpyrazone is used cautiously in patients with renal function impairment and those who are pregnant (category unknown). Colchicine is used with caution in older adults and during pregnancy (pregnancy category C) and lactation.

There is an increased incidence of skin rash when allopurinol and ampicillin are administered concurrently. Concurrent administration of allopurinol and theophylline increases the risk of theophylline toxicity. When angiotensin-converting enzyme inhibitors or the thiazide diuretics are administered with allopurinol, there is an increased risk of hypersensitivity reactions. Administration of allopurinol with aluminum salts may decrease the effectiveness of allopurinol.

Salicylates antagonize probenecid's uricosuric action. Concurrent administration of probenecid increases the effects of acyclovir, barbiturates, benzodiazepines, dapsone, methotrexate, nonsteroidal anti-inflammatory drugs, rifampin, and the sulfonamides.

Sulfinpyrazone may increase the anticoagulant activity of oral anticoagulants. The patient has an increased risk of hypoglycemia when sulfinpyrazone is administered with tolbutamide. Concurrent administration of sulfinpyrazone with verapamil may decrease the effectiveness of verapamil.

Skeletal Muscle Relaxants

Actions of Skeletal Muscle Relaxants

The mode of action of many skeletal muscle relaxants, such as carisoprodol (Soma), baclofen (Lioresal), and chlorzoxazone (Paraflex), is not clearly understood. Many of these drugs do not directly relax skeletal muscles, but their ability to relieve acute painful musculoskeletal conditions may be attributable to their sedative action. Cyclobenzaprine (Flexeril) appears to have an effect on muscle tone, thus reducing muscle spasm.

The exact mode of action of diazepam (Valium), an antianxiety drug (see Chapter 5), in the relief of painful musculoskeletal conditions is unknown. The drug does have a sedative action, which may account for some of its ability to relieve muscle spasm and pain.

Uses of Skeletal Muscle Relaxants

Skeletal muscle relaxants are used in various acute, painful musculoskeletal conditions, such as muscle strains and back pain.

Adverse Reactions of Skeletal Muscle Relaxants

Drowsiness is the most common reaction occurring with the use of skeletal muscle relaxants. Additional adverse reactions are given in the Summary Drug Table: Drugs Used to Treat Musculoskeletal Disorders. Some of the adverse reactions that may occur with the administration of diazepam include drowsiness, sedation, sleepiness, lethargy, constipation or diarrhea, bradycardia or tachycardia, and rash.

Because of the risk of injury caused by drowsiness, the patient is carefully monitored before being allowed to walk or perform self-care activities alone. If drowsiness does occur, then assistance with activities is necessary. If drowsiness is severe, then the health care provider should be notified before the next dose is due.

Contraindications, Precautions, and Interactions of Skeletal Muscle Relaxants

The skeletal muscle relaxants are contraindicated in patients with known hypersensitivity. Baclofen is contraindicated in skeletal muscle spasms caused by rheumatic disorders. Carisoprodol is contraindicated in patients with a known hypersensitivity to meprobamate. Cyclobenzaprine is contraindicated in patients with a recent myocardial infarction, cardiac conduction disorders, and hyperthyroidism. In addition, cyclobenzaprine is contraindicated within 14 days of the administration of a monoamine oxidase inhibitor. Oral dantrolene is contraindicated in patients with active hepatic disease and muscle spasm caused by rheumatic disorders and during lactation. See Chapter 5 for information on diazepam.

The skeletal muscle relaxants are used with caution in patients with a history of cerebrovascular accident, cerebral palsy, Parkinsonism, or seizure disorders and during pregnancy (pregnancy category C) and lactation. Carisoprodol is used with caution in patients with severe liver or kidney disease and during pregnancy (category unknown) and lactation. Cyclobenzaprine is used cautiously in patients with cardiovascular disease and during pregnancy (pregnancy category B) and lactation. Dantrolene is a pregnancy category C drug and is used with caution during pregnancy. See Chapter 5 for information on diazepam.

An increased central nervous system depressant effect occurs when a skeletal muscle relaxant is administered with another central nervous system depressant, such as alcohol, antihistamines, opiates, and sedatives. There is an additive anticholinergic effect when cyclobenzaprine is administered with another drug with anticholinergic effects (e.g., antihistamines, antidepressants, atropine, haloperidol). See Chapter 5 for information on diazepam.

Bisphosphonates

The bisphosphonates are used to treat musculoskeletal disorders such as osteoporosis and Paget disease. This chapter discusses the use of these drugs in the treatment of osteoporosis.

Actions of Bisphosphonates

Alendronate, etidronate, and risedronate act primarily on the bone by inhibiting normal and abnormal bone resorption. This results in increased bone mineral density, reversing the progression of osteoporosis.

Uses of Bisphosphonates

The bisphosphonates are used to treat osteoporosis in postmenopausal women, Paget disease of the bone, and postoperative treatment after total hip replacement (etidronate).

Adverse Reactions of Bisphosphonates

Adverse reactions with the bisphosphonates include nausea, diarrhea, increased or recurrent bone pain, headache, dyspepsia, acid regurgitation, dysphagia, and abdominal pain. An analgesic may be used for headache. The health care provider must be notified of adverse reactions such as the return of bone pain or severe diarrhea.

Contraindications, Precautions, and Interactions of Bisphosphonates

These drugs are contraindicated in patients with known hypersensitivity. Alendronate and risedronate are contraindicated in patients with hypocalcemia. Alendronate is a pregnancy category C drug and is contraindicated during pregnancy. These drugs are contraindicated in patients with significant renal impairment. Concurrent use of these drugs with hormone replacement therapy is not recommended.

These drugs are used cautiously in patients with gastrointestinal disorders or renal function impairment and during pregnancy and lactation.

When administered with ranitidine, alendronate bioavailability is increased. When calcium supplements or antacids are administered with risedronate or alendronate, absorption of the bisphosphonates is decreased. In addition, risedronate absorption is inhibited when the drug is administered with magnesium and aluminum. There is an increased risk of gastrointestinal effects when a bisphosphonate is administered with aspirin.

Corticosteroids

Actions of Corticosteroids

Corticosteroids are hormones secreted from the adrenal cortex. These hormones arise from the cortex of the adrenal gland and are made from the crystalline steroid alcohol cholesterol. Synthetic forms of the natural adrenal cortical hormones are available. The potent anti-inflammatory action of the corticosteroids makes these drugs useful in the treatment of many types of musculoskeletal disorders. The corticosteroids are discussed in Chapter 23.

Uses of Corticosteroids

The corticosteroids may be used to treat rheumatic disorders such as ankylosing spondylitis, rheumatoid arthritis, gout, bursitis (inflammation of the bursa, usually the bursa of the shoulder), and osteoarthritis.

Adverse Reactions of Corticosteroids

Corticosteroids may be given in high doses for some arthritic disorders. Many adverse reactions are associated with high-dose and long-term corticosteroid therapy. A comprehensive list of adverse reactions is provided along with contraindications, precautions, and interactions of the corticosteroids in Chapter 23.

Miscellaneous Drugs

The miscellaneous drugs are used to treat a variety of musculoskeletal disorders. Penicillamine, methotrexate, and hydroxychloroquine are used to treat rheumatoid arthritis in patients who have had an insufficient therapeutic response to or are intolerant of other antirheumatic drugs such as the salicylates and nonsteroidal anti-inflammatory drugs. The Summary Drug Table: Drugs Used to Treat Musculoskeletal Disorders provides additional information about these and other drugs. One compound, hylan G-F 20, listed in the Summary Drug Table is not used for rheumatoid arthritis, but rather for osteoarthritis knee pain. It is a viscous, elastic sterile mixture made of hylan A fluid, hylan B gel, and salt water that is administered directly into the knee.

Actions of Miscellaneous Drugs

The mechanisms of action of penicillamine, methotrexate, and hydroxychloroquine in the treatment of rheumatoid arthritis are unknown.

Uses of Miscellaneous Drugs

Penicillamine, methotrexate, and hydroxychloroquine are used in the treatment of rheumatoid arthritis. Methotrexate is reserved for severe, disabling disease that is not responsive to other treatment.

Adverse Reactions of Miscellaneous Drugs

Hydroxychloroquine may result in irritability, nervousness, anorexia, nausea, vomiting, and diarrhea. This drug also may have adverse effects on the eye, including blurred vision, corneal edema, halos around lights, and retinal damage. Hematologic effects, such as aplastic anemia and leukopenia, may also occur.

The adverse reactions seen with penicillamine include pruritus, rash, anorexia, nausea, vomiting, epigastric pain, bone marrow depression, proteinuria, hematuria, increased skin friability, and tinnitus. Penicillamine may cause a severe toxic reaction.

Methotrexate is a potentially toxic drug that is also used in the treatment of malignancies and psoriasis. Nausea, vomiting, a decreased platelet count, leukopenia (decreased white blood cell count), stomatitis (inflammation of the oral cavity), rash, pruritus, dermatitis, diarrhea, alopecia (loss of hair), and diarrhea may occur with the administration of this drug.

Managing Adverse Reactions of
Miscellaneous Drugs

Patients taking hydroxychloroquine are closely observed for adverse reactions such as skin rash, fever, cough, easy bruising, or unusual bleeding, or symptoms of sore throat, visual changes, mood changes, loss of hair, tinnitus, or hearing loss. Any adverse reactions should be reported immediately. Particularly important are visual changes because irreversible retinal damage may occur. The patient is observed for signs of easy bruising and infection, which may indicate bone marrow depression, an adverse reaction related to the platelets and white blood cells. A decreased platelet count may cause the patient to bleed easily. The mouth is inspected daily for signs of inflammation or ulceration. Stools are also inspected for diarrhea or signs of gastrointestinal bleeding.

Penicillamine has been associated with many adverse reactions, some of which are potentially serious and even fatal. Any patient symptom should be reported to the health care provider. Increased skin friability may occur, which may result in easy breakdown of the skin at pressure sites, such as the hips, elbows, and shoulders. If the patient cannot walk or engage in self-care activities, then the patient's position is changed and pressure sites are inspected for skin breakdown every 2 hours.

Methotrexate is potentially toxic. Therefore, development of adverse reactions, such as thrombocytopenia and leukopenia, are closely monitored. Hematology, liver, and renal function studies are monitored every 1 to 3 months with methotrexate therapy. The health care provider is notified of abnormal hematology, liver function, or kidney function findings. All adverse reactions or suspected adverse reactions should immediately be reported to the health care provider.

Contraindications, Precautions, and Interactions of Miscellaneous Drugs

These drugs are contraindicated in patients with known hypersensitivity. Hydroxychloroquine is contraindicated in patients with porphyria (a group of serious inherited disorders affecting the bone marrow or the liver), psoriasis (chronic skin disorder), and retinal disease (may cause irreversible retinal damage). Methotrexate is contraindicated during pregnancy because it is a pregnancy category X drug and may cause birth defects in the developing fetus. Penicillamine is contraindicated in patients with a history of allergy to penicillin.

Hydroxychloroquine is used cautiously in patients with hepatic disease or alcoholism and during pregnancy (pregnancy category C) and lactation. Methotrexate is used cautiously in patients with renal impairment, women of childbearing age, and older adults or individuals who are chronically ill or debilitated. Penicillamine is used with extreme caution during pregnancy (pregnancy category C) and lactation.

There is an increased risk of toxicity of Methotrexate when administered with a nonsteroidal anti-inflammatory drug, salicylate, oral antidiabetic drug, phenytoin, tetracycline, or probenecid. There is an additive bone marrow depressant effect when administered with other drugs known to depress the bone marrow or with radiation therapy. There is an increased risk for nephrotoxicity when methotrexate is administered with another drug that causes nephrotoxicity. When penicillamine is administered with digoxin, decreased blood levels of digoxin may occur. There is a decreased absorption of penicillamine when the drug is administered with food, iron preparations, and antacids.

Patient Management Issues with Drugs that Affect the Musculoskeletal System

Periodic evaluation is an important part of therapy for musculoskeletal disorders. With some disorders such as acute gout, the patient can be expected to respond to therapy in hours, and the joints are inspected every 1 to 2 hours to identify a response or nonresponse to therapy. At this time, the patient is questioned regarding the relief of pain, as well as adverse drug reactions. In other disorders, response is gradual and may take days, weeks, and even months of treatment. Depending on the drug and the disorder, the evaluation of therapy may be daily or weekly.

Some of these drugs are toxic. The patient is closely observed for adverse reactions. Should any one or more adverse reactions occur, the health care provider is notified before the next dose is due.

A patient with a musculoskeletal disorder may be in acute pain or have longstanding mild to moderate pain, which can be just as difficult to tolerate as severe pain. Along with pain, there may be skeletal deformities, such as the joint deformities seen with advanced rheumatoid arthritis (Fig. 29-3). For many musculoskeletal condi-

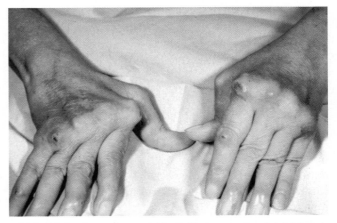

FIGURE 29-3   Severe rheumatoid arthritis may produce joint deformities. (With permission from Rubin E, Farber JL. Pathology, 3rd ed. Philadelphia: Lippincott Williams & Wilkins; 1999.)

tions, drug therapy is a major treatment modality. Therapy with these drugs may keep the disorder under control (e.g., therapy for gout), improve the patient's ability to perform the activities of daily living, or make the pain and discomfort tolerable.

Patients with an arthritis disorder may experience much pain or discomfort and may require assistance with activities, such as walking, eating, and grooming. Patients with osteoporosis may require a brace or corset when out of bed.

Patients with a musculoskeletal disorder often have anxiety related to the symptoms and the chronicity of their disorder. In addition to physical care, these patients often require emotional support, especially when a disorder is disabling and chronic. It is explained to the patient that therapy may take weeks or longer before any benefit is noted.

ALERT

Corticosteroids

When corticosteroid use is discontinued, the dosage must be tapered gradually over several days. If high dosages have been given, then it may take a week or more to taper the dosage.

Educating the Patient and Family About Drugs that Affect the Musculoskeletal System

The information given a patient and family members depends on the type and severity of the musculoskeletal disorder. It must be carefully explained to the patient that treatment for the disorder includes drug therapy, as well as other medical management, such as diet, exercise, limitations or nonlimitations of activity, and periodic physical therapy treatments. Patients need to understand the importance of not taking any nonprescription drugs unless the health care provider has approved their use. Patient Education Box 29-1 includes key points about drugs that affect the musculoskeletal system the patient and family members should know.

Natural Remedies: Glucosamine and Chondroitin

Both glucosamine and chondroitin are used, in combination or alone, to treat arthritis, particularly osteoarthritis. Chondroitin acts as the flexible connecting matrix between the protein filaments in cartilage. Chondroitin can be produced in the laboratory or be derived from natural sources (e.g., shark cartilage). Some studies suggest that if chondroitin sulfate is available to the cell

matrix, synthesis of the matrix can occur. For this reason, it is used to treat arthritis. Although there is not much information on chrondroitin's long-term effects, it is generally not considered to be harmful.

Glucosamine is found in mucopolysaccharides, mucoproteins, and chitin. Chitin is found in various marine invertebrates and other lower animals and members of the plant family. In osteoarthritis, there is a progressive degeneration of cartilage glycosaminoglycans. Oral glucosamine theoretically provides a building block for regeneration of damaged cartilage. The absorption of oral glucosamine is 90% to 98%, making it widely accepted for use. However, chondroitin molecules are very large (50 to 300 times larger than glucosamine), and only 0% to 13% of chondroitin is absorbed. These larger molecules may not be undelivered to cartilage cells. Glucosamine is generally well-tolerated, and no adverse reactions have been reported with its use.

KEY POINTS

● Gold suppresses or prevents, but does not cure, arthritis and synovitis (inflammation of the joints). The exact mechanism of action of the gold compounds (for example, gold sodium thiomalate, aurothioglucose, and auranofin) in the suppression or prevention of inflammation is unknown. Adverse reactions to the gold compounds may occur any time during therapy, as well as many months after therapy has been discontinued, and include dermatitis, stomatitis, pruritus, and chrysiasis.

● Drugs may be used to manage acute attacks of gout or prevent acute attacks (prophylaxis). Allopurinol is used to reduce the production of uric acid, and colchicine is used to reduce inflammation. Sulfinpyrazone and probenecid increase the excretion of uric acid by the kidneys. Probenecid (Benemid) may be given alone or with colchicine as combination therapy for frequent, recurrent attacks of gout. Adverse reactions to these drugs include skin rash, nausea, vomiting, diarrhea, and abdominal pain.

● Skeletal muscle relaxants are used in various acute, painful musculoskeletal conditions, such as muscle strains and back pain. Drowsiness is the most common reaction seen with the use of skeletal muscle relaxants. There is an increased central nervous system depressant effect when the skeletal muscle relaxants are administered with another central nervous system depressant such as alcohol, antihistamines, opiates, and sedatives.

● The bisphosphonates are used to treat musculoskeletal disorders, such as osteoporosis and Paget disease, and act primarily on the bone by inhibiting normal and abnormal bone resorption, thereby increasing bone density. These drugs are used to treat osteoporosis in postmenopausal women, Paget disease of the bone, and postoperative treatment after total hip replacement (etidronate). Adverse reactions include nausea, diarrhea, increased or recurrent bone pain, headache, dys-

PATIENT EDUCATION BOX 29-1

Key Points for Patients Taking Drugs that Affect the Musculoskeletal System:

GOLD COMPOUNDS

❏ Toxic reactions are possible when taking gold compounds. Report adverse reactions to your health care provider as soon as possible.

❏ Contact your health care provider if you note a metallic taste.

❏ Arthralgia (pain in the joints) may occur for 1 to 2 days after the parenteral form is given.

❏ Chrysiasis (gray to blue pigmentation of the skin) may occur, especially on areas exposed to sunlight. Avoid exposure to sunlight or ultraviolet light.

DRUGS USED FOR GOUT

❏ Drink at least 10 glasses of water per day until the acute attack has subsided.

❏ Take this drug with food to minimize gastrointestinal upset.

❏ If you feel drowsy, do not drive or perform other hazardous tasks.

❏ Acute gout: Notify your health care provider if your pain is not relieved in a few days.

❏ Colchicine for acute gout: Take this drug at the intervals prescribed by your health care provider, and stop taking the drug when the pain is relieved or if diarrhea or vomiting occurs. If the pain is not relieved in approximately 12 hours, notify your health care provider.

❏ Allopurinol: Notify your health care provider if a skin rash occurs.

❏ Colchicine: Notify your health care provider if skin rash, sore throat, fever, unusual bleeding or bruising, unusual fatigue, or weakness occurs.

SKELETAL MUSCLE RELAXANTS

❏ This drug may cause drowsiness. Do not drive or perform other hazardous tasks if you feel drowsy.

❏ This drug is for short-term use. Do not use the drug for longer than 2 to 3 weeks.

❏ Avoid alcohol or other depressants while taking this drug.

BISPHOSPHONATES

❏ Alendronate and risedronate: These drugs are taken with 6 to 8 oz of water first thing in the morning. Do not lie down for at least 30 minutes after taking the drug and wait at least 30 minutes before taking any other food or drink. Take the drugs exactly as prescribed. Your health care provider may prescribe alendronate as a once-weekly dose or to be taken daily. Risedronate is taken daily. Take supplemental calcium and vitamin D if dietary intake is inadequate. Take all medications, including vitamin and mineral supplements, at a different time of the day to prevent interference with absorption of the drug.

MISCELLANEOUS DRUGS

❏ Penicillamine: Your health care provider will explain the treatment regimen and adverse reactions before therapy is started. You must know which toxic reactions require contacting your health care provider immediately. Take penicillamine on an empty stomach, 1 hour before or 2 hours after a meal. If other drugs are prescribed, then penicillamine is taken 1 hour apart from any other drug. Observe skin areas over the elbows, shoulders, and buttocks for evidence of bruising, bleeding, or break in the skin (delayed wound healing may occur). If these occur, then do not self-treat the problem, but notify your health care provider immediately. An alteration in taste perception may occur. Taste perception should return to normal within 2 to 3 months.

❏ Methotrexate: Take methotrexate exactly as directed. If a weekly dose is prescribed, then use a calendar or some other method to take the drug on the same day each week. Never increase the prescribed dose of this drug. Mistaken daily use has led to fatal toxicity. Notify your health care provider immediately if you experience any of the following: sore mouth, sores in the mouth, diarrhea, fever, sore throat, easy bruising, rash, itching, or nausea and vomiting. Women of childbearing age should use an effective contraceptive during therapy with methotrexate and for 8 weeks after therapy.

❏ Hydroxychloroquine: Take hydroxychloroquine with food or milk. Contact your health care provider immediately if you experience any of the following: hearing or visual changes, skin rash or severe itching, hair loss, change in the color of the hair (bleaching), changes in the color of the skin, easy bruising or bleeding, fever, sore throat, muscle weakness, or mood changes. It may be several weeks before symptoms are relieved.

---

pepsia, acid regurgitation, dysphagia, and abdominal pain.

● Corticosteroids are hormones secreted from the adrenal cortex. The potent anti-inflammatory action of corticosteroids makes these drugs useful in the treatment of many types of musculoskeletal disorders. Corticosteroids may be given in high doses for some arthritic disorders, and many adverse reactions are associated with high-dose and long-term corticosteroid therapy.

● Miscellaneous drugs are used to treat a variety of musculoskeletal disorders, such as rheumatoid arthritis in patients who have had an insufficient therapeutic response to or are intolerant of other antirheumatic drugs such as salicylates and nonsteroidal anti-inflammatory drugs. Penicillamine, methotrexate, and hydroxychloroquine are used in the treatment of rheumatoid arthritis. Hydroxychloroquine may result in irritability, nervousness, anorexia, nausea, vomiting, and diarrhea. Adverse reactions to penicillamine include pruritus, rash, anorexia, nausea, vomiting, epigastric pain, bone marrow depression, proteinuria, hematuria, increased skin friability, and tinnitus. Methotrexate is a potentially toxic drug that is also used in the treatment of malignancies and psoriasis. Adverse reactions include nausea, vomiting, a decreased platelet count, leukopenia, stomatitis, rash, pruritus, dermatitis, diarrhea, alopecia, and diarrhea.

CASE STUDY

Ms. Leeds is prescribed methotrexate for rheumatoid arthritis that has not responded to other therapies. She is nervous about starting the drug after she was told that the drug can cause many serious adverse reactions.

1. Ms. Leeds wonders what the adverse effects of methotrexate may include. She should be told:
   a. nausea, severe bone marrow depression, leukopenia, blurred vision, and rash
   b. rash, anorexia, hematuria
   c. emesis and Stevens-Johnson syndrome
   d. none of the above

2. Ms. Leeds asks why she is being asked to take methotrexate. She is told:
   a. methotrexate is used to treat rheumatoid arthritis when other treatments are not working
   b. methotrexate is used for patients intolerant of the salicylates and nonsteroidal anti-inflammatory drugs
   c. methotrexate is used primarily in older patients; it is most effective in patients older than 60
   d. a and b

3. Ms. Leeds asks if methotrexate is used to treat anything other than rheumatoid arthritis. You tell her:
   a. methotrexate is also used for dialysis patients
   b. methotrexate is used solely for rheumatoid arthritis treatment
   c. methotrexate is also used to treat malignancies and psoriasis
   d. all of the above

WEBSITE ACTIVITIES

1. Got to the National Library of Medicine website (http://www.nlm.nih.gov), and click on the "Health Information," and then click on "NIH Senior Health." Explore the information on arthritis. What information does this website offer about the causes and risk factors for osteoarthritis?

2. At the same website, what information is available about the symptoms and diagnosis of osteoarthritis?

REVIEW QUESTIONS

1. A patient who is taking gold compound therapy on an outpatient basis should be told to contact the health care provider if what occurs?
   a. decreased appetite
   b. severe headache
   c. metallic taste in mouth
   d. hair loss

2. When taking a skeletal muscle relaxant the most common adverse reaction is:
   a. drowsiness
   b. gastrointestinal bleeding
   c. vomiting
   d. constipation

3. A corticosteroid may be prescribed for what condition?
   a. rheumatoid arthritis
   b. gout
   c. osteoarthritis
   d. all of the above

4. When allopurinol (Zyloprim) is used for the treatment of gout, what adverse effect may occur?
   a. rash
   b. nausea and vomiting
   c. hematologic changes
   d. all of the above

5. What should a patient prescribed risedronate be educated about?
   a. the drug is taken once weekly
   b. take a daily laxative because the drug will likely cause constipation
   c. take the drug in the morning before breakfast and immediately lie down for 30 minutes to facilitate absorption
   d. after taking the drug, remain upright for at least 30 minutes

30 Topical Drugs Used in the Treatment of Skin Disorders

Topical Anti-Infectives
Topical Antibiotic Drugs
Topical Antifungal Drugs
Topical Antiviral Drugs
Adverse Reactions of Topical Anti-Infectives
Contraindications, Precautions, and Interactions of
  Topical Anti-Infectives

Topical Antiseptics and Germicides
Actions of Topical Antiseptics and Germicides
Uses of Topical Antiseptics and Germicides
Adverse Reactions of Topical Antiseptics and
  Germicides
Contraindications, Precautions, and Interactions of
  Topical Antiseptics and Germicides

Topical Corticosteroids
Actions and Uses of Topical Corticosteroids
Adverse Reactions of Corticosteroids
Contraindications, Precautions, and Interactions of
  Corticosteroids

Topical Antipsoriatics
Actions and Uses of Antipsoriatics
Adverse Reactions of Antipsoriatics
Contraindications, Precautions, and Interactions of
  Antipsoriatics

Topical Enzymes
Actions and Uses of Topical Enzymes

Adverse Reactions of Topical Enzymes
Contraindications, Precautions, and Interactions of
  Topical Enzymes

Keratolytics
Actions and Uses of Keratolytics
Adverse Reactions of Keratolytics
Contraindications, Precautions, and Interactions of
  Keratolytics

Topical Local Anesthetics
Actions and Uses of Topical Local Anesthetics
Adverse Reactions of Topical Local Anesthetics
Contraindications, Precautions, and Interactions of
  Topical Local Anesthetics

Patient Management Issues with Topical Drugs
Managing Adverse Reactions of Topical Drugs

Educating the Patient and Family About Topical Drugs

Natural Remedies: Aloe Vera

Key Points

Case Study

Website Activities

Review Questions

KEY TERMS   **antipsoriatics**—drugs used to treat psoriasis
antiseptic—a drug that stops, slows, or prevents the growth of microorganisms
bactericidal—a substance that destroys bacteria
bacteriostatic—the slowing or retarding of the multiplication of bacteria
dermis—the layer of skin below the epidermis that contains small capillaries, which
  supply nourishment to the dermis and epidermis
epidermis—the outermost layer of the skin
germicide—a drug that kills bacteria
immunocompromised—patients with an immune system not fully capable of fighting infection
keratolytic—a drug that removes excess growth of the epidermis (top layer of skin) in disorders such as warts
necrotic—dead, as in dead tissue
proteolysis—the process of hastening the reduction of proteins into simpler substances
purulent exudates—pus-containing fluid
superinfection—an overgrowth of bacterial or fungal microorganisms not affected by the
  antibiotic being administered

CHAPTER OBJECTIVES

On completion of this chapter, students will be able to:

1 Define the chapter's key terms.

2 Describe the general drug actions, uses, adverse reactions, contraindications, precautions, and interactions of topical drugs used in the treatment of skin disorders.

3 Discuss important points to keep in mind when educating the patient or family members about the use of topical drugs used in the treatment of skin disorders.

The skin forms a barrier between the outside environment and the structures located beneath the skin (Fig. 30-1). The **epidermis** is the outermost layer of the skin. Immediately below the epidermis is the dermis. The **dermis** contains small capillaries, which supply nourishment to the dermis and epidermis, sebaceous (oil-secreting) glands, sweat glands, nerve fibers, and hair follicles. Because the skin interacts with the outside environment, it is subject to various types of injury and trauma, as well as changes in the skin itself. Each of the following sections discusses only select topical drugs for various skin conditions. See the Summary Drug Table: Dermatologic Drugs for a more complete listing of the drugs and additional information.

Topical Anti-Infectives

Localized skin infections may require the use of a topical anti-infective. The topical anti-infectives include antibiotic, antifungal, and antiviral drugs.

Topical Antibiotic Drugs

Topical antibiotics exert a direct local effect on specific microorganisms and may be **bactericidal** (a substance that destroys bacteria) or **bacteriostatic** (the slowing or retarding of the multiplication of bacteria). Bacitracin (Baciguent) inhibits the cell wall synthesis. Bacitracin, gentamicin (G-myticin), erythromycin (Emgel), and neomycin are examples of topical antibiotics.

These drugs are used to prevent superficial infections in minor cuts, wounds, skin abrasions, and minor burns. Erythromycin is also used to treat acne vulgaris.

Topical Antifungal Drugs

Antifungal drugs exert a local effect by inhibiting growth of the fungi. Examples of antifungal drugs and their uses are:

- Amphotericin B (Fungizone): used for treatment of mycotic infections (fungal)

- Miconazole (Micatin), ciclopirox (Loprox), and econazole (Spectazole): used for treatment of tinea pedis (athlete's foot), tinea cruris (jock itch), tinea corporis (ringworm) (Fig. 30-2), and superficial candidiasis
- Clioquinol: used for eczema, athlete's foot, and other fungal infections

Topical Antiviral Drugs

Acyclovir (Zovirax) and penciclovir (Denavir) are the only topical antiviral drugs currently available. These drugs inhibit viral replication.

Acyclovir is used in the treatment of initial episodes of genital herpes, as well as herpes simplex virus infections in **immunocompromised** patients (patients with an immune system not fully capable of fighting infection). Penciclovir is used for the treatment of recurrent herpes labialis (cold sores) in adults.

Adverse Reactions of Topical Anti-Infectives

Adverse reactions to topical anti-infectives are usually mild. Occasionally, the patient may experience a skin rash, itching, urticaria (hives), dermatitis, irritation, or redness, which may indicate a hypersensitivity (allergic) reaction to the drug. Prolonged use of topical antibiotic preparations may result in a superficial **superinfection** (an overgrowth of bacterial or fungal microorganisms not affected by the antibiotic being administered).

Contraindications, Precautions, and Interactions of Topical Anti-Infectives

These drugs are contraindicated in patients with known hypersensitivity. Because neomycin toxicity can cause nephrotoxicity and ototoxicity, it is used cautiously in patients with extensive burns or trophic ulceration when extensive absorption can occur.

Topical antibiotics are pregnancy category C drugs and are used cautiously during pregnancy and lactation. Acyclovir and penciclovir are pregnancy category B drugs and are used cautiously during pregnancy and lactation. The pregnancy categories of the antifungals are unknown except for econazole nitrate, which is pregnancy category C, and ciclopirox, which is pregnancy category B; both are used with caution during pregnancy and lactation. There are no significant interactions with the topical anti-infectives.

Topical Antiseptics and Germicides

An **antiseptic** is a drug that stops, slows, or prevents the growth of microorganisms. A **germicide** is a drug that kills bacteria. *(text continued on page 519)*

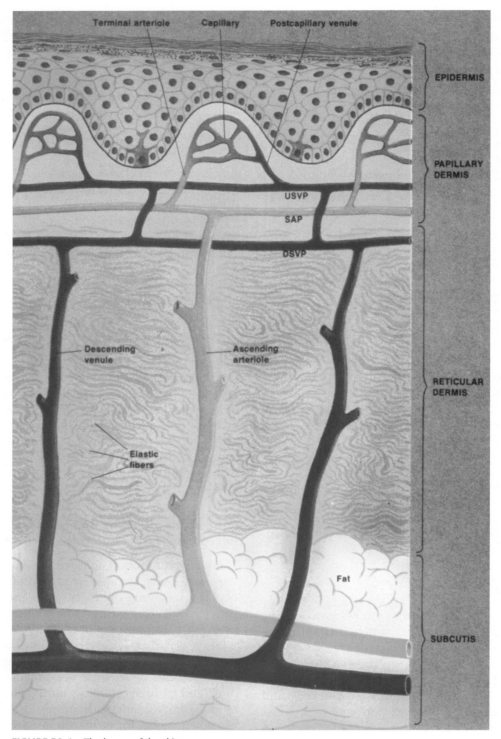

FIGURE 30-1   The layers of the skin.

Generic Name	Trade Name*	Uses	Adverse Reactions	Dosage Ranges
Antibiotic Drugs azelaic acid *az-e-lak'*	Azelex	Acne vulgaris	Mild and transient pruritus, burning, stinging, erythema	Apply twice daily
bacitracin *ba-ci-tra'-sin*	Baciguent, *generic*	Relief of skin infections	Rare; occasionally redness, burning, pruritus, stinging	Apply 1–5 times daily
benzoyl peroxide *been'-zoyl per-ox'-ide*	Acne-5, Benzac, Desquam-X 10% Wash, Dryox Wash, Exact, Loroxide Neutrogena, Acne Mask, *generic*	Mild to moderate acne vulgaris and oily skin	Excessive drying, stinging, peeling, erythema, possible edema, allergic dermatitis	Use once to three times daily
clindamycin, topical *clin'-da-my-sin*	Cleocin T, Clinda-Derm, Clindets, C/T/S, *generi*	Acne vulgaris	Dryness, erythema, burning, peeling, oiliness/oily skin, diarrhea, bloody diarrhea, abdominal pains, colitis	Apply a thin film twice daily to affected area
erythromycin *ee-rith-ro-my'-sin*	Akne-Mycin, Emgel, Erygel	Acne vulgaris	Skin irritation, tenderness, pruritus, erythema, peeling, oiliness and burning sensations	Clean affected area twice daily
gentamicin *jen-ta-my'-sin*	G-myticin, *generic*	Relief of primary skin infections	Mild and transient pruritus, burning, stinging, erythema, photosensitivity	Apply 1–5 times daily to affected area
metronidazole *meh-trow-nye'-dah-zoll*	Metro-Gel, MetroLotion, Noritate	Rosacea	Watery (tearing) eyes, transient redness, mild dryness, burning, skin irritation	Apply a thin film twice daily to affected areas
mupirocin *mew'-pie-ro-sin*	Bactroban	Impetigo, infections caused by *Staphylococcus aureus* and *S. pyogenes*	Ointment: burning, stinging, pain, itching, rash, nausea, erythema, dry skin; Cream: headache, rash, nausea, abdominal pain, burning at application site, dermatitis; Nasal: headache, rhinitis, respiratory disorders, such as pharyngitis, taste perversion, burning, stinging, cough	Ointment: apply 3 times daily for 3–5 d; Cream: apply 3 times daily for 10 d; Nasal: divide the single-use tube between both nostrils and apply twice daily for 5 d

Generic Name	Trade Name*	Uses	Adverse Reactions	Dosage Ranges
neomycin *knee-oh-my'-sin*	Myciguent, *generic*	Relief of skin infections	Mild and transient pruritus, burning, stinging, erythema	Apply 1–3 times daily
sulfacetamide sodium *sul-fah-see'-ta-mide*	Sebizon	Seborrheic dermatitis, seborrhea sicca (dandruff), bacterial infections of the skin	Rare; skin rash, nausea, vomiting	Apply 2–4 times daily
Antifungal Drugs amphotericin B *am-fo-ter'-eye-sin*	Fungizone	Mycotic infections	Rare; drying effect, local irritation, including erythema, pruritus, burning sensation	Apply liberally to lesions 2–4 times daily for 2–4 wk
butenafine HCl *beu-ten'-ah-feen*	Mentax	Dermatologic infections	Burning, stinging, itching, worsening of the condition, contact dermatis, erythema, irritation	Apply once daily for 4 wk
ciclopirox *sic-lo-peer'-ox*	Loprox, Penlac Nail Lacquer	Loprox: tinea pedis (athlete's foot), tinea cruris (jock itch), tinea corporis (ringworm), cutaneous candidiasis; Penlac: mild to moderate onychomycosis of fingernails and toenails	Pruritus, burning, worsening of clinical signs and symptoms, periungual erythema, nail disorders, irritation, ingrown toenail, burning of the skin	Apply to affected areas 1–2 times daily
clioquinol *kli-oh-qwe'-knol*	Generic	Tinea pedis, tinea cruris, and other skin infections caused by ringworm	Burning, itching, erythema, worsening of the condition	Apply thin layer to affected areas BID for 4 wk
econazole nitrate *ee-kon'-a-zole*	Spectazole	Tinea pedis, tinea cruris, tinea corporis, cutaneous candidiasis, tinea versicolor	Local burning, itching, stinging, erythema, pruritic rash	Apply to affected areas 1–2 times daily
gentian violet *jen'-shun*	*Generic*	External treatment of abrasions, minor cuts, surface injuries, superficial fungus, infections of the skin	Local irritation or sensitivity reactions	Apply locally BID

Generic Name	Trade Name*	Uses	Adverse Reactions	Dosage Ranges
haloprogin *ha-lo-pro'-jin*	Halotex	Tinea pedis, tinea cruris, tinea corporis, tinea manuum	Local irritation, burning sensation, vesicle formation, erythema, scaling, itching, pruritus	Apply twice daily for 2–4 wk
ketoconazole *kee-toe-koe'-na-zole*	Nizoral, *generic*	Cream: tinea cruris, tinea corporis, and tinea versicolor; Shampoo: reductions of scaling caused by dandruff	Local burning, itching, stinging, erythema, pruritic rash	Cream: once daily to affected areas for 2 wk; Shampoo: twice a week for 4 wk with at least 3 d between each shampoo
miconazole nitrate *mi-kon'-a-zole*	Fungoid-HC Creme, Lotrimin, Micatin, Monistat-Derm Cream, Tetterine, *generic*	Tinea pedis, tinea cruris, tinea corporis, cutaneous candidiasis	Local irritation, burning, maceration, allergic contact dermatitis	Cover affected areas twice daily
naftifine HCl *naf'-ti-feen*	Naftin	Topical treatment of tinea pedis, tinea cruris, tinea corporis	Burning, stinging, erythema, itching, local irritation, rash, tenderness	Apply BID for 4 wk
nystatin *nye-stat'-in*	Mycostatin, Nystex, *generic*	Mycotic infections caused by *Candida albicans*, and other *Candida* species	Virtually nontoxic and nonsensitizing; well tolerated by all age groups, even with prolonged administration; if irritation occurs, discontinue use	Apply 2–3 times daily until healing is complete
oxiconazole *ox-ee-kon'-ah-zole*	Oxistat	Tinea pedis, tinea cruris, tinea corporis	Pruritus, burning, stinging, irritation, contact dermatitis, scaling, tingling	Apply daily to BID 1 mo
sulconazole nitrate *sue-kon'-ah-zole*	Exelderm	Same as oxiconazole	Pruritus, burning, stinging, irritation	Apply 1–2 times daily for 2 wk
terbinafine HCl *ter-ben'-a-feen*	Lamisil	Same as oxiconazole	Same as oxiconazole	Apply twice daily until infection clears (1–4 wk)
tolnaftate *tole-naf'-tate*	Aftate, Genaspor, Tinactin, Ting, *generic*	Same as oxiconazole	Same as oxiconazole	Apply twice daily for 2–3 wk (4–6 wk may be needed)
Antiviral Drugs acyclovir *ay-sye'-kloe-veer*	Zovirax, *generic*	Herpes genitalis, herpes simplex virus infections	Mild pain with transient burning/ stinging, pruritus, rash, vulvitis, edema or pain at application site	Apply to all lesions q3h 6 times daily for 1 wk

Generic Name	Trade Name*	Uses	Adverse Reactions	Dosage Ranges
penciclovir *pen-sye´-kloe-veer*	Denavir	Herpes labialis (cold sores)	Irritation at application site, headache, mild erythema, rash, taste perversion	Apply q2h for 4 d
Antiseptic and Germicides benzalkonium chloride (BAC) *benz-al-cone´-e-um*	Benza, Mycocide NS, Ony-Clear, Zephiran, *generic*	Asepsis of skin, mucous membranes, and wounds; preoperative preparation of the skin; surgeon's hand and arm soaks; preservation of ophthalmic solutions; irrigations of the eye; vaginal douching	Well tolerated in most individuals; occasionally mild sensitivity reaction	Varies, depending on administration
chlorhexidine gluconate *klor-hex´-e-deen*	Bacto Shield 2, Betasept, Exidine-2 Scrub, Hibiclens	Surgical scrub, skin cleanser, preoperative skin preparation, skin wound cleanser, preoperative showering and bathing	Irritation, dermatitis, photosensitivity (rare), deafness, mild sensitivity reactions	Varies, depending on administration
Povidone–iodine *pov-e-don*	Acu-Dyne, Aerodine, Betadine, *generic*	Microbicidal against bacteria, fungi, viruses, spores, protozoa, yeasts	Dermatitis, irritation, burning, sensitivity reactions	Varies, depending on administration
triclosan *trye´-klo-san*	Clearasil Daily Face Wash	Skin cleanser, and skin degermer	None significant	5 mL on hands or face and rub thoroughly for 30 seconds, rinse thoroughly, pat dry
Corticosteroids, Topical alclometasone dipropionate *al-kloe-met-a-sone die-pro´-pee-oh-nate*	Aclovate	Treatment of various allergic/ immunologic skin problems	Allergic contact dermatitis, burning, dryness, edema, irritation	Apply 1–6 times daily according to directions
amcinonide *am-sin´-oh-nide*	Cyclocort	Same as alclometasone	Same as alclometasone	Apply 1–6 times daily according to directions
augmented betamethasone dipropionate	Diprolene	Same as alclometasone	Same as alclometasone	Apply 1–4 times daily according to directions
betamethasone dipropionate *bay-ta-meth´-a-sone*	Alphatrex, Diprosone, Maxivate, *generic*	Same as alclometasone	Same as alclometasone	Apply 1–4 times daily according to directions

Generic Name	Trade Name*	Uses	Adverse Reactions	Dosage Ranges
betamethasone valerate *bay-ta-meth'-a-sone-val'-eh-rate*	Betatrex, *generic*	Same as alclometasone	Same as alclometasone	Apply 1–4 times daily according to directions
desoximetasone *dess-ox-i-met'-a-sone*	Topicort, *generic*	Same as alclometasone	Same as alclometasone	Apply 1–4 times daily according to directions
dexamethasone sodium phosphate *dex-a-meth'-a-sone*	Decadron Phosphate	Same as alclometasone	Same as alclometasone	Apply 1–4 times daily according to directions
diflorasone diacetate *dye-flor'-a-sone*	Florone, Maxiflor	Same as alclometasone	Same as alclometasone	Apply 1–4 times daily according to directions
fluocinolone acetonide *floo-oh-sin'-oh-lone*	Fluonid, Flurosyn, Synalar, *generic*	Same as alclometasone	Same as alclometasone	Apply 1–4 times daily according to directions
fluocinonide *floo-oh-sin'-oh-nide*	Lidex, *generic*	Same as alclometasone	Same as alclometasone	Apply 1–4 times daily according to directions
flurandrenolide *floor-an-dren'-oh-lide*	Cordran, *generic*	Same as alclometasone	Same as alclometasone	Apply 1–4 times daily according to directions
hydrocortisone *hye-droe-kor'-ti-sone*	Bactine Hydrocortisone, Cort-Dome, Hytone, *generic*	Same as alclometasone	Same as alclometasone	Apply 1–4 times daily according to directions
hydrocortisone buteprate *hye-droe-kor'-ti-sone*	Pandel	Psoriasis and other deep-seated dermatoses	Same as alclometasone	Apply once or twice daily
hydrocortisone butyrate *hye-droe-kor'-ti-sone*	Locoid	Same as alclometasone	Same as alclometasone	Apply 2–3 times daily
triamcinolone acetonide *trye-am-sin'-oh-lone*	Aristocort, Flutex, Kenalog, Triacet, *generic*	Same as alclometasone	Same as alclometasone	Apply 1–4 times daily according to directions
Anti-psoriatic Drugs ammoniated mercury *ah-mo'-ne-at-ed mer-ku-re*	Emersal	Psoriasis	Ammoniated mercury is a potential sensitizer that can cause allergic reactions	Apply 1–2 times daily
anthralin *an-thra'-lin*	Anthra-Derm Dritho Creme, Miconal	Psoriasis	Few; transient irritation of normal skin or uninvolved skin	Apply once per day

Generic Name	Trade Name*	Uses	Adverse Reactions	Dosage Ranges
calcipotriene *cal-cip-o-tri-een*	Dovonex	Psoriasis	Burning, itching, skin irritation, erythema, dry skin, peeling, rash, worsening of psoriasis, dermatitis, hyperpigmentation	Apply twice daily
selenium sulfide *se-le'-ne-um*	Exsel Head and Shoulders Intensive Treatment Dandruff Shampoo, Selsun Blue, *generic*	Treatment of dandruff, seborrheic dermatitis of the scalp, and tinea versicolor	None significant; Rare some skin irritation	Massage 5–10 mL into wet scalp and allow to remain on scalp for 2–3 minutes, rinse
Enzyme Preparations collagenase *koll-ah-gen'-ase*	Santyl, *generic*	For debriding chronic dermal ulcers and severely burned areas	Well tolerated and nonirritating; transient burning sensation may occur	Apply once daily according to directions
enzyme combinations	Accuzyme, Granulderm, Granulex, Panafil	Debridement of necrotic tissue and liquefication of slough in acute and slough in acute and chronic lesions such as decubitus ulcers, varicose and diabetic ulcers, burns, wounds, pilonidal cyst wounds, and miscellaneous trauma of infected wounds	Well-tolerated and nonirritating; transient burning sensation may occur	Apply once or twice daily
Keratolytic Drugs diclofenac sodium *dye-kloe'-fen-ak*	Solaraze	Actinic keratoses	Usually well-tolerated; transient burning sensation, rash, dry skin, scaling, flu syndrome	Apply twice daily
masoprocol *ma-so-pro-kol*	Actinex	Actinic keratoses	Erythema, flaking, dryness, itching, edema, burning, soreness, bleeding, crusting, skin roughness	Apply twice daily

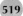

Generic Name	Trade Name*	Uses	Adverse Reactions	Dosage Ranges
salicylic acid *sal-i-sill'-ik*	DuoFilm, Wart Remover, Fostex, Fung-O, Mosco, Panscol	Aids in the removal of excessive keratin in hyperkeratotic skin disorders, including warts, psoriasis, calluses, and corns	Local irritation	Apply as directed in individual product labeling
Local Anesthetics benzocaine *benz-o-kaine'*	Lanacane	For topical anesthesia in local skin disorders	Rare; hypersensitivity, local burning, stinging, tenderness, sloughing	Apply to affected area
dibucaine *di-bu-kaine'*	Nupercainal, *generic*	For topical anesthesia in local skin disorders, local anesthesia of accessible mucous membranes	Same as benzocaine	Topical: apply to affected area as needed; mucous membranes: dosage varies and depends on the area to be anesthetized
lidocaine *lie'-doe-kaine*	ELA-Max, Lidocaine Viscous, Xylocaine, *generic*	For topical anesthesia in local skin disorders, local anesthesia of accessible mucous membranes	Same as benzocaine	Topical: apply to affected area as needed; mucous membranes: dosage varies and depends on the area to be anesthetized
lidocaine HCl *lie'-doe-kaine*	Dentipatch	Topical anesthesia of accessible mucous membranes of the mouth before dental procedures	Rare; local burning, stinging, tenderness	Apply to affected area
butamben picrate *byoo'-tam-ben*	*Generic*	Topical anesthesia	Rare; local burning, stinging, tenderness	Apply to affected area

*The term *generic* indicates the drug is available in generic form.

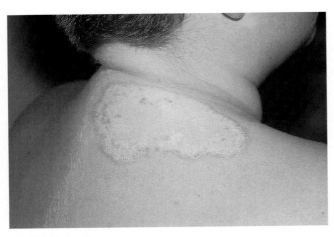

FIGURE 30-2 Ringworm.

Actions of Topical Antiseptics and Germicides

The exact mechanism of action of topical antiseptics and germicides is not well understood. These drugs affect a variety of microorganisms. Some of these drugs have a short duration of action, whereas others have a long duration of action. The action of these drugs may depend on the strength used and the time the drug is in contact with the skin or mucous membrane.

Benzalkonium (Zephiran) is a rapid-acting preparation with a moderately long duration of action. It is active against bacteria and some viruses, fungi, and protozoa. Benzalkonium solutions are bacteriostatic or bactericidal, depending on their concentration.

Chlorhexidine gluconate (Hibiclens) affects a wide range of microorganisms, including Gram-positive and Gram-negative bacteria.

Iodine has anti-infective action against many bacteria, fungi, viruses, yeasts, and protozoa. Povidone iodine (Betadine) is a combination of iodine and povidone, which liberates free iodine. Povidone–iodine is often preferred over iodine solution or tincture because it is less irritating to the skin. Unlike with the use of iodine, treated areas may be bandaged or taped.

Uses of Topical Antiseptics and Germicides

Topical antiseptics and germicides are primarily used to reduce the number of bacteria on skin surfaces. Some of these drugs, such as chlorhexidine gluconate, may be used as a surgical scrub, as a preoperative skin cleanser, for washing the hands before and after caring for patients, and in the home to cleanse the skin. Others may be applied to minor cuts and abrasions to prevent infection. Some of these drugs may also be used on mucous membranes.

Adverse Reactions of Topical Antiseptics and Germicides

Topical antiseptics and germicides have few adverse reactions. Occasionally, an individual may be allergic to the drug, and a skin rash or itching may occur. If an allergic reaction is noted, then the topical drug is discontinued.

Contraindications, Precautions, and Interactions of Topical Antiseptics and Germicides

These drugs are contraindicated in patients with known hypersensitivity. There are no significant precautions or interactions when used as directed.

Topical Corticosteroids

Topical corticosteroids vary in potency, depending on the concentration of the drug (percentage), the vehicle in which the drug is suspended (lotion, cream, aerosol spray), and the area to which the drug is applied (open or denuded skin, unbroken skin, thickness of the skin over the treated area).

Examples of topical corticosteroids include amcinonide (Cyclocort), betamethasone dipropionate (Diprosone), fluocinolone acetonide (Flurosyn), hydrocortisone (Cort-Dome), and triamcinolone acetate (Aristocort).

Actions and Uses of Topical Corticosteroids

Topical corticosteroids exert localized anti-inflammatory activity. When applied to inflamed skin, they reduce itching, redness, and swelling.

These drugs are useful in treating skin disorders, such as psoriasis, dermatitis, rashes, eczema, insect bite reactions, and first- and second-degree burns, including sunburns.

Adverse Reactions of Corticosteroids

Localized reactions may include burning, itching, irritation, redness, dryness of the skin, and secondary infection.

Contraindications, Precautions, and Interactions of Corticosteroids

Topical corticosteroids are contraindicated in patients with known hypersensitivity; as monotherapy for bacterial skin infections; for use on the face, groin, or axilla (only the high-potency corticosteroids); and for ophthalmic use (may cause steroid-induced glaucoma or cataracts). The topical corticosteroids are pregnancy category C drugs and are used cautiously during pregnancy and lactation. There are no significant interactions when administered as directed.

Topical Antipsoriatics

Actions and Uses of Antipsoriatics

Topical **antipsoriatics** are drugs used in the treatment of psoriasis (Fig. 30-3). Topical antipsoriatics help remove the plaques associated with psoriasis (a chronic skin disease manifested by bright red patches covered with silver scales or plaques). Examples of antipsoriatics include anthralin (Anthra-Derm) and calcipotriene (Dovonex).

Adverse Reactions of Antipsoriatics

These drugs may cause burning, itching, and skin irritation. Anthralin may cause skin irritation, as well as temporary discoloration of the hair and fingernails.

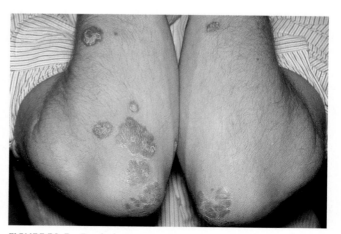

FIGURE 30-3   Psoriasis.

Contraindications, Precautions, and Interactions of Antipsoriatics

These drugs are contraindicated in patients with known hypersensitivity to the drugs. Anthralin and calcipotriene are pregnancy category C drugs and are used cautiously during pregnancy and lactation.

Topical Enzymes

Actions and Uses of Topical Enzymes

A topical enzyme aids in the removal of dead soft tissues by hastening the reduction of proteins into simpler substances. This is called **proteolysis** or a proteolytic action.

The components of certain types of wounds, namely **necrotic** (dead) tissues and **purulent exudates** (pus-containing fluid), prevent effective wound healing. Removal of this type of debris by application of a topical enzyme aids in healing. Examples of conditions that may respond to application of a topical enzyme include second- and third-degree burns, pressure ulcers, and ulcers caused by peripheral vascular disease. An example of a topical enzyme is collagenase (Santyl).

Adverse Reactions of Topical Enzymes

The application of collagenase may cause mild, transient pain. Numbness and dermatitis also may occur. Collagenase has a low incidence of adverse reactions.

Contraindications, Precautions, and Interactions of Topical Enzymes

Topical enzyme preparations are contraindicated in patients with known hypersensitivity, in wounds in contact with major body cavities or where nerves are exposed, and in fungating neoplastic ulcers. These drugs are pregnancy category B drugs and are used cautiously during pregnancy and lactation. Enzymatic activity may be impaired when these agents are administered with several detergents and antiseptics (benzalkonium chloride, hexachlorophene, iodine, and nitrofurazone).

Keratolytics

Actions and Uses of Keratolytics

A **keratolytic** is a drug that removes excess growth of the epidermis (top layer of skin) in disorders such as warts.

These drugs are used to remove warts, calluses, corns, and seborrheic keratoses (benign variously colored skin growths arising from oil glands of the skin). Examples of keratolytics include salicylic acid, masoprocol (Actinex),

and diclofenac (Solaraze). Some strengths of salicylic acid are available as nonprescription products for the removal of warts on the hands and feet.

Adverse Reactions of Keratolytics

These drugs are usually well-tolerated. Occasionally, a transient burning sensation, rash, dry skin, scaling, or flu-like syndrome may occur.

Contraindications, Precautions, and Interactions of Keratolytics

Keratolytics are contraindicated in patients with known hypersensitivity, and for use on moles, birthmarks, or warts with hair growing from them, on genital or facial warts, on warts on mucous membranes, or on infected skin. Prolonged use of the keratolytics in infants or patients with diabetes or impaired circulation is contraindicated. Salicylic acid may cause salicylate toxicity (see Chapter 10) with prolonged use. These drugs are pregnancy category C drugs and are used cautiously during pregnancy and lactation.

Topical Local Anesthetics

A topical anesthetic may be applied to the skin or mucous membranes.

Actions and Uses of Topical Local Anesthetics

Topical anesthetics temporarily inhibit the conduction of impulses from sensory nerve fibers. Examples of local anesthetics include benzocaine (Lanacane), dibucaine (Nupercainal), and lidocaine (Xylocaine). These drugs may be used to relieve itching and pain caused by skin conditions, such as minor burns, fungus infections, insect bites, rashes, sunburn, and plant poisoning, such as poison ivy. Some are applied to mucous membranes as local anesthetics.

Adverse Reactions of Topical Local Anesthetics

Occasionally, local irritation, dermatitis, rash, burning, stinging, and tenderness may occur.

Contraindications, Precautions, and Interactions of Topical Local Anesthetics

These drugs are contraindicated in those with a known hypersensitivity. The topical anesthetics are used cautiously in patients receiving class I anti-arrhythmic drugs, such as tocainide and mexiletine, because the toxic effects are additive and potentially synergistic.

Patient Management Issues with Topical Drugs

These solutions are not kept at the bedside of any patient who is confused or disoriented because the solution may be mistaken for water or another beverage.

The health care provider usually orders the patient to apply topical corticosteroids sparingly. The health care provider also may order the area of application to be covered or left exposed to the air. Some corticosteroids are applied as an occlusive dressing. In such a situation, the drug is applied while the skin is still moist after washing with soap and water, the area is covered with a plastic wrap, sealed with tape or bandage, and the drug left in place for the prescribed period of time.

Certain types of wounds may require special preparations before applying the topical enzyme. The area is cleaned or prepared and the topical enzyme applied as directed by the health care provider. If bleeding occurs with the use of sutilains, then the ointment is discontinued and the health care provider is contacted.

When applying antipsoriatics, care is exercised so that the product is applied only to the psoriatic lesions and not to surrounding skin. Signs of excessive irritation should be reported to the health care provider.

When a topical gel, such as lidocaine viscous, is used for oral anesthesia for the control of pain, the patient is instructed not to eat food for 1 hour after use because local anesthesia of the mouth or throat may impair swallowing and increase the possibility of aspiration.

Managing Adverse Reactions of Topical Drugs

Most topical drugs cause few adverse reactions and, if they occur, discontinuing use of the drug may be all that is necessary to relieve the symptoms. Occasionally, an increased skin sensitivity can occur, causing increased redness, discomfort, and itching. With itching and rash, cool, wet compresses or a bath may help to relieve the itching. Keeping the environment cool may also make the patient more comfortable. Dry skin increases the risk of skin breakdown caused by scratching. The patient can be advised to keep nails short, to use warm water with mild soap for cleaning the skin, and to rinse and dry the skin thoroughly. Bath oils, creams, and lotions may be applied if necessary as long as the health care provider is consulted first. Dry, flaky skin is subject to breakdown and infection. The skin is observed for signs of infection (e.g., redness, heat, pus, and elevated temperature and pulse) and any sign of infection is immediately reported.

> **ALERT**
>
> **Older Adults and Calcipotriene**
> Adults older than 65 years have more skin-related adverse reactions to calcipotriene. Calcipotriene should be used cautiously in older adults.

Educating the Patient and Family About Topical Drugs

Patient Education Box 30-1 includes key points about topical drugs used in the treatment of skin disorders that the patient and family members should know.

Natural Remedies: Aloe Vera

Aloe is used to prevent infection and promote healing of minor burns (e.g., sunburn) and wounds. When used externally, the herb helps repair skin tissue and reduce inflammation. It aids in the healing of dermal ulcers, wounds, and frostbite. In the United States, the food and Drug Administration (FDA) classifies topical aloe as a dietary supplement rather than a drug. A regular ingredient in face and hand creams, lotions, and skin moisturizers, it is also used in diapers, wipes, and bandages to sooth, reduce inflammation, and protect the skin. Aloe gel is naturally thick when taken from the leaf but quickly becomes watery because of the action of enzymes in the plant. Commercially available preparations have additive thickeners to make the aloe appear like the fresh gel. The herb can be applied directly from the fresh leaf by cutting the leaf in half lengthwise and gently rubbing the inner gel directly onto the skin. Commercially prepared products are applied externally as needed. Rare cases of allergy have been reported with the external use of aloe. Although available as an oral juice, its benefits have not been confirmed. Some individuals have reported the oral juice effective in healing and preventing stomach ulcers. The FDA regulates aloe in drink-form. Historically, it was used in the United States as a powerful laxative, and is currently approved as a natural flavoring substance in foods. Although available as a juice that is promoted to help heal and prevent stomach ulcers, no research exists to support this claim.

KEY POINTS

○ Topical anti-infectives include antibiotic, antifungal, and antiviral drugs. Topical antibiotic drugs may be either bactericidal or bacteriostatic, and are used to prevent superficial infections in minor cuts, wounds, skin abrasions, minor burns, and for treatment of acne vulgaris. Antifungal drugs exert a local effect by inhibiting growth of the fungi. Antiviral drugs inhibit viral replication. Adverse reactions to topical anti-infectives are usually mild and may include a skin rash, itching, urticaria (hives), dermatitis, irritation, or redness. These drugs are contraindicated in patients with known hypersensitivity.

◯ Topical antiseptics and germicides affect a variety of microorganisms, although the exact mechanism is not clearly understood. The action of these drugs may depend on the strength used and the time the drug is in contact with the skin or mucous membrane. Topical antiseptics and germicides are primarily used to reduce the number of bacteria on skin surfaces. These drugs have few adverse reactions but are contraindicated in patients with known hypersensitivity.

◯ Topical corticosteroids exert localized anti-inflammatory activity, and when applied to inflamed skin, they reduce itching, redness, and swelling. These drugs are useful in treating skin disorders, such as psoriasis, dermatitis, rashes, eczema, insect bite reactions, and first- and second-degree burns, including sunburns. Localized reactions may include burning, itching, irritation, redness, dryness of the skin, and secondary infection. The topical corticosteroids are contraindicated in patients with known hypersensitivity.

◯ Topical antisporiatics help remove the plaques associated with psoriasis and may cause burning, itching, and skin irritation. Topical antipsoriatics are contraindicated in patients with known hypersensitivity.

◯ A topical enzyme aids in the removal of dead soft tissues by hastening the reduction of proteins into simpler substances. Removal of this type of dead skin debris by application of a topical enzyme aids in healing for certain types of wounds. Collagenase may cause mild, transient pain, numbness, and dermatitis. Topical enzyme preparations are contraindicated in patients with known hypersensitivity, in wounds in contact with major body cavities or where nerves are exposed, and in fungating neoplastic ulcers.

◯ Keratolytics are drugs that remove excess growth of the epidermis (top layer of skin) in disorders such as warts. These drugs are usually well tolerated. The keratolytics are contraindicated in patients with known hypersensitivity, and for use on moles, birthmarks, or warts with hair growing from them, on genital or facial warts, on warts on mucous membranes, or on infected skin.

◯ Topical anesthetics temporarily inhibit the conduction of impulses from sensory nerve fibers. These drugs may be used to relieve itching and pain due to skin conditions, such as minor burns, fungus infections, insect bites, rashes, sunburn, and plant poisoning, such as poison ivy. Occasionally, local irritation, dermatitis, rash, burning, stinging, and tenderness may occur. Topical anesthetics are used cautiously in patients receiving class I anti-arrhythmic drugs and in patients with known hypersensitivity.

CASE STUDY

Mr. Davies, age 42 years, contracted poison ivy while doing yard work. His arms and torso are covered in a rash, and he is concerned that the poison ivy rash is spreading to his face.

1. Mr. Davies wonders about what drug might be effective in treating the itching of his poison ivy rash. His health care provider tells him:
   a. a topical local anesthetic
   b. a topical enzyme
   c. a keralytic
   d. a and c

2. Mr. Davies asks whether aloe vera may be useful in treating his poison ivy. He should be told:
   a. aloe vera is used primarily to treat minor burns and wounds
   b. aloe vera is toxic in the treatment of poison ivy
   c. aloe vera has several important adverse reactions
   d. all of the above

3. Mr. Davies worries his poison ivy may become infected. He asks whether an antiseptic is the same as a germicide. He can be told:
   a. a germicide slows the growth of microorganisms; an antiseptic kills bacteria
   b. a germicide kills bacteria; an antiseptic slows the growth of microorganisms
   c. the terms mean the same thing
   d. none of the above

WEBSITE ACTIVITIES

1. Go to the National Psoriasis Foundation website (www.psoriasis.org), and click on the "Research" tab, and then choose "Clinical Trials." This section describes drugs currently being tested. Choose any one clinical trial and read about it. Write a brief statement about what the trial is testing.

2. At the same website, return to the home page and click on "News and Events," and then "News Stories." Choose any news story about a drug, and write a brief summary about the use of that drug for psoriasis.

REVIEW QUESTIONS

1. What reaction could occur with prolonged use of the topical antibiotics?
   a. water intoxication
   b. superficial superinfection
   c. an outbreak of eczema
   d. cellulitis

2. Which of the following drugs has a proteolytic action?
   a. amcinonide (Cyclocort)
   b. collagenase (Santyl)
   c. bacitracin (Baciguent)
   d. ciclopirox (Loprox)

3. A keratolytic agent would be safe to use on which of the following skin conditions?
   a. moles
   b. birthmarks
   c. facial warts
   d. calluses

4. What type of action do the corticosteroids have when used topically?
   a. bacteriocidal activity
   b. anti-inflammatory activity
   c. antifungal activity
   d. antiviral activity

5. Which of the following drugs is best suited to be used as a topical antiseptic?
   a. amphotericin B
   b. benzocaine
   c. clindamycin
   d. povidone–iodine

31 Otic and Ophthalmic Preparations

KEY TERMS

cycloplegia—paralysis of the ciliary muscle, resulting in an inability to focus the eye
intraocular pressure—the pressure within the eye
miosis—the contraction of the pupil of the eye
miotics—drugs used to help contract the pupil of the eye
mydriasis—dilation of the pupil
mydriatics—drugs that dilate the pupil, constrict superficial blood vessels of the sclera,
    and decrease the formation of aqueous humor
ophthalmic—eye
otic—ear

CHAPTER OBJECTIVES

On completion of this chapter, students will be able to:

1 Define the chapter's key terms.

2 Describe the general drug actions, uses, adverse reactions, contraindications, precautions, and interactions of otic and ophthalmic preparations.

3 Discuss important points to keep in mind when educating the patient or family members about the use of otic and ophthalmic preparations.

The eyes and ears are subject to various disorders, which range from mild to serious. Because the eyes and ears provide an interpretation of our outside environment, any disease or injury that has the potential for partial or total loss of function of these organs must be treated.

Otic Preparations

Actions of Otic Preparations

Various types of preparations are used for the treatment of **otic** (ear) disorders. There are three categories of otic preparations: (1) antibiotics; (2) antibiotic and steroid combinations; and (3) miscellaneous preparations. The miscellaneous preparations usually contain one or more of the following ingredients:

- Benzocaine: a local anesthetic
- Phenylephrine: a vasoconstrictor decongestant
- Hydrocortisone, desonide: corticosteroids for anti-inflammatory and antipruritic effects
- Glycerin: an emollient and a solvent
- Antipyrine: an analgesic

- Acetic acid, boric acid, benzalkonium chloride, aluminum acetate, benzethonium chloride: provide antifungal or antibacterial action
- Carbamide peroxide: aids in removing earwax by softening and breaking up the wax

Examples of otic preparations are listed in the Summary Drug Table: Otic Preparations.

Uses of Otic Preparations

Otic preparations are instilled in the external auditory canal and may be used to relieve pain, treat infection and inflammation, and aid in the removal of earwax (Fig. 31-1). When a patient has an inner ear infection, systemic antibiotic therapy is indicated.

Adverse Reactions of Otic Preparations

When otic drugs are applied topically, the amount of drug that enters the systemic circulation is not sufficient to produce adverse reactions. Prolonged use of otic preparations containing an antibiotic may result in a superinfection (an overgrowth of bacterial or fungal microorganisms not affected by the antibiotic being administered).

Contraindications, Precautions, and Interactions of Otic Preparations

These drugs are contraindicated in patients with a known hypersensitivity. Otic drugs are used with caution during pregnancy and lactation. The pregnancy cat-

egory of these drugs is unknown when they are used as otic drugs. Otic drugs available in dropper bottles may be dangerous if ingested by young children; therefore, the drugs must be stored safely out of the reach of children. Drugs to remove cerumen are not used if ear drainage, discharge, pain, or irritation is present, if the eardrum is perforated, or after ear surgery. Although rare, bone marrow hypoplasia including aplastic anemia has been reported with local application of chloramphenicol. No significant interactions have been reported with use of the otic preparations.

> **ALERT**
>
> **Drugs for Otic Use**
>
> Only preparations labeled as otic are instilled in the ear. The label of the preparation must be checked carefully for the name of the drug and a statement indicating that the preparation is for otic use.

Patient Management Issues with Otic Preparations

Ear disorders may result in symptoms such as pain, a feeling of fullness in the ear, tinnitus, dizziness, or a change in hearing. Before an otic solution is instilled, the patient should be informed that a feeling of fullness may be felt in the ear and that hearing in the treated ear may be impaired while the solution remains in the ear canal.

Educating the Patient and Family About Otic Preparations

The patient and family members are given instructions or a demonstration of the instillation technique of an otic preparation. Patient Education Box 31-1 includes key points about otic preparations that the patient and family members should know.

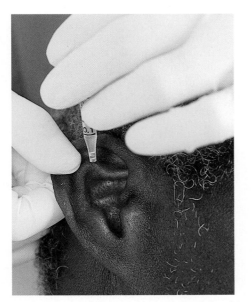

FIGURE 31-1 Instilling ear drops. With the patient's head turned toward the unaffected side, the cartilaginous portion of the outer ear (pinna) is pulled up and back in an adult, and the prescribed number of drops is instilled on the side of the auditory canal. (From Roach SS. Introductory Clinical Pharmacology, 7th ed. Baltimore: Lippincott Williams & Wilkins; 2004.)

Ophthalmic Preparations

Various types of preparations are used for the treatment of ophthalmic disorders such as glaucoma to lower the **intraocular pressure** (the pressure within the eye), bacteria or viral infections of the eye, inflammatory conditions, and symptoms of allergy related to the eye.

Glaucoma is a condition of the eye in which there is an increase in the intraocular pressure, causing progressive atrophy of the optic nerve with deterioration of vision and, if untreated, blindness. The higher the intraocular pressure, the greater the risk of optic nerve damage, visual loss, and blindness. There are two types of glaucoma: angle-closure glaucoma and open-angle,

SUMMARY DRUG TABLE   Otic Preparations

Generic Combinations	Trade Name*	Uses	Adverse Reactions	Dosage Ranges
Steroid and Antibiotic Combinations, Solutions				
1% hydrocortisone, 5 mg neomycin sulfate, 10,000 units polymyxin *B*	Antibiotic Ear Solution, AntibiOtic, Cortisporin Otic, Drotic, Ear-Eze, Otic-Care, Oticair, Otocort, Otosporin	Bacterial infections of the external auditory canal	Few; when used for prolonged periods there is a danger of a superinfection	4 gtt instilled TID, QID
0.5% hydrocortisone, 10,000 units polymyxin B	Otobiotic Otic	Same as hydrocortisone	Same as hydrocortisone	4 gtt instilled TID, QID
Steroid and Antibiotic Combinations, Suspensions				
1% hydrocortisone, 5 mg neomycin sulfate, 10,000 units polymyxin B	AK-Spore, Antibi-Otic, Antibiotic Ear Suspension, Otocort, UAD Otic	Same as hydrocortisone	Same as hydrocortisone	4 gtt instilled TID, QID
1% hydrocortisone, 4.71 mg neomycin sulfate	Coly-Mycin S Otic	Same as hydrocortisone	Same as hydrocortisone	4 gtt instilled TID, QID
1% hydrocortisone, 3.3 mg neomycin sulfate	Cortisporin-TC Otic	Same as hydrocortisone	Same as hydrocortisone	4 gtt instilled TID, QID
2 mg ciprofloxacin, 10 mg hydrocortisone/mL	Cipro HC Otic	Same as hydrocortisone	Same as hydrocortisone	4 gtt instilled TID, QID
Otic Antibiotics				
Chloramphenicol	Chloromycetin Otic	Treatment of superficial infections involving the external auditory canal	Local irritation (itching, burning, angioneurotic edema, urticaria, vesicular and maculopapular dermatitis)	2–3 gtt into the ear TID
Select Miscellaneous Preparations				
1% hydrocortisone, 2% acetic acid, 3% propylene glycol diacetate, 0.015% sodium acetate, 0.02% benzethonium chloride	Acetasol HC, VoSoL HC Otic	Relieve pain, inflammation, and irritation in the external auditory canal	Local irritation, itching, burning	Insert wick, use 3–5 gtt q4–6h, 3 24 h; remove wick, instill 5 gtt TID, QID
1% hydrocortisone, 1% pramoxine HCl, 0.1% chloroxylenol, 3% propylene glycol diacetate and benzalkonium chloride	Cortic	Same as hydrocortisone	Same as hydrocortisone	Insert saturated wick into the ear; leave in for 24 h, keeping moist with 3–5 gtt q4–6h; remove wick and instill 5 gtt TID, QID

Generic Combinations	Trade Name*	Uses	Adverse Reactions	Dosage Ranges
1% hydrocortisone, 2% acetic acid glacial, 3% propylene glycol diacetate, 0.02% benzethonium Cl, 0.015% sodium acetate, 0.2% citric acid	AA-HC Otic	Same as hydrocortisone	Same as hydrocortisone	Insert saturated wick into the ear; leave in for 24 h, keeping moist with 3–5 gtt q4–6h; remove wick and instill 5 gtt TID, QID
1.4% benzocaine, 5.4% antipyrine glycerin	Allergen Ear Drops, Auralgan Otic, Auroto Otic, Ear Drops, Otocalm Ear	Same as hydrocortisone	Same as hydrocortisone	Fill ear canal with 2–4 gtt; insert saturated cotton pledget; repeat TID, QID or q1–2h
20% benzocaine, 0.1% benzethonium chloride, 1% glycerin, PEG 300	Americaine Otic, Otocain	Same as hydrocortisone	Same as hydrocortisone	Instill 4–5 gtt; insert cotton pledget; repeat every 1–2h
10% triethanolamine polypeptide oleate-condensate, 0.5% chlorobutanol in propylene glycol	Cerumenex Drops	Aid in the removal of ear wax	Local irritation, itching, burning	Fill ear canal; insert cotton plug; allow to remain 15–30 min; flush ear
1 mg chloroxylenol, 10 mg hydrocortisone, 10 mg/mL pramoxine HCl	Otomar-HC	Relieve pain and irritation in the external auditory canal	Local irritation, itching, burning	Instill 5 gtt into affected ear TID, QID
2% acetic acid in aluminum acetate solution	Burow's Otic, Otic Domeboro, *generic*	Relieve pain and irritation in the external auditory canal	Local irritation, itching, burning	Insert saturated wick; keep moist for 24 h; instill 4–6 gtt every 2–3 h

*The term *generic* indicates the drug is available in generic form.

or chronic, glaucoma. Box 31-1 describes the two types of glaucoma.

Most of the drug classifications used to treat **ophthalmic** (eye) conditions have already been discussed in previous chapters. The following sections provide a short summary of these drugs in ophthalmic use. The Summary Drug Table: Select Ophthalmic Preparations provides examples of the drugs used to treat ophthalmic problems.

The incidence of adverse reactions associated with ophthalmic drugs is usually small. Because small amounts of the ophthalmic preparation may be absorbed systemically, some of the adverse effects associated with systemic administration of the particular drug may be observed. Some ophthalmic preparations produce momentary stinging or burning on instillation.

Alpha₂ Adrenergic Drugs

Brimonidine tartrate is an alpha₂-adrenergic receptor agonist that acts to reduce aqueous humor production and increase the outflow of aqueous humor. It is used to lower intraocular pressure in patients with open-angle glaucoma or ocular hypertension.

Although adverse reactions are usually mild, treatment with brimonidine tartrate includes oral dryness,

(text continued on page 534)

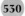

PATIENT EDUCATION BOX 31-1

Key Points for Patients Using Otic Preparations

- ❑ Cold and warm (above body temperature) preparations may cause dizziness or other sensations after being instilled into your ear. Warm preparations before use by holding the container in your hand.
- ❑ Wash your hands thoroughly before cleansing the area around your ear (when necessary) and instilling ear drops or ointment.
- ❑ Instill the prescribed number of drops or amount of ointment in your ear. Do not put the applicator or dropper tip in your ear.
- ❑ Immediately after use, replace the cap or dropper and refrigerate the solution if so stated on the label.
- ❑ If the drops are in a suspension form, shake well for 10 seconds before using.
- ❑ Keep your head tilted or lie on the untreated side for 2 to 3 minutes to allow the solution to remain in contact with your ear. Excess solution and solution running out of your ear can be wiped off with a tissue.
- ❑ Do not insert anything into the ear canal before or after applying the prescribed drug unless advised to do so by your health care provider. At times, a soft cotton plug may be inserted into the affected ear.
- ❑ Complete a full course of treatment with the prescribed drug to achieve satisfactory results.
- ❑ Do not use nonprescription ear products during or after treatment unless such use has been approved by your health care provider.
- ❑ Temporary changes in hearing or a feeling of fullness in the ear may occur for a short time after the drug has been instilled.
- ❑ Notify your health care provider if your symptoms do not improve or become worse.

DRUGS USED TO REMOVE CERUMEN

- ❑ Do not use if ear drainage, discharge, pain, or irritation occurs.
- ❑ Do not use for more than 4 days. If excessive cerumen remains, consult your health care provider.
- ❑ Any wax remaining after the treatment may be removed by gently flushing the ear with warm water using a soft rubber bulb ear syringe.
- ❑ Drugs that loosen cerumen work by softening the dried earwax inside the ear canal. Cerumenex is available by prescription and is not allowed to stay in the ear canal more than 30 minutes before irrigation. When cerumenex is administered, your ear canal is filled with the solution and a cotton plug is inserted. The drug is allowed to remain in your ear for 15 to 30 minutes, and then your ear is flushed with warm water using a soft rubber bulb ear syringe.
- ❑ If you become dizzy, consult a physician.

Box 31-1 **Glaucoma**

The eye's lens, iris, and cornea are continuously bathed and nourished by a fluid called aqueous humor. As aqueous humor is produced, excess fluid normally flows out through a complex network of tissue called trabecular meshwork. An angle is formed where the trabeculum and iris meet. This forms a filtration angle that maintains the normal pressure within the eye by allowing excess aqueous humor to leave the anterior chamber of the eye (Fig. 31-2). In chronic or open-angle glaucoma, the angle that permits the drainage of aqueous humor appears to be normal but does not function properly. In angle-closure glaucoma, the iris blocks the trabecular meshwork and limits the flow of aqueous humor from the anterior chamber of the eye. This limitation of outflow causes an accumulation of intraocular fluid, followed by increased intraocular pressure. Some individuals have an anatomical defect that causes the angle to be more narrow than normal but do not have any symptoms and glaucoma does not develop under normal circumstances. However, certain situations, such as medication that causes dilation of the eye, fear, or pain, that cause the eye to dilate may precipitate an attack. The aim of treatment in glaucoma is to lower the intraoccular pressure. For more information on glaucoma, see Chapter 4.

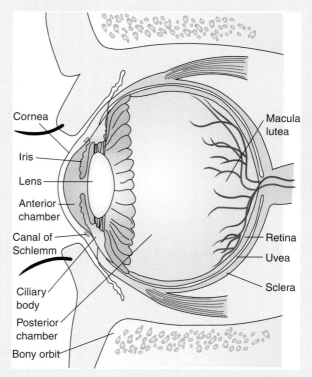

FIGURE 31-2 Cross section of eye. (From Pillitteri A. *Maternal and Child Nursing*, 4th ed. Philadelphia: Lippincott Williams & Wilkins; 2003.)

SUMMARY DRUG TABLE   Select Ophthalmic Preparations

Generic Name	Trade Name*	Uses	Dosage Ranges
Alpha₂ Adrenergic Agonist brimonidine tartrate *brih-moe'-nih-deen*	Alphagan	Lowering intraocular pressure (IOP)	1 gtt in affected eye(s) TID
Sympathomimetics apraclonidine HCl *app-rah-kloe'-nih-deen*	Iopidine	1% solution: control or prevention of postoperative elevations in IOP; 5% solution: short-term therapy in patients receiving maximal medical therapy who require additional IOP reduction	1% solution: 1 gtt in operative eye 1 h before surgery and 1 gtt immediately after surgery; 5% solution: 1–2 gtt in the affected eye(s) TID
dipivefrin HCl (dipivalyl epinephrine) *die-pihv'-eh-frin*	Propine, AKPro, *generic*	IOP	1 gtt into affected eye(s) every 12 h
epinephrine *epp-ih-neff-rin*	Epifrin, Glaucon Solution, *generic*	Open-angle (chronic simple glaucoma); may be used in combination with miotics, beta blockers, or carbonic anhydrase inhibitors	1 drop into affected eye(s) QD, BID
Alpha-Adrenergic Blocking Drugs dapiprazole HCl *dap-ih-pray'-zole*	Rev-Eyes	After ophthalmic examination to reverse the diagnostic mydriasis	2 gtt into the conjunctiva of each eye, followed 5 min later by an additional 2 gtt
Beta-Adrenergic Blocking Drugs betaxolol *bay-tax'-oh-lahl*	Betoptic, Betoptic S, *generic*	Elevated IOP	1–2 gtt in the affected eye(s) BID
carteolol HCl *car'-tee-oh-lahl*	Ocupress, *generic*	Elevated IOP	1 gtt in affected TID
levobetaxolol HCl *lee'-voe-beh-tax'-oh-lahl*	Betaxon	Elevated IOP	1 gtt in affected eye(s) BID
levobunolol HCl *lee'-voe-byoo'-no-lahl*	AKBeta, Betagan Liquifilm, *generic*	Elevated IOP	0.5% solution: 1–2 gtt in affected eye(s) QD; 0.25% solution: 1–2 gtt in affected eye(s) BID
metipranolol HCl *meh-tih-pran'-oh-lahl*	OptiPranolol	Elevated IOP	1–2 gtt in affected eye(s) BID
timolol *ti'-moe-lahl*	Betimol, Timoptic, Timoptic-XE, *generic*	Elevated IOP	1 gtt in affected eye(s) QD, BID Gel: invert the closed container and shake once before each use; administer 1 gtt/day
Miotics, Direct Acting carbachol *car'-bah-kole*	Carboptic, Isopto Carbachol	Glaucoma	1–2 gtt up to TID PRN

Generic Name	Trade Name*	Uses	Dosage Ranges
pilocarpine HCl *pie-low-car'-peen*	Adsorbocarpine, Akarpine, Isopto Carpine, Pilocar, Pilostat, *generic*	Glaucoma, preoperative and postoperative intraocular tension	Solution: 1–2 gtt in affected eye(s) up to 6 times daily; Gel: apply a 0.5-inch ribbon in the lower conjunctival sac of affected eye(s) once daily at HS
pilocarpine nitrate	Pilagan	Elevated IOP	1–2 gtt in affected eye(s) 2–4 times daily
pilocarpine ocular therapeutic system	Ocusert Pilo-20, Ocusert Pilo-40	Elevated IOP	See package insert
Miotics, Cholinesterase Inhibitors demecarium bromide *deh-meh-care'-ee-uhm broe'-mide*	Humorsol	Glaucoma and strabismus	1–2 gtt/wk, up to 1–2 gtt/d
echothiophate iodide *eck-oh-thigh'-oh-fate eye-oh-dide*	Phospholine Iodide	Chronic open-angle glaucoma	2 doses/d in the morning and at HS or 1 dose every other day
Carbonic Anhydrase Inhibitors brinzolamide *brin-zoe'-lah-mide*	Azopt	Elevated IOP	1 gtt in affected eye(s) TID
dorzolamide HCl *dore-zole-lah-mide*	TruSopt	Elevated IOP	1 gtt in affected eye(s) TID
Prostaglandin Agonist latanoprost *lah-tan'-oh-prahst*	Xalatan	Elevated IOP	1 gtt in affected eye(s) QD in the evening
travoprost	Travatan	Elevated IOP	1 gtt in affected eye(s) QD in the evening
bimatoprost	Lumigan	Elevated IOP	1 gtt in affected eye(s) QD in the evening
unoprostone isopropyl *yoo-noh-prost'-ohn*	Rescula	Elevated IOP	1 gtt in affected eye(s) BID
Combinations Used to Treat Glaucoma pilocarpine and epinephrine	E-Pilo-1, E-Pilo-2, E-Pilo-4, E-Pilo-6, P_1E_1, P_4E_1	Glaucoma	1–2 gtt in the affected eye(s) 1–4 times daily
dorzolamide HCl and timolol maleate *dore-zole'-ah-mide*	Cosopt	Elevated IOP	1 gtt into the affected eye(s) BID
Mast Cell Stabilizer nedocromil sodium *neh-doe-kroe'-mill*	Alocril	Allergic conjunctivitis	1–2 gtt in each eye BID
pemirolast potassium *peh-mihr-oh'-last*	Alamast	Allergic conjunctivitis	1–2 gtt in each eye QID

Generic Name	Trade Name*	Uses	Dosage Ranges
Nonsteroidal Anti-Inflammatory Drugs			
diclofenac sodium *di-klo'-fen-ak*	Voltaren, *generic*	Postoperative inflammation after cataract surgery	1 drop QID
flurbiprofen sodium *flure-bi'-pro-fen*	Ocufen, *generic*	Inhibition of intraoperative miosis	1 gtt q 30 min beginning 2 h before surgery (total of 4 gtt)
ketorolac tromethamine *ke-tor'-o-lac*	Acular	Relief of ocular itching due to seasonal allergies	1 drop QID
Corticosteroids			
dexamethasone phosphate *dex-a-meth'-a-sone*	AK-Dex, Maxidex, *generic*	Treatment of inflammatory conditions of the conjunctiva, lid, cornea, anterior segment of the eye	Solution: 1–2 gtt qh during the day and q2h at night, reduced to 1 gtt q4h when response noted, then 1 gtt TID–QID; Ointment: thin coating in lower conjunctival sac 3–4 times/d
fluorometholone *flure-oh-meth'-oh-lone*	Flarex, Fluor-Op, *generic*	Treatment of inflammatory conditions of the conjunctiva, lid, cornea, anterior segment of the eye	Suspension: 1–2 gtt 2–4 times/d, may increase to 2 gtt q2h; Ointment: thin coating in lower conjunctival sac 1–3 times/d (up to 1 application q4h)
loteprednol etabonate *low-teh'-pred'-nol ett-ab'-ohn-ate*	Alrex, Lotemax	Allergic conjunctivitis	1–2 gtt QID
prednisolone *pred-niss'-oh-lone*	AK-Pred, Pred Forte, Pred Mild, *generic*	Treatment of inflammatory conditions of the conjunctiva, lid, cornea, anterior segment of the eye	1–2 gtt qh during the day and q2h at night, reduced to 1 drop q4h, then 1 gtt TID or QID; Suspensions: 1–2 gtt 2–4 times daily
Antibiotics			
bacitracin *bass-i-tray'-sin*	AK-Tracin	Treatment of eye infections	See package insert
erythromycin *er-ith-roe-mye'-sin*	Ilotycin, *generic*	Treatment of eye infections	See package insert
gentamicin *jen-ta-mye'-sin*	Garamycin, *generic*	Treatment of eye infections	See package insert
tobramycin *toe-bra-mye'-sin*	Tobrex, *generic*	Treatment of eye infections	See package insert
Sulfonamides			
sodium sulfacetamide *sul-fa-see'-ta-mide*	AK-Sulf, *generic*	Treatment of conjunctivitis, corneal ulcer, other superficial eye infections	1–2 gtt q1–3h

Generic Name	Trade Name*	Uses	Dosage Ranges
Silver silver nitrate *nye-trate*	*Generic*	Prevention of ophthalmia neonatorum	2 gtt of 1% solution in each eye
Antiviral Drugs idoxuridine *eye-dox-yoor'-i-deen*	Herplex	Treatment of herpes simplex keratitis	1 gtt qh during the day and q2h at night
vidarabine *vye-dare'-a-been*	Vira-A	Treatment of herpes simplex keratitis and conjunctivitis	0.5 inch of ointment into lower conjunctival sac 5 times/d at 3-h intervals
Antifungal Drugs natamycin *na-ta-mye'-sin*	Natacyn	Treatment of fungal infections of the eye	1 gtt q1–2h
Vasoconstrictors/Mydriatics oxymetazoline hydrochloride *ox-i-met-az'-oh-leen*	OcuClear, Visine L. R.	Relief of redness of eye caused by minor irritation	1–2 gtt q3–4h up to QID
phenylephrine hydrochloride *fen-ill-ef'-rin*	AK-Dilate 2.5%, Neo-Synephrine 10%	0.12% for relief of redness of eye caused by minor irritation; 2.5% and 10% treatment of uveitis, glaucoma; refraction procedures, before eye surgery	0.12% 1–2 gtt up to 4 times/d; 2.5% and 10%, 1 gtt
tetrahydrozoline hydrochloride *tet-ra-hyd-drozz'-a-leen*	Murine Plus Eye Drops, Visine, *generic*	Relief of redness of eye caused by minor irritation	1–2 gtt up to 4 times/d
Cycloplegic/Mydriatics atropine sulfate *a'-troe-peen*	Isopto-Atropine, *generic*	Eye refraction, treatment of acute inflammatory conditions of iris, uveal tract	1–2 gtt up to 4 times/d
homatropine hydrobromide *hoe-ma'-troe-peen*	Isopto Homatropine	Eye refraction, treatment of inflammatory conditions of uveal tract	1–2 gtt q3–4h
Artificial Tears benzalkonium chloride *benz-al-koe'-nee-um*	Artificial Tears	Treatment of dry eyes	1–2 gtt 3–4 times/d
glycerin, sodium chloride	Eye-Lube-A	Treatment of dry eyes	1–2 gtt 3–4 times/d

*The term *generic* indicates the drug is available in generic form.

ocular hyperemia, burning and stinging, headache, visual blurring, foreign body sensation, fatigue, drowsiness, ovular allergic reactions, and ocular pruritus.

This drug is contraindicated in patients with hypersensitivity and in patients taking the monoamine oxidase inhibitors. Patients should wait at least 15 minutes after instilling brimonidine before inserting soft contact lenses because the preservative in the drug may be absorbed by soft contact lenses. It is used cautiously during pregnancy (pregnancy category B) and lactation and in patients with cardiovascular disease, depression, cerebral or coronary insufficiency, orthostatic hypotension, or Raynaud phenomenon. When brimonidine is used with central nervous system depressants such as alcohol, barbiturates, opiates, sedatives, or anesthetics, there is a risk for an additive central nervous system depressant effect. The drug is used cautiously in combination with the beta blockers, antihypertensive drugs, and cardiac glycosides because a synergistic effect may occur.

Sympathomimetic Drugs

Sympathomimetics have alpha (α)-adrenergic and beta (β)-adrenergic activity (see Chapter 4 for a detailed discussion of adrenergic drugs). These drugs lower intraocular pressure by increasing the outflow of aqueous humor in the eye and are used to treat glaucoma. Apraclonidine is used to control or prevent postoperative elevations in intraocular pressure. The Summary Drug Table: Select Ophthalmic Preparations provides additional information about these drugs.

These drugs may cause transient local reactions such as burning and stinging, eye pain, brow ache, headache, allergic lip reactions, and ocular irritation. With prolonged use, adrenochrome (a red pigment contained in epinephrine) deposits may occur in the conjunctiva and cornea. Although rare, systemic reactions may occur such as headache, palpitations, tachycardia, extrasystoles, cardiac arrhythmia, hypertension, and faintness. Dipivefrin appears to be better-tolerated and has fewer adverse reactions than the other sympathomimetic drugs used to lower intraocular pressure.

These drugs are contraindicated in patients with hypersensitivity to the drug. Epinephrine is contraindicated in patients with narrow-angle glaucoma, or patients with a narrow angle but no glaucoma, or aphakia (absence of the crystalline lens of the eye). Epinephrine should not be used while wearing soft contact lenses (discoloration of the lenses may occur).

Sympathomimetic drugs are used cautiously during pregnancy (epinephrine and apraclonidine, pregnancy category C; dipivefrin, pregnancy category B) and lactation and in patients with hypertension, diabetes, hyperthyroidism, heart disease, cerebral arteriosclerosis, or bronchial asthma. Some of these drugs contain sulfites that may cause allergic-like reactions (hives, wheezing, anaphylaxis) in patients with sulfite sensitivity. See Chapter 4 for information on interactions.

Alpha-Adrenergic Blocking Drugs

Dapiprazole acts by blocking the β-adrenergic receptor in smooth muscle and produces miosis through an effect on the dilator muscle of the iris. Dapiprazole is used primarily after ophthalmic examinations to reverse the diagnostic **mydriasis** (dilation of the pupil).

Dapiprazole may cause burning in the eye, ptosis (drooping of the upper eyelid), lid edema, itching, corneal edema, brow ache, photophobia, dryness of the eye, tearing, and blurring of vision.

The drug is contraindicated in patients with hypersensitivity, in conditions in which pupil constriction is not desirable, such as in acute iritis (inflammation of the iris), and in the treatment of intraocular pressure in open-angle glaucoma. This drug is used cautiously during pregnancy (pregnancy category B) and lactation. No significant drug interactions have been reported.

Beta-Adrenergic Blocking Drugs

The β-adrenergic blocking drugs decrease the rate of production of aqueous humor and thereby lower the intraocular pressure. These drugs are used in the treatment of glaucoma.

Adverse reactions associated with the β-adrenergic blocking drugs include eye irritation, burning, tearing, conjunctivitis, decreased night vision, ptosis, abnormal corneal staining, and corneal sensitivity. Systemic reactions, although rare, include arrhythmias, palpitation, headache, nausea, and dizziness. See Chapter 4 for additional systemic adverse reactions.

β-adrenergic blocking drugs are contraindicated in patients with bronchial asthma, obstructive pulmonary disease, sinus bradycardia, heart block, cardiac failure, or cardiogenic shock, and in patients with hypersensitivity to the drug or any components of the drug. These drugs are pregnancy category C and are used cautiously during pregnancy and lactation and in patients with cardiovascular disease, diabetes (may mask the symptoms of hypoglycemia), and hyperthyroidism (may mask symptoms of hyperthyroidism). A patient taking β-adrenergic blocking drugs for ophthalmic reasons may experience increased or additive effects when the drugs are administered with the oral beta blockers. Co-administration of timolol maleate and calcium antagonists may cause hypotension, left ventricular failure, and conduction disturbances within the heart. There is a potential additive hypotensive effect when the beta-blocking ophthalmic drugs are administered with the phenothiazines.

Direct Acting Miotics

Miotics contract the pupil of the eye, a condition called **miosis**, resulting in an increase in the space through which the aqueous humor flows. This increased space and improved flow results in a decrease in the intraocular pressure. Miotics may be used in the treatment of glaucoma (see Chapter 4). The miotics were, for a number of years, the drug of choice for glaucoma. These drugs have lost that first choice treatment status to the β-adrenergic blocking drugs.

Direct-acting miotics may cause stinging on instillation, transient burning, tearing, headache, brow ache, and decreased night vision. Systemic adverse reactions include hypotension, flushing, breathing difficulties, nausea, vomiting, diarrhea, cardiac arrhythmias, and frequent urge to urinate.

These drugs are contraindicated in patients with hypersensitivity to the drug and in conditions in which constriction is undesirable (e.g., iritis, uveitis, and acute inflammatory disease of the anterior chamber). The drugs are used cautiously in patients with corneal abrasion, pregnancy (pregnancy category C), lactation, cardiac failure, bronchial asthma, peptic ulcer, hyperthyroidism, gastrointestinal spasm, urinary tract infection, Parkinson disease, recent myocardial infarction, hypotension, or hypertension. These drugs are also used cautiously in patients with angle-closure glaucoma because miotics can occasionally precipitate angle-closure glaucoma by increasing the resistance to aqueous flow from posterior to anterior chamber. See Chapter 4 for information on interactions.

Cholinesterase Inhibitor Miotics

The cholinesterase inhibitors are more potent and longer acting than the direct-acting miotics and are used to treat open-angle glaucoma. When administered into the eye, these drugs produce intense miosis (constriction of the pupil) and muscle contractions, causing a decreased resistance to aqueous outflow.

Adverse reactions and systemic toxicity are more common in the cholinesterase inhibitor ophthalmic preparations than in the direct-acting miotics. Ophthalmic adverse reactions include the development of iris cysts, burning, lacrimation, lid muscle twitching, conjunctivitis and ciliary redness, brow ache, headache, activation of latent iritis or uveitis (an inner-eye inflammation), retinal detachment, and conjunctival thickening. Systemic adverse reactions include nausea, vomiting, abdominal cramps, diarrhea, urinary incontinence, fainting, salivation, difficulty breathing, and cardiac irregularities. Iris cysts may form, enlarge, and obstruct vision. The iris cyst usually shrinks on discontinuation of use of the drug or after a reduction in strength of the drops or frequency of instillation.

Cholinesterase inhibitors are contraindicated in patients with hypersensitivity to the drug or any components of the drug. Some of these products contain sulfites, and patients with sulfite sensitivity may experience allergic-type reactions. The drugs are also contraindicated in patients with any active inflammatory disease of the eye and during pregnancy (demecarium, pregnancy category X; echothiophate iodine, pregnancy category C) and lactation. The cholinesterase inhibitors are used cautiously in patients with myasthenia gravis (may cause additive adverse effects), before and after surgery, and in patients with chronic angle-closure (narrow angle) glaucoma or those with narrow angles (may cause papillary block and increase the angle blockage). When the cholinesterase inhibitors are administered with systemic anticholinesterase drugs, there is a risk for additive effects. Individuals, such as farmers, warehouse workers, or gardeners, working with carbamate or organophosphate insecticides or pesticides are at risk for systemic effects of the cholinesterase inhibitors from absorption of the pesticide or insecticide through the respiratory tract or the skin. Individuals working with pesticides or insecticides containing carbamate or organophosphate and taking a cholinesterase inhibitor should be advised to wear respiratory masks, change clothes frequently, and wash exposed clothes thoroughly.

Carbonic Anhydrase Inhibitors

Except for dorzolamide and brinzolamide, carbonic anhydrase inhibitors are administered systemically. Carbonic anhydrase is an enzyme found in many tissues of the body, including the eye. Inhibition of carbonic anhydrase in the eye decreases aqueous humor secretion, resulting in a decrease of intraocular pressure.

These drugs are used in the treatment of elevated intraocular pressure seen in open-angle glaucoma.

Adverse reactions associated with use of the carbonic anyhydrase inhibitors include ocular burning, stinging, or discomfort immediately after administration, bitter taste, ocular allergic reaction, blurred vision, tearing, dryness, dermatitis, foreign body sensation, ocular discomfort, photophobia, and headache.

Use of the carbonic anhydrase inhibitors is contraindicated in patients with known hypersensitivity and during pregnancy (pregnancy category C) and lactation. The drugs are used cautiously in patients with renal and hepatic impairment. When high doses of the salicylates are administered concurrently, toxic levels of the carbonic anhydrase inhibitors have been reported. See Chapter 19 for more information on interactions of carbonic anhydrase inhibitors.

Prostaglandin Agonists

Prostaglandin agonists act to lower intraocular pressure by increasing the outflow of aqueous humor through the trabecular meshwork. Prostaglandin agonists are used to lower intraoccular pressure in patients with open-angle glaucoma and ocular hypertension in patients who do not tolerate other intraoccular pressure-lowering medications or have an insufficient response to these medications.

Adverse reactions associated with the prostaglandin agonists include blurred vision, burning and stinging, foreign body sensation, itching, increased pigmentation of the iris, dry eye, excessive tearing, lid discomfort and pain, and photophobia.

Prostaglandin agonists are contraindicated in patients with hypersensitivity, and during pregnancy (pregnancy category C). These drugs are used cautiously in lactating women and in patients with active intraocular inflammation, those wearing contact lenses (contact lenses must be removed and left out for at least 15 minutes after administration of the drug), and those with macular edema.

Mast Cell Stabilizers

Mast cell stabilizers currently for ophthalmic use are nedocromil and pemirolast. Mast cell stabilizers act by inhibiting the antigen-induced release of inflammatory mediators (e.g., histamine) from human mast cells. These drugs are used for the prevention of eye itching caused by allergic conjunctivitis.

Although mild, the adverse reactions associated with the mast cell inhibitors include headache, rhinitis, unpleasant taste, asthma, and cold/flu symptoms. These drugs may also cause ocular burning or irritation, dry eye, eye redness, foreign body sensation, and ocular discomfort.

These drugs are contraindicated in patients with hypersensitivity. Mast cell stabilizers are used cautiously in patients who wear contact lenses (preservative may be absorbed by the soft contact lenses) and during pregnancy (pemirolast is pregnancy category C; nedocromil is pregnancy category B) and lactation. There have been no significant drug–drug interactions associated with these drugs.

Nonsteroidal Anti-Inflammatory Drugs

Nonsteroidal anti-inflammatory drugs inhibit prostaglandin synthesis (see Chapter 10 for a discussion), thereby exerting anti-inflammatory action. These drugs are used to treat postoperative inflammation after cataract surgery (diclofenac), for the relief of itching of the eyes caused by seasonal allergies (ketorolac), and during eye surgery to prevent miosis (flurbiprofen).

The most common adverse reactions associated with nonsteroidal anti-inflammatory drugs include transient burning and stinging on instillation and other minor ocular irritation.

These drugs are contraindicated in individuals with known hypersensitivity. Nonsteroidal anti-inflammatory drug flurbiprofen is contraindicated in patients with herpes simplex keratitis. Diclofenac and ketorolac are contraindicated in patients who wear soft contact lenses (may cause ocular irritation). Nonsteroidal anti-inflammatory drugs are used cautiously during pregnancy (pregnancy category C, flurbiprofen, ketorolac; pregnancy category B, diclofenac) and lactation. Nonsteroidal anti-inflammatory drugs are used cautiously in patients with bleeding tendencies. When used topically, there is less risk of interactions with drugs or other substances. There is a possibility of a cross-sensitivity reaction when nonsteroidal anti-inflammatory drugs are administered to patients allergic to the salicylates. Corticosteroids and antibiotics are used cautiously in patients with sulfite sensitivity because an allergic-type reaction may result. Co-administration of idoxuridine with solutions containing boric acid may cause irritation. Sulfonamides are incompatible with silver nitrate.

Corticosteroids

Corticosteroids possess anti-inflammatory activity. They are used for inflammatory conditions, such as allergic conjunctivitis, keratitis, herpes zoster keratitis, and inflammation of the iris. Corticosteroids also may be used after injury to the cornea or after corneal transplants to prevent rejection.

Adverse reactions associated with administration of the corticosteroid ophthalmic preparations include elevated intraocular pressure with optic nerve damage, loss of visual acuity, cataract formation, delayed wound healing, secondary ocular infection, exacerbation of corneal infections, dry eyes, ptosis, blurred vision, discharge, ocular pain, foreign body sensation, and pruritus.

Corticosteroid ophthalmic preparations are contraindicated in patients with acute superficial herpes simplex keratitis, fungal disease of the eye, or viral diseases of the eye, and after removal of a superficial corneal foreign body. Corticosteroid ophthalmic preparations are used cautiously in patients with infectious conditions of the eye. These drugs are pregnancy category C drugs and are used cautiously during pregnancy and lactation. Prolonged use of the corticosteroids may result in elevated intraocular pressure and optic nerve damage.

Antibiotics, Sulfonamides, and Silver

Antibiotics have antibacterial activity. Sulfonamides possess a bacteriostatic effect against a wide range of Gram-positive and Gram-negative microorganisms. Silver possesses antibacterial activity against Gram-positive and Gram-negative microorganisms. Antibiotics are used in the treatment of eye infections. Sulfonamides are used in the treatment of conjunctivitis, corneal ulcer, and other superficial infections of the eye. See the Summary Drug Table: Select Ophthalmic Preparations and Chapter 25 for additional information on the sulfonamides. Silver protein is occasionally used in the treatment of eye infections. Silver nitrate is occasionally used to prevent gonorrheal ophthalmia neonatorum (gonorrhea infection of the newborn's eyes). Ophthalmic tetracycline and erythromycin have largely replaced the use of silver nitrate in newborns.

Antibiotic and sulfonamide ophthalmics are usually well-tolerated, and few adverse reactions occur. Occasional transient irritation, burning, itching, stinging, inflammation, or blurring of vision may occur. With prolonged or repeated use, a superinfection may occur.

Antibiotic and sulfonamide ophthalmics are contraindicated in patients with hypersensitivity. These drugs are also contraindicated in patients with epithelial herpes simplex keratitis, varicella, mycobacterial infection of the eye, and fungal diseases of the eye. There are no significant precautions or interactions when the drugs are administered as directed by the health care provider.

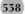

Antiviral Drugs

Antiviral drugs interfere with viral reproduction by altering DNA synthesis. These drugs are used for the treatment of herpes simplex infections of the eye, treatment of immunocompromised patients with cytomegalovirus retinitis, and prevention of cytomegalovirus retinitis in patients undergoing transplantation.

The use of the antiviral ophthalmics may cause occasional irritation, pain, pruritus, inflammation, or edema of the eyes or lids; allergic reactions; foreign body sensation; photophobia; and corneal clouding.

These drugs are contraindicated in patients with hypersensitivity to the drug and are used cautiously in immunocompromised patients and during pregnancy and lactation. Some of these solutions contain boric acid and may result in a precipitate that causes irritation.

Antifungal Drugs

Antifungal drugs act against a variety of yeast and fungi. Natamycin is the only ophthalmic antifungal in use.

Adverse reactions are rare. Occasional local irritation to the eye may occur. Natamycin is contraindicated in patients with hypersensitivity. It is a pregnancy category C drug and is used cautiously during pregnancy and lactation.

Vasoconstrictors/Mydriatics

Vasoconstrictors and **mydriatics** dilate the pupil (mydriasis), constrict superficial blood vessels of the sclera, and decrease the formation of aqueous humor. Depending on the specific drug and strength, these drugs may be used before eye surgery in the treatment of glaucoma, for relief of minor eye irritation, and to dilate the pupil for examination of the eye.

Adverse reactions include transitory stinging on initial instillation, blurring of vision, mydriasis, increased redness, irritation, discomfort, and increased intraocular pressure. Systemic adverse reactions include headache, brow ache, palpitations, tachycardia, arrhythmias, hypertension, myocardial infarction, and stroke.

These drugs are contraindicated in individuals with hypersensitivity and in patients with narrow-angle glaucoma or anatomically narrow angle and no glaucoma, and in patients with sulfite sensitivity (some of these products contain sulfite). The drugs are used cautiously in patients with hypertension, diabetes, hyperthyroidism, cardiovascular disease, and arteriosclerosis. Local anesthetics can increase absorption of topical drugs. Systemic adverse reactions may occur more frequently when these drugs are administered with the β-adrenergic blocking drugs. When mydriatics (drugs that dilate the pupil) are administered with monoamine oxidase inhibitors or as long as 21 days after monoamine oxidase inhibitors administration, exaggerated adrenergic effects may occur.

Cycloplegic Mydriatics

Cycloplegic mydriatics cause mydriasis and **cycloplegia** (paralysis of the ciliary muscle, resulting in an inability to focus the eye). These drugs (see Chapter 4) are used in the treatment of inflammatory conditions of the iris and uveal tract of the eye and for examination of the eye.

Local adverse reactions associated with administration of the cycloplegic mydriatics include increased intraocular pressure, transient stinging or burning, and irritation with prolonged use (e.g., conjunctivitis, edema, exudates). Systemic adverse reactions include dryness of the mouth and skin, blurred vision, photophobia, corneal staining, tachycardia, headache, parasympathetic stimulation, and somnolence.

These drugs are contraindicated in patients with a hypersensitivity and in patients with glaucoma. Some of these preparations contain sulfite, and individuals who are allergic to sulfites may have allergic-like symptoms. The cycloplegic mydriatics are used cautiously in elderly patients and during pregnancy (pregnancy category C) and lactation. No significant interactions have been reported when the drugs are given topically.

Artificial Tear Solutions

These products lubricate the eyes. Inactive ingredients may be found in some preparations. Examples of these drugs include preservatives, antioxidants, which prevent deterioration of the product, and drugs that slow drainage of the drug from the eye into the tear duct. Examples of the types of eye preparations are found in the Summary Drug Table: Select Ophthalmic Preparations. Artificial tear solutions are used for conditions such as dry eyes and eye irritation caused by inadequate tear production.

Adverse reactions are rare, but on occasion redness or irritation may occur. Artificial tears are contraindicated in patients with hypersensitivity. No precautions or interactions have been reported.

Patient Management Issues with Ophthalmic Preparations

Before being placed in the eye, ophthalmic solutions and ointments can be warmed by hand for a few minutes. Ophthalmic ointments are applied to the eyelids or dropped into the lower conjunctival sac; ophthalmic solutions are dropped into the middle of the lower conjunctival sac (Fig. 31-3). When two eye drops are prescribed for use at the same time, it is important to wait at least 5 minutes before instilling the second drug. This help prevents dilution of the drug and loss of some therapeutic effect from tearing.

Some ophthalmic drugs produce blurring of vision, which can result in falls and other injuries. Patients

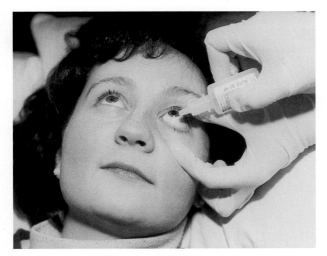

FIGURE 31-3 Instilling eye medication. While the patient looks upward, the lower lid is gently pulled down and the correct number of drops is instilled into the lower conjunctival sac. (From Roach SS. *Introductory Clinical Pharmacology*, 7th ed. Baltimore: Lippincott Williams & Wilkins, 2004.)

should be warned to be careful getting out of bed when their vision is impaired by these drugs.

Managing Adverse Reactions of Ophthalmic Preparations

Although adverse reactions are rare, these drugs can cause visual impairment such as blurring of vision and local irritation and burning. These reactions usually resolve in a few minutes. However, if visual impairment does not resolve or occurs as a consequence of an eye disorder, the patient needs help walking and with other activities of daily living. Visual impairment that does not clear within 30 minutes after therapy should be reported to the health care provider.

Educating the Patient and Family About Ophthalmic Preparations

The patient or a family member requires instruction in the technique of instilling an ophthalmic preparation. In addition, Patient Education Box 31-2 includes key points about ophthalmic preparations the patient and family members should know.

Natural Remedies: Bilberry

Bilberry, also known as whortleberry, blueberry, trackleberry, and huckleberry, is a shrub with blue flowers that appear in early spring and ripen in July and August. Although bilberry is given to improve capillary strength and flexibility and as an antioxidant, the most beneficial use appears to be in promoting healthy eyes. Bilberry is thought to increase production of the enzymes responsible for energy production in the eye and promote capillary blood flow in the eyes, hands, and feet. Bilberry extract has been shown to increase the flexibility of the cell walls of both red blood cells and endothelial cells, making the cells better able to stretch and squeeze through tighter spaces. With increased flexibility in the red blood cells, more oxygen reaches the tissues, including the retina of the eye. A component of bilberry also speeds the regeneration of rhodopsin (visual purple), which is a critical protein found in the rods of the eye.

Bilberry fruit is a safe food herb with no known adverse reactions or toxicity. There are no known contraindications to its use as directed.

KEY POINTS

⦿ Various preparations are used for the treatment of otic disorders. Three categories are antibiotics, antibiotic and steroid combinations, and miscellaneous preparations. Otic preparations are instilled in the external auditory canal and may be used to relieve pain, treat infection and inflammation, and aid in the removal of earwax. Prolonged use of otic preparations containing an antibiotic may result in a superinfection. Otic drugs are used with caution during pregnancy and lactation.

⦿ Various types of preparations are used for the treatment of ophthalmic disorders such as glaucoma (to lower the intraocular pressure), bacterial or viral infections of the eye, inflammatory conditions, and symptoms of allergy related to the eye. The incidence of adverse reactions associated with ophthalmic drugs is usually small. Because small amounts of the ophthalmic preparation may be absorbed systemically, some of the adverse effects associated with systemic administration of the particular drug may occur. Some ophthalmic preparations produce momentary stinging or burning on instillation.

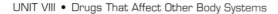

PATIENT EDUCATION BOX 31-2

Key Points for Patients Using Ophthalmic Preparations

❑ Eye preparations may cause a momentary stinging or burning sensation; this is normal.

❑ Temporary blurring of vision may occur. Avoid activities requiring clear vision until vision returns to normal.

❑ If more than one topical ophthalmic drug is being used, administer the drugs at least 5 to 10 minutes apart or as directed by the health care provider.

❑ Complete a full course of treatment with the prescribed drug to achieve satisfactory results.

❑ Do not rub your eyes, and keep your hands away from your eyes.

❑ Do not use nonprescription eye products during or after treatment unless your health care provider approves.

❑ Some of these preparations cause sensitivity (photophobia) to light; to minimize this, wear sunglasses.

❑ Notify your health care provider if your symptoms do not improve or if they worsen.

❑ Brimonidine patients should wait at least 15 minutes after instilling brimonidine before inserting soft contact lenses.

PROSTAGLANDIN AGONISTS

❑ Remove contact lenses before administration and leave them out at least 15 minutes before reinserting them.

❑ The color of your iris may change because of an increase of the brown pigment and cause different eye coloration. This may be more noticeable in patients with blue, green, gray–brown or other light-colored eyes.

CASE STUDY

Ms. Stone, age 76 years, has glaucoma and is prescribed timolol (Timoptic) eye drops. The initial assessment of Ms. Stone reveals that she also has severe arthritis and appears to have difficulty following instructions.

1. What other information should be obtained from Ms. Stone before beginning treatment?
   a. whether she feels comfortable administering the eye drops
   b. whether there is a family member who may be able to assist her should her arthritis make inserting the drops into her eye difficult
   c. whether Ms. Stone lives alone
   d. all of the above

2. Ms. Stone looks perplexed about proper use of timolol. She wonders whether the number of drops she inserts into her eye matters. She should be told:
   a. it is important to try to insert the prescribed amount in each eye
   b. there is no precise measure; Ms. Stone should attempt to insert enough that her eye feels moist from the medication
   c. Ms. Stone should insert a drop, rub her eye, and insert another drop
   d. none of the above

3. Ms. Stone wonders whether there are any potential adverse reactions to timolol. You tell her:
   a. burning, tearing, and decreased night vision are known adverse reactions
   b. there are no known adverse reactions
   c. adverse reactions exist only when timolol is combined with antidiabetic drugs
   d. a and c

WEBSITE ACTIVITIES

1. Go to the American Optometric Association website (http://www.aoa.org) and click on the tab "Eye Conditions and Concerns," and then "Eye Diseases." Go to the information on conjunctivitis. What are the three main types of conjunctivitis? What are the symptoms of conjunctivitis?

2. At the same website, return to the "Eye Diseases" page and go to "Dry Eye." What are the symptoms of dry eye? What are possible treatments?

REVIEW QUESTIONS

1. What is the rationale for warming an otic solution that has been refrigerated before instilling the drops into a patient's ear?
   a. the drug becomes thick when refrigerated, and warming liquefies the solution
   b. it helps to prevent dizziness on instillation
   c. a cold solution can significantly increase the patient's blood pressure
   d. a cold solution could damage the tympanic membrane

2. Which of the following adverse reactions might occur in a patient receiving prolonged treatment with an antibiotic otic drug?
   a. congestive heart failure
   b. superinfection
   c. anemia
   d. hypersensitivity reactions

3. An ophthalmic solution is instilled into the:
   a. inner canthus
   b. upper conjunctival sac
   c. lower conjunctival sac
   d. upper canthus

4. Which of the following instructions would be included for a patient prescribed an ophthalmic solution?
   a. squeeze your eyes tightly after the solution is instilled
   b. immediately wipe your eye using pressure to squeeze out excess medication
   c. after the drug is instilled, remain upright with your head bent slightly forward for approximately 2 minutes
   d. temporary stinging or burning may be felt at the time the drug is inserted in your eye

32 Fluids and Electrolytes

Solutions Used in the Management of Body Fluids
Blood Plasma
Plasma Protein Fractions
Protein Substrates
Energy Substrates
Plasma Expanders
Intravenous Replacement Solutions
Patient Management Issues
Educating the Patient and Family

Electrolytes
Bicarbonate (HCO$_3^-$)
Calcium (Ca^{++})
Magnesium (Mg^{++})

Potassium (K$^+$)
Sodium (Na$^+$)
Combined Electrolyte Solutions
Patient Management Issues
Educating the Patient and Family

Total Parenteral Nutrition

Key Points

Case Study

Website Activities

Review Questions

KEY TERMS

electrolyte—an electrically charged particle (ion) that is essential for normal cell function and is involved in various metabolic activities

extravasation—escape of fluid from a vessel into surrounding tissues

fluid overload—a condition when the body's fluid requirements are met and the administration of fluid occurs at a rate that is greater than the rate at which the body can use or eliminate the fluid

half-normal saline—solution containing 0.45% NaCl

hypocalcemia—low blood calcium

hypokalemia—low blood potassium

hyponatremia—low blood sodium

normal saline—solution containing 0.9% NaCl

protein substrates—amino acid preparations that act to promote the production of proteins and are essential to life

substrate—a substance that is the basic component of an organism

---

CHAPTER OBJECTIVES

On completion of this chapter, students will be able to:

1 Define the chapter's key terms.

2 Describe the general drug actions, uses, adverse reactions, contraindications, precautions, and interactions of fluids and electrolytes.

3 Discuss important points to keep in mind when educating the patient or family members about the use of fluids and electrolytes.

The composition of body fluids remains relatively constant despite the many demands placed on the body each day. On occasion, these demands cannot be met, and electrolytes and fluids must be given in an attempt to restore equilibrium. The solutions used in the management of body fluids discussed in this chapter include

blood plasma, plasma protein fractions, protein substrates, energy substrates, plasma proteins, electrolytes, and miscellaneous replacement fluids.

Electrolytes are electrically charged particles (ions) that are essential for normal cell function and are involved in various metabolic activities. This chapter discusses the use of electrolytes to replace one or more electrolytes that may be lost by the body.

Solutions Used in the Management of Body Fluids

Blood Plasma

Blood plasma is the liquid part of blood, containing water, sugar, electrolytes, fats, gases, proteins, bile pigment, and clotting factors. Human plasma, also called human pooled plasma, is obtained from donated blood. Although whole blood must be typed and cross-matched because it contains red blood cells carrying blood type and Rh factors, human plasma does not require this procedure. Therefore, plasma can be given quickly in acute emergencies.

Plasma administered intravenously is used to increase blood volume when severe hemorrhage has occurred and it is necessary to partially restore blood volume while waiting for whole blood to be typed and cross-matched. Another use of plasma is in treating conditions when plasma alone has been lost, as may occur with severe burns.

No interactions have been reported in the use of blood plasma.

Solutions used in the management of body fluids are contraindicated in patients with hypersensitivity to any component of the solution. Blood plasma is considered a pregnancy category C drug and is used cautiously during pregnancy and lactation.

Plasma Protein Fractions

Plasma protein fractions include human plasma protein fraction 5% and normal serum albumin 5% (Albuminar-5, Buminate 5%) and 25% (Albuminar-25, Buminate 25%). Plasma protein fraction 5% is an intravenous solution containing 5% human plasma proteins. Serum albumin is obtained from donated whole blood and is a protein found in plasma. The albumin fraction of human blood acts to maintain plasma colloid osmotic pressure and as a carrier of intermediate metabolites in the transport and exchange of tissue products. It is critical in regulating the volume of circulating blood. When blood is lost from shock, such as in hemorrhage, the person has a reduced plasma volume. When blood volume is reduced, albumin quickly restores the volume in most situations.

Plasma protein fractions are used to treat hypovolemic (low blood volume) shock that occurs as the result of burns, trauma, surgery, and infections, or in conditions in which shock is not currently present but likely to occur. Plasma protein fractions are also used to treat hypoproteinemia (a deficiency of protein in the blood), as might occur in patients with nephrotic syndrome and hepatic cirrhosis, as well as other diseases or disorders. A blood type and cross-match is not needed when plasma protein fractions are given.

Adverse reactions are rare when plasma protein fractions are administered, but nausea, chills, fever, urticaria, and hypotensive episodes may occur occasionally.

Plasma proteins are contraindicated in those with a history of allergic reactions to albumin, severe anemia, or cardiac failure; in the presence of normal or increased intravascular volume; and in patients on cardiopulmonary bypass. Plasma protein fractions are

used cautiously in patients who are in shock or dehydrated, and in those with congestive cardiac failure or liver or kidney failure. These solutions are pregnancy category C drugs and are used cautiously during pregnancy and lactation.

Protein Substrates

A **substrate** is a substance that is the basic component of an organism. **Protein substrates** are amino acid preparations that act to promote the production of proteins (anabolism). Amino acids are necessary to promote synthesis of structural components, reduce the rate of protein breakdown (catabolism), promote wound healing, and act as buffers in extracellular and intracellular fluids. Crystalline amino acid preparations are hypertonic solutions of balanced essential and nonessential amino acid concentrations that provide substrates for protein synthesis or act to conserve existing body protein.

Amino acids promote the production of proteins, enhance tissue repair and wound healing, and reduce the rate of protein breakdown. Amino acids are used in certain disease states, such as severe kidney and liver disease, as well as in total parenteral nutrition solutions (see the last section of this chapter). Total parenteral nutrition may be used in patients with conditions such as impairment of gastrointestinal absorption of protein, in patients with an increased requirement for protein, as seen in those with extensive burns or infections, and in patients with no available oral route for nutritional intake.

Use of protein substrates (amino acids) may result in nausea, fever, flushing of the skin, metabolic acidosis or alkalosis, and decreased phosphorus and calcium blood levels.

Solutions used in the management of body fluids are contraindicated in patients with hypersensitivity to any component of the solution. These solutions are pregnancy category C drugs and are used cautiously during pregnancy and lactation.

Energy Substrates

Energy substrates include dextrose solutions and fat emulsion. Solutions used to supply energy and fluid include dextrose (glucose) in water or sodium chloride, alcohol in dextrose, and intravenous fat emulsion. Dextrose is available in various strengths in a fluid, which may be water or saline. Dextrose and dextrose in alcohol are available in various strengths in water. Dextrose solutions also are available with electrolytes, for example, Plasma-Lyte 56 and 5% Dextrose.

An intravenous fat emulsion contains soybean or safflower oil and a mixture of natural triglycerides, predominately unsaturated fatty acids. No more than 60% of the patient's total caloric intake should come from fat emulsion, with carbohydrates and amino acids comprising the remaining 40% or more of caloric intake.

Dextrose is a carbohydrate used to provide a source of calories and fluid. Alcohol (in dextrose) also provides calories.

Intravenous fat emulsion is used in the prevention and treatment of essential fatty acid deficiency. It also provides nonprotein calories for those receiving total parenteral nutrition when calorie requirements cannot be met by glucose. Fat emulsion is used as a source of calories and essential fatty acids for patients requiring parenteral nutrition for extended periods (usually more than 5 days).

The most common adverse reaction associated with the administration of fat emulsion is sepsis caused by administration equipment and thrombophlebitis caused by vein irritations. Less frequently occurring adverse reactions include dyspnea, cyanosis, hyperlipidemia, hypercoagulability, nausea, vomiting, headache, flushing, increase in temperature, sweating, sleepiness, chest and back pain, slight pressure over the eyes, and dizziness.

The energy substrates are contraindicated in patients with hypersensitivity to any component of the solution. Dextrose solutions are contraindicated in patients with diabetic coma with excessively high blood sugar. Concentrated dextrose solutions are contraindicated in patients with increased intracranial pressure, delirium tremens (if patient is dehydrated), hepatic coma, or glucose–galactose malabsorption syndrome. Alcohol dextrose solutions are contraindicated in patients with epilepsy, urinary tract infections, alcoholism, and diabetic coma.

Alcohol dextrose solutions are used cautiously in patients with hepatic and renal impairment, vitamin deficiency (may cause or potentate vitamin deficiency), diabetes, or shock; during postpartum hemorrhage; and after cranial surgery. Dextrose solutions are used cautiously in patients receiving a corticosteroid or corticotropin. Dextrose and alcohol dextrose solutions are incompatible with blood (may cause hemolysis).

Intravenous fat emulsions are contraindicated in conditions that interfere with normal fat metabolism (e.g., acute pancreatitis) and in patients allergic to eggs. Intravenous fat emulsions are used with caution in those with severe liver impairment, pulmonary disease, anemia, and blood coagulation disorders. These solutions are pregnancy category C drugs and are used cautiously during pregnancy and lactation.

Plasma Expanders

The intravenous solutions of plasma expanders include hetastarch (Hespan), low-molecular-weight dextran (Dextran 40), and high-molecular-weight dextran (Dextran 70, Dextran 75).

Plasma expanders are used to expand plasma volume when shock is caused by burns, hemorrhage, surgery, and other trauma, and for prophylaxis of venous thrombosis and thromboembolism. When used in the treatment of shock, plasma expanders are not a substitute for whole blood or plasma, but they are of value as emergency measures until those substances can be used.

Use of hetastarch, a plasma expander, may cause vomiting, a mild temperature elevation, itching, and allergic reactions. Allergic reactions are evidenced by wheezing, edema around the eyes (periorbital edema), and urticaria. Other plasma expanders may result in mild cutaneous eruptions, generalized urticaria, hypotension, nausea, vomiting, headache, dyspnea, fever, tightness of the chest, bronchospasm, wheezing, and, rarely, anaphylactic shock.

Plasma expanders are contraindicated in patients with hypersensitivity to any component of the solution and those with severe bleeding disorders, severe cardiac failure, renal failure with oliguria, or anuria. Plasma expanders are used cautiously in patients with renal disease, congestive heart failure, pulmonary edema, and severe bleeding disorders. Plasma expanders are pregnancy category C drugs and are used cautiously during pregnancy and lactation.

Intravenous Replacement Solutions

Intravenous replacement solutions are a source of electrolytes and water for hydration and used to facilitate amino acid utilization and maintain electrolyte balance.

Dextrose and electrolyte solutions such as Plasma-Lyte R and 5% dextrose are used as a parenteral source of electrolytes, calories, or water for hydration. Invert sugar–electrolyte solutions, such as Multiple Electrolytes and Travert 5% and 10%, contain equal parts of dextrose and fructose and are used as a source of calories and hydration.

Patient Management Issues

Before intravenous use of fluids and electrolytes, the patient's blood pressure, pulse, and respiratory rate are taken to provide a baseline, which is especially important when the patient is receiving blood plasma, plasma expanders, or plasma protein fractions for shock or other serious disorders. Ongoing measurements are important, also. A patient in shock and receiving a plasma expander may require monitoring of the blood pressure and pulse rate every 5 to 15 minutes, whereas the patient receiving dextrose 3 days after surgery may require monitoring every 30 to 60 minutes.

ALERT

Infusion with a Fat Solution

During the first 30 minutes of infusion of a fat solution, the patient is carefully observed for difficulty in breathing, headache, flushing, nausea, vomiting, or signs of a hypersensitivity reaction. If any of these reactions occur, the infusion is discontinued and the health care provider is notified immediately.

One adverse reaction common to all solutions administered by the parenteral route is **fluid overload**, that is, the administration of more fluid than the body is able to handle. Patients receiving intravenous solutions are observed at frequent intervals for signs of fluid overload. If signs of fluid overload (Box 32-1) are observed, the intravenous infusion rate is slowed and the health care provider is notified immediately.

ALERT

Older Adults and Increased Risk of Fluid Overload

Older adults are at increased risk for fluid overload because of the increased incidence of cardiac disease and decreased renal function that may accompany old age. Careful monitoring for signs and symptoms of fluid overload is extremely important when administering fluids to older adults.

Educating the Patient and Family

The patient and family members are given a brief explanation of the reason for and the method of administration of an intravenous solution. Sometimes, patients or family members tamper with or adjust the rate of flow of intravenous administration sets. They need to understand the importance of not touching the intravenous administration set or the equipment used to administer intravenous fluids.

Electrolytes

Along with a disturbance in fluid volume (e.g., loss of plasma, blood, or water) or a need for parenteral nutrition, an electrolyte imbalance may exist. An electrolyte is an electrically charged substance essential to the normal functioning of all cells. Electrolytes circulate in the blood at specific levels where they are available for use when needed by the cells. An electrolyte imbalance occurs when the concentration of an electrolyte in the blood is either too high or too low. In some instances, an electrolyte imbalance may be present without an appreciable disturbance in fluid balance. For example, a patient taking a diuretic is able to maintain fluid balance by an adequate oral intake of water, which replaces the water lost through diuresis. However, the patient is likely to be unable to replace the potassium that is also lost during diuresis. When the potassium concentration in the blood is too low, as may occur with the use of a diuretic, an imbalance may occur that requires the addition of potassium. Commonly used electrolytes are listed in the Summary Drug Table: Electrolytes.

Bicarbonate (HCO_3^-)

This electrolyte plays a vital role in the acid–base balance of the body. Bicarbonate may be given intravenously as sodium bicarbonate ($NaHCO_3$) in the treatment of metabolic acidosis, a state of imbalance that may be seen in diseases or situations such as severe shock, diabetic acidosis, severe diarrhea, extracorporeal circulation of blood, severe renal disease, and cardiac arrest. Oral sodium bicarbonate is used as a gastric and urinary alkalinizer. It may be used as a single drug or may be found as one of the ingredients in some antacid preparations. It is also useful in treating severe diarrhea accompanied by bicarbonate loss.

Bicarbonate is no longer used as the first-line treatment during cardiopulmonary resuscitation after cardiac arrest. Recent evidence suggests little benefit, and the drug may actually be detrimental to resuscitation. According to the American Heart Association, bicarbonate is used when all other treatment options have failed.

In some instances, excessive oral use may produce nausea and vomiting. Some individuals may use sodium bicarbonate (baking soda) for the relief of gastric disturbances, such as pain, discomfort, symptoms of

---

Box 32-1 Signs and Symptoms of Fluid Overload

- Headache
- Weakness
- Blurred vision
- Behavioral changes (confusion, disorientation, delirium, drowsiness)
- Weight gain
- Isolated muscle twitching
- Hyponatremia
- Rapid breathing
- Wheezing
- Coughing
- Rise in blood pressure
- Distended neck veins
- Elevated central venous pressure
- Convulsions

SUMMARY DRUG TABLE   Electrolytes

Generic Name	Trade Name*	Uses	Adverse Reactions	Dosage Ranges
calcium acetate	PhosLo	Control of hyperphosphatemia in end-stage renal disease	See Box 32-2	3–4 tablets PO with each meal
calcium carbonate	Calcium-600, Caltrate, Oyster Shell Calcium Tums, Tums E-X, Tums Ultra, *generic*	Dietary supplement for prevention or treatment of calcium deficiency, osteoporosis, osteomalacia, rickets, latent tetany	Rare; see Box 32-2 for signs of hypercalcemia	500–2000 mg/d PO
calcium citrate	Citracal, Citracal Liquitab, *generic*	Same as calcium carbonate; premenstrual syndrome	Same as calcium carbonate	500–2000 mg/d PO
calcium gluconate	*Generic*	Same as calcium carbonate; premenstrual syndrome	Same as calcium carbonate	500–2000 mg/d PO
calcium lactate	*Generic*	Same as calcium carbonate	Same as calcium carbonate	500–2000 mg/d PO
oral electrolyte mixtures	Infalyte Oral Solution, Naturalyte, Pedialyte, Pedialyte Electrolyte, Pedialyte Freezer Pops, Rehydralyte, Resol	Maintenance of water and electrolytes after corrective parenteral therapy of severe diarrhea; maintenance to replace mild to moderate fluid losses when food and liquid intake are discontinued, to restore fluid and minerals lost in diarrhea and vomiting in infants and children	Rare	Individualize dosage following the guidelines on the product labeling
magnesium	Almora, Magonate, Mag-Ox 400, Magtrate, Mag-200, Slow-Mag, Uro-Mag, *generic*	Dietary supplement, hypermagnesemia	Rare; see Box 32-2 for signs of hypomagnesemia	54–483 mg/d PO
potassium replacements	Effer-K, K 10, Kaon Cl, K-Dur, Klor-Con, K-Lyte, K-Tab, Micro-K, Slow-K, *generic*	Hypokalemia	See Box 32-2; most common: nausea, vomiting, diarrhea, flatulence, abdominal discomfort, skin rash	40–150 mEq/d PO
sodium chloride	*Generic*	Prevention or treatment of extracellular volume depletion, dehydration, sodium depletion, aid in the prevention of heat prostration	Nausea, vomiting, diarrhea, abdominal cramps, edema, irritability, restlessness, weakness, hypertension tachycardia, fluid accumulation, pulmonary edema, respiratory arrest (see Box 32-2)	Individualize dosage

*The term *generic* indicates the drug is available in generic form.

indigestion, and gas. Prolonged use of oral sodium bicarbonate or excessive doses of intravenous sodium bicarbonate may result in systemic alkalosis.

Bicarbonate is contraindicated in patients losing chloride by continuous gastrointestinal suction or through vomiting, in patients with metabolic or respiratory alkalosis, hypocalcemia, renal failure, or severe abdominal pain of unknown cause, and in those on sodium-restricted diets. Bicarbonate is used cautiously in patients with congestive heart failure or renal impairment and with glucocorticoid therapy. Bicarbonate is a pregnancy category C drug and is used cautiously during pregnancy.

Oral administration of bicarbonate may decrease the absorption of ketoconazole. Increased blood levels of quinidine, flecainide, or sympathomimetics may occur when these agents are taken with bicarbonate. There is an increased risk of crystalluria when bicarbonate is taken with the fluoroquinolones. Possible decreased effects of lithium, methotrexate, chlorpropamide, salicylates, and tetracyclines may occur when these drugs are taken with sodium bicarbonate. Sodium bicarbonate is not used within 2 hours of enteric-coated drugs; the protective enteric coating may disintegrate before the drug reaches the intestine.

Calcium (Ca^{++})

Calcium is necessary for the functioning of nerves and muscles, the clotting of blood (see Chapter 18), the building of bones and teeth, and other physiologic processes. Examples of calcium salts are calcium gluconate and calcium carbonate.

Calcium may be given for the treatment of **hypocalcemia** (low blood calcium), which may be seen in patients with parathyroid disease or after accidental removal of the parathyroid glands during surgery of the thyroid gland. Calcium may also be given during cardiopulmonary resuscitation, particularly after open heart surgery, when epinephrine fails to improve weak or ineffective myocardial contractions. Calcium may be used as adjunct therapy of insect bites or stings to reduce muscle cramping, such as occurs with black widow spider bites. Calcium may also be recommended for those eating a diet low in calcium or as a dietary supplement when there is an increased need for calcium, such as during pregnancy.

Irritation of the vein, tingling, a metallic or chalky taste, and "heat waves" may occur when calcium is given intravenously. Rapid intravenous administration (calcium gluconate) may result in bradycardia, vasodilation, decreased blood pressure, cardiac arrhythmias, and cardiac arrest. Oral administration may result in gastrointestinal disturbances. Use of calcium chloride may cause peripheral vasodilation, temporary decline in blood pressure, and a local burning. Box 32-2 gives adverse reactions associated with hypercalcemia and hypocalcemia.

Calcium is contraindicated in patients with hypercalcemia or ventricular fibrillation and in patients taking digitalis. Calcium is used cautiously in patients with cardiac disease. Hypercalcemia may occur when calcium is taken with the thiazide diuretics. When calcium is used with atenolol, there is a decrease in the effect of atenolol, possibly resulting in decreased beta blockade. There is an increased risk of digitalis toxicity when digitalis preparations are administered with calcium. The clinical effect of verapamil may be decreased when the drug is used with calcium. Concurrent ingestion of spinach or cereal may decrease the absorption of calcium supplements.

Magnesium (Mg^{++})

Magnesium plays an important role in the transmission of nerve impulses. It is also important in the activity of many enzyme reactions, such as carbohydrate metabolism.

Magnesium sulfate is used as replacement therapy in hypomagnesemia. Magnesium sulfate is used in the prevention and control of seizures in obstetric patients with pregnancy-induced hypertension, also referred to as eclampsia and preeclampsia. It may also be added to total parenteral nutrition mixtures.

Adverse reactions seen with magnesium administration are rare. If they do occur, they are most likely related to overdose and may include flushing, sweating, hypotension, depressed reflexes, muscle weakness, and circulatory collapse (see Box 32-2).

Magnesium sulfate is contraindicated in patients with heart block or myocardial damage and in women with pregnancy-induced hypertension during the 2 hours before delivery. Magnesium is a pregnancy category A drug, and studies indicate no increased risk of fetal abnormalities if the agent is used during pregnancy. Nevertheless, caution is used when using magnesium during pregnancy. In addition, magnesium chloride is contraindicated in patients with renal impairment or marked myocardial disease and those in a coma. Magnesium (sulfate) is used with caution in patients with renal function impairment. Prolonged respiratory depression and apnea may occur when magnesium is administered with the neuromuscular blocking agents.

Potassium (K$^+$)

Potassium is necessary for the transmission of impulses; the contraction of smooth, cardiac, and skeletal muscles; and other important physiologic processes. Potassium as a drug is available as potassium chloride (KCl) and potassium gluconate.

Potassium may be given for **hypokalemia** (low blood potassium). Examples of causes of hypokalemia are a

---

Box 32-2 **Signs and Symptoms of Electrolyte Imbalances**

Calcium

Normal laboratory values: 4.5–5.3 mEq/L or 9–11 mg/dL*

Hypocalcemia

Hyperactive reflexes, carpopedal spasm, perioral paresthesias, positive Trousseau sign, positive Chvostek sign, muscle twitching, muscle cramps, tetany (numbness, tingling, and muscular twitching usually of the extremities), laryngospasm, cardiac arrhythmias, nausea, vomiting, anxiety, confusion, emotional lability, convulsions

Hypercalcemia

Anorexia, nausea, vomiting, lethargy, bone tenderness or pain, polyuria, polydipsia, constipation, dehydration, muscle weakness and atrophy, stupor, coma, cardiac arrest

Magnesium

Normal laboratory values: 1.5–2.5 mEq/L or 1.8–3 mg/dL*

Hypomagnesemia

Leg and foot cramps, hypertension, tachycardia, neuromuscular irritability, tremor, hyperactive deep tendon reflexes, confusion, disorientation, visual or auditory hallucinations, painful paresthesias, positive Trousseau sign, positive Chvostek sign, convulsions

Hypermagnesemia

Lethargy, drowsiness, impaired respiration, flushing, sweating, hypotension, weak to absent deep tendon reflexes

Potassium

Normal laboratory values: 3.5–5 mEq/L*

Hypokalemia

Anorexia, nausea, vomiting, mental depression, confusion, delayed or impaired thought processes, drowsiness, abdominal distention, decreased bowel sounds, paralytic ileus, muscle weakness or fatigue, flaccid paralysis, absent or diminished deep tendon reflexes, weak irregular pulse, paresthesias, leg cramps, ECG changes

Hyperkalemia

Irritability, anxiety, listlessness, mental confusion, nausea, diarrhea, abdominal distress, gastrointestinal hyperactivity, paresthesias, weakness and heaviness of the legs, flaccid paralysis, hypotension, cardiac arrhythmias, electrocardiograph (ECG) changes

Sodium

Normal laboratory values: 132–145 mEq/L*

Hyponatremia

Cold clammy skin, decreased skin turgor, apprehension, confusion, irritability, anxiety, hypotension, postural hypotension, tachycardia, headache, tremors, convulsions, abdominal cramps, nausea, vomiting, diarrhea

Hypernatremia

Fever, hot dry skin, dry sticky mucous membranes, rough dry tongue, edema, weight gain, intense thirst, excitement, restlessness, agitation, oliguria or anuria

---

* These laboratory values may not concur with the normal range of values in all hospitals and laboratories. The hospital policy manual or laboratory values sheet should be consulted for the normal ranges of all laboratory tests.

---

marked loss of gastrointestinal fluids (severe vomiting, diarrhea, nasogastric suction, draining intestinal fistulas), diabetic acidosis, marked diuresis, and severe malnutrition.

Nausea, vomiting, diarrhea, abdominal pain, and phlebitis have been seen with oral and intravenous use of potassium. Adverse reactions related to hypokalemia or hyperkalemia are listed in Box 32-2.

If **extravasation** (escape of fluid from a vessel into surrounding tissues) of the intravenous solution should occur, local tissue necrosis (death of tissue) may occur. If extravasation occurs, the health care provider should be contacted immediately and the infusion slowed to a rate that keeps the vein open.

Potassium is contraindicated in patients who are at risk for experiencing hyperkalemia, such as those with renal failure, oliguria, or azotemia (the presence of nitrogen-containing compounds in the blood), anuria, severe hemolytic reactions, untreated Addison disease (see Chapter 23), acute dehydration, heat cramps, and any

form of hyperkalemia. Potassium is used cautiously in patients with renal impairment or adrenal insufficiency, heart disease, metabolic acidosis, or prolonged or severe diarrhea. Concurrent use of potassium with angiotensin-converting enzyme inhibitors may result in elevated serum potassium. Potassium-sparing diuretics and salt substitutes used with potassium can produce severe hyperkalemia. The use of digitalis with potassium increases the risk of digoxin toxicity.

Sodium (Na$^+$)

Sodium is essential for the maintenance of normal heart action and in the regulation of osmotic pressure in body cells. Sodium, as sodium chloride, may be given intravenously. A solution containing 0.9% sodium chloride is called **normal saline**, and a solution containing 0.45% NaCl is called **half-normal saline**. Sodium also is available combined with dextrose, such as dextrose 5% and sodium chloride 0.9%.

Sodium is used to treat **hyponatremia** (low blood sodium). Examples of causes of hyponatremia are excessive diaphoresis, severe vomiting or diarrhea, excessive diuresis, and draining intestinal fistulas.

Sodium as the salt (e.g., NaCl) has no adverse reactions except those related to overdose (see Box 32-2). In some instances, excessive oral use may cause nausea and vomiting.

Sodium is contraindicated in patients with hypernatremia or fluid retention and when the administration of sodium or chloride could be detrimental. Sodium is used cautiously in surgical patients and those with circulatory insufficiency, hypoproteinemia, urinary tract obstruction, congestive heart failure, edema, or renal impairment. Sodium is a pregnancy category C drug and is used cautiously during pregnancy.

Combined Electrolyte Solutions

Combined electrolyte solutions are available for oral and intravenous use. The intravenous solutions contain various electrolytes and dextrose.

Intravenous solutions are used to replace fluid and electrolytes that have been lost and to provide calories by means of their carbohydrate content. Examples of intravenous electrolyte solutions are dextrose 5% with 0.9% sodium chloride, lactated Ringer's injection, Plasma-Lyte, and 10% Travert (invert sugar—a combination of equal parts of fructose and dextrose), and Electrolyte No. 2. The health care provider selects the type of combined electrolyte solution to meet the patient's needs.

Oral electrolyte solutions contain a carbohydrate and various electrolytes. Examples of combined oral electrolyte solutions are Pedialyte and Rehydralyte. Oral electrolyte solutions are most often used to replace lost electrolytes, carbohydrates, and fluid in conditions such as severe vomiting or diarrhea.

Patient Management Issues

When bicarbonate is given in the treatment of metabolic acidosis, the drug may be added to the intravenous fluid or given as a prepared intravenous sodium bicarbonate solution. The patient is observed for signs of clinical improvement, and the blood pressure, pulse, and respiratory rate are monitored every 15 to 30 minutes or as ordered by the health care provider. Extravasation of the drug requires selection of another needle site because the drug is irritating to the tissues.

Before, during, and after the use of calcium, blood pressure, pulse, and respiratory rate are monitored every 30 minutes until the patient's condition has stabilized. After administration of calcium, the patient is observed for signs of hypercalcemia (see Box 32-2).

ALERT

Overloading of Calcium Ions

Systemic overloading of calcium ions in the systemic circulation results in acute hypercalcemic syndrome. Symptoms of hypercalcemic syndrome include elevated plasma calcium, weakness, lethargy, severe nausea and vomiting, coma, and, if left untreated, death. Any signs of hypercalcemic syndrome must be reported immediately to the health care provider.

Patients receiving oral potassium should have their blood pressure and pulse monitored every 4 hours, especially during early therapy. The patient is also observed for signs of hyperkalemia (see Box 32-2), which would indicate that the dose of potassium is too high. Signs of hypokalemia may also occur during therapy and may indicate that the dose of potassium is too low and must be increased. In some instances, frequent laboratory monitoring of the serum potassium may be ordered.

Potassium is irritating to the tissues. If extravasation occurs, the intravenous administration is immediately ended and the health care provider is notified. An acutely ill patient and a patient with severe hypokalemia will require monitoring of the blood pressure and pulse rate every 15 to 30 minutes during the time of the intravenous infusion. Intake and output is measured every 8 hours. The infusion rate is slowed to keep the vein open, and the health care provider is notified if an irregular pulse is noted.

When magnesium sulfate is ordered to treat convulsions or severe hypomagnesemia, the patient requires constant observation. The patient's blood pressure, pulse, and respiratory rate are obtained immediately before the drug is administered, as well as every 5 to 10 minutes during the time of intravenous infusion or after the drug is given direct intravenously. Urine output of at least 100 mL every 4 hours is essential. Voiding less than 100 mL of urine every 4 hours is reported to the health care provider.

The patient is observed for early signs of hypermagnesemia (see Box 32-2) and the health care provider is contacted immediately if this imbalance is suspected.

When sodium is administered by intravenous infusion, the patient is observed during and after administration for signs of hypernatremia (see Box 32-2). Patients receiving a 3% or 5% sodium chloride solution by intravenous infusion are observed closely for signs of pulmonary edema (dyspnea, cough, restlessness, bradycardia). If any one or more of these symptoms should occur, the intravenous infusion is slowed to keep the vein open, and the health care provider is contacted immediately.

Electrolyte disturbances can cause varying degrees of confusion, muscular weakness, nausea, vomiting, and cardiac irregularities (see Box 32-2 for specific symptoms). Serum electrolyte blood levels have a very narrow therapeutic range. Careful monitoring is needed to determine if blood levels are above or below normal. Maintaining blood levels of the various electrolytes within the normal range usually controls adverse reactions.

Oral sodium bicarbonate tablets are taken with a full glass of water. If the urine remains acidic, the health care provider is notified because an increase in the dose of the drug may be necessary. Intravenous sodium bicarbonate is given in emergency situations, such as metabolic acidosis or certain types of drug overdose, when alkalization of the urine is necessary to hasten drug elimination.

When given orally, potassium may cause gastrointestinal distress. Therefore, it is given immediately after meals or with food and a full glass of water. Oral potassium must not be crushed or chewed.

ALERT

Concentrated Potassium Solutions

Concentrated potassium solutions are for intravenous mixtures only and should never be used undiluted. Direct intravenous injection of potassium could result in sudden death. When potassium is given intravenously, it is always diluted in 500 to 1000 mL of an intravenous solution

---

Magnesium sulfate may be ordered intramuscularly, intravenously, or by intravenous infusion diluted in a specified type and amount of intravenous solution. When ordered to be given intramuscularly, this drug is given undiluted as a 50% solution for adults and a 20% solution for children. Magnesium sulfate is given deep intramuscularly in a large muscle mass, such as the gluteus muscle.

ALERT

Older Adults and Magnesium Dosage

Older adults may need a reduced dosage of magnesium because of decreased renal function. Serum magnesium levels should be closely monitored when magnesium is administered to older adults.

Managing Adverse Reactions of Electrolytes

When electrolyte solutions are administered, adverse reactions are most often related to overdose. Correcting the imbalance by decreasing the dosage or discontinuing the solution usually works, and the adverse reactions subside within a short period of time. Frequent serum electrolyte levels are used to monitor blood levels.

If gastrointestinal disturbances occur from oral administration, taking the drug with meals may decrease the nausea. If weakness or muscular cramping occurs,

the patient should be assisted with walking and self-care activities to prevent falls or other injury.

Some electrolytes may cause cardiac irregularities. The pulse rate should be checked at regular intervals, usually every 4 hours or more often if an irregularity in the heart rate is observed. Depending on the patient's condition, cardiac monitoring may be indicated when administering the electrolytes (particularly when administering potassium or calcium). For example, if potassium is administered to a patient with cardiac disease, a cardiac monitor is needed to continuously monitor the heart rate and rhythm during therapy.

Educating the Patient and Family

Because overdose (which can be serious) may occur if the patient does not adhere to the prescribed dosage and schedule, it is most important that the patient completely understands how much and when to take the drug.

The health care provider may order periodic laboratory and diagnostic tests for some patients receiving oral electrolytes. The patient is encouraged to keep all appointments for these tests, as well as health care provider or clinic visits. Patients with a history of using sodium bicarbonate (baking soda) as an antacid are warned that overuse can result in alkalosis and could disguise a more serious problem. Those with a history of using salt tablets (sodium chloride) are advised not to do so during hot weather unless the health care provider recommends it. Excessive use of salt tablets can result in a serious electrolyte imbalance.

Patient Education Box 32-1 includes key points about electrolytes the patient and family members should know.

Total Parenteral Nutrition

When normal eating is not possible or is inadequate to meet an individual's nutritional needs, intravenous nutritional therapy or total parenteral nutrition is required. Products used to meet the intravenous nutritional requirements of a patient include protein substrates (amino acids), energy substrates (dextrose and fat emulsions), fluids, electrolytes, and trace minerals (see the Summary Drug Table: Electrolytes).

Total parenteral nutrition is used to prevent nitrogen and weight loss or to treat negative nitrogen (mineral component in protein and amino acids) balance (a situation in which more nitrogen is used by the body than is taken in) when:

- the oral, gastrostomy, or jejunostomy route cannot or should not be used
- gastrointestinal absorption of protein is impaired by obstruction

- inflammatory disease or antineoplastic therapy prevents normal gastrointestinal functioning
- bowel rest is needed (e.g., after bowel surgery)
- metabolic requirements for protein are significantly increased (e.g., in hypermetabolic states such as serious burns, infections, or trauma)
- morbidity and mortality may be reduced by replacing amino acids lost from tissue breakdown (e.g., renal failure)
- tube feeding alone cannot provide adequate nutrition

Total parenteral nutrition may be administered through a peripheral vein or through a central venous catheter. Peripheral total parenteral nutrition is used for patients requiring parenteral nutrition for relatively short periods of time (no more than 5–14 days) and when the central venous route is not possible or necessary. Peripheral total parenteral nutrition is used when the patient's caloric needs are minimal and can be partially met by normal means (through the alimentary tract); it prevents protein catabolism (breakdown of cells) in patients who have adequate body fat and no clinically significant protein malnutrition. These solutions may be used alone or combined with dextrose (5% or 10%) solutions.

Total parenteral nutrition through a central vein is indicated in patients to promote protein synthesis in those who are severely hypercatabolic, severely depleted of nutrients, or require long-term nutritional parenteral nutrition. For example, amino acids combined with hypertonic dextrose and intravenous fat emulsions are infused through a central venous catheter to promote protein synthesis. Vitamins, trace minerals, and electrolytes may be added to the total parenteral nutrition mixture to meet the patient's individual needs. The daily dose depends on a patient's daily protein requirement, metabolic state, and clinical responses. Various laboratory studies and assessments are required before and during administration of total parenteral nutrition.

ALERT

Hyperglycemia

Hyperglycemia is the most common metabolic complication of total parenteral nutrition. A too rapid infusion of amino acid–carbohydrate mixtures may result in hyperglycemia, glycosuria, mental confusion, and loss of consciousness. Blood glucose levels may be obtained every 4 to 6 hours to monitor for hyperglycemia and guide the dosage of dextrose and insulin (if required). To minimize these complications, the health care provider may decrease the rate of administration, reduce the dextrose concentration, or administer insulin.

To prevent a rebound hypoglycemic reaction from the sudden withdrawal of total parenteral nutrition containing a concentrated dose of dextrose, the rate of administration is slowly reduced or the concentration of dextrose gradually decreased.

KEY POINTS

● Blood plasma is the liquid part of blood. Human plasma is obtained from donated blood and can be given in acute emergencies because it does not require a donor match. Plasma is considered a pregnancy class C drug, with no known adverse reactions.

○ Plasma protein fractions are critical in regulating the volume of circulating blood. Plasma protein fractions are used to treat hypovolemic (low blood volume) shock that occurs as the result of burns, trauma, surgery, and infections. Plasma protein fractions do not require a donor match. Adverse reactions are rare, but nausea, chills, fever, urticaria, and hypotensive episodes may occasionally be seen. Plasma proteins are contraindicated in those with a history of allergic reactions to albumin, severe anemia, or cardiac failure; in the presence of normal or increased intravascular volume; and in patients on cardiopulmonary bypass.

○ Protein substrates are amino acid preparations that promote the production of proteins (anabolism). Amino acids promote the production of proteins, enhance tissue repair and wound healing, and reduce the rate of protein breakdown. Amino acids are used in certain disease states, such as severe kidney and liver disease, as well as in total parenteral nutrition solutions. Plasma expanders are used cautiously in patients with renal disease, congestive heart failure, pulmonary edema, and severe bleeding disorders.

○ Energy substrates include dextrose solutions and fat emulsion. Intravenous fat emulsion is used in the prevention and treatment of essential fatty acid deficiency. The most common adverse reaction associated with fat emulsion is sepsis caused by administration equipment and thrombophlebitis caused by vein irritations from concurrently administering hypertonic solutions. Dextrose solutions are contraindicated in patients with diabetic coma with excessively high blood sugar, concentrated dextrose solutions in patients with increased intracranial pressure, delirium tremens, hepatic coma, or glucose–galactose malabsorption syndrome, and alcohol dextrose solutions in patients with epilepsy, urinary tract infections, alcoholism, and diabetic coma.

○ Plasma expanders are used to expand plasma volume when shock is caused by burns, hemorrhage, surgery, and other trauma, and for prophylaxis of venous thrombosis and thromboembolism. Use of hetastarch may cause vomiting, a mild temperature elevation, itching, and allergic reactions. Allergic reactions are evidenced by wheezing, edema around the eyes, and urticaria. Plasma expanders are contraindicated in patients with hypersensitivity to any component of the solution and those with severe bleeding disorders, severe cardiac failure, renal failure with oliguria, or anuria.

○ Intravenous replacement solutions are a source of electrolytes and water for hydration and used to facilitate amino acid utilization and maintain electrolyte balance. Dextrose and electrolyte solutions are used as a parenteral source of electrolytes, calories, or water for hydration.

○ Bicarbonate plays a vital role in the acid–base balance of the body. Bicarbonate may be given intra-venously as sodium bicarbonate, which may be given intravenously in the treatment of metabolic acidosis, a state of imbalance that may occur in severe shock, diabetic acidosis, severe diarrhea, extracorporeal circulation of blood, severe renal disease, and cardiac arrest. Excessive oral use may cause nausea and vomiting. Prolonged use of oral sodium bicarbonate or excessive doses of intravenous sodium bicarbonate may result in systemic alkalosis. Bicarbonate is contraindicated in patients losing chloride by continuous gastrointestinal suction or through vomiting, in patients with metabolic or respiratory alkalosis, hypocalcemia, renal failure, or severe abdominal pain of unknown cause, and in those on sodium-restricted diets.

○ Calcium may be given for the treatment of hypocalcemia, which may occur in patients with parathyroid disease or after removal of the parathyroid glands, and during cardiopulmonary resuscitation when epinephrine fails to improve weak or ineffective myocardial contractions. Irritation of the vein, tingling, a metallic or chalky taste, and "heat waves" may occur when calcium is given intravenously. Calcium is contraindicated in patients with hypercalcemia or ventricular fibrillation and in patients taking digitalis. Calcium is used cautiously in patients with cardiac disease.

○ Magnesium is used as replacement therapy in hypomagnesemia. Magnesium sulfate is used in the prevention and control of seizures in obstetric patients with pregnancy-induced hypertension. Adverse reactions seen with magnesium administration are rare. Magnesium sulfate is contraindicated in patients with heart block or myocardial damage and in women with pregnancy-induced hypertension during the 2 hours before delivery.

○ Potassium is necessary for the transmission of impulses; the contraction of smooth, cardiac, and skeletal muscles; and other important physiologic processes. It is also given for hypokalemia. Nausea, vomiting, diarrhea, abdominal pain, and phlebitis have been seen with oral and intravenous use of potassium. Potassium is contraindicated in patients who are at risk for experiencing hyperkalemia, such as those with renal failure, oliguria, or azotemia, anuria, severe hemolytic reactions, untreated Addison disease, acute dehydration, heat cramps, and any form of hyperkalemia.

○ Sodium is essential for the maintenance of normal heart action and in the regulation of osmotic pressure in body cells. Sodium is used to treat hyponatremia. Sodium has no adverse reactions except in overdose situations and is contraindicated in patients with hypernatremia or fluid retention and when the administration of sodium or chloride could be detrimental.

○ Combined electrolyte solutions are available for oral and intravenous use. Intravenous solutions are used to replace fluid and electrolytes that have been lost and to provide calories by means of their carbohydrate content.

○ Total parenteral nutrition is used to prevent nitrogen and weight loss or to treat negative nitrogen balance. Peripheral total parenteral nutrition is used for patients requiring parenteral nutrition for relatively short periods of time and when the central venous route is not possible or necessary. Peripheral total parenteral nutrition is used when the patient's caloric needs are minimal and can be partially met by normal means.

CASE STUDY

Mr. Kendall is prescribed an oral potassium chloride liquid. He has questions about the drug and why it was prescribed.

1. Mr. Kendall asks why his health care provider chose potassium chloride liquid. He should be told:
   a. potassium is important in physiologic processes, such as helping the cardiac muscle contract
   b. he can ask his health care provider for more specifics
   c. potassium helps relieve hyperkalemia
   d. a and b

2. Mr. Kendall wonders if adverse reactions may occur with this drug. He should be told:
   a. there are no known adverse reactions
   b. nausea and vomiting sometimes occur with potassium chloride
   c. headache, fatigue, and confusion are common adverse reactions
   d. none of the above

WEBSITE ACTIVITIES

1. Go to the Kids Health website (http://www.kidshealth.org) and enter as "Parents." Conduct a search on "electrolytes," and read the article entitled "Electrolytes." How is the test of electrolytes performed? How long does it take to get the results?

2. Return to the search page at the same website and search for "calcium." Read the article entitled "Nutrients Your Child Needs: Calcium, Iron, Fiber." How much calcium does a child need? How is calcium related to osteoporosis and bone mass?

REVIEW QUESTIONS

1. Which of the following is a symptom of fluid overload?
   a. tinnitus
   b. hypotension
   c. decreased body temperature
   d. behavioral changes

2. Which of the following symptoms may result from hypocalcemia?
   a. tetany
   b. constipation
   c. muscle weakness
   d. hypertension

3. Sodium is used:
   a. to treat hyponatremia
   b. to treat hypokalemia
   c. to treat hypocalcemia
   d. none of the above

4. Which of the following symptoms is most likely related to hypernatremia?
   a. fever, increased thirst
   b. cold, clammy skin
   c. decreased skin turgor
   d. hypotension

5. Which of the following is the most common metabolic complication of total parenteral nutrition?
   a. hypomagnesemia
   b. hypermagnesemia
   c. hypoglycemia
   d. hyperglycemia

Answers to Case Study Questions and Review Questions

Chapter 1

REVIEW QUESTIONS

1. a	2. b	3. d	4. d	5. a
6. c	7. b	8. c	9. d	10. d

Chapter 2

REVIEW QUESTIONS

1. d	2. c	3. a	4. b	5. b
6. d	7. a			

Chapter 3

CASE STUDY

1. b	2. c	3. d

REVIEW QUESTIONS

1. d	2. a	3. c	4. a	5. b

Chapter 4

CASE STUDY

1. b	2. c	3. d

REVIEW QUESTIONS

1. c	2. a	3. b	4. b	5. d

Chapter 5

CASE STUDY

1. b	2. c	3. a

REVIEW QUESTIONS

1. a	2. b	3. d	4. c	5. d
6. c	7. c	8. b	9. c	10. a

Chapter 6

CASE STUDY

1. b	2. b	3. d

REVIEW QUESTIONS

1. a	2. d	3. d	4. b	5. a
6. b				

Chapter 7

CASE STUDY

1. b	2. a	3. d

REVIEW QUESTIONS

1. b	2. d	3. b	4. c	5. a

Chapter 8

CASE STUDY

1. b	2. a	3. d

REVIEW QUESTIONS

1. b	2. c	3. d	4. a	5. d

Chapter 9

CASE STUDY

1. b	2. d	3. a

REVIEW QUESTIONS

1. a	2. d	3. a	4. b

Chapter 10

CASE STUDY

1. a	2. b	3. c

REVIEW QUESTIONS

1. a	2. c	3. a	4. d	5. b

Chapter 11

CASE STUDY

1. a	2. c	3. a

REVIEW QUESTIONS

1. a	2. b	3. c	4. c

Chapter 12

CASE STUDY

1. a.	2. d	3. d

REVIEW QUESTIONS

1. d	2. c	3. a	4. c	5. b

Chapter 13

CASE STUDY

1. a   2. a   3. b

REVIEW QUESTIONS

1. b   2. d   3. b   4. a   5. a

Chapter 14

CASE STUDY

1. a   2. b   3. a   4. c

REVIEW QUESTIONS

1. b   2. c   3. a   4. a

Chapter 15

CASE STUDY

1. c   2. b   3. a

REVIEW QUESTIONS

1. a   2. b   3. c   4. b

Chapter 16

CASE STUDY

1. c   2. b   3. b

REVIEW QUESTIONS

1. c   2. b   3. a   4. b   5. a

Chapter 17

CASE STUDY

1. d   2. b   3. a

REVIEW QUESTIONS

1. a   2. a   3. b   4. c   5. d

Chapter 18

CASE STUDY

1. c   2. a   3. b

REVIEW QUESTIONS

1. b   2. a   3. b   4. a   5. a

Chapter 19

CASE STUDY

1. b   2. b   3. d

REVIEW QUESTIONS

1. b   2. c   3. b   4. d   5. c

Chapter 20

CASE STUDY

1. d   2. d   3. a

REVIEW QUESTIONS

1. a   2. d   3. c   4. d   5. c

Chapter 21

CASE STUDY

1. d   2. b   3. a

REVIEW QUESTIONS

1. c   2. c   3. a   4. b   5. d

Chapter 22

CASE STUDY

1. b   2. d   3. c

REVIEW QUESTIONS

1. c   2. d   3. c   4. a   5. c

Chapter 23

CASE STUDY

1. d   2. a   3. d

REVIEW QUESTIONS

1. b   2. c   3. a   4. c   5. b

Chapter 24

CASE STUDY

1. a   2. a   3. d

REVIEW QUESTIONS

1. d   2. a   3. a   4. c

Chapter 25

CASE STUDY

1. d   2. d   3. a

REVIEW QUESTIONS

1. b   2. b   3. c   4. c   5. a
6. d   7. a

Chapter 26

CASE STUDY

1. c   2. a   3. d

REVIEW QUESTIONS

1. d   2. a   3. a   4. d   5. b
6. c

Chapter 27

CASE STUDY

1. b   2. b   3. a

REVIEW QUESTIONS

1. b   2. a   3. c   4. a

Chapter 28

CASE STUDY

1. b   2. d   3. a

REVIEW QUESTIONS

1. d   2. a   3. b   4. b   5. d

Chapter 29

CASE STUDY

1. a   2. d   3. c

REVIEW QUESTIONS

1. c   2. a   3. d   4. d   5. d

Chapter 30

CASE STUDY

1. a   2. a   3. b

REVIEW QUESTIONS

1. b   2. b   3. d   4. b   5. d

Chapter 31

CASE STUDY

1. d   2. a   3. a

REVIEW QUESTIONS

1. b   2. b   3. c   4. d

Chapter 32

CASE STUDY

1. d   2. b

REVIEW QUESTIONS

1. d   2. a   3. a   4. a   5. d

Abbreviations

A

aa	of each
abd	abdomen, abdominal
ABG	arterial blood gas
ac	before meals
ADH	antidiuretic hormone
ADL	activities of daily living
ad lib	as much as desired
ADT	alternate-day therapy
AIDS	acquired immunodeficiency syndrome
ALT	alanine aminotransferase
AMA	against medical advice
AMI	acute myocardial infarction
AODM	adult-onset diabetes mellitus
ARC	AIDS-related complex
ASAP	as soon as possible
ASHD	arteriosclerotic heart disease
AST	aspartate aminotransferase

B

BE	barium enema; base excess
bid	twice a day
bili	bilirubin
BM	bowel movement
BMR	basal metabolic rate
B&O	belladonna and opium
BP	blood pressure
BPH	benign prostatic hypertrophy
BRP	bathroom privileges
BUN	blood urea nitrogen

C

c̄	with
Ca	cancer; calcium
C&A	Clinitest and Acetest
CAD	coronary artery disease
caps	capsules
CBC	complete blood count
CC	chief complaint
CCU	Coronary Care Unit
CHF	congestive heart failure
CHO	carbohydrate
chol	cholesterol
CLL	chronic lymphocytic leukemia
CNS	central nervous system
C/O	complains of
COPD	chronic obstructive pulmonary disease

CPK	creatine phosphokinase
CRF	chronic renal failure
C&S	culture and sensitivity
CTZ	chemoreceptor trigger zone
CVA	cerebrovascular accident
CVP	central venous pressure
CXR	chest x-ray

D

/d	per day
d	daily
DC (D/C)	discontinue
Diff	differential blood count
DJD	degenerative joint disease
DM	diabetes mellitus
DOE	dyspnea on exertion
DT	delirium tremens
Dx	diagnosis

E

ECG	electrocardiogram
ECT	electroconvulsive therapy
EENT	eyes, ears, nose, and throat
EKG	electrocardiogram
ENT	eyes, nose, and throat
ER	emergency room
ESR	erythrocyte sedimentation rate (sed rate)
et	and

F

F	Fahrenheit
FBS	fasting blood sugar
fl	fluid
fx	fracture; fraction

G

g	gram
GB	gallbladder
GERD	gastroesophageal reflux disease
GFR	glomerular filtration rate
GI	gastrointestinal
gtt	drop
GU	genitourinary

H

h	hour
HA	headache

Hct	hematocrit
Hgb	hemoglobin
hs	hour of sleep
HTN	hypertension
Hx	history

I

ICU	intensive care unit
IM	intramuscular
I&O	intake and output
IOP	intraocular pressure
IPPB	intermittent positive pressure breathing
IU	international units
IV	intravenous
IVP	intravenous pyelogram
IVPB	intravenous piggyback

J

JRA	juvenile rheumatoid arthritis

K

K	potassium
KUB	kidney, ureters, and bladder
KVO	keep vein open

L

LDH	lactic dehydrogenase
LDL	low-density lipoproteins
LOC	level of consciousness
LP	lumbar puncture
lytes	electrolytes

M

mcg	microgram
MI	myocardial infarction (heart attack)
mL	milliliter
MOM	milk of magnesia
MS	morphine sulfate; multiple sclerosis; mitral stenosis

N

N	normal
NG	nasogastric
NPO	nothing by mouth
NS	normal saline
NGT	nitroglycerin
NVD	nausea, vomiting, diarrhea; neck vein distension

O

O_2	oxygen
OD	right eye
OOB	out of bed
OR	operating room
OU	both eyes
OTC	over the counter (nonprescription)
OS	left eye

P

PAT	paroxysmal atrial tachycardia
PBI	protein-bound iodine
PC	after meals
PERRLA	pupils equal, round, react to light and accommodation
PERL	pupils equal and react to light
PID	pelvic inflammatory disease
PKU	phenylketonuria
PND	paroxysmal nocturnal dyspnea
PO	by mouth
postop	after surgery
preop	before surgery
prn	as needed
PT	physical therapy; prothrombin time
PZI	protamine zinc insulin

Q

qd	every day
qh	every hour (q2h, q3h, etc.—every 2 hours, every 3 hours, etc.)
qid	four times per day
qod	every other day

R

RA	rheumatoid arthritis; right atrium
RBC	red blood cell
REM	rapid eye movement
RF	rheumatoid factor
RHD	rheumatic heart disease; renal hypertensive disease
ROM	range of motion
RR	recovery room

S

s̄	without
SC	subcutaneous
sed rate	erythrocyte sedimentation rate (ESR)
SGOT	serum glutamic oxaloacetic transaminase
SGPT	serum glutamic pyruvic transaminase
SL	sublingual
SOB	shortness of breath
SR	sedimentation rate (ESR)
STAT	as soon as possible

T

t	temperature
T_3	triiodothyronine
T_4	thyroxine
T&A	tonsillectomy and adenoidectomy
TB	tuberculosis
TEDS	elastic stockings
TIA	transient ischemic attack
tid	three times per day
TKO	to keep open
TLC	tender loving care

TM	tympanic membrane		**V**	
TPN	total parenteral nutrition		VS	vital signs
TPR	temperature, pulse, respiration			
TSH	thyroid-stimulating hormone		**W**	
			WNL	within normal limits
U			Wt	weight
UGI	upper gastrointestinal			
ung	ointment			
URI	upper respiratory infection			
UTI	urinary tract infection			

C   Glossary

A

absence seizures: previously referred to as petit mal seizures; characterized by a brief loss of consciousness, during which physical activity ceases, and may last a few seconds and happen multiple times per day

abstinence syndrome: symptoms that occur if a drug causing physical or psychological dependence is suddenly discontinued

acetylcholine: a neurotransmitter in the parasympathetic nervous system required for memory and thinking

acetylcholinesterase: a neurotransmitter that inactivates acetylcholine

achalasia: failure to relax; usually referring to the smooth muscle fibers of the gastrointestinal tract, especially failure of the lower esophagus to relax when swallowing, causing difficulty swallowing and a feeling of fullness in the sternal region

action potential: an electrical impulse that passes from cell to cell in the myocardium, stimulating fibers to shorten and causing muscular contraction (systole)

active immunity: type of immunity that occurs when the person is exposed to a disease and the disease develops, and the body makes antibodies to provide future protection against the disease

acute pain: pain that is of short duration and lasts less than 3 to 6 months and can be from mild to severe

addiction: a compulsive desire or craving to use a drug or chemical with a resultant physical dependence

additive drug reaction: a reaction that occurs when the combined effect of two drugs is equal to the sum of each drug given alone

adrenal insufficiency: a critical deficiency of the mineralocorticoids and the glucocorticoids that requires immediate treatment

adrenergic blocking drugs: drugs that impede certain sympathetic nervous system functions

adrenergic drugs: drugs with effects similar to those that occur in the body when the adrenergic nerves are stimulated

adverse reaction: undesirable drug effect

aerobic: organisms that require oxygen to live

affective domain: refers to one's attitudes, feelings, beliefs, and opinions

afferent nerve fiber: a sensory nerve that carries an impulse toward the brain

agonist: drug that binds with a receptor to produce a therapeutic response

agonist–antagonist: drug with both agonist and antagonist properties

agranulocytosis: a decrease or lack of granulocytes (a type of white blood cell)

akathisia: extreme restlessness and increased motor activity

alanine aminotransferase (ALT): an enzyme found predominately in the liver; high levels may indicate liver damage

aldosterone: hormone secreted by the adrenal cortex and contributing to an increase in blood pressure

allergic reaction: a drug reaction that occurs because the individual's immune system views the drug as a foreign substance

alopecia: abnormal loss of hair; baldness

Alzheimer disease: a disease of the elderly causing progressive deterioration of mental and physical abilities

amebiasis: invasion of the body by the ameba *Entamoeba histolytica*

amenorrhea: absence or suppression of menstruation

anabolism: tissue-building process

anaerobic: organisms that do not require oxygen to live

analeptics: drugs that stimulate the respiratory center

analgesia: absence of pain

analgesic: a drug that relieves pain

anaphylactic reaction: a sudden, severe hypersensitivity reaction with symptoms that progress rapidly and may result in death if not treated

anaphylactic shock: a severe form of hypersensitivity reaction

anaphylactoid reaction: unusual or exaggerated allergic reaction

androgens: hormones that stimulate activity of the accessory male sex organs; testosterone and its derivatives

anemia: a decrease in the number of red blood cells (RBCs), a decrease in the amount of hemoglobin in RBCs, or a decrease in the number of RBCs and hemoglobin

anesthesia: a loss of feeling or sensation

anesthesiologist: a physician with special training in administering anesthetics

anesthetist: a nurse with special training who is qualified to administer anesthetics

angina pectoris (angina): acute pain in the chest resulting from decreased blood supply to the heart muscle

angioedema: localized wheals or swellings in subcutaneous tissues or mucous membranes, which may be caused by an allergic response; also called angioneurotic edema

angiotensin-converting enzyme: a naturally occurring enzyme that converts angiotensin I to angiotensin II, which is a powerful vasoconstrictor

anorexia: loss of appetite

anorexiant: a drug used to suppress the appetite

antacids: drugs that neutralize or reduce the acidity of stomach and duodenal contents

antagonist: a drug that joins with a receptor to prevent the action of an agonist at that receptor

anthelmintic: a drug used to treat helminthiasis (worms)

antianxiety drugs: drugs used to treat anxiety

antibacterial: active against bacteria

antibody: molecule with the ability to bind with a specific antigen responsible for the immune response

anticonvulsants: drugs used for the management of convulsive disorders

antidepressants: drugs used to treat depression

antiemetic: drug that is used to treat or prevent nausea

antiflatulent: drug that works against flatus (gas)

antigen: a substance that the immune system perceives as foreign and that causes production of antibodies

antigen–antibody response: the reaction of specific circulating antibodies to a specific antigen

antihistamine: a drug used to counteract the effects of histamine on body organs and structures

anti-infective: another word for antibacterial; drugs used to treat infections and bacteria

antineoplastic drugs: drugs used for cure, control, or palliative (relief of symptoms) treatment of malignancies

antipsoriatics: drugs used to treat psoriasis

antipsychotic drugs: drugs used to treat psychotic disorders

antipyretic: a drug that lowers an elevated body temperature

antiseptic: an agent that stops, slows, or prevents the growth of microorganisms

antitubercular drugs: drugs used to treat active cases of tuberculosis

antitussive: a drug used to relieve coughing

antivenin: an antitoxin specific for an animal or insect venom

antivertigo: a drug used to treat or prevent vertigo

anxiety: a feeling of apprehension, worry, or uneasiness that may or may not be based on reality

anxiolytics: term used to describe the antianxiety drugs

aplastic anemia: a blood disorder caused by damage to the bone marrow resulting in a marked reduction in the number of red blood cells and some white blood cells

arrhythmia: a disturbance or irregularity in the heart rate or rhythm, or both; also called dysrhythmia

assessment: the collection of subjective and objective data

asthenia: weakness; loss of strength

asthma: a reversible obstructive disease of the lower airway

ataxia: a loss of control of voluntary movements, especially producing an unsteady gait

atelectasis: reduction of air in the lung

atherosclerosis: a disorder in which lipid deposits accumulate on the lining of the blood vessels, eventually producing degenerative changes and obstruction of blood flow

atrial fibrillation: a cardiac arrhythmia characterized by rapid contractions of the atrial myocardium, resulting in an irregular and often rapid ventricular rate

attention deficit hyperactivity disorder: a disorder manifested by a short attention span, hyperactivity, impulsiveness, and emotional lability

attenuated: weakened, as in the antigen strain used for vaccine development

aura: sense preceding a sudden attack, as in the aura that occurs before a convulsion

auscultation: the process of listening for sounds within the body

autonomic nervous system: a division of the peripheral nervous system concerned with functions essential to the life of the organism and not consciously controlled (e.g., blood pressure, heart rate, gastrointestinal activity)

azotemia: retention of excessive amounts of nitrogenous compounds in the blood caused by failure of the kidney to remove urea from the blood

B

bacterial resistance: ability of bacteria to produce substances that inactivate or destroy impact of a drug

bactericidal: a drug or agent that destroys or kills bacteria

bacteriostatic: drugs that slow or retard the multiplication of bacteria

bigeminy: an irregular pulse rate consisting or two beats followed by a pause before the next two paired beats

bile acid sequestrants: these drugs bind to bile acids to form an insoluble substance that cannot be absorbed by the intestine, so it is excreted in the feces

biliary colic: pain caused by the pressure of passing gallstones

bipolar disorder: a psychiatric disorder characterized by severe mood swings from extreme hyperactivity to depression (manic–depressive disease)

blepharospasm: a twitching or spasm of the eyelid

blockade effect: the action of antiarrhythmic drugs blocking stimulation of beta receptors of the heart by adrenergic neurohormones

blood pressure: the force of the blood against the walls of the arteries

blood–brain barrier: a meshwork of tightly packed cells in the walls of the brain's capillaries that screen out certain substances and potentially harmful molecules from crossing into the brain

bone marrow suppression: a decreased production of all blood cells

booster: the administration of an additional dose of the vaccine to "boost" the production of antibodies to a level that will maintain the desired immunity

bowel prep: the use of drugs preoperatively to reduce the number of bacteria normally present in the intestine

brachial plexus block: type of regional anesthesia produced by injection of a local anesthetic into the brachial plexus

brachial plexus: a network of spinal nerves affecting the arm, forearm, and the hand

bradycardia: slow heart rate, usually at a rate less than 60 beats per minute

bronchodilator: a drug used to relieve bronchospasm associated with respiratory disorders

bronchospasm: spasm or constriction of the bronchi resulting in difficulty breathing

buccal: within the cheek

bulla: blister or skin vesicle filled with fluid

bursa: pad-like sac found in connecting tissue usually located in the joint area

C

candidiasis: infection of the skin or mucous membrane with a species of *Candida*

cardiac arrhythmia: irregular heartbeat

cardiac output: the amount of blood leaving the left ventricle

catabolism: tissue-depleting process

catalyst: substance that accelerates a chemical reaction without itself undergoing a change

cell-mediated immunity: the process of T lymphocytes and macrophages (large cells that surround, engulf, and digest microorganisms and cellular debris) working together to destroy an antigen

central nervous system: one of two main divisions of the nervous system consisting of the brain and spinal cord

cervical mucorrhea: increased cervical discharge

cheilosis: cracking of the edges of the lips

chelating agent: a substance that selectively and chemically binds the ion of a metal to itself, thus aiding in the elimination of the metallic ion from the body

chemoreceptor trigger zone: a group of nerve fibers in the brain that when stimulated by chemicals, such as drugs or toxic substances, sends impulses to the vomiting center of the brain

chemotherapy: drug therapy with a chemical, often used when referring to treatment with an antineoplastic drug

cholesterol: a fat-like substance produced mostly in the liver of animals

cholinergic blocking drugs: drugs that impede certain parasympathetic nervous system functions

cholinergic crisis: cholinergic drug toxicity

cholinergic drugs: drugs that mimic the activity of the parasympathetic nervous system

chorea: continuous rapid, jerky, involuntary movements

choreiform movements: involuntary muscular twitching of the limbs or facial muscles

chronic pain: pain that lasts longer than 6 months and ranges in intensity from mild to severe

chrysiasis: grey to blue pigmentation of the skin that may occur from gold deposits in tissues

chylomicrons: small particles of fat in the blood

cinchonism: a group of symptoms associated with quinine toxicity or poisoning, including tinnitus, dizziness, headache, gastrointestinal disturbances, and visual disturbances

cognitive domain: refers to intellectual activities such as thought, recall, decision-making, and drawing conclusions

conduction block: type of regional anesthesia produced by injection of a local anesthetic into or near a nerve trunk

conjunctivitis: inflammation of the conjunctiva (mucous membrane lining the inner surfaces of the eye)

controlled substances: drugs with a high potential for abuse that are controlled by special regulations

convulsions: paroxysm (occurring suddenly) of involuntary muscular contractions and relaxations; another term for seizure

corticosteroids: hormones secreted from the adrenal cortex that contain potent anti-inflammatory action; the collective name for the glucocorticoids and mineralocorticoids

coughing: the forceful expulsion of air from the lungs

Crohn disease: inflammation of the terminal portion of the ileum

cross-allergenicity: allergy to drugs in the same or related groups

cross-sensitivity: see cross-allergenicity

cryptorchism: failure of the testes to descend into the scrotum

crystalluria: formation of crystals in the urine

culture and sensitivity tests: culturing performed to grow bacteria along with tests of their sensitivity to specific drugs

cumulative drug effect: a drug effect that occurs when the body has not fully metabolized a dose of a drug before the next dose is given

Cushing syndrome: a disease caused by the overproduction of endogenous glucocorticoids

cyanosis: blue, gray, or dark purple discoloration of the skin caused by abnormal amounts of reduced hemoglobin in the blood

cycloplegia: paralysis of the ciliary muscle resulting in an inability to focus the eye

cystinuria: the presence of cystine, an amino acid, in the urine

cytomegalovirus (CMV): any of a group of herpes viruses infecting humans, monkeys, or rodents; the human CMV is found in the salivary glands and causes cytomegalic inclusion disease

D

debridement: removal of all foreign material and dead or damaged tissue from a wound or infected lesion

decaliter: 10 liters or 10,000 mL

decongestant: a drug that reduces the swelling of nasal passages

dehydration: loss of too much water from the body

delirium tremens: signs and symptoms of withdrawal from a drug or chemical, including tremors, weakness, anxiety, restlessness, excessive perspiration, nausea, and vomiting

dementia: decrease in cognitive functioning (memory, decision making, speech, etc.)

depolarization: the movement of a stimulus passing along the nerve; the positive ions move from outside the cell into the cell, and the negative ions move from inside the cell to outside the cell

depression: a common psychiatric disorder characterized by feelings of intense sadness, helplessness, and worthlessness, and by impaired functioning

dermis: the layer of skin below the epidermis that contains small capillaries, which supply nourishment to the dermis and epidermis

diabetes insipidus: a disease resulting in the failure of the pituitary to secrete vasopressin or from the surgical removal of the pituitary gland

diabetes mellitus: a chronic disorder characterized by either insufficient insulin production in the beta cells of the pancreas or by cellular resistance to insulin

diabetic ketoacidosis: a potentially life-threatening deficiency of insulin (hypoinsulinism), resulting in severe hyperglycemia and requiring prompt diagnosis and treatment

diaphoresis: increased sweating or perspiration

digitalization: administration of digitalis at intervals to produce and maintain a therapeutic blood level

diluent: a fluid that dilutes

diplopia: double vision

diuretic: a drug that increases the secretion of urine (water, electrolytes, and waste products) by the kidneys

drug error: any incident in which a patient receives the wrong dose, the wrong drug, a drug by the wrong route, or a drug given at the incorrect time

drug idiosyncrasy: any unusual or abnormal reaction to a drug

drug tolerance: a decreased response to a drug, requiring an increase in dosage to achieve the desired effect

dyscrasia: a morbid general state resulting from the presence of abnormal material in the blood

dyskinesia: impairment of voluntary movement

dysphoric: extreme or exaggerated sadness, anxiety, or unhappiness

dyspnea: labored or difficult breathing; shortness of breath

dystonia: prolonged muscle contractions that may cause facial grimacing and twisting of the neck into unnatural positions

dystonic movements: muscular spasms most often affecting the tongue, jaw, eyes, and neck

dysuria: painful or difficult urination

E

edema: accumulation of excess water in the body

efferent: carrying away from a central organ or section

ejection fraction: the amount of blood that the ventricle ejects per beat in relationship to the amount of blood available to eject

electrolyte: an electrically charged particle (ion) that is essential for normal cell function and is involved in various metabolic activities

emesis: the expelled gastric contents; vomitus

emetic: drug that induces vomiting

endogenous: substances normally manufactured by the body

endorphins: naturally occurring analgesic produced by the body in response to certain stimulus (e.g., exercise)

enkephalins: neurotransmitter within the brain involved with pain perception, mood, movement, and behavior

epidermis: outermost layer of the skin

epidural: drug administration is performed when a catheter is placed into the epidural space outside of the dura matter of the brain and spinal cord

epidural block: type of regional anesthesia produced by injection of a local anesthetic into the space surrounding the dura of the spinal cord

epigastric distress: discomfort in the abdomen

epilepsy: a permanent, recurring seizure disorder

epilepticus: an emergency situation characterized by continual seizure activity with no interruptions

epiphysis: a center of ossification (conversion of tissue to bone) at each extremity of long bone

epistaxis: nosebleed

ergotism: an overdose of ergonovine

erythrocytes: red blood cells; one of several formed elements in the blood

Escherichia coli: a nonpathogenic colon bacillus; when found outside of the colon may cause infection

essential hypertension: hypertension without a known cause

estradiol: the most potent of the three endogenous estrogens

estriol: one of three endogenous estrogens

estrogens: female hormones influenced by the anterior pituitary gland

estrone: one of three endogenous estrogens

euthyroid: normal thyroid function

exacerbation: increase in severity

exfoliative dermatitis: red rash in which scaling occurs after the erythema

exogenous: normally occurring outside of the organism or community

expectorant: drug that aids in raising thick, tenacious mucus from the respiratory tract

expectoration: the elimination of thick, tenacious mucus from the respiratory tract by spitting it up

extrapulmonary: occurring outside of the respiratory system (e.g., lungs)

extrapyramidal effects: a group of adverse reactions occurring on the extrapyramidal portion of the nervous system causing abnormal muscle movements, especially akathisia and dystonia

extravasation: escape of fluid from a blood vessel into surrounding tissue

F

fat-soluble: dissolves in fat

febrile: related to fever (elevated body temperature)

fibrolytic: a drug that dissolves clots already formed within the vessel walls

filtrate: fluid removed from the blood through kidney function

first dose effect: an unusually strong therapeutic effect experienced by some patients with the first doses of a medication

fluid overload: a condition when the body's fluid requirements are met and the administration of fluid occurs at a rate that is greater than the rate at which the body can use or eliminate the fluid

folinic acid or leucovorin rescue: the technique of administering leucovorin after a large dose of methotrexate to rescue normal cells and allow them to survive

fungicidal: able to destroy fungi

fungistatic: able to slow or retard the multiplication of fungi

fungus: a colorless plant that lacks chlorophyll

G

gallstone-solubilizing: gallstone-dissolving

gastric stasis: failure to move food normally out of the stomach

gastroesophageal reflux disease: a reflux or backup of gastric contents into the esophagus

general anesthesia: provision of a pain-free state for the entire body

germicide: a drug or agent that kills bacteria

gingival hyperplasia: overgrowth of gum tissue

gingivitis: inflammation of the gums

ginkgo biloba: an herb that appears to increase blood flow to the brain

ginseng: an herb used to improve energy and mental performance

glaucoma: a group of diseases of the eye characterized by increased intraocular pressure; results in changes within the eye, visual field defects, and eventually blindness (if left untreated)

globulin: proteins present in blood serum or plasma that contain antibodies

glossitis: inflammation of the tongue

glucagons: a hormone produced by the alpha cells of the pancreas that increases blood sugar by stimulating the conversion of glycogen to glucose in the liver

glucocorticoids: a hormone essential to life produced by the adrenal cortex

glucometer: a device used to monitor blood glucose levels

goiter: enlargement of the thyroid gland causing a swelling in the front part of the neck, usually caused by a lack of iodine in the diet

gonad: glands responsible for sexual activity and characteristics

gonadotropins: hormones that promote growth and function of the gonads

gout: a form of arthritis in which uric acid accumulates in increased amounts in the blood and often is deposited in the joints

granulocytopenia: a reduction or decrease in the number of granulocytes (a type of white blood cell)

gynecomastia: breast enlargement in the male

H

habituation: a desire to continually use a drug or chemical for the desired effect with no physical dependence but some psychological dependence

half-normal saline: solution containing 0.45% NaCl

hallucinogen: drug capable of producing a state of delirium characterized by visual or sensory disturbances

heart failure: denoted by the area of the initial ventricle dysfunction: left-sided (left ventricular) dysfunction and right-sided (right ventricular) dysfunction; because both sides work together, both sides are affected in heart failure

Helicobacter pylori: bacteria that causes a type of chronic gastritis and peptic and duodenal ulcers

helminthiasis: invasion of the body by helminths (worms)

helminth: a type of parasitic worm

hemolytic anemia: disorder characterized by chronic premature destruction of red blood cells

hemostasis: a process that stops bleeding in a blood vessel

hepatotoxic: capable of producing liver damage

herb: plant used in medicine or as seasoning

high-density lipoproteins (HDL): macromolecules that carry cholesterol from peripheral cells to the liver, where it is metabolized and excreted

hirsutism: excessive growth of hair or hair growth in unusual places, usually in women

histamine: a substance in various body tissues, such as the heart, lungs, gastric mucosa, and skin, that is produced in response to injury

HMG-CoA reductase inhibitor: an enzyme that is a catalyst in the manufacture of cholesterol

humoral immunity: antibody-mediated immune response of the body

hydrochloric acid: a substance the stomach secretes that aids in the digestive process

hyperglycemia: high blood glucose (sugar) level

hyperinsulinism: elevated levels of insulin in the body

hyperkalemia: high blood level of potassium

hyperlipidemia: an increase in the lipids in the blood

hypersecretory: excessive gastric secretion of hydrochloric acid

hypersensitivity: being allergic to a drug

hypersensitivity reaction: allergic reaction to a drug or other substance

hyperstimulation syndrome: sudden ovarian enlargement with accumulation of serous fluid in the peritoneal cavity

hypertension: high blood pressure; usually defined as a systolic pressure above 140 mm Hg or a diastolic pressure above 90 mm Hg

hyperthyroidism: an increase in the amount of thyroid hormones secreted

hypnotic: a drug that induces sleep

hypocalcemia: low blood calcium

hypoglycemia: low blood glucose (sugar) level

hypoinsulinism: low levels of insulin in the body

hypokalemia: low blood level of potassium

hyponatremia: low blood sodium level

hypotension, orthostatic: a decrease in blood pressure occurring after standing in one place for an extended period

hypotension, postural: a decrease in blood pressure after a sudden change in body position

hypotension: abnormally low blood pressure

hypothyroidism: a decrease in the amount of thyroid hormones secreted

hypoxia: inadequate oxygen at the cellular level

I

idiosyncrasy: unusual or abnormal drug response

immune globulin: solutions obtained from human blood containing antibodies that have been formed by the body to specific antigens

immunity: the ability of the body to identify and resist microorganisms that are potentially harmful

immunocompromised: patients with an immune system not fully capable of fighting infection

infiltration: the collection of fluid in a tissue

inhalation: route of administration in which drug droplets, vapor, or gas is inhaled and absorbed through the mucous membranes of the respiratory tract

inotropic: affecting the force of muscular contractions

insulin: a hormone produced by the pancreas that helps maintain blood glucose levels within normal limits

intermittent claudication: a group of symptoms characterized by pain in the calf muscle of one or both legs, caused by walking and relieved by rest

intradermal: route of administration in which the drug is injected into skin tissue

intramuscular: route of administration in which the drug is injected into muscle tissue

intraocular pressure: the pressure within the eye

intravenous: route of administration in which the drug is injected into a vein

intrinsic factor: a substance produced by cells in the stomach that is necessary for the absorption of vitamin B_{12} in the intestine

iodism: excessive amounts of iodine in the body

iritis: inflammation of the iris of the eye

iron deficiency anemia: condition that results when the body does not have enough iron to supply the body's needs

ischemic: marked by reduced blood flow caused by arterial narrowing or blockage or other causes

isolated systolic hypertension: a condition of only an elevated systolic pressure

J

jacksonian seizure: a focal seizure that begins with an uncontrolled stiffening or jerking of the body such as the finger, mouth, hand, or foot that may progress to a generalized seizure

jaundice: yellow discoloration of the skin

K

keratolytic: a drug that removes excess growth of the epidermis (top layer of skin) in disorders such as warts

ketoacidosis: a type of metabolic acidosis caused by an accumulation of ketone bodies in the blood

ketonuria: presence of ketones in the blood

L

laryngospasm: spasm of the larynx resulting in dyspnea and noisy respirations

learning: acquiring new knowledge or skills

left ventricular dysfunction: also called left ventricular systolic dysfunction; the most common form of heart failure

leprosy: a chronic, communicable disease spread by prolonged intimate contact with an infected person

lethargic: sluggish, difficult to rouse

leukopenia: a decrease in the white blood cells or leukocytes; a symptom of bone marrow suppression

leukotrienes: substances that are released by the body during the inflammatory process and constrict the bronchia

lipids: fats or fat-like substances in the blood

lipodystrophy: atrophy of subcutaneous fat

lipoprotein: a lipid-containing protein

local anesthesia: provision of a pain-free state in a specific area

local infiltration anesthesia: anesthesia produced by injecting a local anesthetic drug into tissues

low-density lipoproteins (LDL): macromolecules that carry cholesterol from the liver to the body cells

lumen: the inside diameter of a vessel such as an artery

lupus erythematosus: A chronic inflammatory connective tissue disease affecting the skin, joints, kidneys, nervous system, and mucous membranes. A butterfly rash or erythema may be seen on the face, particularly across the nose

M

malaise: discomfort, uneasiness

malignant hypertension: hypertension in which the diastolic pressure usually exceeds 130 mm Hg

megacolon: dilatation and hypertrophy of the colon

megaloblastic anemia: a type of anemia that results from a deficiency of folic acid and certain other causes; characterized by the presence of large, abnormal, immature erythrocytes circulating in the blood

melasma: discoloration of the skin

melena: blood in the stools

merozoites: cells formed as the result of asexual reproduction

methemoglobinemia: clinical condition in which more than 1% of hemoglobin in the blood has been oxidized to the ferric form

micturition: voiding of urine

mineralocorticoids: a hormone essential to life produced by the adrenal cortex

miosis: the contraction of the pupil of the eye

miotics: drugs used to help contract the pupil of the eye

motivation: the desire for, or seeing the need for, something

musculoskeletal: the bone and muscular structure of the body

myasthenia gravis: a disease that causes fatigue of skeletal muscles because of the lack of acetylcholine released at the nerve endings of parasympathetic nerve fibers

Mycobacterium leprae: the bacteria that cause leprosy

Mycobacterium tuberculosis: the bacteria that cause tuberculosis

mycotic infection: a superficial or deep infection caused by a fungi disease in humans that may be yeast-like or mold-like

mycotic: pertaining to a fungus or fungal infection

mydriasis: dilation of the pupil

mydriatics: drugs that dilate the pupil, constrict superficial blood vessels of the sclera, and decrease the formation of aqueous humor

myocardial infarction: heart attack

myoclonic seizures: sudden, forceful contractions involving the musculature of the trunk, neck, and extremities

myopia: near-sightedness

myxedema: condition caused by hypothyroidism or deficiency of thyroxine and characterized by swelling of the face, periorbital tissues, hands, and feet.

N

narcolepsy: a chronic disorder that results in recurrent attacks of drowsiness and sleep during daytime

nausea: an unpleasant gastric sensation usually preceding vomiting

nebulization: the dispersing of liquid medication in a mist of extremely fine particles to be inhaled into the deeper parts of the respiratory tract

necrosis: death of tissue (as adjective, necrotic)

necrotic: dead, as in dead tissue

nephron: long tubular structure that is the functional part of the kidney

nephrotoxic: harmful to the kidney

nephrotoxicity: damage to the kidneys by a toxic substance

neurogenic bladder: altered bladder function caused by a nervous system abnormality

neurohypophysis: posterior lobe of the pituitary gland

neuroleptanalgesia: a state of general quietness achieved through a combination of analgesic and neuroleptic drugs

neuroleptic malignant syndrome: a rare reaction to antipsychotic drugs characterized by a combination of extrapyramidal effects, hyperthermia, and autonomic disturbance

neuroleptic: drug that causes an altered state of consciousness (i.e., antipsychotic)

neuromuscular blockade: acute muscle paralysis and apnea

neurotoxicity: damage to the nervous system of a toxic substance

neurotransmitter: a chemical substance, also called a neurohormone, released at nerve endings to help transmit nerve impulses

neutropenia: abnormally small number of neutrophil cells (type of white blood cell)

nonpathogenic: not disease-causing

nonprescription drugs: drugs designated by the FDA to be obtained without a prescription

nonproductive cough: a dry, hacking cough that produces no secretions

nonsteroidal: not a steroid

normal flora: nonpathogenic microorganisms within or on the body

normal saline: solution containing 0.9% NaCl

nystagmus: an involuntary and constant movement of the eyeball

O

oliguria: a decrease in urinary output

on-off phenomenon: associated with long-term levodopa treatment, a patient may alternate suddenly between improved clinical status and loss of therapeutic effect

onychomycosis: nail fungus condition

ophthalmic: pertaining to the eye

opioids: narcotic analgesics obtained from the opium plant

opportunistic infection: infection resulting from microorganisms commonly found in the environment, which normally do not cause an infection unless there is an impaired immune system

oral mucositis: inflammation of the oral mucous membranes

orthostatic hypotension: a feeling of light-headedness and dizziness after standing in one place for a long period, caused by a drop in blood pressure

osteoarthritis: a noninflammatory joint disease resulting in degeneration of the articular cartilage and changes in the synovial membrane

osteomalacia: a softening of the bones

osteoporosis: a loss of calcium from the bones, resulting in a decrease in bone density

otic: pertaining to the ear

ototoxic: harmful to the ear

ototoxicity: damage to the organs of hearing by a toxic substance

overactive bladder: involuntary contractions of the detrusor or bladder muscle

overt: not hidden, clearly evident

oxytocic drugs: used before birth to induce uterine contractions similar to those of normal labor

oxytocin: an endogenous hormone produced by the posterior pituitary gland

P

pain: an unpleasant sensory and emotional experience associated with actual or potential tissue damage

palliative: therapy designed to treat symptoms, not to produce a cure

pancytopenia: a reduction in all cellular elements of the blood

paralytic ileus: paralysis of the bowel resulting in lack of movement of the bowel contents

parasite: an organism living in or on another organism (the host) without contributing to the survival or well-being of the host

parasympathetic nervous system: part of the autonomic nervous system concerned with conserving body energy (e.g., slowing the heart rate, digesting food, and eliminating waste)

parenteral: a general term for drug administration in which the drug is injected inside the body

paresthesia: an abnormal sensation such as numbness, tingling, prickling, or heightened sensitivity

Parkinsonism: refers to the symptoms of Parkinson disease, as well as Parkinson-like symptoms that may be seen with the use of certain drugs, head injuries, and encephalitis (e.g., fine tremors, slowing of the voluntary movements, and muscular weakness)

Parkinson disease: a degenerative disorder of the central nervous system; also known as paralysis agitans

partial agonist: a category of narcotic analgesic that binds to a receptor, but the response is limited (i.e., is not as great as with the agonist).

passive immunity: a type of immunity occurring from the administration of ready-made antibodies from another individual or animal

patency: being open or exposed

pathogenic: disease producing

patient-controlled analgesia: a method of pain relief that allows patients to administer their own analgesic by means of an intravenous pump system

penicillinase: an enzyme that inactivates penicillin

peripheral nervous system: all nerves outside of the brain and spinal cord, connecting all parts of the body with the central nervous system

peripheral: pertaining to the outward surface; away from the center

pernicious anemia: a type of megaloblastic anemia that results from a deficiency of intrinsic factor

petechiae: tiny purple or red spots that appear on the skin as a result of pinpoint hemorrhages within the outer layers of the skin

pharmaceutic phase: the dissolution of the drug

pharmacodynamics: a drug's actions and effects within the body

pharmacogenetic disorder: a genetically determined abnormal response to normal doses of a drug

pharmacokinetics: activities occurring within the body after a drug is administered, including absorption, distribution, metabolism, and excretion

pharmacology: the study of drugs and their action on living organisms

pheochromocytoma: tumor of the adrenal medulla characterized by hypersecretion of epinephrine and norepinephrine

phenylketonuria (PKU): a congenital disease caused by a defect in the metabolism of phenylalanine (an amino acid); results from the lack of an enzyme necessary for the conversion of phenylalanine into tyrosine; untreated, the condition leads to mental retardation

phlebitis: inflammation of a vein

photophobia: an aversion to or intolerance of light

photosensitivity: abnormally heightened reactivity of the skin to sunlight

physical dependence: a compulsive need to use a substance repeatedly to avoid mild to severe withdrawal symptoms

plasma expanders: intravenous solutions used to expand plasma volume in shock caused by burns, hemorrhage, or other trauma

polarization: the point at which positive ions on the outside and negative ions on the inside of the cell membrane are in equilibrium

polydipsia: excessive thirst

polyphagia: eating large amounts of food

polypharmacy: taking a large number of drugs (may be prescribed or over-the-counter drugs)

polyposis: numerous polyps

positive inotropic action: the increased force of the contraction of the muscle (myocardium) of the heart through the use of cardiotonic drugs

postural hypotension: a feeling of light-headedness and dizziness after suddenly changing from a lying to a sitting or standing position, or from a sitting to a standing position

preanesthetic drug: a drug given before the administration of anesthesia

prepubertal: before puberty

prescription drugs: drugs the federal government has designated as potentially harmful unless supervised by a licensed health care provider

proarrhythmic effect: the development of a new arrhythmia or the worsening of an existing arrhythmia caused by an antiarrhythmic drug

productive cough: a cough that expels secretions from the lower respiratory tract

progestins: natural or synthetic substances that cause changes similar to those of progesterone

prophylaxis: a drug or treatment designed for prevention of a condition or symptom

prostaglandins: a fatty acid derivative found in almost every tissue of the body and body fluid that affects the uterus and other smooth muscles; also thought to increase the sensation of peripheral pain receptors to painful stimuli

prostatic hypertrophy: abnormal enlargement of the prostate gland

protein substrates: amino acids essential to life

proteolysis: the process of hastening the reduction of proteins into simpler substances

prothrombin: a substance that is essential for the clotting of blood

proton pump inhibitors: drugs with antisecretory properties

pruritus: itching

pseudomembranous colitis: a common bacterial superinfection

psychological dependence: a compulsion to use a substance to obtain a pleasurable experience

psychomotor domain: refers to physical skills or tasks

psychomotor seizures: most often occur in children younger than 3 years of age through adolescence; may involve an aura with perceptual alterations, such as hallucinations or a strong sense of fear

psychotherapeutic drug: used to treat disorders of the mind

psychotic disorder: a disorder, such as schizophrenia, characterized by extreme personality disorganization and a loss of contact with reality

psychotropic drug: another term for psychotherapeutic drugs

ptosis: drooping of the upper eyelid

purpura: condition characterized by various degrees of hemorrhaging into the skin and/or mucous membranes producing ecchymoses (bruises) and petechiae (small red patches) on the skin

purulent exudates: pus-containing fluid

R

rales: abnormal lung sounds often described as crackles

rebound: causing the opposite of the desired effect

receptor: a specialized macromolecule that binds to the drug molecule, altering the function of the cell and producing the therapeutic response

refractory period: the period between transmissions of nerve impulses along a nerve fiber

regional anesthesia: anesthesia produced by injecting a local anesthetic around nerves to limit the pain signals sent to the brain

REM: (rapid eye movement) the dreaming stage of sleep

remission: periods of partial or complete disappearance of signs and symptoms

repolarization: the movement back to the original state of positive and negative ions after a stimulus passes along the nerve fiber; the positive ions are on the outside and the negative ions on the inside of the nerve cell

retinitis: inflammation of the retina of the eye

Reye syndrome: acute and potentially fatal disease of childhood; associated with a previous viral infection; characterized by vomiting and lethargy, progressing to coma

rhabdomyolysis: a rare condition in which muscle damage results in the release of muscle cell contents into the bloodstream

rheumatic fever: a disease associated with a delayed response to a previous streptococcal infection in the body and characterized by fever and pain in the joints

rheumatoid arthritis: a chronic disease characterized by inflammatory changes within the body's connective tissue

rhinitis: inflammation of the nasal passages resulting in increased nasal secretions

S

salicylates: drugs that have analgesic, antipyretic, and anti-inflammatory effects

salicylism: a condition produced by salicylate toxicity

secondary failure: a gradual increase in blood sugar levels that can be caused by an increase in the severity of diabetes or a decreased response to a drug

secondary hypertension: hypertension in which a direct cause can be identified

sedative: a drug producing a relaxing, calming effect

seizure: a periodic attack of disturbed cerebral function

shock: a life-threatening condition occurring when the supply of arterial blood flow and oxygen to the cells and tissues is inadequate

somatic nervous system: branch of the peripheral nervous system that controls sensation and voluntary movement

somatotropic hormone: growth hormone produced by the anterior pituitary gland

somnolence: prolonged drowsiness; sleepiness

soporific: substance or procedure that causes sleep; a hypnotic drug

spinal anesthesia: a type of regional anesthesia produced by injecting a local anesthetic drug into the subarachnoid space of the spinal cord

sprue: a disease characterized by weakness, anemia, weight loss, and malabsorption of essential nutrients

standard precautions: a set of actions recommended by CDC for preventing contact with potentially infectious body fluids, such as wearing gloves

status epilepticus: an emergency situation characterized by continual seizure activity with no interruptions

Stevens-Johnson syndrome: serious allergic reaction to a drug which initially exhibits reactions easily confused with less severe disorders, with fever, cough, muscular aches and pains, headache, and lesions of the skin, mucous membranes, and eyes

stomatitis: inflammation of the mouth

striae: lines or bands elevated above or depressed below surrounding tissue, or differing in color or texture

subcutaneous: route of administration in which the drug is injected just below the layer of skin

sublingual: route of administration in which the drug is placed under the tongue for absorption

substrate: a substance that is the basic component of an organism

sulfonylurea: a type of drug used to lower blood sugar in persons with noninsulin-dependent diabetes

superinfection: an overgrowth of bacterial or fungal microorganism not affected by the antibiotic being administered

sympathetic nervous system: branch of the autonomic nervous system that regulates the expenditure of energy and has key effects in stressful situations

sympathomimetics: drugs that mimic the activities or actions of the sympathetic nervous system

synergism: a drug interaction that occurs when drugs produce an effect that is greater than the sum of their separate actions

T

tachycardia: heart rate above 100 beats/minute

tardive dyskinesia: a syndrome consisting of potentially irreversible, involuntary dyskinetic movements of the tongue, face, mouth, jaw, and sometimes the extremities

teratogen: any substance that causes abnormal development of the fetus

testosterone: the most prominent male sex hormone that acts to stimulate development of the male reproductive organ and the secondary sex characteristics

tetany: nervous condition characterized by sharp flexion of the wrist and ankle joints, muscle twitching, cramps, and possible convulsions, usually caused by abnormal levels of calcium, vitamin D, and alkalosis

theophyllinization: process of giving the patient a higher initial dose, called a loading dose, of theophylline to bring blood levels to a therapeutic range more quickly

therapeutic response: the intended (beneficial) effect of a drug

thrombocytopenia: a decrease in the thrombocytes; a symptom of bone marrow suppression

thrombolytic drugs: drugs designed to dissolve blood clots that have already formed within a blood vessel

thrombosis: the formation of a clot

thrombus: a blood clot (plural: thrombi)

thyroid storm: a severe form of hyperthyroidism also known as thyrotoxicosis

thyrotoxicosis: severe hyperthyroidism that is characterized by symptoms such as high fever, extreme tachycardia, and altered mental status (also called thyroid storm)

thyroxine: a hormone manufactured and secreted by the thyroid gland

tinea corporis: ringworm

tinea cruris: jock itch

tinea pedis: athlete's foot

tinnitus: ringing in the ears

tolerance: patient condition in which increasingly larger dosages are required to obtain the desired effect

tonic–clonic seizure: an alternate contraction (tonic phase) and relaxation (clonic phase) of muscles, a loss of consciousness, and abnormal behavior

toxic: harmful drug effect

toxin: a poisonous substance produced by some bacteria

toxoid: a toxin that is weakened but still capable of stimulating the formation of antitoxins

transdermal: route of administration in which the drug is absorbed through the skin from a patch

transdermal system: a convenient form of drug administration in which the drug is impregnated in a pad and absorbed through the skin

transient ischemic attack (TIA): temporary interference with blood supply to the brain causing symptoms related to the portion of the brain affected (e.g., temporary blindness, aphasia, dizziness, numbness, difficulty swallowing or paresthesias); may last from a few moments to several hours, after which no residual neurologic damage is evident

transsacral block: type of regional anesthesia produced by injection of a local anesthetic into the epidural space at the level of the sacrococcygeal notch

trigeminy: an irregular pulse rate consisting of three beats followed by a pause before the next three beats

triglycerides: a type of lipids in the blood

triiodothyronine: a hormone manufactured and secreted by the thyroid gland

tuberculosis: a disease caused by *Mycobacterium tuberculosis*

tyramine: substance found in most cheeses and in beer, bean pods, yeast, wine, and chicken liver; individuals taking the antidepressant MAOIs and eating foods containing tyramine may experience severe hypertension

U

unit dose: a single dose of a drug packaged ready for patient use

universal precautions: guidelines set forth by the Centers for Disease Control (CDC) to control the spread of disease

urge incontinence: accidental loss of urine caused by a sudden and unstoppable need to urinate

urinary frequency: frequent urination day and night

urinary tract infection: an infection caused by pathogenic microorganisms of one or more structures of the urinary tract

urinary urgency: sudden strong need to urinate

urticaria: hives; itchy wheals on the skin resulting from contact with or ingestion of an allergic substance or food

uterine atony: marked relaxation of the uterine muscle

uterine relaxants: drugs used to manage preterm labor by decreasing uterine activity

uveitis: a nonspecific term for any intraocular inflammatory disorder

V

vaccine: substance with either weakened or killed antigens developed for the purpose of creating resistance to disease

vasoconstriction: a narrowing of the blood vessel

vasodilation: an increase in the size of blood vessels, primarily small arteries and arterioles

vasopressor: a drug that raises the blood pressure because it constricts blood vessels

venous: pertaining to the veins

vertigo: an abnormal feeling of spinning or rotation motion that may occur with motion sickness and other disorders

vesicant: an adverse drug reaction resulting in tissue necrosis, which is caused by the infiltration or extravasation of the drug out of a blood vessel and into soft tissue

vestibular neuritis: inflammation of the vestibular nerve to the inner ear

virilization: acquisition of male sexual characteristics by a woman

vitamin: organic substance needed by the body in small amounts for normal growth and nutrition

volatile liquid: a liquid that evaporates on exposure to the air

vomiting: forceful expulsion of gastric contents through the mouth

von Willebrand disease: a congenital bleeding disorder manifested at an early age by epistaxis and easy bruising; symptoms usually decrease in severity with age

W

water-soluble: dissolves in water

withdrawal: a syndrome of physical and psychological symptoms caused by abruptly stopping use of a drug in a dependent patient

X

xanthine derivatives: drugs that stimulate the central nervous system and result in bronchodilation

Z

Z-track: a technique of intramuscular injection used with drugs that are irritating to subcutaneous tissues

D MedWatch

U.S. Department of Health and Human Services

MedWatch

The FDA Safety Information and Adverse Event Reporting Program

For VOLUNTARY reporting of adverse events and product problems

Page _____ of _____

Form Approved: OMB No. 0910-0291, Expires: 03/31/05
See OMB statement on reverse.

FDA USE ONLY

Triage unit sequence #

A. PATIENT INFORMATION

1. Patient Identifier	2. Age at Time of Event:	3. Sex	4. Weight
In confidence	or _____ Date of Birth:	☐ Female ☐ Male	_____ lbs or _____ kgs

B. ADVERSE EVENT OR PRODUCT PROBLEM

1. ☐ Adverse Event   and/or   ☐ Product Problem *(e.g., defects/malfunctions)*

2. **Outcomes Attributed to Adverse Event** *(Check all that apply)*

☐ Death: _____ *(mo/day/yr)*

☐ Life-threatening

☐ Hospitalization - initial or prolonged

☐ Disability

☐ Congenital Anomaly

☐ Required Intervention to Prevent Permanent Impairment/Damage

☐ Other: _____

3. Date of Event *(mo/day/year)*	4. Date of This Report *(mo/day/year)*

5. **Describe Event or Problem**

6. **Relevant Tests/Laboratory Data, Including Dates**

7. **Other Relevant History, Including Preexisting Medical Conditions** *(e.g., allergies, race, pregnancy, smoking and alcohol use, hepatic/renal dysfunction, etc.)*

PLEASE TYPE OR USE BLACK INK

C. SUSPECT MEDICATION(S)

1. **Name** *(Give labeled strength & mfr/labeler, if known)*

#1 _____

#2 _____

2. Dose, Frequency & Route Used	3. Therapy Dates *(If unknown, give duration)* from/to *(or best estimate)*
#1	#1
#2	#2

4. Diagnosis for Use *(Indication)*

#1 _____

#2 _____

5. Event Abated After Use Stopped or Dose Reduced?

#1 ☐ Yes ☐ No ☐ Doesn't Apply

#2 ☐ Yes ☐ No ☐ Doesn't Apply

6. Lot # *(if known)*	7. Exp. Date *(if known)*
#1	#1
#2	#2

8. Event Reappeared After Reintroduction?

#1 ☐ Yes ☐ No ☐ Doesn't Apply

#2 ☐ Yes ☐ No ☐ Doesn't Apply

9. NDC# *(For product problems only)*

_____ – _____

10. Concomitant Medical Products and Therapy Dates *(Exclude treatment of event)*

D. SUSPECT MEDICAL DEVICE

1. **Brand Name**

2. **Type of Device**

3. **Manufacturer Name, City and State**

4. Model #	Lot #	5. Operator of Device
Catalog #	Expiration Date *(mo/day/yr)*	☐ Health Professional ☐ Lay User/Patient ☐ Other: _____
Serial #	Other #	

6. If Implanted, Give Date *(mo/day/yr)*	7. If Explanted, Give Date *(mo/day/yr)*

8. **Is this a Single-use Device that was Reprocessed and Reused on a Patient?**
☐ Yes ☐ No

9. **If Yes to Item No. 8, Enter Name and Address of Reprocessor**

10. **Device Available for Evaluation?** *(Do not send to FDA)*
☐ Yes ☐ No ☐ Returned to Manufacturer on: _____ *(mo/day/yr)*

11. **Concomitant Medical Products and Therapy Dates** *(Exclude treatment of event)*

E. REPORTER *(See confidentiality section on back)*

1. Name and Address	Phone #

2. Health Professional?	3. Occupation	4. Also Reported to:
☐ Yes ☐ No		☐ Manufacturer ☐ User Facility ☐ Distributor/Importer

5. **If you do NOT want your identity disclosed to the manufacturer, place an "X" in this box:** ☐

FDA

Mail to: **MedWatch**
5600 Fishers Lane
Rockville, MD 20852-9787

-or-

FAX to:
1-800-FDA-0178

FORM FDA 3500 (12/03)   Submission of a report does not constitute an admission that medical personnel or the product caused or contributed to the event.

ADVICE ABOUT VOLUNTARY REPORTING

Report adverse experiences with:

- Medications *(drugs or biologics)*
- Medical devices *(including in-vitro diagnostics)*
- Special nutritional products *(dietary supplements, medical foods, infant formulas)*
- Cosmetics
- Medication errors

Report product problems - quality, performance or safety concerns such as:

- Suspected counterfeit product
- Suspected contamination
- Questionable stability
- Defective components
- Poor packaging or labeling
- Therapeutic failures

Report SERIOUS adverse events. An event is serious when the patient outcome is:

- Death
- Life-threatening *(real risk of dying)*
- Hospitalization *(initial or prolonged)*
- Disability *(significant, persistent or permanent)*
- Congenital anomaly
- Required intervention to prevent permanent impairment or damage

Report even if:

- You're not certain the product caused the event
- You don't have all the details

How to report:

- Just fill in the sections that apply to your report
- Use section C for all products except medical devices
- Attach additional blank pages if needed
- Use a separate form for each patient
- Report either to FDA or the manufacturer *(or both)*

Confidentiality: The patient's identity is held in strict confidence by FDA and protected to the fullest extent of the law. FDA will not disclose the reporter's identity in response to a request from the public, pursuant to the Freedom of Information Act. The reporter's identity, including the identity of a self-reporter, may be shared with the manufacturer unless requested otherwise.

If your report involves a serious adverse event with a device and it occurred in a facility outside a doctor's office, that facility may be legally required to report to FDA and/or the manufacturer. Please notify the person in that facility who would handle such reporting.

Important numbers:

- 1-800-FDA-0178 -- To FAX report
- 1-800-FDA-1088 -- To report by phone or for more information
- 1-800-822-7967 -- For a VAERS form for vaccines

To Report via the Internet:

http://www.fda.gov/medwatch/report.htm

FORM FDA 3500 (12/03) (Back)

Drugs and Health Care Information Sources on the World Wide Web

Alzheimer's Disease Education & Referral Center
http://www.alzheimers.org

American Academy of Allergy, Asthma and Immunology
http://www.aaaai.org

American Diabetes Association
http://www.diabetes.org

American Heart Association (AHA)
http://www.americanheart.org

American Optometric Association
http://www.aoa.org

Centers for Disease Control and Prevention
http://www.cdc.gov

Centers for Disease Control Travel's Health
http://www.cdc.gov/travel

Cystic Fibrosis Foundation
http://www.cff.org

Epilepsy Foundation of America
http://www.efa.org

Kids Health
http://www.kidshealth.org

Mayo Clinic's public health information
http://www.mayoclinic.com

Medline (NIH)
http://medlineplus.gov

MedWatch
http://www.fda.gov/medwatch/index.html

National Center for Complementary and Alternative Medicine
http://nccam.nih.gov

National Center for Health Statistics
http://www.cdc.gov/nchs/fastats

National Comprehensive Cancer Network
http://www.nccn.org

National High Blood Pressure Education Program (NHBPEP)
http://www.nhlbi.nih.gov/about/nhbpep/index.htm

National Institute on Drug Abuse
http://www.steroidabuse.org

National Institutes of Health
http://health.nih.gov

National Library of Medicine
http://www.nlm.nih.gov

National Psoriasis Foundation
http://www.psoriasis.org

National Sleep Foundation
http://www.sleepfoundation.org

U.S. Department of Labor Occupational Safety & Health Administration (OSHA)
http://www.osha.gov

U.S. Food and Drug Administration
http://www.fda.gov

University of Pennsylvania's health encyclopedia
http://pennhealth.com/hi.html

Vaccine Adverse Event Reporting System
http://www.vaers.org

Select Herbs and Natural Products Used for Medicinal Purposes

Common Name	Scientific Name	Uses	Adverse Reactions	Significant Considerations
Aloe vera	*Aloe vera*	Inhibits infection and promotes healing of minor burns and wounds	None significant if used as directed; may cause burning sensation in wound	Rare reports of delayed healing when used in the gel form on a wound; taken internally, aloe gel may have laxative effect
Bilberry	*Vaccinium myrtillus*	Vision enhancement and eye health, microcirculation, spider veins and varicose veins, capillary strengthening before surgery	No adverse effects have been reported in clinical studies	None significant
Black Cohosh, (black snakeroot, squawroot)	*Cimicifuga racemosa*	Management of some symptoms of menopause and as an alternative to hormone replacement therapy; may be beneficial for hypercholesterolemia or peripheral vascular disease	Overdose causes nausea, dizziness, nervous system and visual disturbances, decreased pulse rate and increased perspiration	Should not be used during pregnancy; possible interactions with hormone therapy
Chamomile	*Matricaria chamomilla*	As a tea for gastrointestinal disturbances, as a sedative, and as an anti-inflammatory agent	Possible contact dermatitis and, in rare instances, anaphylaxis	Chamomile is a member of the ragweed family and those allergic to ragweed should not take the herb
Chondroitin	Chondroitin sulfate, chondroitin sulfuric acid, chonsurid	Arthritis	None significant if used as directed	Because chondroitin is concentrated in cartilage, theoretically it produces no toxic or teratogenic effects
Cranberry	*Vaccinium macrocarpon*	Urinary tract infection (UTI)	Large doses can produce gastrointestinal symptoms (e.g., diarrhea)	None significant
Echinacea (American coneflower, black susans)	*Echinacea angustifolia*	Prevents and shortens symptoms and duration of upper respiratory infections (URIs) including colds	Rare; nausea and mild gastrointestinal (GI) upsets	Should not be used by individuals with autoimmune diseases such as tuberculosis, collagenosis, multiple sclerosis, AIDS, and HIV infection

Common Name	Scientific Name	Uses	Adverse Reactions	Significant Considerations
Ephedra (sea grape, ma-huang, yellow horse)	*Ephedra sinica*	Relieves colds, improves respiratory function, headaches, diuretic effects	Skin eruptions, hypertension, irregular heart rate, psychosis	Ephedra should only be used after consulting with the physician; many restrictions apply and the herb can cause serious reactions; do not use with cardiac glycosides, monoamine oxidase inhibitor halothane, guanethidine, (MAOIs) or oxytocin; do not use with St. John's wort or in weight loss formulas
Garlic	*Allium sativum*	Lowers blood sugar, cholesterol, and lipids	May cause abnormal blood glucose levels	Increased risk of bleeding in patients taking the coumarins, salicylates, or antiplatelet drugs
Ginger (ginger root, black ginger)	*Zingiber officinale*	Antiemetic, cardiotonic, antithrombotic, antibacterial, antioxidant, antitussive, anti-inflammatory, GI disturbances, lower cholesterol, prophylaxis for nausea and vomiting, colic, bronchitis	Excessive doses may cause CNS depression and interfere with cardiac functioning or anticoagulant activity	Theoretically, ginger could enhance the effects of the antiplatelet drugs, such as coumarin
Ginkgo (maiden hair tree, kew tree)	*Ginkgo biloba*	Raynaud disease, cerebral insufficiency, anxiety, stress, tinnitus, dementias, circulatory problems, asthma	Rare if used as directed; possible effects include headache, dizziness, heart palpitations, GI effects, rash, allergic dermatitis	Do not take with antidepressant drugs, such as the MAOIs, or the antiplatelet drugs such as coumarin, unless advised to do so by the primary care provider
Ginseng	*Panax quinquefolius, Panax ginseng*	Popular but unproven uses: antineoplastic, enhances immune function, improves cardiovascular or CNS function	Most common: nervousness, excitation, hypoglycemia; rare: diffuse mammary nodularity, vaginal bleeding	Taking ginseng in combination with stimulants such as caffeine is not advised; do not use for longer than 3 mo (some herbalists recommend use for 1 mo followed by nonuse for 2 mo)
Goldenseal	*Hydrastis canadensis*	Antiseptic for skin (topical), astringent for mucous membranes (mouthwash), wash for inflamed eyes, sinus infections, peptic ulcers, colitis, gastritis	Large doses may cause dry or irritated mucous membranes and injury to the gastrointestinal system; may reduce the beneficial bacteria in the intestines	Should not be taken for more than 3–7 days

Common Name	Scientific Name	Uses	Adverse Reactions	Significant Considerations
Glucosamine (chitosamine)	2-Amino-2-deoxyglucose	Antiarthritic in osteoarthritis;	Well-tolerated	No direct toxic effects have been reported
Green tea	*Camellia sinensis*	Reduces cancer, lowers lipid levels, helps prevent dental caries, antimicrobial and antioxidative effects	Contains caffeine (may cause mild stimulant effects such as anxiety, nervousness, heart irregularities, restlessness, insomnia, and digestive irritation)	Contains caffeine and should be avoided during pregnancy, by individuals with hypertension, anxiety, eating disorders, insomnia, diabetes, and ulcers
Kava (kawa, kava-kava, awa yanggona)	*Piper methysticum*	Mild to moderate anxiety and as a sedative	Scaly skin rash, disturbances in visual accommodation, habituation	Limit use to no more than 3 mo
Lemon balm (balm, melissa, sweet balm)	*Melissa officinalis*	Graves disease, sedative, antispasmodic, cold sores (topical)	None significant	None significant
Passion flower (passion fruit, granadilla, water lemon, apricot vine)	*Passiflora incarnata*	Promotes sleep, treatment for pain and nervous exhaustion	None if used as directed; excessively large doses may cause CNS depression	May interact with anticoagulants and MAOIs
Saw palmetto (cabbage palm, fan palm, scrub palm)	*Serenoa repens*	Symptoms of benign prostatic hyperplasia	Generally well-tolerated; occasional gastrointestinal effects	May interact with hormones such as oral contraceptive drugs and hormone replacement therapy
St. John's wort (Klamath weed, goatweed, rosin rose)	*Hypericum perforatum*	Antidepressant and antiviral	Usually mild; may cause dry mouth, dizziness, constipation, other GI symptoms, photosensitivity	May decrease efficacy of theophylline, warfarin, and digoxin; use with other prescriptions is not recommended
Tea tree oil	*Melaleuca alternifolia*	Topical antimicrobial	Contact dermatitis	For topical use only; do not take orally
Valerian	*Valeriana officinalis*	Restlessness, sleep disorders	Rare if used as directed.	May interact with the barbiturates (e.g., phenobarbital), the benzodiazepines (e.g., diazepam), and the opiates (e.g., morphine)
Willow bark (weidenrinde, white willow, purple osier willow, crack willow)	*Salix alba, S. purpurea, S. fragilis*	Analgesic	Adverse reactions are those associated with the salicylates	Do not use with aspirin or other NSAIDs; do not use in patients with peptic ulcers and other medical conditions in which the salicylates are contraindicated

Index

Page numbers followed by b indicate box; those followed by t indicate table; those in *italics* indicate figure.